AF711907

Clinical Neuropsychology and Cognitive Neurology of Parkinson's Disease and Other Movement Disorders

CLINICAL NEUROPSYCHOLOGY AND COGNITIVE NEUROLOGY OF PARKINSON'S DISEASE AND OTHER MOVEMENT DISORDERS

Edited by
Alexander I. Tröster, Ph.D., ABPP-CN
Barrow Neurological Institute, Phoenix, Arizona, USA

OXFORD
UNIVERSITY PRESS

OXFORD
UNIVERSITY PRESS

Oxford University Press is a department of the University of Oxford. It furthers the University's objective of excellence in research, scholarship, and education by publishing worldwide.

Oxford New York
Auckland Cape Town Dar es Salaam Hong Kong Karachi
Kuala Lumpur Madrid Melbourne Mexico City Nairobi
New Delhi Shanghai Taipei Toronto

With offices in
Argentina Austria Brazil Chile Czech Republic France Greece
Guatemala Hungary Italy Japan Poland Portugal Singapore
South Korea Switzerland Thailand Turkey Ukraine Vietnam

Oxford is a registered trademark of Oxford University Press in the UK and certain other countries.

Published in the United States of America by
Oxford University Press
198 Madison Avenue, New York, NY 10016

© Oxford University Press 2015

All rights reserved. No part of this publication may be reproduced, stored in a retrieval system, or transmitted, in any form or by any means, without the prior permission in writing of Oxford University Press, or as expressly permitted by law, by license, or under terms agreed with the appropriate reproduction rights organization. Inquiries concerning reproduction outside the scope of the above should be sent to the Rights Department, Oxford University Press, at the address above.

You must not circulate this work in any other form
and you must impose this same condition on any acquirer.

Library of Congress Cataloging-in-Publication Data
Clinical neuropsychology and cognitive neurology of Parkinson's disease and other movement disorders / edited by Alexander I. Tröster.
p. ; cm.
Includes bibliographical references and index.
ISBN 978-0-19-981237-0
I. Tröster, Alexander I., editor.
[DNLM: 1. Parkinson Disease—complications. 2. Cognition Disorders—etiology. 3. Mental Disorders—etiology. 4. Movement Disorders—complications. 5. Neurobehavioral Manifestations. 6. Parkinson Disease—psychology. WL 359]
RC382
616.8′33—dc23
2014012805

To the Memory of Early Mentors
William W. Beatty and Nelson Butters

Contents

Contributors

Roy N. Alcalay
Columbia University Medical Center
New York, NY

Melissa J. Armstrong
University of Maryland School of Medicine
Baltimore, MD

Eirik Auning
Akershus University Hospital
Lorenskog, Norway

Dag Aarsland
Karolinska Institute
Stockholm, Sweden

Barbara Borroni
University of Brescia
Brescia, Italy

Brenna A. Cholerton
University of Washington
Seattle, WA

Eiron Cudaback
University of Washington
Seattle, WA

Luc Defebvre
Lille University Medical Center
Lille, France

Mahlon R. DeLong
Emory University
Atlanta, GA

Günther Deuschl
Christian-Albrechts-University
Kiel, Germany

Roseanne D. Dobkin
Rutgers-Robert Wood Johnson Medical School
Piscataway, NJ

Kathy Dujardin
Lille University Medical Center
Lille, France

Julie A. Fields
Mayo Clinic College of Medicine
Rochester, MN

Jennifer G. Goldman
Rush University Medical Center
Chicago, IL

Astrid Haram
University of Oslo
Oslo, Norway

Marjan Jahanshahi
Institute of Neurology
The National Hospital for Neurology and Neurosurgery
London, UK

Carme Junque
University of Barcelona and Institute of Biomedical Research August Pi i Sunyer
Barcelona, Spain

Jaime Kulisevsky
Sant Pau Hospital and Sant Pau Institute of Biomedical Research
Universitat Autònoma de Barcelona
Barcelona, Spain

Irene Litvan
University of California, San Diego
La Jolla, CA

Delia Lorenz
Christian-Albrechts-University
Kiel, Germany

Kelly E. Lyons
University of Kansas Medical Center
Kansas City, KS

Laura Marsh
Michael E. Debakey VA Medical Center and Baylor College of Medicine
Houston, TX

Kathleen S. Montine
University of Washington
Seattle, WA

Thomas J. Montine
University of Washington
Seattle, WA

Alessandro Padovani
University of Brescia
Brescia, Italy

Javier Pagonabarraga
Sant Pau Hospital and Sant Pau Institute of Biomedical Research
Universitat Autònoma de Barcelona
Barcelona, Spain

Arvid Rongve
Haugesund Hospital
Haugesund, Norway

Arshia Sadreddin
Barrow Neurological Institute
Phoenix, AZ

Ben Schmand
University of Amsterdam
Amsterdam, The Netherlands

Madeleine E. Sharp
Columbia University Medical Center
New York, NY

Ioan Stroescu
NeuroCog Trials, Inc.
Durham, NC

Adriana M. Strutt
Baylor College of Medicine
Houston, TX

Mariam Torkamani
Institute of Neurology
The National Hospital for Neurology and Neurosurgery
London, UK

Alexander I. Tröster
Barrow Neurological Institute
Phoenix, AZ

Michele K. York
Baylor College of Medicine and Michael E. Debakey VA Medical Center
Houston, TX

Daniel Weintraub
University of Pennsylvania
Philadelphia, PA

Thomas Wichmann
Emory University
Atlanta, GA

Preface

In his original work, James Parkinson, despite acknowledging the presence of melancholia in the eponymous disease, observed it to spare the intellect. Charcot's observations, to the contrary, seemed not to greatly influence medicine or psychology's view of the disease, and the cause of the condition's motor symptoms and their treatment remained almost the sole focus of research in Parkinson's disease for more than a century. Only in the middle of 20th century did the advent of postencephalitic parkinsonism and surgical treatments of parkinsonism spur neurobehavioral research. The concomitant growth of clinical neuropsychology and the psychometric approach, perhaps largely driven by work with veterans of the World Wars, saw this method of inquiry increasingly applied to Parkinson's disease. By the 1960s neurobehavioral studies began documenting the effects of the "silver bullet" treatment at the time: levodopa. Neurobehavioral studies' sophistication grew in tandem with cognitive psychology, and by the 1970s and 1980s more emphasis was placed on understanding cognitive mechanisms underlying neurobehavioral alterations in Parkinson's disease. By the 1980s the robust advances in Alzheimer's disease diagnosis brought with them studies about the neurobehavioral differentiation of that disease from Parkinson's disease and greater interest in dementia in Parkinson's disease. Further technological advances in neuroimaging and surgical treatments, such as deep brain stimulation and an expansion of the pharmacotherapeutic armamentarium informed by enhanced understanding of molecular biology, spurred a growth in neurobehavioral studies of the neural correlates of cognitive and behavioral outcomes of various interventions. In parallel, animal studies enhanced our understanding of the behavioral role of the basal ganglia.

A true explosion in neurobehavioral studies of Parkinson's disease occurred in the last decade, however. Several factors seem to have prompted this: a realization that motor symptoms can, in the majority of persons, be treated very well for a considerable time; the observation that neurobehavioral symptoms, rather than motor symptoms, are often the determinants of quality of life, disability, institutionalization, and premature mortality; and the realization of some of the implications of decades-old evidence that Parkinson's disease affects neurotransmitter systems other than just the dopaminergic one. Among neurobehavioral studies, epidemiologic approaches highlighted that cognitive and behavioral issues are much more common than once thought and neuropsychological studies demonstrated that the cognitive and behavioral changes are more heterogeneous and occur earlier in the disease than previously appreciated. Indeed, subtle cognitive and behavioral changes, and even frank psychiatric disturbance, may already occur during the lengthy disease prodrome. Neurobehavioral conditions may thus be of prognostic significance and require early treatment and prevention. The large amount of work into the neurobehavioral features of Parkinson's disease has indirectly benefited similar research into the atypical parkinsonism (such as multiple system atrophy, corticobasal degeneration and progressive supranuclear palsy) and other movement disorders such as Huntington's disease, essential tremor, and dystonia. Not only are the neurobehavioral features of these disorders being described in increasing detail, but the pathophysiology and treatment of these features is being better understood, thereby enabling the amelioration of the quality of life of persons with such disorders.

This book is intended as a collection of works that summarizes the current state of knowledge about the neurobehavioral features of various movement disorders. The rapid accumulation of research in this field makes it increasingly difficult for one or two people to author a comprehensive text in an expert manner. The team assembled for this volume succeeds in expertly covering a diversity of facets such as the pathology; neuroimaging; assessment; and treatment of an ever growing set of neurobehavioral features of movement disorders, including cognitive impairment and dementia, depression, apathy, anxiety, psychosis, and impulse control disorders. Covering mostly Parkinson's disease given that this condition has attracted the most neuropsychological research among movement disorders, the book, however, also contains chapters that highlight the rapid advances being made in research into neurobehavioral features in other movement disorders. The book also covers fundamental knowledge about basal ganglia function and dysfunction, assessment and evaluation techniques applicable to a range of movement disorders and quality of life, the very construct that all the research and clinical practice ultimately tries to optimize.

In bringing this book to fruition, I dearly thank the contributors who worked so hard and endured my editorial whims, Joan Bossert and Louis Gulino at Oxford University Press who encouraged me to pursue this project and shepherded the volume through an utterly professional editorial and production process, and finally, but certainly not least, Kristy and Madison, who not only tolerated dwindling family time despite a promise of "no more books" but also provided staunch support throughout.

Alexander I. Tröster, Ph.D., ABPP-CN
Phoenix, Arizona

PART ONE

GENERAL ISSUES IN THE CLINICAL NEUROPSYCHOLOGY AND COGNITIVE NEUROLOGY OF PARKINSON'S DISEASE AND OTHER MOVEMENT DISORDERS

1 Basal Ganglia Circuits

Structure, Function, and Dysfunction

Thomas Wichmann and Mahlon R. DeLong

INTRODUCTION

The basal ganglia are key subcortical structures involved in the control of behavior, and basal ganglia dysfunction is implicated in a variety of movement and other neuropsychiatric disorders, including Parkinson's disease (PD), Huntington's disease, and Tourette's syndrome. These structures receive input from the cerebral cortex, thalamus, and midbrain, and send output back to the frontal lobe via the thalamus. Concepts of the organization and function of the basal ganglia circuits have undergone considerable change over the past decades. The basal ganglia were previously regarded as playing a role in *funneling* information from widespread cortical areas to the motor cortex, thereby playing a major role in various aspects of movement, including action selection and movement initiation (Kemp & Powell, 1971). This concept has now been largely replaced with a schema of *parallel* processing of cortical inputs by a family of segregated circuits that traverse the basal ganglia. Each of these circuits is centered on specific cortical areas that send projections to their respective basal ganglia domains, which, in turn, return information via the thalamus back to the cortical areas of origin (Alexander, DeLong, & Strick, 1986). Diseases of the basal ganglia can be profitably viewed as "circuit disorders," that result in mixtures of motor, behavioral, cognitive, and emotional disturbances.

This chapter is focused on the progress made in refining our understanding of the anatomic and physiologic features of the basal ganglia circuits, and of their role in the pathophysiology of PD. Knowledge of circuit structure, function, and dysfunction is also crucial for the neurosurgical targeting of these circuits for ablation and deep brain stimulation (DBS) procedures, which are carried out for a wide variety of movement disorders as well as other neurologic and psychiatric conditions. Indeed, the renaissance in functional surgery that began with treatments of PD over two decades ago resulted in part from the advances in our understanding of the functional organization of the basal ganglia and associated areas and of the pathophysiology of parkinsonism, based on studies in animal models of these diseases.

BASAL GANGLIA-THALAMOCORTICAL CIRCUITS

The current "segregated circuit" model of basal ganglia function is based on anatomic, physiologic, and imaging data (Figure 1-1). Combined single cell/behavioral studies in primates have identified somatotopically organized regions of the putamen, subthalamic nucleus (STN), and globus pallidus, each containing neurons whose activity is related to movements of specific body parts. These areas interact anatomically and are called the "motor circuit." The finding of specificity and somatotopic organization throughout the nodes of the motor circuit is consistent with the anatomical evidence of highly topographic connections between them.

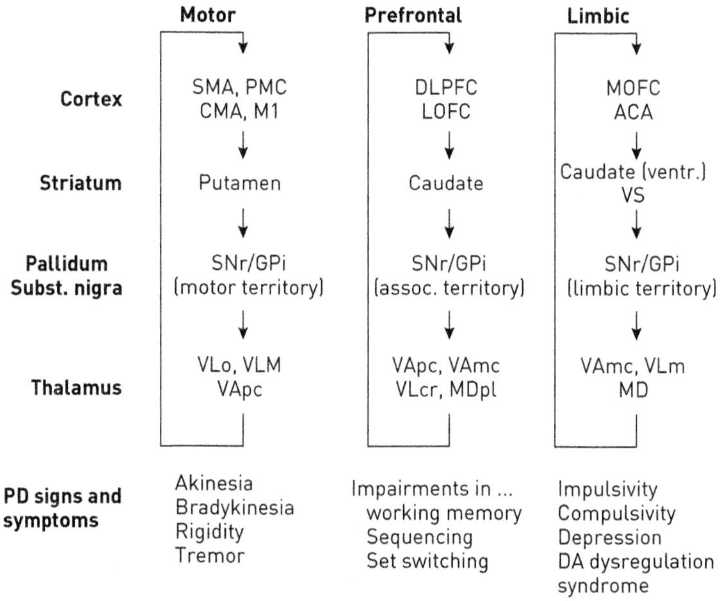

FIGURE 1-1

Circuit anatomy of the major motor and nonmotor cortex-basal ganglia-thalamocortical circuits. PD signs and symptoms that are presumed to arise from dysfunction of these circuits are indicated as well. Abbreviations: ACA, anterior cingulate area; CMA, cingulate motor area; DLPFC, dorsolateral prefrontal cortex; LOFC, lateral orbitofrontal cortex; M1, primary motor cortex; MD, mediodorsal nucleus of the thalamus; MDpl, mediodorsal nucleus of thalamus, pars lateralis; MOFC, medial orbitofrontal cortex; PMC, premotor cortex; SMA, supplementary motor area; VApc, ventral anterior nucleus of thalamus, pars parvocellularis; VAmc, ventral anterior nucleus of thalamus, pars magnocellularis; VLm, ventrolateral nucleus of thalamus, pars medialis; VLo, ventrolateral nucleus of thalamus, pars oralis; VLcr, ventrolateral nucleus of thalamus, pars caudalis, rostral division. See text for other abbreviations. Reproduced, with permission, from Wichmann & Delong (2006b).

Primate recording and behavioral studies lead initially to the identification of two separate cortical–subcortical loops, a "motor" loop centered on the posterior (postcommissural) putamen, and an "associative" loop centered on the caudate nucleus and the precommissural putamen, each projecting to different portions of the pallidum, and, via the thalamus, to precentral motor fields and prefrontal cortex, respectively (see Figure 1-1 and DeLong & Georgopoulos, 1981; DeLong, Georgopoulos, & Crutcher, 1983). Subsequent anatomic and physiologic studies gave rise to the current schema of the basal ganglia as components of *multiple* parallel and largely closed cortical–subcortical circuits, in which information is sent from different cortical areas to spatially separate domains of the basal ganglia, processed, and integrated with other inputs, and then returned to the frontal cortical area of origin via the thalamus (Alexander & Crutcher, 1990; Alexander, Crutcher, & DeLong, 1990; Alexander et al., 1986; Middleton & Strick, 2000; A. Parent & Hazrati, 1995). Based on the presumed function(s) of the cortical regions involved "motor," "oculomotor," "prefrontal" (or "associative,") and "limbic" circuits were distinguished (Alexander & Crutcher, 1990; Alexander et al., 1986; Alexander et al., 1990; S.N. Haber, Kunishio, Mizobuchi, & Lynd-Balta, 1995; A. Parent, 1990). Each of these circuits has been shown, in turn, to consist of multiple subcircuits, centered on specific cortical subregions (Hoover & Strick, 1993; Turner, Grafton, Votaw, Delong, & Hoffman, 1998). Although the segregation of information between the larger circuits is well accepted, the degree to which segregation is maintained between the subcircuits (within the same larger circuit) is still uncertain. Evidence points to the presence of some instances of open-loop projections with a degree of convergence and "funneling" (Joel & Weiner, 1994). As will be discussed later, there is also evidence that limbic input may reach the other loops via a number of routes.

Basal ganglia disorders may be associated with abnormalities in one or more of the larger segregated circuits. The motor signs and symptoms of PD, for example, largely result from disturbances in the motor circuit (see Figure 1-1). As shown in Figure 1-2, this circuit originates from pre- and postcentral sensory-motor fields. It then engages motor portions of the basal ganglia, including the postcommissural putamen, the posterior external pallidum, dorsolateral STN, and the ventral posterolateral internal pallidal segment of the globus pallidus (GPi). The motor projections from GPi reach the ventrolateral nucleus in the thalamus (VL), which then projects back to the precentral motor fields (Hoover & Strick, 1993; Inase & Tanji, 1995; Schell & Strick, 1984). As discussed, there is strong evidence that a topographic segregation is maintained during the processing of sensorimotor information flowing from cortical motor areas to the sensorimotor areas of the basal ganglia (Nambu, 2011).

In contrast to the movement abnormalities that are associated with disturbances in the motor circuit, disturbances in the associative and limbic circuits are associated with some of the nonmotor signs of PD (Figure 1-1). For example, impulsivity, compulsivity, emotional disturbances, and the dopamine dysregulation syndrome, are thought to result from disturbances within the "limbic" circuit. This circuit originates from the anterior cingulate and medial orbitofrontal

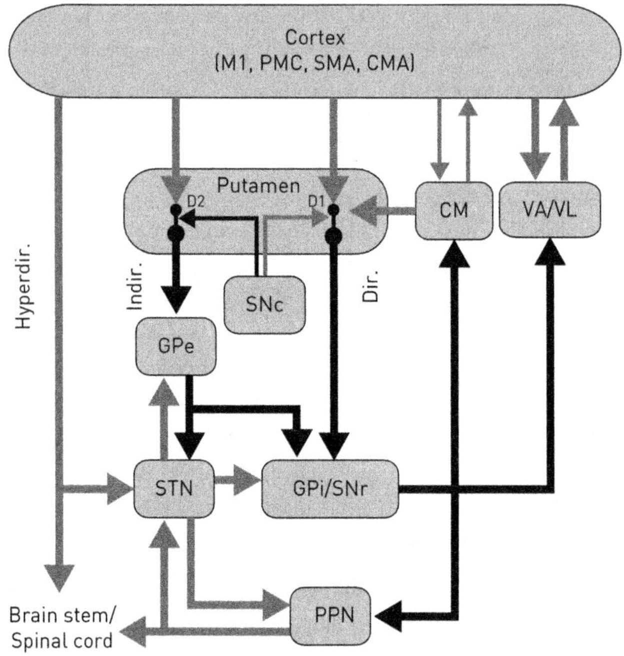

FIGURE 1-2
Connections between basal ganglia nuclei, thalamus and cortex. Black arrows indicate inhibitory connections; gray arrows indicate excitatory connections. Abbreviations: CM, centromedian nucleus of thalamus; CMA, cingulate motor area; Dir., direct pathway; D1, D2, dopamine receptor subtypes; Indir., indirect pathway; M1, primary motor cortex; Pf, parafascicular nucleus of the thalamus; PMC, premotor cortex; PPN, pedunculopontine nucleus; SMA, supplementary motor area. See text for other abbreviations. Reproduced, with permission, from Galvan and Wichmann (2008).

cortices, passes through the ventral striatum, the medial and caudal STN, the ventral and rostromedial GPi and rostrodorsal SNr, the paramedian portion of the mediodorsal nucleus (MD), and the magnocellular ventral anterior (VA) nucleus of the thalamus, and then projects back to the anterior cingulate and medial orbitofrontal cortices.

Disturbances in the associative circuit are believed to account for elements of the executive dysfunction in PD (Figure 1-1), including those affecting working memory, sequencing, and switching of sets. This circuit originates in the dorsolateral prefrontal and lateral orbitofrontal cortex, engages the caudate nucleus and associative portions of GPi and SNr, as well as the magno- and parvocellular portions of VA, the rostral division of the pars caudalis of VL, and the lateral MD, and then projects back to the cortical regions of origin.

CIRCUIT COMPONENTS

In each of the aforementioned circuits, the striatum is a key entry point for cortical and thalamic inputs to the basal ganglia (Voorn, Vanderschuren, Groenewegen, Robbins, & Pennartz, 2004). Rodent experiments indicate that corticostriatal projections arise from neurons in cortical layers 2–6, which also project to other cortical neurons in either hemisphere (so-called intratelencephalic (IT) neurons) and from cortical neurons, mostly found in cortical layer 5B, whose axons become the pyramidal tract (PT neurons) (Shepherd, 2013) In rodents, PT neurons innervate multiple targets (striatum, thalamus, subthalamic nucleus, midbrain, pontine nuclei, and other areas) as they descend to their ultimate target in the brainstem or spinal cord (Kita & Kita, 2012). Based on these findings, it has been proposed (Lei, Jiao, Del Mar, & Reiner, 2004) that PT neurons innervate striatal medium spiny projection neurons (MSNs) that project to GPe (so-called indirect pathway, see later), whereas projections from IT neurons reach predominately the GPi and SNr (so-called "direct" pathway, see later). However, the PT/IT neuron dichotomy and branching pattern has not been confirmed in primates (see, e.g., M. Parent & Parent, 2006). Instead, it has been shown that the electrophysiologic and functional properties of cortical PT neurons in the primate M1 differ from those of corticostriatal neurons, with no evidence of PT collaterals innervating the striatum (Bauswein, Fromm, & Preuss, 1989; Pasquereau & Turner, 2011; Turner & DeLong, 2000).

In addition to the striatum, the STN, a key node of the indirect pathway, also receives segregated and topographically specific projections from cortical motor and nonmotor areas. The cortical projection to the STN and the subsequent STN projections to the GPi/SNr have been referred to as the "hyperdirect" pathway, emphasizing the possibility that this pathway may provide a fast route for cortical input to modulate the inhibitory activity of the basal ganglia output nuclei (Hartmann-von Monakow, Akert, & Kunzle, 1978; Nambu et al., 2000; Nambu, Tokuno, & Takada, 2002), and, potentially, even the thalamus via a direct (excitatory) subthalamo–thalamic projection (Rico et al., 2010). This concept is supported by anatomical data suggesting a collateral or direct projection to STN neurons from PT neurons, as well as physiologic data indicating short-latency responses of pallidal cells to cortical stimulation that are eliminated by inhibition of STN activity (Nambu et al., 2000).

The GPi and SNr are the major source of basal ganglia GABAergic inhibitory output to the thalamus and brainstem. GPi and SNr output neurons fire tonically at very high rates, providing a continuous inhibition of the thalamic and brainstem targets (Chevalier, Vacher, Deniau, & Desban, 1985; Deniau & Chevalier, 1985). This feature figures prominently in all models of basal ganglia function, which view the phasic release of inhibition as being facilitatory to behavior and assigns a role of tonic inhibition to the suppression of action (see later).

According to models developed in the late 1980s, the striatum and GPi/SNr are linked via two anatomically distinct pathways (Albin, Young, & Penney, 1989; DeLong, 1990). The "direct" pathway arises from MSNs that project monosynaptically to neurons in GPi and SNr, whereas the "indirect" pathway arises from other MSNs that project to the external segment of the globus pallidus (GPe), which then projects to GPi and SNr, both directly and via the STN. The STN sends excitatory, glutamatergic projections to both GPi and SNr.

Indirect pathway MSNs express predominately dopamine D2 receptors, whereas direct pathway MSNs express D1 receptors. From an anatomical point of view, the concept of strictly segregated direct and indirect pathways is almost certainly too simple, since single-cell tracing studies have shown that some striatal output neurons project to both, GPe and GPi, thus demonstrating that these neurons do not strictly belong to either the "direct" or "indirect" pathway. However, recent optogenetic studies of the effects of selectively activating these pathways have demonstrated that they have contrasting effects on basal ganglia output and behavior, with activation of the indirect MSNs leading to akinesia/bradykinesia, and activation of direct MSNs leading to increased motility, thus supporting the concept that striatal output pathways can be grossly divided into direct and indirect projections (Kravitz et al., 2010). Furthermore, some of the most prominent basal ganglia diseases are known to affect the balance of activity of the direct and indirect pathways, and pharmacological treatments aiming at restoring balance, have proven successful in treating disorders such as PD. For example, interventions that reduce the activity of indirect pathway MSNs, such as selective D2/D3 receptor agonists, are effective treatments for parkinsonian symptoms and signs.

Collaterals from pallido- and nigrothalamic projections also reach the centromedian and parafascicular (CM/Pf) nuclei of the thalamus. These projections are components of a massive thalamostriatal feedback system (Nanda, Galvan, Smith, & Wichmann, 2009; Sidibe, Bevan, Bolam, & Smith, 1997; Smith, Raju, Pare, & Sidibe, 2004). Like thalamocortical projections, the CM/Pf-striatal projections are topographically arranged in primates. The CM receives somatotopically organized motor input from the basal ganglia and projects similarly to the motor portions of putamen and STN, whereas Pf inputs and outputs are related to associative and limbic territories of the basal ganglia (Sadikot, Parent, & Francois, 1992; Smith & Parent, 1986; Smith et al., 2004). In addition to their feedback function, the intralaminar nuclei are believed to provide saliency information to the striatum, which may be important for procedural learning, action selection, and other functions (Minamimoto, Hori, & Kimura, 2005; 2009). These functions are thought to prominently involve striatal aspiny cholinergic interneurons (see later).

In addition to their thalamic projections, the basal ganglia output nuclei also project to brainstem areas, such as the superior colliculus and pedunculopontine nucleus (PPN, see Harnois & Filion, 1982; Mena-Segovia, Bolam, & Magill, 2004; Rye, Lee, Saper, & Wainer, 1988). The PPN is a component of the brainstem locomotor region, which plays a role in the regulation of gait and balance, whereas the superior colliculus is involved in the control of saccades and head/neck movements (Hikosaka, 2007; Kaneda, Isa, Yanagawa, & Isa, 2008; Liu & Basso, 2008; May et al., 2009). The projections from the basal ganglia output nuclei to the brainstem are phylogenetically older than those to the thalamus. Connections between the basal ganglia and the brainstem are present at the earliest stages of evolutionary development in vertebrates, such as the lamprey (Stephenson-Jones, Samuelsson, Ericsson, Robertson, & Grillner, 2011). There is evidence that the descending pathways of the basal ganglia are also divisible into parallel loop systems, similar to those that project to thalamus and cortex (Redgrave, Prescott, & Gurney, 1999).

OTHER ASPECTS OF BASAL GANGLIA CIRCUITS

Limbic basal ganglia connectivity: How emotional states and reward influence motor function and impact motor and executive function has been a key question for decades. Although the cortical-basal ganglia loops are largely segregated, limbic information may reach the other circuits via several routes. Limbic cortical areas, as well as subcortical limbic structures, such as the amygdala, project not only to the ventral (limbic) striatum, but also to "striosomes" within the territory of other corticosubcortical loops. Striosomes together with the surrounding extrastriosomal "matrix" are striatal compartments that can be delineated by staining for immunocytochemical markers such as acetylcholinesterase (Graybiel & Ragsdale, 1978). Striosomal MSNs project directly to dopaminergic neurons of the SNc, which, in turn, project back to large areas of the striatum and, thereby, distribute the limbic information to nonlimbic basal ganglia circuits (S. N. Haber, Fudge, & McFarland, 2000). Thus far, this anatomically based hypothesis is not directly supported by physiologic data, but it is obviously clinically important to clarify striosomal function(s) because striosomal involvement has been implicated in a number of neurologic disorders, including Huntington's disease, levodopa-induced dyskinesias, dystonia, and drug addiction (Crittenden & Graybiel, 2011).

Another interface between the limbic system and the other circuits that has received recent attention involves the lateral habenula (Hikosaka, Sesack, Lecourtier, & Shepard, 2008). Tract tracing studies in primates indicate that projections from the sensorimotor, associative, and limbic portions of GPi project to the lateral habenula (Pare & Smith, 2009), conveying reward-related signals to it (Hong & Hikosaka, 2008). The lateral habenula, in turn, sends glutamatergic projections to the dopaminergic neurons in the ventral tegmental area (VTA). The lateral habenula has also been implicated in other functions, such as the regulation of memory and attention (Lecourtier & Kelly, 2007).

Basal Ganglia and Cerebellar Connectivity

Interactions between basal ganglia and cerebellar systems have long been known to exist at the cortical level (see, for instance, Akkal, Dum, & Strick, 2007), but it was believed until recently that the cortical-subcortical loops that involve basal ganglia and cerebellum remain separate throughout their respective subcortical courses. However, studies published in the last decade showed that, in rodents and primates, the cerebellum interacts with the basal ganglia via a bi-synaptic pathway that involves the thalamus and terminates in the striatum (Bostan, Dum, & Strick, 2013; Bostan & Strick, 2010; Hoshi, Tremblay, Feger, Carras, & Strick, 2005; Ichinohe, Mori, & Shoumura, 2000). In addition, the basal ganglia can influence the cerebellum via connections from the STN to the pontine nuclei, which project to the cerebellar cortex (Bostan, Dum, & Strick, 2010). These connections have potential relevance for our understanding of the pathophysiology of conditions that have traditionally been considered as "basal ganglia disorders."

For example, cerebellar output appears to be involved in the generation of parkinsonian tremor and other aspects of parkinsonism (Wu & Hallett, 2013) as well as some forms of dystonia (Argyelan et al., 2009; Calderon, Fremont, Kraenzlin, & Khodakhah, 2011; Carbon et al., 2008; Jinnah & Hess, 2006; Neychev, Fan, Mitev, Hess, & Jinnah, 2008). The recently identified connections between the cerebellum and nonmotor circuits of the basal ganglia suggest that interactions between basal ganglia and cerebellum may also play a role in nonmotor aspects of behavior (Villanueva, 2012)

BASAL GANGLIA FUNCTIONS

Action Selection

There is a general consensus that the basal ganglia play a role in action selection, enabling appropriate actions and inhibiting undesired, potentially competing, actions (e.g., Mink, 1996; Redgrave et al., 1999). Such decisions may help the organism to prioritize feeding, predator avoidance, courtship, and other behaviors. According to this view, competing impulses for action are projected to the striatum from the cerebral cortex. The connectivity of the basal ganglia allows for motivation and salience to influence the strength of motor programs that encode competing actions, and the selection of the most appropriate behavior in a given context (see also later). It is believed that action selection is a fundamental aspect of basal ganglia function and present at the earliest stages of vertebrate evolution (Grillner, Robertson, & Stephenson-Jones, 2013; Stephenson-Jones et al., 2011). Over the course of evolution, with the development of cortex and of the connections between cortex and basal ganglia, the circuitry appears to have been expanded for additional functions, in particular the processing of complex cognitive, emotional, and motor information.

It is generally believed that the basal ganglia participate in action selection at the level of the striatum, where the dopaminergic, CM/Pf, and cholinergic inputs may shape corticostriatal transmission to favor those inputs that are associated with maximal reward, or where lateral inhibitory connections inside of the striatum (mediated via GABAergic interneurons and local collaterals of the GABAergic projection neurons) may facilitate behavioral programs for desired actions and suppress programs for unintended actions.

The anatomic dichotomy of direct and indirect striatal pathways is implicated in several aspects of movement, including action selection or movement scaling. According to the classic circuit model of the basal ganglia (Figure 1-2), excitatory cortical activation of MSNs that give rise to the GABAergic direct pathway reduces the output of the basal ganglia to related thalamocortical projection neurons, whereas activation of indirect pathway MSNs leads to the opposite outcome. Indirect pathway activation will, thus, lead to suppression of movement, whereas activation of the direct pathway results in disinhibition of thalamocortical projections, activation of cortex, and facilitation of the movement. The balance between the proposed opposing actions of the direct and indirect pathways on GPi/SNr neurons may determine the overall amount of movement, or may select or limit the extent or duration of individual movements (Albin et al., 1989; Gurney, Prescott, & Redgrave, 2001; Mink & Thach, 1993; Nambu, Mori, Stuart, & Wiesendanger, 2004).

A Role of the Basal Ganglia in the On-Line Control of Movement?

There has been a strong assumption that the basal ganglia are involved in motor control, because diseases of the basal ganglia such as PD, disrupt voluntary movements, and physiologic and imaging studies have convincingly demonstrated that basal ganglia neurons respond to movement. There is, however, little experimental support for a direct and critical role of the basal ganglia in the on-line control of movements (including the selection, focusing, or scaling of individual actions). For example, the timing of changes in movement-related changes in neuronal activity in the basal ganglia, when examined in relation to a stimulus-triggered movement, lags behind that in the cerebellum and cortex (e.g., Mitchell, Richardson, Baker, & DeLong, 1987; Wichmann, Bergman, & DeLong, 1994). Moreover, lesions of the motor portions of GPi (pallidotomy), which interrupt basal ganglia motor output, have relatively little negative effect on movement initiation or execution of learned motor skills in normal animals or in patients with movement disorders, although the learning of new motor skills may be impaired (Desmurget & Turner, 2008; Marsden & Obeso, 1994; Obeso et al., 2009), and they may affect movement speed and "vigor" (Shadmehr & Krakauer, 2008; Turner & Desmurget, 2010). It is evident from the available data that the basal ganglia play a role in action selection, but that they are not involved in the "on-line" control of movement parameters. Cortical mechanisms may play a major role in monitoring the choices between currently available options and the real time demands for action, and its selection and initiation (Cisek, 2007). In this sense, the basal ganglia are neither a repository of innate behaviors or habits but rather, are primarily involved in aspects of associative learning and reinforcement.

Learning/Habit Formation

The evidence for a role of the basal ganglia in goal-directed movements, the formation of habits, has increased greatly, based on electrophysiologic studies, lesion studies and neuroimaging studies.

The release of dopamine at the highly plastic corticostriatal synapse plays an essential role in these procedural-learning functions. The firing pattern of dopaminergic neurons in the SNc that provide most dopaminergic terminals in the striatum signals discrepancies between the expectation of rewards and actual rewards (Hollerman & Schultz, 1998; Tanaka et al., 2004; Waelti, Dickinson, & Schultz, 2001). Additional learning-related signals are supplied to the striatum by neurons of CM/Pf whose discharge patterns appear to provide saliency information to the striatum, particularly to cholinergic striatal interneurons which, in turn, interact with striatal dopamine release (e.g., Cragg, 2006; Threlfell et al., 2012).

Based on findings in animals and humans (Miyachi, Hikosaka, & Lu, 2002; Redgrave et al., 2010) it has been proposed that portions of the associative circuit (the rostral putamen and caudate nucleus) is engaged in the acquisition of new behaviors, whereas the more posterior putamen is involved in the automatic execution of previously learned behaviors. The apparent differential involvement of caudate nucleus and putamen in cue-driven (early) stages of learning or in the execution of fully learned behaviors, respectively, may explain why the early striatal dopamine loss in parkinsonism, which affects the putamen more strongly than the caudate nucleus, lessens an individual's ability to carry out behavioral sequences "automatically" and may force greater reliance on voluntary control and external cues (Redgrave et al., 2010).

Response Inhibition

Potentially related to the strong inhibitory output of the basal ganglia, these structures may act to inhibit movement execution when necessary in response to external cues (Aron & Poldrack, 2006; Band & van Boxtel, 1999; Liddle et al., 2009; Verbruggen & Logan, 2009). Involvement of the basal ganglia in response inhibition is supported by the observation that lesions in the basal ganglia produce deficits in response inhibition (as measured with stop-signal reaction time tasks) that are similar in extent to those produced by prefrontal cortical damage (Rieger, Gauggel, & Burmeister, 2003). Dysfunction in this network may be important in the pathophysiology of a variety of disorders, including, in particular, attention deficit hyperactivity disorder (ADHD, see, e.g., Armstrong & Munoz, 2003; Aron & Poldrack, 2005; Casey et al., 1997; Dickstein, Bannon, Castellanos, & Milham, 2006; Groman, James, & Jentsch, 2009; Robbins, 2007). Imaging and other studies have suggested that the response inhibition network includes not only the basal ganglia, but also several frontal and prefrontal regions (particularly the right inferior prefrontal cortex and the pre-supplementary motor area [pre-SMA]) (Aron, Behrens, Smith, Frank, & Poldrack, 2007; Dickstein et al., 2006).

The STN may have a particularly prominent role in this inhibitory network because it is anatomically positioned to rapidly increase inhibitory pallidal and nigral output, which may then act to block thalamocortical transmission (Aron, Durston, et al., 2007; Aron & Poldrack, 2006; Chambers, Garavan, & Bellgrove, 2009; Eagle & Baunez, 2010; Eagle et al., 2008; Isoda & Hikosaka, 2008; Kuhn et al., 2004; Mink, 1996; Nambu et al., 2002). Consistent with such a role, studies of the effects of STN lesions in rats showed impairments of response inhibition in conflict situations (Baunez et al., 2001; Baunez, Nieoullon, & Amalric, 1995; Baunez & Robbins, 1997). The STN may also play a role in inhibiting automatic eye movements when switching to voluntary eye movements (Hikosaka & Isoda, 2008). Similar evidence is available with regard to a basal ganglia role in inhibiting limb movements (but see Tunik, Houk, & Grafton, 2009). Furthermore, STN-DBS treatment in patients with PD has been found to interfere with response inhibition functions, as measured in cognitive and motor tasks (Ballanger et al., 2009; Frank, Samanta,

Moustafa, & Sherman, 2007; Hershey et al., 2004; Jahanshahi et al., 2000; Ray et al., 2009; Schroeder et al., 2002; Witt et al., 2004).

Areas of the basal ganglia other than the STN may also be involved in response inhibition functions. For instance, lesions of the rodent striatum increase stop-signal reaction times (Dalley, Cardinal, & Robbins, 2004; Eagle & Robbins, 2003), and imaging and other studies have led to speculation that disturbances of response inhibition in the associative portions of the striatum may play a role in the development of features of ADHD (e.g., Booth et al., 2005; Casey et al., 1997).

Control of bimanual movements. Because parkinsonian patients have significant problems with the performance of bimanual movements, especially antiphase movements (Song, Yoo, Park, & Park, 2010; Wu, Wang, Hallett, Li, & Chan, 2010), many studies have been designed to examine the role of the basal ganglia in these movements. For example, it was shown that DBS of the STN reduces the impact of motivation on the performance of bimanual movements (Sauleau, Eusebio, Vandenberghe, Nuttin, & Brown, 2009), and that changes in the activation patterns of the STN and globus pallidus may be involved in, or be reflective of, age-related declines in the performance of bimanual switching tasks (Coxon et al., 2010). In a task involving temporally uncoupled bimanual finger movements, functional magnetic resonance imaging (fMRI) studies showed increased activation within right premotor and dorsolateral prefrontal, bilateral inferior parietal, basal ganglia, and cerebellar areas, identifying the basal ganglia as part of a larger bimanual movement circuitry (Meister, Foltys, Gallea, & Hallett, 2010) that is disturbed in PD (Wu et al., 2010).

Nonmotor Functions

The behavioral contribution of the associative and limbic basal ganglia loops remain poorly understood. Some of the functions of the nonmotor circuits were already mentioned earlier. Given the anatomic similarities between the motor and nonmotor circuits, the operations performed at individual nodes of the motor and nonmotor circuits are likely to be similar. For instance, it is possible that the basal ganglia play a role in the competitive role of directed attention or resolution of conflicting cognitive and emotional aspects of behavior, acting, thus, in a manner analogous to action selection.

PATHOPHYSIOLOGY OF PARKINSON'S DISEASE

The cardinal motor features of PD, that is, the triad of akinesia/bradykinesia, tremor at rest and muscular rigidity (jointly called parkinsonism), result from decreased dopaminergic transmission in the motor portions of the basal ganglia, due to progressive loss of dopaminergic neurons in the SNc. Other features of the disease such as depression, autonomic dysfunction, sleep disorders, aspects of cognitive impairment, and dopamine-unresponsive gait/balance disturbances are now ascribed to progressive pathologic changes outside of the dopaminergic system (Braak et al., 2003; Lim & Lang, 2010).

Although PD clearly encompasses nondopaminergic pathology, an appreciation of the consequences of dopamine depletion remains central to our understanding of the cardinal motor features of the disease. Dopamine is lost throughout the brain, but the earliest and greatest changes are found in the posterior "motor" portion of the putamen, which later spreads to also involve the more anterior (nonmotor) putamen and caudate nucleus (e.g., Kish, Shannak, & Hornykiewicz, 1988). The striatal (and perhaps extrastriatal) loss of dopamine leads to major downstream activity changes in the other basal ganglia nuclei. Thus, studies in animals with experimental dopamine depletion and in humans with PD have provided evidence for significant abnormalities of activity of neurons within the direct and indirect striatal output pathways. Initially, firing-rate changes in the basal ganglia, including a reduction of firing in GPe and an increase of firing in the STN and GPi/SNr were felt to be highly important (Bergman, Wichmann, Karmon, & DeLong, 1994; Crossman, Mitchell, & Sambrook, 1985; Dogali et al., 1994; Filion, Tremblay, & Bedard, 1988; Galvan & Wichmann, 2008; Lozano et al., 1996; Miller & DeLong, 1987; Schwartzman & Alexander, 1985; Vitek et al., 1993), leading to a model in which reduced dopaminergic transmission at corticostriatal synapses would disinhibit indirect pathway MSNs and reduce facilitation of direct pathway MSNs. The increased activity along the indirect pathway would lead to inhibition of GPe, and subsequent disinhibition of STN and GPi/SNr. The resulting increased (inhibitory) activity in GPi and SNr would be further amplified by the reduction of activity along the direct pathway. Increased basal ganglia output was thought to result in excessive inhibition of thalamocortical neuronal activity, and the hypokinetic features of PD.

However, it is now thought that firing-pattern abnormalities in the basal ganglia and associated areas of thalamus and cortex play may play a more prominent role than rate changes (Galvan & Wichmann, 2008; Rubin, McIntyre, Turner, & Wichmann, 2012). The pattern changes include an increased tendency of basal ganglia neurons to discharge in bursts (Bergman et al., 1994; Filion & Tremblay, 1991; Hammond, Bergman, & Brown, 2007; Miller & DeLong, 1987; Wichmann & DeLong, 2006), oscillatory firing patterns (Brown, 2006, 2007; Eusebio & Brown, 2007; Galvan & Wichmann, 2008; Gatev, Darbin, & Wichmann, 2006; Hammond et al., 2007; Timmermann & Fink, 2009; Timmermann, Florin, & Reck, 2007; Weinberger, Hutchison, & Dostrovsky, 2009; Wichmann & DeLong, 2006), and increased neuronal synchrony (Bergman et al., 1994; Hammond et al., 2007). Of these, the presence of synchronized neuronal oscillations in the beta-range of frequencies (10-30Hz), and the failure to generate gamma-band oscillations (30-60Hz) before and during movement are believed to play a major role, based on recordings of local field potentials from the basal ganglia in surgically treated parkinsonian patients, or recordings of EEG in such patients (Brown, 2007; Gatev et al., 2006; Hammond et al., 2007; Weinberger et al., 2009). Other recently identified changes are an increased coherence of the oscillatory activity between cortex and basal ganglia, and between STN and GPi, particularly affecting the alpha-, theta-, and beta-bands (P. J. Magill, Bolam, & Bevan, 2000; P. J. Magill,

Bolam, & Bevan, 2001; Sharott et al., 2005; Shimamoto et al., 2013; Williams et al., 2002). The emergence of unusual cross-frequency coupling phenomena, such as the entrainment of the amplitude of cortical gamma-band activity to the phase of concomitant beta activity (de Hemptinne et al., 2013; Shimamoto et al., 2013) has also been observed. It is important to realize that it has been difficult to firmly link any of the described rate or pattern changes to the emergence of parkinsonian signs.

Imaging studies have also been used to assess abnormalities in basal ganglia activity patterns in PD. Spatial covariance mapping has been extensively used to examine resting state metabolism in PD patients and in parkinsonian monkeys (e.g., Spetsieris & Eidelberg, 2011). These studies have resulted in the identification of distinct covariance patterns associated with the motor and cognitive manifestations of the disease. One such pattern, the "PD-related pattern" (PDRP) is associated with increased pallido-thalamic and pontine metabolic activity and reductions in premotor cortex, supplemental motor area, and parietal association regions with increased putamenal and decreased motor cortical activity. The PDRP correlates mainly with bradykinesia and rigidity (Antonini et al., 1998), whereas other spatial covariance patterns are correlated with the severity of tremor (Habeck et al., 2005; Mure et al., 2011), or with memory and executive control in PD patients.

Dopamine loss in nonmotor areas of the striatum and other basal ganglia may contribute to the nonmotor symptoms and signs of the disease. It has been proposed that the gradually increasing involvement of the nonmotor caudate nucleus in the dopamine deficit may lead to progressive disruption of automatic or habitual behaviors, with a greater reliance on volitional control of actions (Redgrave et al., 2010). Impaired executive functions, decreased motivation (apathy, depression), and impulsivity could also be manifestations of frontal-subcortical circuit dysfunction in PD, perhaps not just involving the dopamine system in the striatum, but also other transmitter systems in the basal ganglia (such as the serotonergic and the norepinephrine system), or changes at other nodes of the cortico-basal ganglia network of connections. As an example for the (at least partial) nondopaminergic origin of nonmotor signs and symptoms of PD, the spatial covariance pattern associated with memory and executive control is not altered by dopaminergic medications or DBS (Brooks & Pavese, 2011; Huang et al., 2007).

CONCLUSION

Our concepts of the functional organization and role of the basal ganglia as key components of cortical-subcortical and brainstem networks has undergone considerable change over the past decades, replacing the earlier concept of a role in the selection and funneling of motor commands from diverse cortical areas to the motor cortex. Although the proposed schema of parallel processing of cortical motor, associative, and limbic information through separate domains in the basal ganglia-thalamocortical networks remains largely valid, there is evidence of some degree of convergence within the individual larger circuits, and for the transmission of limbic information through various routes to the motor and associative loops. The recently identified connectivity between the basal ganglia and cerebellar cortical-subcortical loops has opened fresh insight into the interactions between these two loop systems in motor and cognitive functioning. This may eventually contribute to a better understanding of the clinical features of movement and cognitive disorders.

Although the basal ganglia appear to play a role in action-selection, reward-based, and goal-directed learning, they do not appear to be involved per se in the storage of motor programs (procedural learning) or on-line action selection, which are most likely critical cortical functions. There is growing evidence as well of a role of the basal ganglia in the arrest of ongoing behavior and switching to a new task (a form of set shifting), via the "hyperdirect" pathway. The role(s) of the basal ganglia circuits in cognition and emotion are less well defined, but these may be similar to those outlined for movement, given the role of these phylogenetically recent additions to the basic circuit modules.

Diseases of the basal ganglia, such as PD, reflect a complex mix of motor, cognitive, and limbic disturbances that result, at least in part, from disturbances of the respective basal ganglia-thalamocortical networks. It is worth mentioning, however, that the clinical aspects of movement disorders such as PD do not necessarily reflect dysfunction of the basal ganglia loops but also dysfunction and compensation within connected downstream networks. This is reflected most clearly in the effectiveness of surgical procedures that interrupt basal ganglia output pathways by ablation (as in pallidotomy) or deep brain stimulation (of GPi or STN) in relieving much of the clinical burden of movement disorders. Obviously, these procedures do not restore networks to the normal state, yet they are able, by blocking or overriding abnormal network activity, to restore an astonishing degree of behavioral normality to the individual.

ACKNOWLEDGMENTS

The preparation of this chapter was supported through grants from the NIH/NINDS (R01-NS054976, R01-NS071074 and P50-NS071669 (TW)), and by NIH/NCRR grant RR-000165 (Yerkes National Primate Center).

REFERENCES

Akkal, D., Dum, R. P., & Strick, P. L. (2007). Supplementary motor area and presupplementary motor area: targets of basal ganglia and cerebellar output. *Journal of Neuroscience, 27*(40), 10659–10673. doi: 10.1523/JNEUROSCI.3134-07.2007

Albin, R. L., Young, A. B., & Penney, J. B. (1989). The functional anatomy of basal ganglia disorders. *Trends in Neuroscience, 12*, 366–375.

Alexander, G. E., & Crutcher, M. D. (1990). Functional architecture of basal ganglia circuits: neural substrates of parallel processing. *Trends in Neuroscience, 13*, 266–271.

Alexander, G. E., Crutcher, M. D., & DeLong, M. R. (1990). Basal ganglia-thalamocortical circuits: parallel substrates for motor, oculomotor, 'prefrontal' and 'limbic' functions. *Progress in Brain Research, 85*, 119–146.

Alexander, G. E., DeLong, M. R., & Strick, P. L. (1986). Parallel organization of functionally segregated circuits linking basal ganglia and cortex. *Annual Review of Neuroscience, 9*, 357–381.

Antonini, A., Moeller, J. R., Nakamura, T., Spetsieris, P., Dhawan, V., & Eidelberg, D. (1998). The metabolic anatomy of tremor in Parkinson's disease. *Neurology, 51*(3), 803–810.

Argyelan, M., Carbon, M., Niethammer, M., Ulug, A. M., Voss, H. U., Bressman, S. B., . . . Eidelberg, D. (2009). Cerebellothalamocortical connectivity regulates penetrance in dystonia. *Journal of Neuroscience, 29*(31), 9740–9747. doi: 10.1523/JNEUROSCI.2300-09.2009

Armstrong, I. T., & Munoz, D. P. (2003). Inhibitory control of eye movements during oculomotor countermanding in adults with attention-deficit hyperactivity disorder. *Experimental Brain Research, 152*(4), 444–452. doi: 10.1007/s00221-003-1569-3

Aron, A. R., Behrens, T. E., Smith, S., Frank, M. J., & Poldrack, R. A. (2007). Triangulating a cognitive control network using diffusion-weighted magnetic resonance imaging (MRI) and functional MRI. *Journal of Neuroscience, 27*(14), 3743–3752. doi: 10.1523/JNEUROSCI.0519-07.2007

Aron, A. R., Durston, S., Eagle, D. M., Logan, G. D., Stinear, C. M., & Stuphorn, V. (2007). Converging evidence for a fronto-basal-ganglia network for inhibitory control of action and cognition. *Journal of Neuroscience, 27*(44), 11860–11864. doi: 10.1523/JNEUROSCI.3644-07.2007

Aron, A. R., & Poldrack, R. A. (2005). The cognitive neuroscience of response inhibition: relevance for genetic research in attention-deficit/hyperactivity disorder. *Biology & Psychiatry, 57*(11), 1285–1292. doi: 10.1016/j.biopsych.2004.10.026

Aron, A. R., & Poldrack, R. A. (2006). Cortical and subcortical contributions to Stop signal response inhibition: role of the subthalamic nucleus. *Journal of Neuroscience, 26*(9), 2424–2433. doi: 10.1523/JNEUROSCI.4682-05.2006

Ballanger, B., van Eimeren, T., Moro, E., Lozano, A. M., Hamani, C., Boulinguez, P., . . . Strafella, A. P. (2009). Stimulation of the subthalamic nucleus and impulsivity: release your horses. *Annals of Neurology, 66*(6), 817–824. doi: 10.1002/ana.21795

Band, G. P., & van Boxtel, G. J. (1999). Inhibitory motor control in stop paradigms: review and reinterpretation of neural mechanisms. *Acta Psychologica (Amst), 101*(2-3), 179–211. doi: S0001-6918(99)00005-0 [pii]

Baunez, C., Humby, T., Eagle, D. M., Ryan, L. J., Dunnett, S. B., & Robbins, T. W. (2001). Effects of STN lesions on simple vs choice reaction time tasks in the rat: preserved motor readiness, but impaired response selection. *European Journal of Neuroscience, 13*(8), 1609–1616.

Baunez, C., Nieoullon, A., & Amalric, M. (1995). In a rat model of parkinsonism, lesions of the subthalamic nucleus reverse increases of reaction time but induce a dramatic premature responding deficit. *Journal of Neuroscience, 15*(10), 6531–6541.

Baunez, C., & Robbins, T. W. (1997). Bilateral lesions of the subthalamic nucleus induce multiple deficits in an attentional task in rats. *European Journal of Neuroscience, 9*(10), 2086–2099.

Bauswein, E., Fromm, C., & Preuss, A. (1989). Corticostriatal cells in comparison with pyramidal tract neurons: contrasting properties in the behaving monkey. *Brain Research, 493*, 198–203.

Bergman, H., Wichmann, T., Karmon, B., & DeLong, M. R. (1994). The primate subthalamic nucleus. II. Neuronal activity in the MPTP model of parkinsonism. *Journal of Neurophysiology, 72*(2), 507–520.

Booth, J. R., Burman, D. D., Meyer, J. R., Lei, Z., Trommer, B. L., Davenport, N. D.,...Mesulam, M. M. (2005). Larger deficits in brain networks for response inhibition than for visual selective attention in attention deficit hyperactivity disorder (ADHD). *Journal of Child Psychology & Psychiatry, 46*(1), 94–111. doi: 10.1111/j.1469-7610.2004.00337.x

Bostan, A. C., Dum, R. P., & Strick, P. L. (2010). The basal ganglia communicate with the cerebellum. *Proceedings of the National Academy of Science (USA), 107*(18), 8452–8456. doi: 10.1073/pnas.1000496107

Bostan, A. C., Dum, R. P., & Strick, P. L. (2013). Cerebellar networks with the cerebral cortex and basal ganglia. *Trends in Cognitive Science, 17*(5), 241–254. doi: 10.1016/j.tics.2013.03.003

Bostan, A. C., & Strick, P. L. (2010). The cerebellum and basal ganglia are interconnected. *Neuropsychology Review, 20*(3), 261–270. doi: 10.1007/s11065-010-9143-9

Braak, H., Del Tredici, K., Rub, U., de Vos, R. A., Jansen Steur, E. N., & Braak, E. (2003). Staging of brain pathology related to sporadic Parkinson's disease. *Neurobiology of Aging, 24*(2), 197–211.

Brooks, D. J., & Pavese, N. (2011). Imaging biomarkers in Parkinson's disease. *Progress in Neurobiology, 95*(4), 614–628. doi: 10.1016/j.pneurobio.2011.08.009

Brown, P. (2006). Bad oscillations in Parkinson's disease. In P. Riederer, H. Reichmann, M. B. Youdim & M. Gerlach (Eds.), *Journal of Neural Transmission. Supplemental* (Vol. 70, pp. 27–30). Vienna: Springer.

Brown, P. (2007). Abnormal oscillatory synchronisation in the motor system leads to impaired movement. *Current Opinions in Neurobiology, 17*(6), 656–664. doi: S0959-4388(07)00136-5 [pii] 10.1016/j.conb.2007.12.001

Calderon, D. P., Fremont, R., Kraenzlin, F., & Khodakhah, K. (2011). The neural substrates of rapid-onset Dystonia-Parkinsonism. *Nature Neuroscience, 14*(3), 357–365. doi: 10.1038/nn.2753

Carbon, M., Ghilardi, M. F., Argyelan, M., Dhawan, V., Bressman, S. B., & Eidelberg, D. (2008). Increased cerebellar activation during sequence learning in DYT1 carriers: an equiperformance study. *Brain, 131*(Pt 1), 146–154. doi: 10.1093/brain/awm243

Casey, B. J., Castellanos, F. X., Giedd, J. N., Marsh, W. L., Hamburger, S. D., Schubert, A. B.,...Rapoport, J. L. (1997). Implication of right frontostriatal circuitry in response inhibition and attention-deficit/hyperactivity disorder. *Journal of the American Academy of Child & Adolescent Psychiatry, 36*(3), 374–383. doi: 10.1097/00004583-199703000-00016

Chambers, C. D., Garavan, H., & Bellgrove, M. A. (2009). Insights into the neural basis of response inhibition from cognitive and clinical neuroscience. *Neuroscience & Biobehavior Review, 33*(5), 631–646. doi: 10.1016/j.neubiorev.2008.08.016

Chevalier, G., Vacher, S., Deniau, J. M., & Desban, M. (1985). Disinhibition as a basic process in the expression of striatal functions. I. The striato-nigral influence on tecto-spinal/tecto-diencephalic neurons. *Brain Research, 334*(2), 215–226.

Cisek, P. (2007). Cortical mechanisms of action selection: the affordance competition hypothesis. *Philosophical Transactions of the Royal Society of London B Biological Science, 362*(1485), 1585–1599. doi: 10.1098/rstb.2007.2054

Coxon, J. P., Goble, D. J., Van Impe, A., De Vos, J., Wenderoth, N., & Swinnen, S. P. (2010). Reduced basal ganglia function when elderly switch between coordinated movement patterns. *Cerebral Cortex, 20*(10), 2368–2379. doi: 10.1093/cercor/bhp306

Cragg, S. J. (2006). Meaningful silences: how dopamine listens to the ACh pause. *Trends in Neuroscience, 29*(3), 125–131.

Crittenden, J. R., & Graybiel, A. M. (2011). Basal Ganglia disorders associated with imbalances in the striatal striosome and matrix compartments. *Frontiers in Neuroanatomy, 5*, 59. doi: 10.3389/fnana.2011.00059

Crossman, A. R., Mitchell, I. J., & Sambrook, M. A. (1985). Regional brain uptake of 2-deoxyglucose in N-methyl-4-phenyl-1,2,3,6-tetrahydropyridine (MPTP)-induced parkinsonism in the macaque monkey. *Neuropharmacology, 24*(6), 587–591.

Dalley, J. W., Cardinal, R. N., & Robbins, T. W. (2004). Prefrontal executive and cognitive functions in rodents: neural and neurochemical substrates. *Neuroscience & Biobehavior Review, 28*(7), 771–784. doi: 10.1016/j.neubiorev.2004.09.006

de Hemptinne, C., Ryapolova-Webb, E. S., Air, E. L., Garcia, P. A., Miller, K. J., Ojemann, J. G.,... Starr, P. A. (2013). Exaggerated phase-amplitude coupling in the primary motor cortex in Parkinson disease. *Proceedings of the National Academy of Science, U S A, 110*(12), 4780–4785. doi: 10.1073/pnas.1214546110

DeLong, M. R. (1990). Primate models of movement disorders of basal ganglia origin. *Trends in Neuroscience, 13*, 281–285.

DeLong, M. R., & Georgopoulos, A. P. (1981). Motor functions of the basal ganglia. In J. M. Brookhart, V. B. Mountcastle, V. B. Brooks & S. R. Geiger (Eds.), *Handbook of physiology. The nervous system. Motor control* (Sect. 1, Vol. II, Pt. 2, pp. 1017–1061). Bethesda, MD: American Physiological Society.

DeLong, M. R., Georgopoulos, A. P., & Crutcher, M. D. (1983). Cortico-basal ganglia relations and coding of motor preformance. In J. Massion, J. Paillard, W. Schultz & M. Wiesendanger (Eds.), *Neural coding of motor performance* (pp. 30–40). Heidelberg: Springer-Verlag Berlin.

Deniau, J. M., & Chevalier, G. (1985). Disinhibition as a basic process in the expression of striatal functions. II. The striato-nigral influence on thalamocortical cells of the ventromedial thalamic nucleus. *Brain Research, 334*, 227–233.

Desmurget, M., & Turner, R. S. (2008). Testing basal ganglia motor functions through reversible inactivations in the posterior internal globus pallidus. *Journal of Neurophysiology, 99*(3), 1057–1076. doi: 10.1152/jn.01010.2007

Dickstein, S. G., Bannon, K., Castellanos, F. X., & Milham, M. P. (2006). The neural correlates of attention deficit hyperactivity disorder: An ALE meta-analysis. *Journal of Child Psychology & Psychiatry, 47*(10), 1051–1062.

Dogali, M., Beric, A., Sterio, D., Eidelberg, D., Fazzini, E., Takikawa, S.,... Kolodny, E. H. (1994). Anatomic and physiological considerations in pallidotomy for Parkinson's disease. *Stereotactic & Functional Neurosurgery, 62*(1-4), 53–60.

Eagle, D. M., & Baunez, C. (2010). Is there an inhibitory-response-control system in the rat? Evidence from anatomical and pharmacological studies of behavioral inhibition. *Neuroscience & Biobehavioral Review, 34*(1), 50–72. doi: 10.1016/j.neubiorev.2009.07.003

Eagle, D. M., Baunez, C., Hutcheson, D. M., Lehmann, O., Shah, A. P., & Robbins, T. W. (2008). Stop-signal reaction-time task performance: role of prefrontal cortex and subthalamic nucleus. *Cerebral Cortex, 18*(1), 178–188. doi: 10.1093/cercor/bhm044

Eagle, D. M., & Robbins, T. W. (2003). Inhibitory control in rats performing a stop-signal reaction-time task: Effects of lesions of the medial striatum and d-amphetamine. *Behavioral Neuroscience, 117*(6), 1302–1317. doi: 10.1037/0735-7044.117.6.1302

Eusebio, A., & Brown, P. (2007). Oscillatory activity in the basal ganglia. *Parkinsonism & Related Disorders, 13*(Suppl 3), S434–436. doi: 10.1016/S1353-8020(08)70044-0

Filion, M., & Tremblay, L. (1991). Abnormal spontaneous activity of globus pallidus neurons in monkeys with MPTP-induced parkinsonism. *Brain Research, 547*(1), 142–151.

Filion, M., Tremblay, L., & Bedard, P. J. (1988). Abnormal influences of passive limb movement on the activity of globus pallidus neurons in parkinsonian monkeys. *Brain Research, 444*(1), 165–176.

Frank, M. J., Samanta, J., Moustafa, A. A., & Sherman, S. J. (2007). Hold your horses: impulsivity, deep brain stimulation, and medication in parkinsonism. *Science, 318*(5854), 1309–1312. doi: 10.1126/science.1146157

Galvan, A., & Wichmann, T. (2008). Pathophysiology of parkinsonism. *Clinical Neurophysiology, 119*(7), 1459–1474. doi: 10.1016/j.clinph.2008.03.017

Gatev, P., Darbin, O., & Wichmann, T. (2006). Oscillations in the basal ganglia under normal conditions and in movement disorders. *Movement Disorders, 21*(10), 1566–1577. doi: 10.1002/mds.21033

Graybiel, A. M., & Ragsdale, C. W., Jr. (1978). Histochemically distinct compartments in the striatum of human being, monkey, and cat demonstrated by the acetylcholinesterase staining method. *Proceedings of the National Academy of Science (USA), 75,* 5723–5726.

Grillner, S., Robertson, B., & Stephenson-Jones, M. (2013). The evolutionary origin of the vertebrate basal ganglia and its role in action-selection. *Journal of Physiology* doi: 10.1113/jphysiol.2012.246660

Groman, S. M., James, A. S., & Jentsch, J. D. (2009). Poor response inhibition: at the nexus between substance abuse and attention deficit/hyperactivity disorder. *Neuroscience & Biobehavior Review, 33*(5), 690–698. doi: 10.1016/j.neubiorev.2008.08.008

Gurney, K., Prescott, T. J., & Redgrave, P. (2001). A computational model of action selection in the basal ganglia. II. Analysis and simulation of behaviour. *Biological Cybernetics, 84*(6), 411–423.

Habeck, C., Krakauer, J. W., Ghez, C., Sackeim, H. A., Eidelberg, D., Stern, Y., & Moeller, J. R. (2005). A new approach to spatial covariance modeling of functional brain imaging data: Ordinal trend analysis. *Neural Computation, 17*(7), 1602–1645.

Haber, S. N., Fudge, J. L., & McFarland, N. R. (2000). Striatonigrostriatal pathways in primates form an ascending spiral from the shell to the dorsolateral striatum. *Journal of Neuroscience, 20*(6), 2369–2382.

Haber, S. N., Kunishio, K., Mizobuchi, M., & Lynd-Balta, E. (1995). The orbital and medial prefrontal circuit through the primate basal ganglia. *Journal of Neuroscience, 15,* 4851–4867.

Hammond, C., Bergman, H., & Brown, P. (2007). Pathological synchronization in Parkinson's disease: networks, models and treatments. *Trends in Neuroscience, 30*(7), 357–364.

Harnois, C., & Filion, M. (1982). Pallidofugal projections to thalamus and midbrain: a quantitative antidromic activation study in monkeys and cats. *Experimental Brain Research, 47*(2), 277–285.

Hartmann-von Monakow, K., Akert, K., & Kunzle, H. (1978). Projections of the precentral motor cortex and other cortical areas of the frontal lobe to the subthalamic nucleus in the monkey. *Experimental Brain Research, 33,* 395–403.

Hershey, T., Revilla, F. J., Wernle, A., Gibson, P. S., Dowling, J. L., & Perlmutter, J. S. (2004). Stimulation of STN impairs aspects of cognitive control in PD. *Neurology, 62*(7), 1110–1114.

Hikosaka, O. (2007). Basal ganglia mechanisms of reward-oriented eye movement. *Annals of the New York Academy of Science, 1104,* 229–249.

Hikosaka, O., & Isoda, M. (2008). Brain mechanisms for switching from automatic to controlled eye movements. *Progress in Brain Research, 171,* 375–382. doi: 10.1016/S0079-6123(08)00655-9

Hikosaka, O., Sesack, S. R., Lecourtier, L., & Shepard, P. D. (2008). Habenula: Crossroad between the basal ganglia and the limbic system. *Journal of Neuroscience, 28*(46), 11825–11829. doi: 10.1523/JNEUROSCI.3463-08.2008

Hollerman, J. R., & Schultz, W. (1998). Dopamine neurons report an error in the temporal prediction of reward during learning. *Nature Neuroscience, 1*(4), 304–309.

Hong, S., & Hikosaka, O. (2008). The globus pallidus sends reward-related signals to the lateral habenula. *Neuron, 60*(4), 720–729. doi: 10.1016/j.neuron.2008.09.035

Hoover, J. E., & Strick, P. L. (1993). Multiple output channels in the basal ganglia. *Science, 259,* 819–821.

Hoshi, E., Tremblay, L., Feger, J., Carras, P. L., & Strick, P. L. (2005). The cerebellum communicates with the basal ganglia. *Nature Neuroscience, 8*(11), 1491–1493.

Huang, C., Mattis, P., Tang, C., Perrine, K., Carbon, M., & Eidelberg, D. (2007). Metabolic brain networks associated with cognitive function in Parkinson's disease. *Neuroimage, 34*(2), 714–723. doi: 10.1016/j.neuroimage.2006.09.003

Ichinohe, N., Mori, F., & Shoumura, K. (2000). A di-synaptic projection from the lateral cerebellar nucleus to the laterodorsal part of the striatum via the central lateral nucleus of the thalamus in the rat. *Brain Research, 880*(1-2), 191–197. doi: S0006-8993(00)02744-X [pii]

Inase, M., & Tanji, J. (1995). Thalamic distribution of projection neurons to the primary motor cortex relative to afferent terminal fields from the globus pallidus in the macaque monkey. *Journal of Comparative Neurology, 353*(3), 415–426.

Isoda, M., & Hikosaka, O. (2008). Role for subthalamic nucleus neurons in switching from automatic to controlled eye movement. *Journal of Neuroscience, 28*(28), 7209–7218. doi: 10.1523/JNEUROSCI.0487-08.2008

Jahanshahi, M., Ardouin, C. M., Brown, R. G., Rothwell, J. C., Obeso, J., Albanese, A.,... Limousin-Dowsey, P. (2000). The impact of deep brain stimulation on executive function in Parkinson's disease. *Brain, 123*(Pt 6), 1142–1154.

Jinnah, H. A., & Hess, E. J. (2006). A new twist on the anatomy of dystonia: the basal ganglia and the cerebellum? *Neurology, 67*(10), 1740–1741.

Joel, D., & Weiner, I. (1994). The organization of the basal ganglia-thalamocortical circuits: open interconnected rather than closed segregated. *Neuroscience, 63*(2), 363–379.

Kaneda, K., Isa, K., Yanagawa, Y., & Isa, T. (2008). Nigral inhibition of GABAergic neurons in mouse superior colliculus. *Journal of Neuroscience, 28*(43), 11071–11078. doi: 10.1523/JNEUROSCI.3263-08.2008

Kemp, J. M., & Powell, T. P. S. (1971). The connexions of the striatum and globus pallidus: Synthesis and speculation. *Philosophical Transactions of the Royal Society of London—Series B: Biological Sciences, 262,* 441–457.

Kish, S. J., Shannak, K., & Hornykiewicz, O. (1988). Uneven pattern of dopamine loss in the striatum of patients with idiopathic Parkinson's disease. *New England Journal of Medicine, 318,* 876–880.

Kita, T., & Kita, H. (2012). The subthalamic nucleus is one of multiple innervation sites for long-range corticofugal axons: A single-axon tracing study in the rat. *Journal of Neuroscience, 32*(17), 5990–5999. doi: 10.1523/JNEUROSCI.5717-11.2012

Kravitz, A. V., Freeze, B. S., Parker, P. R., Kay, K., Thwin, M. T., Deisseroth, K., & Kreitzer, A. C. (2010). Regulation of parkinsonian motor behaviours by optogenetic control of basal ganglia circuitry. *Nature, 466*(7306), 622–626. doi: 10.1038/nature09159

Kuhn, A. A., Williams, D., Kupsch, A., Limousin, P., Hariz, M., Schneider, G. H., . . . Brown, P. (2004). Event-related beta desynchronization in human subthalamic nucleus correlates with motor performance. *Brain, 127*(Pt 4), 735–746.

Lecourtier, L., & Kelly, P. H. (2007). A conductor hidden in the orchestra? Role of the habenular complex in monoamine transmission and cognition. *Neuroscience Biobehavior Review, 31*(5), 658–672. doi: 10.1016/j.neubiorev.2007.01.004

Lei, W., Jiao, Y., Del Mar, N., & Reiner, A. (2004). Evidence for differential cortical input to direct pathway versus indirect pathway striatal projection neurons in rats. *Journal of Neuroscience, 24*(38), 8289–8299.

Liddle, E. B., Scerif, G., Hollis, C. P., Batty, M. J., Groom, M. J., Liotti, M., & Liddle, P. F. (2009). Looking before you leap: A theory of motivated control of action. *Cognition, 112*(1), 141–158. doi: 10.1016/j.cognition.2009.03.006

Lim, S. Y., & Lang, A. E. (2010). The nonmotor symptoms of Parkinson's disease—an overview. *Movement Disorders, 25*(Suppl 1), S123–130. doi: 10.1002/mds.22786

Liu, P., & Basso, M. A. (2008). Substantia nigra stimulation influences monkey superior colliculus neuronal activity bilaterally. *Journal of Neurophysiology, 100*(2), 1098–1112. doi: 10.1152/jn.01043.2007

Lozano, A., Hutchison, W., Kiss, Z., Tasker, R., Davis, K., & Dostrovsky, J. (1996). Methods for microelectrode-guided posteroventral pallidotomy. *Journal of Neurosurgery, 84*(2), 194–202.

Magill, P. J., Bolam, J. P., & Bevan, M. D. (2000). Relationship of activity in the subthalamic nucleus-globus pallidus network to cortical electroencephalogram. *Journal of Neuroscience, 20*(2), 820–833.

Magill, P. J., Bolam, J. P., & Bevan, M. D. (2001). Dopamine regulates the impact of the cerebral cortex on the subthalamic nucleus-globus pallidus network. *Neuroscience, 106*(2), 313–330.

Marsden, C. D., & Obeso, J. A. (1994). The functions of the basal ganglia and the paradox of stereotaxic surgery in Parkinson's disease. *Brain, 117*, 877–897.

May, P. J., McHaffie, J. G., Stanford, T. R., Jiang, H., Costello, M. G., Coizet, V., . . . Redgrave, P. (2009). Tectonigral projections in the primate: a pathway for pre-attentive sensory input to midbrain dopaminergic neurons. *European Journal of Neuroscience, 29*(3), 575–587. doi: 10.1111/j.1460-9568.2008.06596.x

Meister, I. G., Foltys, H., Gallea, C., & Hallett, M. (2010). How the brain handles temporally uncoupled bimanual movements. *Cerebral Cortex, 20*(12), 2996–3004. doi: 10.1093/cercor/bhq048

Mena-Segovia, J., Bolam, J. P., & Magill, P. J. (2004). Pedunculopontine nucleus and basal ganglia: distant relatives or part of the same family? *Trends in Neuroscience, 27*(10), 585–588.

Middleton, F. A., & Strick, P. L. (2000). Basal ganglia and cerebellar loops: Motor and cognitive circuits. *Brain Research Reviews, 31*(2-3), 236–250.

Miller, W. C., & DeLong, M. R. (1987). Altered tonic activity of neurons in the globus pallidus and subthalamic nucleus in the primate MPTP model of parkinsonism. In M. B. Carpenter & A. Jayaraman (Eds.), *The basal ganglia II* (pp. 415–427). New York, NY: Plenum Press.

Minamimoto, T., Hori, Y., & Kimura, M. (2005). Complementary process to response bias in the centromedian nucleus of the thalamus. *Science, 308*(5729), 1798–1801.

Minamimoto, T., Hori, Y., & Kimura, M. (2009). Roles of the thalamic CM-PF complex-Basal ganglia circuit in externally driven rebias of action. *Brain Research Bulletin, 78*(2-3), 75–79. doi: 10.1016/j.brainresbull.2008.08.013

Mink, J. W. (1996). The basal ganglia: focused selection and inhibition of competing motor programs. *Progress in Neurobiology, 50*(4), 381–425.

Mink, J. W., & Thach, W. T. (1993). Basal ganglia intrinsic circuits and their role in behavior. *Current Opinion in Neurobiology, 3*(6), 950–957.

Mitchell, S. J., Richardson, R. T., Baker, F. H., & DeLong, M. R. (1987). The primate globus pallidus: Neuronal activity related to direction of movement. *Experimental Brain Research, 68*, 491–505.

Miyachi, S., Hikosaka, O., & Lu, X. (2002). Differential activation of monkey striatal neurons in the early and late stages of procedural learning. *Experimental Brain Research, 146*(1), 122–126.

Mure, H., Hirano, S., Tang, C. C., Isaias, I. U., Antonini, A., Ma, Y., ... Eidelberg, D. (2011). Parkinson's disease tremor-related metabolic network: characterization, progression, and treatment effects. *Neuroimage, 54*(2), 1244–1253. doi: 10.1016/j.neuroimage.2010.09.028

Nambu, A. (2011). Somatotopic organization of the primate basal ganglia. *Frontiers in Neuroanatomy, 5*, 26. doi: 10.3389/fnana.2011.00026

Nambu, A., Mori, S., Stuart, D. G., & Wiesendanger, M. (2004). A new dynamic model of the cortico-basal ganglia loop. *Progress in Brain Research, 143*, 461–466).

Nambu, A., Tokuno, H., Hamada, I., Kita, H., Imanishi, M., Akazawa, T., ... Hasegawa, N. (2000). Excitatory cortical inputs to pallidal neurons via the subthalamic nucleus in the monkey. *Journal of Neurophysiology, 84*(1), 289–300.

Nambu, A., Tokuno, H., & Takada, M. (2002). Functional significance of the cortico-subthalamo-pallidal 'hyperdirect' pathway. *Neuroscience Research, 43*(2), 111–117.

Nanda, B., Galvan, A., Smith, Y., & Wichmann, T. (2009). Effects of stimulation of the centromedian nucleus of the thalamus on the activity of striatal cells in awake rhesus monkeys. *European Journal of Neuroscience, 29*(3), 588–598.

Neychev, V. K., Fan, X., Mitev, V. I., Hess, E. J., & Jinnah, H. A. (2008). The basal ganglia and cerebellum interact in the expression of dystonic movement. *Brain, 131*(Pt 9), 2499–2509. doi: 10.1093/brain/awn168

Obeso, J. A., Jahanshahi, M., Alvarez, L., Macias, R., Pedroso, I., Wilkinson, L., ... Rothwell, J. C. (2009). What can man do without basal ganglia motor output? The effect of combined unilateral subthalamotomy and pallidotomy in a patient with Parkinson's disease. *Experimental Neurology, 220*(2), 283–292. doi: 10.1016/j.expneurol.2009.08.030

Pare, J. F., & Smith, Y. (2009). Functional segregation of basal ganglia circuits through the lateral habenula in primates. *Society for Neuroscience Abstracts*, 828.823.

Parent, A. (1990). Extrinsic connections of the basal ganglia. *Trends in Neuroscience, 13*, 254–258.

Parent, A., & Hazrati, L. N. (1995). Functional anatomy of the basal ganglia. I. The cortico-basal ganglia-thalamo-cortical loop. *Brain Research Reviews, 20*(1), 91–127.

Parent, M., & Parent, A. (2006). Single-axon tracing study of corticostriatal projections arising from primary motor cortex in primates. *Journal of Comparative Neurology, 496*(2), 202–213.

Pasquereau, B., & Turner, R. S. (2011). Primary motor cortex of the parkinsonian monkey: differential effects on the spontaneous activity of pyramidal tract-type neurons. *Cerebral Cortex, 21*(6), 1362–1378. doi: 10.1093/cercor/bhq217

Ray, N. J., Jenkinson, N., Brittain, J., Holland, P., Joint, C., Nandi, D., . . . Aziz, T. Z. (2009). The role of the subthalamic nucleus in response inhibition: evidence from deep brain stimulation for Parkinson's disease. *Neuropsychologia, 47*(13), 2828–2834. doi: 10.1016/j.neuropsychologia.2009.06.011

Redgrave, P., Prescott, T. J., & Gurney, K. (1999). The basal ganglia: a vertebrate solution to the selection problem? *Neuroscience, 89*(4), 1009–1023.

Redgrave, P., Rodriguez, M., Smith, Y., Rodriguez-Oroz, M. C., Lehericy, S., Bergman, H., . . . Obeso, J. A. (2010). Goal-directed and habitual control in the basal ganglia: implications for Parkinson's disease. *National Review of Neuroscience, 11*(11), 760–772. doi: 10.1038/nrn2915

Rico, A. J., Barroso-Chinea, P., Conte-Perales, L., Roda, E., Gomez-Bautista, V., Gendive, M., . . . Lanciego, J. L. (2010). A direct projection from the subthalamic nucleus to the ventral thalamus in monkeys. *Neurobiology of Disease, 39*(3), 381–392. doi: 10.1016/j.nbd.2010.05.004

Rieger, M., Gauggel, S., & Burmeister, K. (2003). Inhibition of ongoing responses following frontal, nonfrontal, and basal ganglia lesions. *Neuropsychology, 17*(2), 272–282.

Robbins, T. W. (2007). Shifting and stopping: fronto-striatal substrates, neurochemical modulation and clinical implications. *Philosophical Transactions of the Royal Society B: Biological Sciences, 362*(1481), 917–932. doi: 10.1098/rstb.2007.2097

Rubin, J. E., McIntyre, C. C., Turner, R. S., & Wichmann, T. (2012). Basal ganglia activity patterns in parkinsonism and computational modeling of their downstream effects. *European Journal of Neuroscience, 36*(2), 2213–2228. doi: 10.1111/j.1460-9568.2012.08108.x

Rye, D. B., Lee, H. J., Saper, C. B., & Wainer, B. H. (1988). Medullary and spinal efferents of the pedunculopontine tegmental nucleus and adjacent mesopontine tegmentum in the rat. *Journal of Comparative Neurology, 269*(3), 315–341.

Sadikot, A. F., Parent, A., & Francois, C. (1992). Efferent connections of the centromedian and parafascicular thalamic nuclei in the squirrel monkey: a PHA-L study of subcortical projections. *Journal of Comparative Neurology, 315*(2), 137–159.

Sauleau, P., Eusebio, A., Vandenberghe, W., Nuttin, B., & Brown, P. (2009). Deep brain stimulation modulates effects of motivation in Parkinson's disease. *Neuroreport, 20*(6), 622–626. doi: 10.1097/WNR.0b013e32832aa928

Schell, G. R., & Strick, P. L. (1984). The origin of thalamic inputs to the arcuate premotor and supplementary motor areas. *Journal of Neuroscience, 4*(2), 539–560.

Schroeder, U., Kuehler, A., Haslinger, B., Erhard, P., Fogel, W., Tronnier, V. M., . . . Ceballos-Baumann, A. O. (2002). Subthalamic nucleus stimulation affects striato-anterior cingulate cortex circuit in a response conflict task: a PET study. *Brain, 125*(Pt 9), 1995–2004.

Schwartzman, R. J., & Alexander, G. M. (1985). Changes in the local cerebral metabolic rate for glucose in the 1-methyl-4-phenyl-1,2,3,6-tetrahydropyridine (MPTP) primate model of Parkinson's disease. *Brain Research, 358*(1-2), 137–143.

Shadmehr, R., & Krakauer, J. W. (2008). A computational neuroanatomy for motor control. *Experimental Brain Research, 185*(3), 359–381. doi: 10.1007/s00221-008-1280-5

Sharott, A., Magill, P. J., Harnack, D., Kupsch, A., Meissner, W., & Brown, P. (2005). Dopamine depletion increases the power and coherence of beta-oscillations in the cerebral cortex and subthalamic nucleus of the awake rat. *European Journal of Neuroscience, 21*(5), 1413–1422.

Shepherd, G. M. (2013). Corticostriatal connectivity and its role in disease. *National Review of Neuroscience, 14*(4), 278–291. doi: 10.1038/nrn3469

Shimamoto, S. A., Ryapolova-Webb, E. S., Ostrem, J. L., Galifianakis, N. B., Miller, K. J., & Starr, P. A. (2013). Subthalamic nucleus neurons are synchronized to primary motor cortex local field potentials in Parkinson's disease. *Journal of Neuroscience, 33*(17), 7220–7233. doi: 10.1523/JNEUROSCI.4676-12.2013

Sidibe, M., Bevan, M. D., Bolam, J. P., & Smith, Y. (1997). Efferent connections of the internal globus pallidus in the squirrel monkey: I. Topography and synaptic organization of the pallidothalamic projection. *Journal of Comparative Neurology, 382*(3), 323–347.

Smith, Y., & Parent, A. (1986). Differential connections of caudate nucleus and putamen in the squirrel monkey (Saimiri sciureus). *Neuroscience, 18*(2), 347–371.

Smith, Y., Raju, D. V., Pare, J. F., & Sidibe, M. (2004). The thalamostriatal system: a highly specific network of the basal ganglia circuitry. *Trends in Neuroscience, 27*(9), 520–527.

Song, Y. G., Yoo, K. S., Park, K. W., & Park, J. H. (2010). Coordinative and limb-specific control of bimanual movements in patients with Parkinson's disease and cerebellar degeneration. *Neuroscience Letters, 482*(2), 146–150. doi: 10.1016/j.neulet.2010.07.021

Spetsieris, P. G., & Eidelberg, D. (2011). Scaled subprofile modeling of resting state imaging data in Parkinson's disease: methodological issues. *Neuroimage, 54*(4), 2899–2914. doi: 10.1016/j.neuroimage.2010.10.025

Stephenson-Jones, M., Samuelsson, E., Ericsson, J., Robertson, B., & Grillner, S. (2011). Evolutionary conservation of the basal ganglia as a common vertebrate mechanism for action selection. *Current Biology, 21*(13), 1081–1091. doi: 10.1016/j.cub.2011.05.001

Tanaka, S. C., Doya, K., Okada, G., Ueda, K., Okamoto, Y., & Yamawaki, S. (2004). Prediction of immediate and future rewards differentially recruits cortico-basal ganglia loops. *Nature Neuroscience, 7*(8), 887–893.

Threlfell, S., Lalic, T., Platt, N. J., Jennings, K. A., Deisseroth, K., & Cragg, S. J. (2012). Striatal dopamine release is triggered by synchronized activity in cholinergic interneurons. *Neuron, 75*(1), 58–64. doi: 10.1016/j.neuron.2012.04.038

Timmermann, L., & Fink, G. R. (2009). Modulating pathological oscillatory activity in Parkinson's disease: What's the rhythm? *Experimental Neurology, 215*(2), 209–211. doi: 10.1016/j.expneurol.2008.04.003

Timmermann, L., Florin, E., & Reck, C. (2007). Pathological cerebral oscillatory activity in Parkinson's disease: a critical review on methods, data and hypotheses. *Expert Review of Medical Devices, 4*(5), 651–661. doi: 10.1586/17434440.4.5.651

Tunik, E., Houk, J. C., & Grafton, S. T. (2009). Basal ganglia contribution to the initiation of corrective submovements. *Neuroimage, 47*(4), 1757–1766. doi: 10.1016/j.neuroimage.2009.04.077

Turner, R. S., & DeLong, M. R. (2000). Corticostriatal activity in primary motor cortex of the macaque. *Journal of Neuroscience, 20*(18), 7096–7108.

Turner, R. S., & Desmurget, M. (2010). Basal ganglia contributions to motor control: a vigorous tutor. *Current Opinions in Neurobiology, 20*(6), 704–716. doi: 10.1016/j.conb.2010.08.022

Turner, R. S., Grafton, S. T., Votaw, J. R., Delong, M. R., & Hoffman, J. M. (1998). Motor subcircuits mediating the control of movement velocity: a PET study. *Journal of Neurophysiology, 80*(4), 2162–2176.

Verbruggen, F., & Logan, G. D. (2009). Models of response inhibition in the stop-signal and stop-change paradigms. *Neuroscience Biobehavior Review, 33*(5), 647–661. doi: 10.1016/j.neubiorev.2008.08.014

Villanueva, R. (2012). The cerebellum and neuropsychiatric disorders. *Psychiatry Research, 198*(3), 527–532. doi: 10.1016/j.psychres.2012.02.023

Vitek, J. L., Kaneoke, Y., Turner, R., Baron, M., Bakay, R., & DeLong, M. (1993). Neuronal activity in the internal (GPi) and external (GPe) segments of the globus pallidus (GP) of parkinsonian patients is similar to that in the MPTP-treated primate model of parkinsonism. *Society of Neuroscience Abstracts, 19,* 1584.

Voorn, P., Vanderschuren, L. J., Groenewegen, H. J., Robbins, T. W., & Pennartz, C. M. (2004). Putting a spin on the dorsal-ventral divide of the striatum. *Trends Neurosci, 27*(8), 468–474. doi: 10.1016/j.tins.2004.06.006

Waelti, P., Dickinson, A., & Schultz, W. (2001). Dopamine responses comply with basic assumptions of formal learning theory. *Nature, 412*(6842), 43–48.

Weinberger, M., Hutchison, W. D., & Dostrovsky, J. O. (2009). Pathological subthalamic nucleus oscillations in PD: Can they be the cause of bradykinesia and akinesia? *Experimental Neurology, 219*(1), 58–61. doi: 10.1016/j.expneurol.2009.05.014

Wichmann, T., Bergman, H., & DeLong, M. R. (1994). The primate subthalamic nucleus. I. Functional properties in intact animals. *Journal of Neurophysiology, 72*(2), 494–506.

Wichmann, T., & DeLong, M. R. (2006). Basal ganglia discharge abnormalities in Parkinson's disease. *Journal of Neural Transmission Supplment, 70,* 21–25.

Williams, D., Tijssen, M., Van Bruggen, G., Bosch, A., Insola, A., Di Lazzaro, V., . . . Brown, P. (2002). Dopamine-dependent changes in the functional connectivity between basal ganglia and cerebral cortex in humans. *Brain, 125,* 1558–1569.

Witt, K., Pulkowski, U., Herzog, J., Lorenz, D., Hamel, W., Deuschl, G., & Krack, P. (2004). Deep brain stimulation of the subthalamic nucleus improves cognitive flexibility but impairs response inhibition in Parkinson disease. *Archives of Neurology, 61*(5), 697–700.

Wu, T., & Hallett, M. (2013). The cerebellum in Parkinson's disease. *Brain, 136*(Pt 3), 696–709. doi: 10.1093/brain/aws360

Wu, T., Wang, L., Hallett, M., Li, K., & Chan, P. (2010). Neural correlates of bimanual anti-phase and in-phase movements in Parkinson's disease. *Brain, 133*(Pt 8), 2394–2409. doi: 10.1093/brain/awq151

2 Neurocognitive Screening and Assessment in Parkinsonism

Jaime Kulisevsky and Javier Pagonabarraga

INTRODUCTION

Although restricted in the past to the examination and management of motor disabilities, physicians attending patients with movement disorders are currently aware of the importance of detecting and managing the plethora of mental disturbances that affect these patients. Mood symptoms, psychotic phenomena, and cognitive disturbances have all been observed to have a great impact on quality of life (Schrag, Jahanshahi, & Quinn, 2000). Among them, the assessment of cognitive dysfunction seems especially important given the early and progressive nature of this complication, as well as the difficulty of capturing the severity of the problem by medical history alone.

The neuropsychological examination of patients with parkinsonism could also be useful in the differential diagnosis between Parkinson's disease (PD) and atypical parkinsonisms, and the delineation of different cognitive profiles in PD could offer the possibility of identifying patients with the highest risk of developing dementia earlier in the disease process.

For diseases in which dysfunction of basal ganglia has been clearly defined, frontal-striatal cognitive defects would be expected to represent the main substrate leading to global cognitive dysfunction. Recent evidence, however, has shown that in PD and other parkinsonian disorders, deterioration of cognitive functions seems to be associated with a more diffuse cortical and subcortical dysfunction (Lyoo et al., 2008; Williams-Gray et al., 2009).

In this chapter we will first review the broad features of cognitive impairment in PD, and the available cognitive screening tools that may help us to detect cognitive impairments earlier and to capture them in more detail. Then, we will compare the patterns of cognitive dysfunction in multiple system atrophy (MSA), progressive supranuclear palsy (PSP), and corticobasal degeneration (CBD). A better knowledge of the cognitive defects that characterize each disease will aid us in their differential diagnosis, and in a better understanding of those problems that impair patient's daily life.

NEUROCOGNITIVE ASSESSMENT IN PARKINSON'S DISEASE (PD)

Cognitive impairment (CI) is integral to Parkinson's disease (PD) (Cooper, Sagar, Jordan, Harvey, & Sullivan, 1991; Goldman, Baty, Buckles, Sahrmann, & Morris, 1998). Although most nondemented PD (PD-ND) patients exhibit relatively subtle cognitive deficits, the point prevalence of dementia associated with PD (PDD) is around 25–30% (Aarsland, Zaccai, & Brayne, 2005)—six times greater than in the general population (Hobson & Meara, 2004)—and the cumulative prevalence of dementia at 15—20 years of follow-up varies between 60–80% (Aarsland et al., 2001; Buter et al., 2008; Halliday, Hely, Reid, & Morris, 2008).

Phenomenology of Cognitive Impairment in PD and Associated Clinical Features

Regarding the phenomenology of cognitive symptoms in PD, patients report difficulties in maintaining attention while reading, during prolonged mental effort, or when they have to perform simultaneous mental operations (i.e., multitask). They commonly complain of word-finding difficulties that may slow speech fluency—"tip-of-the-tongue phenomenon"—a symptom related to defects in semantic verbal fluency present in some patients from the first years of the disease (Matison, Mayeux, Rosen, & Fahn, 1982). Complaints of recollection of recent episodic events are also common and relate to early impairment in free-recall of verbal and visual material (Bronnick, Alves, Aarsland, Tysnes, & Larssen, 2011). Difficulties in performing dual-tasks, planning activities, and organizing daily life (correspondence, finances, work projects) may be perceived very soon by patients, and have been associated with executive dysfunction (McKinlay, Grace, Dalrymple-Alford, & Roger, 2010). Despite the early occurrence of deficits in visual perception (i.e., contrast sensitivity), no clear abnormalities of motion perception or visual recognition are reported by patients in the nondementia stages (Mosimann et al., 2004).

As the cognitive deficits evolve, memory and executive symptoms are more frequent, and become apparent to both patients and their caregivers. In the transition to dementia, language problems may arise, and PD patients encounter problems understanding and producing language, and develop a tendency to lose the thread of conversation (Galvin, Pollack, & Morris, 2006). Language problems in mid- to advanced stages of the disease are characterized by impaired sentence comprehension, poor verb production, and diminished semantic activation (Bastiaanse & Leenders, 2009). In a longitudinal clinico-pathological study (Galvin et al., 2006) and comparative neuropsychological studies (Noe et al., 2004), confrontation naming is clearly affected in PDD patients, at a similar degree to that found in Alzheimer's disease (AD) and dementia with Lewy bodies (DLB).

Different neuropsychiatric disturbances have been associated with the development of cognitive impairment in PD. The presence of apathy, anxiety, and depression may act as confounding factors in the assessment of cognition in PD, since it has been evidenced that each one of these symptoms affects the attentional resources necessary for encoding new information, leading to memory and executive deficits (Butterfield, Cimino, Oelke, Hauser, & Sanchez-Ramos, 2010; Starkstein et al. 1989; Troster et al., 1995). Apathy, however, can be understood as a cognitive symptom itself, being the behavioral manifestation of inefficient cognitive strategies connecting different regions of the prefrontal cortex, anterior cingulate cortex, and striatum (Varanese, Perfetti, Ghilardi, & DiRocco, 2011). Moreover, apathy has been suggested to herald cognitive decline and dementia in PD (Dujardin, Sockeel, Delliaux, Destée, & Defebvre, 2009). Hallucinations are frequent, progressive, and have a great impact on quality of life when they become well structured and the patient loses the insight into the unreal nature of the phenomenon (Goetz, Leurgans, Pappert, Raman, & Stemer, 2001). Studies focused on the neuropsychological correlates of hallucinations in PD have shown that the progression in severity of hallucinations is associated with posterior cortical defects superimposed on a progressive frontal-striatal cognitive impairment (Llebaria et al., 2010).

Neuropsychological Characteristics of Cognitive Impairment and Dementia in PD

Cognitive impairment in PD can be present from the earliest disease stages, and can be detected in untreated "de novo" patients, even when traditional instruments measuring global cognitive function (such as the MMSE and Mattis Dementia Rating scale) are within the normal range (Muslimovic, Post, Speelman, & Schmand, 2005; Aarsland et al., 2009). At these early stages, cognitive impairment is characterized by subtle changes that are not generally apparent to the patient or clinician. Muslimovic et al., (2005) studied in detail a "de novo" cohort of 115 PD patients (age 66.2±10 years, disease duration 18.8± 10 months, education 11.7± 2 years) and observed that, compared to well-matched healthy subjects, almost all PD patients performed significantly worse in tests measuring executive dysfunction, almost 50% of the sample showed visuospatial deficits, and 45% had memory deficits. Interestingly, a subset of patients (20% of the sample) already presented language defects in confrontation naming tests (Muslimovic et al., 2005). A more detailed description of the neuropsychological differences observed shows that cognitive impairment in nondemented patients is characterized by impairments in psychomotor speed (Digit Symbol Test), attention/working memory (Digit span backward), measures of set-shifting, planning, and abstract reasoning (Wisconsin Card Sorting test, Tower of London, WAIS similarities), verbal (Rey Auditory Verbal Learning test; RAVLT) and visual (Faces Immediate Recognition test) recall, visuospatial abilities (Line Orientation test), and language (Boston Naming Test). The largest effects of impairment were observed generally in the memory domain, particularly on tests of immediate and delayed free-recall, and the tests that most effectively differentiated patients from controls were the RAVLT, Tower of London, Wechsler Memory Scale (WMS-III) Faces Immediate Recognition test, and Rivermead Behavioural Memory Test-Immediate Story Recall (RBMT), that correctly classified 77% of the cases. Overall, 24% of the sample exhibited cognitive dysfunction, defined as impaired performance on at least three neuropsychological tests (Muslimovic et al., 2005).

The same authors observed that cognitive performance of newly diagnosed PD patients decreased significantly over 3 years, particularly on measures of psychomotor speed and attention and to a lesser extent on tests of memory, visuospatial skills, and executive functions. About 50% of the patients showed cognitive decline and 9% developed dementia. The clinical features that best predicted cognitive change were age at disease onset and axial motor impairment (Muslimovic, Post, Speelman, De Haan, & Schmand, 2009). In another study examining cognitive impairment in "de-novo" PD patients, impairment was evidenced on all neuropsychological tests administered compared to controls, and, as in the study by Muslimovic et al. (2005), the largest effect sizes were found for verbal recall and psychomotor speed (Aarsland et al., 2009). In two other longitudinal studies, however, cognitive test performance was seen to be relatively stable in PD after a follow-up of 14 and 18 months (Azuma, Cruz, Bayles, Tomoeda, & Montgomery Jr, 2003; Troster, Woods, & Morgan, 2007).

The profile of deficits in attention, executive functions, free-recall and visuospatial abilities has been replicated in many studies, and consistent results have also been found in the comparison of cognitive profiles between PD and AD patients, with PD patients showing more evident defects in executive and visuospatial tasks, and AD patients showing more severe memory and language problems (Huber, Shuttleworth, & Freidenberg, 1989; Starkstein et al., 1996). Detailed neuropsychological studies, however, have shown that cognitive defects are not homogeneous. The CamPaIGN cohort (Williams-Gray et al., 2009) study further clarified the profile of cognitive dysfunction in early PD by showing that early conversion to dementia is linked to the differential impairment in cognitive tasks with a posterior cortical basis (semantic verbal fluency, copying intersecting pentagons). The relevance of posterior cortical defects had been previously highlighted by studies that showed intrusion errors and recognition memory defects suggestive of temporal rather than prefrontal dysfunction in 15–20% of non-demented patients in the early to middle stages of the disease. (Weintraub et al., 2004; Whittington, Podd, & Stewart-Williams, 2006). The relevance of posterior cortical dysfunction in PD is also evident from the observation that defects such as naming and copying indicate the transition from MCI to PDD

(Pagonabarraga et al., 2008). In addition, in a recent study of carriers of the E46K mutation of the α-synuclein gene (PARK 1), early development of dementia was associated with salient visuospatial alterations, suggesting that posterior cortical dysfunction might be a distinct early feature leading to clinically relevant cognitive impairment in these patients (Zarranz et al., 2004).

Over time, progression of cognitive impairment is explained by deterioration of the previously affected cognitive domains, but new symptoms and new cognitive defects seem to have a special impact on the conversion to dementia. In a longitudinal clinico-pathological study, patients that converted to dementia were characterized by language defects apparent both clinically (symptoms of aphasia) and neuropsychologically (confrontation naming) (Galvin et al., 2006). Furthermore, in a comparative study of PD, AD, and dementia with Lewy bodies (DLB), the three groups showed the same degree of confrontation naming defects (Galvin et al., 2006). Two meta-analyses of the impairments of verbal fluency (Henry & Crawford, 2004) and recognition memory (Whittington, Podd, & Kan, 2000) in PD provide evidence of a shift in the pattern of cognitive alterations when patients convert to dementia. Whereas in the predementia stage PD patients are more likely to show impaired phonemic verbal fluency and preserved recognition memory, when they develop dementia they also show defects in semantic verbal fluency (which, consistent with confrontation naming deficits, appears more affected than phonemic fluency (Henry & Crawford, 2004)) and in recognition memory (Whittington et al., 2000). In conclusion, cognitive dysfunction in PDD patients seems to be characterized by the addition of impairments in cognitive tasks with a predominantly posterior cortical basis to a progressive impairment in tasks with a frontal-striatal basis seen in early and midstage PD.

Tools for the Assessment of Cognitive Functions in Parkinson's Disease

Estimates of cognitive impairment (CI) and dementia in PD are largely dependent on the diagnostic measures used (Riedel et al., 2008). When trying to identify the tasks and neuropsychological scales that best capture the cognitive changes that appear throughout the course of the disease, it is important to review both which cognitive domains are measured by each scale and the clinimetric properties shown by the scales.

Assessment of cognition in PD can be carried out by using tasks that measure narrow cognitive functions, or by using comprehensive neuropsychological batteries that capture multiple cognitive domains. In research studies focusing on specific cognitive functions (set-shifting, attention, psychomotor speed, verbal memory, visuoperception), the use of more specific tasks is preferred. By contrast, in daily neurological practice and in studies trying to identify different cognitive profiles, track progression of cognitive dysfunction, or evaluate the efficacy of a particular drug on cognition, the use of neuropsychological batteries seems a better option.

Assessment of Specific Cognitive Domains

In 2007, the Movement Disorders Society proposed a set of cognitive tests that consistently and accurately capture cognitive impairment in PD, and have adequate clinimetric/psychometric properties (Dubois et al., 2007). Executive functions are subdivided into different cognitive aspects and tests assessing working memory, conceptualization, set activation, set shifting, and set maintenance/resistance to interference were recommended. The memory tests assessed mainly declarative verbal memory by word list recall. Visuospatial abilities to be assessed include visuoconstructional and visuoperceptual (less dependent on prefrontal activation) functions. Confrontation naming seems useful to assess language in PD (Table 2-1). Due to the increasing prevalence of impulse control disorders in treated PD patients, the assessment of more medially based cognitive functions seems necessary to complete the evaluation of those cortical areas that may predispose to addictive behaviors. Impulsivity (Isaias et al., 2008; Poletti et al., 2011; Robert et al., 2009) and decision-making (Pagonabarraga et al., 2007) defects seem to underlie these behaviors, so the systematic assessment of these two functions is warranted.

Cognitive Screening Tools in Parkinson's Disease

Different screening tests have been used in the study of cognitive functions in PD. Initially, brief assessment of cognition was based on nonspecific screening

Table 2-1 Proposed set of cognitive tests for a comprehensive assessment of cognition in PD

Cognitive domain	*Test*
Executive function	- Digit span, Digit Ordering Test
- Working memory	- Similarities (WAIS-III)
- Conceptualization	- Verbal fluencies (C,F,L)
- Set activation	- Trail Making Test
- Set shifting	- Wisconsin Card Sorting Test
- Set maintenance / resistance to interference	- Stroop Test
Memory	- Rey Auditory Verbal Learning Test (RAVLT)
Language	- Buschke Free and Cued Recall Test
Visuospatial abilities	- Boston Naming Test
Medial prefrontal functions	- Benton Line Orientation Test
- Decision making	- Clock copying tasks
- Impulsivity	- VOSP (Visual Object and Spatial Perception Battery)
	- Benton Face Recognition Test
	- Iowa Gambling Task
	- Cambridge Gambling Test
	- Barrat Impulsivity Scale (BIS)

scales assessing global cognitive function, but in the past five years, various attempts to harmonize results within different research groups have resulted in the development of several new PD-specific scales. These new scales await further evaluation and validation before a decision might be made about which scales are most suitable for assessing cognitive status and cognitive change over time in PD patients.

The scales most frequently used to assess global cognitive function in PD are the Mini-Mental State Examination (MMSE), Mattis Dementia Rating Scale (MDRS), Cambridge Cognitive Assessment (CAMCOG), and Montreal Cognitive Assessment (MoCA), none of which was developed specifically for use in PD. The Frontal Assessment Battery (FAB) aims to assess prefrontal cognitive functions rather than global cognitive function, and although it has been extensively administered in PD populations, it, too, is not a PD-specific instrument. The PD-specific scales recently developed that have received increasing attention are the Scales for Outcomes in Parkinson's Disease-Cognition (SCOPA-COG), Parkinson's Disease-Cognitive Rating Scale (PD-CRS), and the Parkinson Neuropsychometric Dementia Assessment (PANDA).

The characteristics and psychometric properties of each of these scales were recently reviewed (Kulisevsky & Pagonabarraga, 2009), and we summarize here the most salient and clinically relevant characteristics of these instruments.

Mini-Mental State Examination

The Mini-Mental State Examination (MMSE) is a brief scale originally used to detect dementia in AD, which is now widely used in a variety of dementias because it is easily and rapidly administered in the office or at the bedside (Folstein, Folstein, & McHugh, 1975). The reliability of the MMSE for diagnosing dementia in cognitive disorders other than AD has not yet been established, and PD-ND patients may score well in the normal range of the scale (Mamikonyan et al., 2009). In recent studies, the MMSE revealed low sensitivity for the diagnosis of both PD-MCI and PDD (Hoops et al., 2009), and no data regarding the validation of the MMSE in PD populations have so far been reported.

Mattis Dementia Rating Scale

The Mattis Dementia Rating Scale (MDRS) is a test of global cognitive function that sensitively measures the degree of frontal-subcortical deficits in patients with neurodegenerative diseases (Monsch et al., 1995). Compared with the MMSE, the MDRS is a more sensitive tool to detect frontal lobe dysfunction in PDD (Aarsland et al., 2003). One of the main limitations of the MDRS is its length, and the estimated administration time in the general population is 20–45 minutes. In a recent study, a cut-off score of ≤123 on the MDRS total score yielded high sensitivity (92.7%) and specificity (91.4%) for detecting dementia in PD (Llebaria et al., 2008).

Cambridge Cognitive Assessment

The Cambridge Cognitive Assessment (CAMCOG) is the cognitive section of the Cambridge Examination of Mental Disorders (Roth et al., 1986). Applying the cut-off score for dementia in the general population (≤80), the CAMCOG was shown to accurately diagnose dementia in PD with high sensitivity (95%) and specificity (94%) (Hobson & Meara, 1999). The same study demonstrated higher sensitivity and specificity for the CAMCOG in diagnosing PDD than the MMSE. One disadvantage of the CAMCOG is the lengthy administration time (25–30 minutes), and even normal aging is associated with significantly poorer scores (Athey, Porter, et al., 2005).

Frontal Assessment Battery

The Frontal Assessment Battery (FAB) is a short, bedside, cognitive battery assessing frontal-lobe function. The FAB was validated in normal control subjects and in patients with frontal-lobe dysfunction in different degenerative diseases (PD, multiple system atrophy, corticobasal degeneration, frontotemporal dementia [FTD], and progressive supranuclear palsy [PSP]) (Dubois, Slachevsky, Litvan, & Pillon, 2000). The scale displayed strong concurrent validity and good internal consistency and inter-rater reliability (test-retest reliability was not assessed), and allowed accurate discrimination between controls and patient groups. Regression analysis showed that 69.7% of PSP and FTD patients were correctly classified, reflecting the ability of the FAB to capture the CI characteristic of pathologies with predominantly medial-prefrontal dysfunction (Dubois et al., 2000). Validation studies have stressed the usefulness of the FAB in the differential diagnosis of AD and FTD (Lipton et al., 2005), but no studies have formally assessed the discriminative properties of the scale in screening or describing PD-MCI or PDD.

Cognitive Scales Specific to Parkinson's Disease

SCales for Outcomes of PArkinson's Disease—Cognition (SCOPA-COG)

This scale was designed to allow comparison of patient groups and assessment of temporal changes in cognitive functioning. The scale has demonstrated good internal consistency, test-retest reliability, construct validity, and good discriminative properties in groups of subjects classified by dementia status or disease severity (Marinus et al., 2003). The SCOPA-COG has been described as a short, reliable, and valid instrument that is sensitive to the specific cognitive deficits in PD. The main acknowledged limitation of the scale is that, among the initial cognitive domains included in the scale (orientation, attention, memory/learning, executive functions, visuospatial functions, verbal functions, and thinking and reasoning), items assessing posterior cortical functions were removed and only those assessing frontal-subcortical defects were selected. Results obtained in the validation study of the SCOPA-COG have been replicated in a prospective study involving application of the scale to 400 PD patients and 150 control subjects (Verbaan et al., 2007).

PArkinson Neuropsychometric Dementia Assessment

The PArkinsonNeuropsychometric Dementia Assessment (PANDA) is a new, short test specifically designed to screen for CI in patients with PD. The final version of the PANDA can be administered in 8–10 minutes (Kalbe et al., 2008). Although the PANDA displays appropriate discriminative characteristics between control subjects and PD patients, appropriate clinimetric evaluation of the scale (acceptability, construct validity, reliability) (Kalbe et al., 2008) remains to be completed. The PANDA, like several of the other scales, assesses only frontal-subcortical cognitive functions.

Parkinson's Disease—Cognitive Rating Scale (PD-CRS)

The Parkinson's Disease—Cognitive Rating Scale (PD-CRS) is a new cognitive scale specifically designed to capture the whole spectrum of cognitive functions impaired over the course of PD (Pagonabarraga et al., 2008). The PD-CRS displayed very good acceptability, internal consistency, and test-retest and inter-rater reliability. Strong concurrent validity was apparent between PD-CRS total scores and the MDRS (ICC = 0.84), although it was modest between PD-CRS and the MMSE (ICC = 0.43).

The final version of the PD-CRS includes seven tasks assessing frontal-subcortical functions (sustained attention, working memory, alternating and action verbal fluencies, clock drawing, and immediate and delayed free-recall verbal memory), and two tasks assessing posterior cortical functions (confrontation naming, clock copying).

Discriminative analyses showed that the scale does not capture cognitive differences between control subjects and cognitively intact PD patients. However, it differentiates between cognitively intact PD patients and both PD-MCI and PDD patients, and between patients with PD-MCI and PDD. Remarkably, the posterior cortical items selectively differentiated PDD from PD-ND. A cut-off total score of ≤64 on the PD-CRS yielded high sensitivity (94%), specificity (94%), PPV (91%), and NPV (96%) (Pagonabarraga et al., 2008). Administration time for the PD-CRS is around 15 minutes in PD-ND patients and 25 minutes in PDD patients. Patient performance on the PD-CRS showed that PDD is characterized by the addition of posterior cortical dysfunction upon a predominant and progressive frontal-subcortical impairment. The inclusion of frontal-subcortical and posterior cortical items enables characterization of the different patterns of CI over the course of the disease.

Recently published validation and responsiveness data indicate the PD-CRS is a useful tool to identify PD-MCI and to track cognitive changes in PD-ND patients (Fernandez de Bobadilla et al., 2013). A PD-CRS total score </=81 of 134 was the optimal cut-off point for identifying MCI (sensitivity, 79%; specificity,

80%; positive predictive value, 59%; negative predictive value, 91%). A range of change from 10 to 13 points on the PD-CRS total score was indicative of clinically significant change. (Fernandez de Bobadilla et al., 2013).

Montreal Cognitive Assessment (MoCA)

The MoCA is a brief screening instrument developed to identify subjects with mild cognitive impairment (MCI) and AD in the general population. In this population, and in PD patients (Zadikoff et al., 2008), the MoCA has been shown to be more sensitive than the MMSE in identifying MCI. The MoCA takes about 10 minutes to administer and includes tests assessing executive function, attention, visuospatial skills (clock drawing, cube copy), short-term verbal free recall, and a three-item confrontation naming task. In PD, however, well-designed studies have shown the MoCA to have relatively poor accuracy in identifying MCI (MoCA<24/30; sensitivity 70%, specificity 75%) (Hoops et al., 2009), but the scale worked as well as the SCOPA-COG in screening for dementia in PD (MoCA<21/30; sensitivity 81%, specificity 95%) (Dalrymple-Alford et al., 2010) (Table 2-2).

MEASURING THE FUNCTIONAL IMPACT OF COGNITIVE IMPAIRMENT IN PD

Functional decline caused by cognitive worsening is a core criterion for the diagnosis of PDD (Emre et al., 2007). However, the amount of cognitive change needed to interfere significantly with the patient's ability to implement instrumental activities of daily living (IADL) in PD is largely unknown. When accurately measured, certain degree of functional impairment can be identified in PD-MCI subjects (Rosenthal et al., 2010). The usual inventories are known to at least partly reflect motor disabilities, (Shulman et al., 2008) and at present there is no "gold standard" available for IADL assessment in ND-PD (Litvan et al., 2012).

The lack of a valid and reliable instrument to screen and monitor functional changes related to cognitive impairment negatively influence clinical management and the design of up-coming cognitive trials in PD-MCI patients. Besides cognitive measures, therapeutic trials require changes in IADL performance to be used as co-primary outcomes to document that cognitive changes associated with an investigational drug are clinically relevant. Although the Pill Questionnaire has been proposed for detecting functional impairment in PDD (Emre et al., 2007), the sole use of the Pill Questionnaire to identify individuals with mild cognitive impairment is not recommended because of its low sensitivity (Reginold et al., 2012).

A recently validated PD-specific instrument designed to rate the functional impact of cognitive impairment in PD patients (Kulisevsky et al., 2013) can adequately complement neuropsychological ratings and can be readily used in clinical trials.

Table 2-2 Quality assessment of cognitive scales for PD

Scale	*Scale objective*	*Internal consistency*	*Test-retest reliability*	*Intra-rater reliability*	*Content validity*	*Construct validity*	*Acceptability*	*Administration time*
MoCA	Screening of CI in PD	NA	NA	NA	++	+++	–	7-10 minutes
SCOPA-COG	Group comparisons in research and assessment of CI change	+++	+++	NA	+	+++	+	10-15 minutes No different times provided for PD-ND and PDD
PANDA	Screening of CI in PD	NA	? 6-month interval; No ICC or κ_w used	NA	++	+++	–	8–10 minutes No different times provided for PD-ND and PDD
PD-CRS	Research purposes, interventional trials, detection of cognitive patterns, screening of dementia	+++	++++	++++	+++ Inclusion of cortical-type-items	+++	+	PD-ND 17 minutes PDD 25 minutes

PD: Parkinson's disease; CI: Cognitive impairment; PD-ND: Non-demented PD; PDD: PD with dementia; ICC: intraclass correlation coefficient; κ_w: weighted kappa. Results for internal consistency: +++ Cronbach'salfa = 0.71–0.90; Reliability: + poor (ICC or $\kappa_w \leq 0.40$), ++ (0.41–0.60), +++ (0.61–0.80), ++++ (>0.80); Construct validity: + Poor (correlation coefficient ≤0.40), ++ moderate to good (CC 0.41–0.70), +++ good (CC > 0.70); Acceptability:–not assessed or poor (>5% missing values, or ceiling/floor effects), + good (<5% missing values, no ceiling/floor effects); NA: non-available; ? = no appropriate statistics.

Parkinson's Disease-Cognitive Functional Rating Scale (PD-CFRS)

The PD-Cognitive Functional Rating Scale (PD-CFRS) (Kulisevsky et al., 2013) is a 5-minute questionnaire addressed to explore a wide range of functional aspects suspected to be sensible to cognitive impairment in PD, minimizing the motor impact of the disease. The scale is administered to a knowledgeable informant in interview form by 12 items selected to cover the spectrum of instrumental cognitive changes seen in PD over the last two weeks before the evaluation. All 12 questions explore with some examples, whether the patient has had trouble in performing an activity (0 = none; 1 = some of the time; 2 = most of the time; 8 = the subject has never done the activity in the past) such as handling money, domestic economy, arranging holidays or meetings, handling personal mail, controlling drug treatment schedule, organizing daily activities, handling home electrical appliances, understanding how to use public transport, solving unforeseen events, explaining things he/she want to say, understanding the things he/she read, and handling the cell phone.

The maximum score, obtained by the sum of the ratings, is 24. Whenever there are "eights" in the record sheet indicating an activity never done in the past, the mean of all the items answered 0 = 2 is calculated, and this mean value (either 0, 1, or 2) is scored in those items answered with an eight.

A PD-CFRS cut-off score of >/=3 was found to be optimal for detecting functional impairment in PD-MCI patients. A prospective multicenter responsiveness study showed that an increase of 2 points in the PD-CFRS after 6 months was associated with a clinically significant worsening of the cognitive functional status.

NEUROCOGNITIVE ASSESSMENT IN OTHER DEGENERATIVE PARKINSONIAN DISORDERS

Patients with progressive supranuclear palsy (PSP), multiple system atrophy (MSA), and corticobasal degeneration (CBD) develop early and progressively disabling cognitive defects that encompass both frontal-striatal dysfunctions and cognitive alterations dependent on other cortical areas (see also chapters by Armstrong and Litvan, Borroni and Padovani, and Dujardin and Defebvre, in this volume).

Progressive Supranuclear Palsy

Behavioral and cognitive changes occur in 50 to 90% of patients with PSP, often within the first year of the disease (Kaat, Chiu, Boon, & van Swieten, 2011). In cross-sectional studies, frequency of dementia in PSP is about 55% (Menza, Cocchiola, & Golbe, 1995). Cognitive changes were initially reported by Albert et al. and characterized as a prototypical "subcortical dementia" (Albert, Feldman, et al., 1974). This pattern of deficits could be clearly differentiated from that in "cortical dementia," usually involving aphasia, apraxia, and/or agnosia. The cognitive features described in PSP were similar to those observed in patients with frontal lobe lesions. Specifically, the "subcortical dementia" described by Albert et al. was characterized by forgetfulness, slowing of thought processes, emotional or personality changes (apathy, depression, irritability), and impaired ability to manipulate acquired knowledge (Albert, Feldman, & Willis, 1974). PSP patients have dramatically slowed information processing speed, early and severe executive dysfunction with problems in orienting attentional resources, difficulty in planning and shifting conceptual sets, and prominent recall deficits with moderate forgetfulness (Grafman, Litvan, & Stark, 1995). These cognitive defects can be also found in PD patients and other bradykinetic-rigid syndromes, but patients with PSP show a greater decline in attention, processing speed, set-shifting, and categorization abilities than PD or MSA (Soliveri et al., 2000). Executive dysfunction is clearly altered in PSP, with impairment in most tests sensitive to frontal lobe dysfunction. In particular, PSP patients show impairment in tasks of working memory, reasoning, problem solving, conceptualization, planning, and social cognition (Robbins et al., 1994). Characteristically, PSP patients show also perseverative errors during performance of executive tasks, as well as deficits of response inhibition that are less often seen in PD or MSA. Similar to patients with focal prefrontal lesions, PSP patients show decreased ability to inhibit previously learned cognitive responses, whereas PD patients show deficits in the maintenance of new cognitive programs (Partiot, Verin, & Dubois, 1996). This dissociation between the predominant executive dysfunction features in PD and PSP has been linked to differential involvement of the medial prefrontal cortex (associated with impaired response inhibition), and dysfunction of circuits connecting the striatum with the dorsolateral prefrontal cortex (associated with impairment in set maintenance) (Dillon & Pizzagalli, 2007). Thus, in PSP there seems to be a more diffuse impairment of prefrontal-based cognitive functions compared to PD. Recent data have shown neocortical degeneration in the prefrontal cortex in PSP, beyond the well-established degeneration of subcortical nuclei (Donker Kaat et al., 2007).

Neuroimaging studies have shown PSP to affect both the presynaptic and postsynaptic aspects of the dopaminergic and cholinergic neurotransmitter systems, that project their efferents to the prefrontal cortex and lead to early and clinically relevant cognitive dysfunction (Shinotoh et al., 1999). Volumetric MRI studies have shown that PSP patients have greater loss of grey-matter volume in both the medial and lateral aspects of the prefrontal cortex compared with MSA and PD, and this atrophy correlates with the degree of executive dysfunction but not with motor dysfunction (Paviour, Price, Johanshahi, Lees, & Fox, 2006).

Behavioral changes are also a frequent and characteristic feature in PSP. In the first descriptive study of neuropsychiatric symptoms in PSP, almost all patients suffered from moderate to severe apathy (91%), and 36% exhibited disinhibition. Depression (18%), anxiety (18%), and irritability (9%) were infrequent, and hallucinations or delusions were not reported (Litvan, Mega, Cummings, & Fairbanks, 1996). Apathy was significantly associated with executive dysfunction, suggesting that both cognitive dysfunction and apathy in PSP are mediated by degeneration in similar prefrontal areas or by dysfunction of similar frontal-subcortical connections (Cordato, Halliday, Caine, & Morris, 2006). The significance of apathy in PSP is amplified by the fact that PSP can be discriminated from PD and AD by its more severe apathy and lesser depression (Levy et al., 1998). The relationship between apathy and disinhibition emphasizes the important role of the dysfunction of the orbitofrontal and medial frontal circuits in the behavioral disturbances of PSP, which has been documented in recent studies showing frontal atrophy on volumetric MRI studies to correlate with behavioral changes in PSP (Cordato et al., 2002).

Multiple System Atrophy

Original descriptions of patients with MSA emphasized the movement disorders characteristic of the disease, and even now, only a minority of studies have accorded importance to the associated cognitive and behavioral disturbances. Even though dementia is an exclusion criterion for the diagnosis of MSA (Gilman et al., 2008), several studies have reported prominent cognitive defects in patients with MSA when compared with control subjects (Kawai et al., 2008).

The first study to prospectively address the issue of cognitive function in MSA by means of comprehensive neuropsychological testing was published in 1992 by Robbins et al. (1992). The neuropsychological profile presented by MSA patients in that study was characterized by a prominent frontal-lobe-like syndrome (with significant deficits in all three of the frontal and verbal fluency test administered), in the absence of consistent impairments in language, visual perception, and memory or learning. Nevertheless, neuropsychological performance was heterogeneous: one group of patients had a high degree of intellectual competence despite severe physical disability; another group had deficits restricted to tests sensitive to frontal-lobe dysfunction; yet another group exhibited a broader range of impairment, with clear defects on executive tasks, memory, and language (Robbins et al., 1992). Recently, a case of MSA presenting with prominent semantic language deficits has been reported (Apostolova et al., 2006).

Patients with MSA are impaired on tests of verbal fluency, working memory, attentional set-shifting, set acquisition, planning, free recall verbal memory, and response inhibition (Pillon et al., 1995). Compared to PD and PSP, dysexecutive defects in MSA are of similar severity as in PD, but less severe than in PSP (Bak, Crawford, Hearn, Mathuranath, & Hodges, 2005; Testa et al., 1993). In the only longitudinal study reported to date, PD and MSA patients showed a similar overall cognitive profile and performance level at baseline, except for a greater impairment of verbal fluency in MSA. However, after a mean follow-up of 21 months, patients with MSA deteriorated significantly more than those with PD (Soliveri et al., 2000).

When parkinsonian symptoms or cerebellar symptoms are predominant, MSA patients are classified as MSA-P and MSA-C, respectively. A recent comparative study of the cognitive defects in MSA-P (mean disease duration 3.2 years) and MSA-C (mean disease duration 2.6 years), showed MSA-P patients to present with more severe and widespread cognitive dysfunction, with impairments on verbal fluency, executive function, visuospatial, and constructional tests (Kawai et al., 2008). Patients with MSA-C showed milder impairment restricted to visuospatial and constructional functions. Interestingly, the authors correlated the neuropsychological impairment in MSA-P with decreased perfusion in the prefrontal cortex and posterior parietal lobes (^{99m}Tc-Ethylcysteine dimmer SPECT), whereas cognitive impairment in MSA-C correlated with cerebellar hypoperfusion(Kawai et al., 2008).

In accordance with these findings, three groups of patients with MSA have been identified based on different degrees of cognitive impairment and a different pattern of glucose metabolism defects as assessed by fluorodeoxyglucose PET (Lyoo et al., 2008). Patients in the one group had significantly shorter disease duration, frequent memory defects and frontal executive dysfunction, with hypometabolism in the frontal cortex. Patients in the other two groups displayed multiple cognitive deficits, more severe motor deficits, and showed hypometabolism not only in the frontal, but also in the parieto-temporal cortex and bilateral caudate nucleus. These findings emphasize the frequent and progressive nature of cognitive defects in MSA, and that cognitive impairment in MSA is related to cortical hypometabolism beginning in the frontal cortex and spreading to the parieto-temporal cortex (Lyoo et al., 2008). In recent years, several neuroimaging studies have clearly demonstrated that cortical atrophy in MSA is more severe than previously thought. MSA is associated with volume loss in widespread cortical regions, particularly involving the lateral prefrontal cortex, but also the orbitofrontal cortex, posterior parietal cortex, hippocampus, insula, caudate nucleus, putamen, primary sensorimotor cortex, corpus callosum, and supplementary motor area (Brenneis et al., 2003; Konagaya, Konagaya, Sakai, Matsuoka, & Hashizume, 2002).

Corticobasal Degeneration

Corticobasal degeneration (CBD) is currently recognized as a progressive neurodegenerative disease that typically presents with asymmetrical parkinsonism and cognitive dysfunction. In the initial clinical descriptions of CBD, however, symptoms of higher-order cortical dysfunction were restricted to ideomotor and limb-kinetic apraxia, and, in some cases, the development of alien hand syndrome (Rinne, Lee, Thompson, & Marsden, 1994).

In the 1990s, detailed neuropsychological analysis of autopsy-proven cases showed not only that cognitive deficits were common in CBD, but that they may be present from the early stages of the disease and possibly aid in differential diagnosis (Bergeron, Davis, & Lang, 1998). Analyzing the natural history of 14 patients with autopsy-proven CBD, Wenning et al. observed that 64% of them presented with ideomotor apraxia and 36% with features of "cortical-type" dementia at first visit (Wenning et al., 1998). On disease evolution, the development of lateralized and focal cognitive syndromes (e.g., aphasia in 36%) and a progressive frontal syndrome led to the diagnosis of dementia in 6 out of 14 patients (43%). Moreover, 58% of the patients suffered from apathy, irritability, or disinhibited behavior (Wenning et al., 1998). Additional data about the importance of cognitive defects in CBD come from subsequent larger clinical series showing that 25% (36/147) of CBD patients presenting with predominant motor symptoms develop dementia during the course of the disease (Kompoliti et al., 1998). Further clinico-pathological studies have broadened the clinical spectrum of CBD, which can present with various clinical syndromes. Beyond the classical corticobasal syndrome (unilateral and asymmetric parkinsonism, dystonia, ideomotor apraxia, and myoclonus), CBD may also present either with progressive nonfluent aphasia, speech apraxia, a PSP-like syndrome (vertical supranuclear gaze palsy, early postural instability) or posterior cortical atrophy syndrome (Wadia & Lang, 2007). Typical frontotemporal dementia symptoms have been also described in CBD at disease onset, even in the absence of associated features of classical corticobasal syndrome (Boeve, Lang, & Litvan, 2003). The pattern and severity of cognitive dysfunction in CBD is highly variable between patients, but the most characteristic impairments are asymmetric limb apraxia (usually ideomotor and limb-kinetic, with defects in posture imitation, symbolic gesture execution, and object utilization), constructional and visuospatial difficulties, executive dysfunction, acalculia, and progressive nonfluent aphasia (Graham, Bak, & Hodges, 2003) (Table 2-3).

The most frequent cognitive symptom in CBD is apraxia, being present in up to 70% of patients (Soliveri, Piacentini, & Girotti, 2005). Limb apraxia in CBD is asymmetric and most often ideomotor in nature. Ideomotor apraxia impairs the ability of using tools and mimicking tools use, but recognition of the pattern and temporal sequence of actions when performed by others is preserved (Leiguarda, Lees, Merello, Starkstein, & Marsden, 1994). Limb-kinetic apraxia

Table 2-3 Pattern of cognitive and behavioral disturbances in CBD

- Cognitive dysfunction:
  - Limb apraxia (ideomotor, limb-kinetic, ideational)
  - Constructional apraxia
  - Visuospatial difficulties (line orientation, figure rotation, motion perception)
  - Executive dysfunction (medial and lateral prefrontal cortex deficits)
  - Acalculia
  - Progressive nonfluent aphasia
  - Speech apraxia
- Behavioral disturbances:
  - 75% Depression
  - 40% Apathy
  - 20% Irritability
  - 20% Agitation
  - <10% Disinhibition

(usually coexisting with ideomotor apraxia) has been reported less often in CBD, and can be differentiated from ideomotor apraxia because it is more distal, unilateral, impairs only the production of fine finger movements and hand postures, and affect all kind of movement, regardless of its instrumental purpose (impairment of transitive and intransitive movements) (Leiguarda et al., 2003). Visuoperceptual difficulties, especially the difficulty perceiving the spatial relationships among visual stimuli, likely underlies the constructional apraxia observed in CBD, especially in patients with predominant right hemispheric fronto-parietal degeneration (Sawle, Brooks, Marsden, & Frackowiak, 1991). In CBD, constructional apraxia is evidenced by progressive impairment in drawing and writing, and these features are frequently obvious at presentation or early in the disease (Mimura, White, & Albert, 1997).

Aphasia and speech difficulties are common in CBD and represent a good clinical marker for the differential diagnosis of CBD from PD, PSP, and MSA (Frattali, Grafman, Patronas, Maklouf, & Litvan, 2000). Aphasia has been observed in 44% of autopsy-proven CBD cases (Graham et al., 2003). Language disturbances in CBD resemble those in FTD patients with a nonfluent progressive aphasia (Frattali et al., 2000). Neuropsychological studies assessing language in CBD have shown that most patients (65%) develop progressive aphasia during the course of the illness. In particular, at baseline, language is more impaired in CBD patients with a primarily cognitive presentation, though the evolution to aphasia over the disease is s common to both primarily motor and cognitive forms of CBD (McMonagle, Blair, & Kertesz 2006).

Impairments on tests of frontal-lobe function are also a consistent finding in CBD (Soliveri et al., 1999). Measures of working memory, set-shifting, set acquisition, resistance to interference, conceptualization, mental flexibility, and social judgment, have been shown to be early and severely affected in the disease (Pillon et al., 1995). Visuospatial skills are usually impaired, with poor performance on tests of line orientation, mental rotation of figures, and perception of motion, reflecting a predominant dysfunction of the dorsal occipitoparietal cortex rather than a dysfunction of the ventral visual stream, that is more involved in the perception of shapes, colors, and object identification (Soliveri et al., 1999).

Finally, findings of memory impairment in CBD are inconsistent, with some studies reporting episodic memory defects, but other reporting unaltered memory. Less disputed is that episodic (unlike semantic memory) is more preserved in CBD compared to AD, suggesting that dysfunction of semantic networks mediated by anterior and lateral temporal cortex, rather than hippocampal/medial temporal degeneration, may account for the memory defects seen in CBD (Massman, Kreiter, Jankovic, & Doody, 1996).

CONCLUSIONS

Degenerative parkinsonian disorders are no longer seen as monolithic, isolated motor syndromes. Instead, it is widely appreciated that degenerative parkinsonian syndromes frequently involve disabling cognitive disorders, the earliest manifestations of which may be present from the beginnings of the disease. Whereas executive dysfunction is common to PD, PSP, MSA, and CBD, the addition of cognitive deficits dependent on cortical compromise help to distinguish between some of these nosological entities. PSP patients, for example, not only develop working memory defects, but manifest severe apathy and defects in cognitive inhibition more dependent on the medial prefrontal lobe. In CBD, language deficits, ideomotor, and limb-kinetic apraxia are early clinical markers of the disease, and both PD and MSA are characterized by initial predominant dysexecutive symptoms with the subsequent addition of cognitive disturbances more dependent on temporo-parietal structures. For none of these disorders, however, have specific cognitive instruments been developed, and no clear cut-offs have been described for diagnosing cognitive or behavioral disorders in atypical parkinsonian syndromes. To integrate appropriate neuropsychological examinations in the assessment of parkinsonian disorders seems currently mandatory so as not to overlook clinical disease aspects that may have a high clinical impact on the patient's daily life.

REFERENCES

Aarsland, D., Andersen, K., Larson, J.P., Lolk, A., Nielsen, H., & Kragh-Sorensen, P. (2001). Risk of dementia in Parkinson's disease: A community-based, prospective study. *Neurology* 56(6), 730–736.

Aarsland, D., Bronnick, K., Larsen, J. P., Tysnes, O. B., Alves, G.; Norwegian Parkwest Study Group. (2009). Cognitive impairment in incident, untreated Parkinson disease: the Norwegian ParkWest study. *Neurology, 72*(13), 1121–1126.

Aarsland, D., Litvan, I., Salmon, D., Galasko, D., Wentzel-Larsen, T., & Larsen J. (2003). "Performance on the dementia rating scale in Parkinson's disease with dementia and dementia with Lewy bodies: comparison with progressive supranuclear palsy and Alzheimer's disease. *Journal of Neurology, Neurosurgery, and Psychiatry, 74*(9), 1215–1220.

Aarsland, D., Zaccai, J., & Brayne C. (2005). A systematic review of prevalence studies of dementia in Parkinson's disease. *Movement Disorders, 20*(10), 1255–1263.

Albert, M. L., Feldman, R. G., & Willis, A. L. (1974). The "subcortical dementia" of progressive supranuclear palsy. *Journal of Neurology, Neurosurgery and Psychiatry, 37*(2), 121–130.

Apostolova, L. G., Klement, I., Bronstein Y., Vinters, H. V., & Cumings, J. L. (2006). Multiple system atrophy presenting with language impairment. *Neurology, 67*(4), 726–727.

Athey, R. J., Porter, R. W.,Walker R.W. (2005). Cognitive assessment of a representative community population with Parkinson's disease (PD) using the Cambridge Cognitive Assessment-Revised (CAMCOG-R). *Age & Ageing, 34*(3), 268–273.

Azuma, T., R. Cruz, F., Bayles, K. A., Tomoeda, C. K., & Montgomery Jr, E.B. (2003). A longitudinal study of neuropsychological change in individuals with Parkinson's disease. *International Journal of Geriatric Psychiatry, 18*(12), 1115–1120.

Bak, T. H., Crawford, L. M., Hearn, V. C., Mathuranath, P. S., & Hodges, J. R. (2005). Subcortical dementia revisited: similarities and differences in cognitive function between progressive supranuclear palsy (PSP), corticobasal degeneration (CBD) and multiple system atrophy (MSA). *Neurocase, 11*(4), 268–273.

Bastiaanse, R., & Leenders, K. L. (2009). Language and Parkinson's disease. *Cortex, 45*(8), 912–914.

Bergeron, C., Davis, A., & Lang, A. E. (1998). Corticobasal ganglionic degeneration and progressive supranuclear palsy presenting with cognitive decline. *Brain Pathology, 8*(2), 355–365.

Boeve, B. F., Lang, A. E., & Litvan, I. (2003). Corticobasal degeneration and its relationship to progressive supranuclear palsy and frontotemporal dementia. *Annals of Neurology, 54*(Suppl 5), S15–19.

Brenneis, C., Seppi, K., Schocke, M. F., Müller, J., Luginger, E., Bösch, S., . . . Wenning G. K. (2003). Voxel-based morphometry detects cortical atrophy in the Parkinson variant of multiple system atrophy. *Movement Disorders, 18*(10), 1132–1138.

Bronnick, K., Alves, G., Aarsland, D., Tysnes, O. B., & Larssen, J. P. (2011). Verbal memory in drug-naive, newly diagnosed Parkinson's disease. The retrieval deficit hypothesis revisited. *Neuropsychology, 25*(1), 114–124.

Buter, T. C., van den Hout, A., Matthews, F. E., Larsen, J. P., Brayne, C., & Aarsland, D. (2008). Dementia and survival in Parkinson disease: a 12-year population study. *Neurology, 70*(13), 1017–1022.

Butterfield, L. C., Cimino, C. R., Oelke, L. E., Hauser, R. A., & Sanchez-Ramos, J. (2010). The independent influence of apathy and depression on cognitive functioning in Parkinson's disease. *Neuropsychology, 24*(6), 721–730.

Cooper, J. A., Sagar, H. J., Jordan, N., Harvey, N. S., & Sullivan, E. V. (1991). Cognitive impairment in early, untreated Parkinson's disease and its relationship to motor disability. *Brain, 114* (Pt 5), 2095–2122.

Cordato, N. J., Halliday, G. M., Caine, D., & Morris, J. G. (2006). Comparison of motor, cognitive, and behavioral features in progressive supranuclear palsy and Parkinson's disease. *Movement Disorders, 21*(5), 632–638.

Cordato, N. J., Pantelis, C., Halliday, G. M., Velakoulis, D., Wood, S. J., Stuart, G. W., . . . Morris, J. G. (2002). Frontal atrophy correlates with behavioural changes in progressive supranuclear palsy. *Brain, 125*(Pt 4), 789–800.

Dalrymple-Alford, J. C., MacAskill, M. R., Naskas, C. T., Livingston, L., Graham, C., Crucian, C. P., . . . Anderson, T. J. (2010). The MoCA: well-suited screen for cognitive impairment in Parkinson disease. *Neurology, 75*(19), 1717–1725.

Dillon, D. G., & Pizzagalli, D. A. (2007). Inhibition of action, thought, and emotion: A selective neurobiological review. *Applied Preventive Psychology, 12*(3), 99–114.

Donker Kaat, L., Boon, A. J., Kamphorst, W., Ravid, R., Duivenvoorden, H. J., & van Swieten, J. C. (2007). Frontal presentation in progressive supranuclear palsy. *Neurology, 69*(8), 723–729.

Dubois, B., Burn, D., Goetz, C., Aarsland, D., Brown, R. G., Broe, G. A., . . . Emre, M. (2007). Diagnostic procedures for Parkinson's disease dementia: recommendations from the movement disorder society task force. *Movement Disorders, 22*(16), 2314–2324.

Dubois, B., Slachevsky, A., Litvan, I., & Pillon, B. (2000). The FAB: A frontal assessment battery at bedside. *Neurology, 55*(11), 1621–1626.

Dujardin, K., Sockeel, P., Delliaux, M., Destée, A., & Defebvre, L. (2009). Apathy may herald cognitive decline and dementia in Parkinson's disease. *Movement Disorders, 24*(16), 2391–2397.

Emre, M., Aarsland, D., Brown, R., Burn, D. J., Duyckaerts, C., Mizuno, Y., . . . Dubois, B. (2007). Clinical diagnostic criteria for dementia associated with Parkinson's disease. *Movement Disorders, 22*(12), 1689–1707; quiz 1837.

Fernandez de Bobadilla, R., Pagonabarraga, J., Martínez-Horta, S., Pascual-Sedano, B., Campolongo, A., & Kulisevsky, J. (2013). Parkinson's disease-cognitive rating scale: Psychometrics for mild cognitive impairment. *Movement Disorders, 28*(10), 1376–1383.

Folstein, M. F., Folstein, S. E., & McHugh, P. R. (1975). "Mini-mental state." A practical method for grading the cognitive state of patients for the clinician. *Journal of Psychiatric Research, 12*(3), 189–198.

Frattali, C. M., Grafman, J., Patronas N., Maklouf, F., & Litvan, I. (2000). Language disturbances in corticobasal degeneration. *Neurology, 54*(4), 990–992.

Galvin, J. E., Pollack, J., & Morris, J. C. (2006). Clinical phenotype of Parkinson disease dementia. *Neurology, 67*(9), 1605–1611.

Gilman, S., Wenning, G. K., Low, P. A., Brooks, D. J., Mathias, C. J., Trojanowski, J. Q., . . . Vidailhet, M. (2008). Second consensus statement on the diagnosis of multiple system atrophy. *Neurology, 71*(9), 670–676.

Goetz, C. G., Leurgans, S., Pappert, E. J., Raman, R., & Stemer, A.. (2001). Prospective longitudinal assessment of hallucinations in Parkinson's disease. *Neurology, 57*(11), 2078–2082.

Goldman, W. P., Baty, J. D., Buckles, V. D., Sahrmann, S., & Morris, J. C. (1998). Cognitive and motor functioning in Parkinson disease: subjects with and without questionable dementia. *Archives of Neurology, 55*(5), 674–680.

Grafman, J., Litvan, I., & Stark, M. (1995). Neuropsychological features of progressive supranuclear palsy. *Brain & Cognition, 28*(3), 311–320.

Graham, N. L., Bak, T. H., Hodges, J. R. (2003). Corticobasal degeneration as a cognitive disorder. *Movement Disorders, 18*(11), 1224–1232.

Halliday, G., Hely, M., Reid, W., & Morris, J. (2008). The progression of pathology in longitudinally followed patients with Parkinson's disease. *Acta Neuropathologica, 115*(4), 409–415.

Henry, J. D. & Crawford, J. R. (2004). Verbal fluency deficits in Parkinson's disease: a meta-analysis. *Journal of the International Neuropsychology Society, 10*(4), 608–622.

Hobson, P. & Meara, J. (1999). The detection of dementia and cognitive impairment in a community population of elderly people with Parkinson's disease by use of the CAMCOG neuropsychological test. *Age & Ageing, 28*(1), 39–43.

Hobson, P. & Meara, J. (2004). Risk and incidence of dementia in a cohort of older subjects with Parkinson's disease in the United Kingdom. *Movement Disorders, 19*(9), 1043–1049.

Hoops, S., Nazem, S., Siderowf, A. D., Duda, J. E., Xie, S. X., Stern, M. B., & Weintraub, D. (2009). Validity of the MoCA and MMSE in the detection of MCI and dementia in Parkinson disease. *Neurology, 73*(21), 1738–1745.

Huber, S. J., Shuttleworth, E. C., & Freidenberg, D. L. (1989). Neuropsychological differences between the dementias of Alzheimer's and Parkinson's diseases. *Archives of Neurology, 46*(12), 1287–1291.

Isaias, I. U., Siri, C., Cilia, R., DeGaspari, D., Pezzoli, G., & Antonini, A. (2008). The relationship between impulsivity and impulse control disorders in Parkinson's disease. *Movement Disorders, 23*(3), 411–415.

Kaat, D. L., Chiu, W. Z., Boon, A. J., & van Swieten, J. C. (2011). Recent advances in progressive supranuclear palsy: a review. *Currents in Alzheimer Research, 8*(3), 295–302.

Kalbe, E., Calabrese, P., Kohn, N., Hilker, R., Riedel, O., Wittchen, H.U.,... Kessler, J.(2008). Screening for cognitive deficits in Parkinson's disease with the Parkinson neuropsychometric dementia assessment (PANDA) instrument. *Parkinsonism & Related Disorders, 14*(2), 93–101.

Kawai, Y., Suenaga, M., Takeda, A., Ito, M., Watanabe, H., Tanaka, F., ... Sobue, G. (2008). Cognitive impairments in multiple system atrophy: MSA-C vs MSA-P. *Neurology, 70*(16 Pt 2), 1390–1396.

Kompoliti, K., Goetz, C. G., Boeve, B.E., Maraganore, D.M., Ahlskog, J.E., Marsden, C.D., . . . Riley, D.E. (1998). Clinical presentation and pharmacological therapy in corticobasal degeneration. *Archives of Neurology, 55*(7), 957–961.

Konagaya, M., Konagaya, Y., Sakai, M., Matsuoka, Y., & Hashizume, Y. (2002). Progressive cerebral atrophy in multiple system atrophy. *Journal of Neurological Science, 195*(2), 123–127.

Kulisevsky, J., Fernandez de Bobadilla, R., Pagonabarraga, J., Martínez-Horta, S., Campolongo, A., García-Sánchez, C., . . . Villa-Bonoma, C. (2013). Measuring functional impact of cognitive impairment: Validation of the Parkinson's Disease Cognitive Functional Rating Scale. *Parkinsonism & Related Disorders,* 19(9), 812–817.

Kulisevsky, J. & Pagonabarraga, J. (2009). Cognitive impairment in Parkinson's disease: tools for diagnosis and assessment. *Movement Disorders, 24*(8), 1103–1110.

Leiguarda, R., Lees, A. J., Merello, M., Starkstein, S., & Marsden, C. D. (1994). The nature of apraxia in corticobasal degeneration. *Journal of Neurology, Neurosurgery and Psychiatry, 57*(4), 455–459.

Leiguarda, R. C., Merello, M., Nouzeilles, M. I., Belej, J., Rivero, A., & Noqués, M. (2003). Limb-kinetic apraxia in corticobasal degeneration: clinical and kinematic features. *Movement Disorders, 18*(1), 49–59.

Levy, M. L., Cummings, J. L., Fairbanks, L. A., Masterman, D. Miller, B. L., Craig, A.H.,... Litvan I. (1998). Apathy is not depression. *Journal of Neuropsychiatry & Clinical Neuroscience, 10*(3), 314–319.

Lipton, A. M., Ohman, K. A., Womack, K. B., Hynan, L. S., Ninman, E. T., & Lacritz, L. H. (2005). Subscores of the FAB differentiate frontotemporal lobar degeneration from AD. *Neurology, 65*(5), 726–731.

Litvan, I., Goldman, J. G., Tröster, A. I., Schmand, B. A., Weintraub, D., Petersen, R. C., . . . Emre, M. (2012). Diagnostic criteria for mild cognitive impairment in Parkinson's disease: Movement Disorder Society Task Force guidelines. *Movement Disorders, 27*(3), 349–356.

Litvan, I., Mega, M. S., Cummings, J. L., & Fairbanks, L. (1996). Neuropsychiatric aspects of progressive supranuclear palsy. *Neurology, 47*(5), 1184–1189.

Llebaria, G., Pagonabarraga, J., Kulisevsky, J., García-Sánchez, C., Pascual-Sedano, B., Gironell, A., & Martínéz-Corral, M. (2008). Cut-off score of the Mattis Dementia Rating Scale for screening dementia in Parkinson's disease. *Movement Disorders, 23*(11), 1546–1550.

Llebaria, G., Pagonabarraga, J., Martínez-Corral, M., García-Sánchez, C., Pascual-Sedano, B., Gironell, A., & Kulisevsky, J. (2010). Neuropsychological correlates of mild to severe hallucinations in Parkinson's disease. *Movement Disorders, 25*(16), 2785–2791.

Lyoo, C. H., Jeong, Y., Ryu, Y. H., Lee, S. Y., Song, T. J., Lee, J. H., ... Lee, M.S.(2008). Effects of disease duration on the clinical features and brain glucose metabolism in patients with mixed type multiple system atrophy. *Brain, 131*(Pt 2), 438–446.

Mamikonyan, E., Moberg, P. J.,Siderowf, A., Duda, J. E., Have, T. T., Hurtig, H. I.,... Weintraub, D. (2009). Mild cognitive impairment is common in Parkinson's disease patients with normal Mini-Mental State Examination (MMSE) scores. *Parkinsonism & Related Disorders, 15*(3), 226–231.

Marinus, J., Visser, M., Verwey, N. A., Verhey, F. R., Middlekoop, H. A., Stigglebout, A. M., & van Hilten, J. J. (2003). Assessment of cognition in Parkinson's disease. *Neurology, 61*(9), 1222–1228.

Massman, P. J., Kreiter, K. T., Jankovic, J., & Doody, R. S. (1996). Neuropsychological functioning in cortical-basal ganglionic degeneration: Differentiation from Alzheimer's disease. *Neurology, 46*(3), 720–726.

Matison, R., Mayeux, R., Rosen, J., & Fahn, S. (1982). "Tip-of-the-tongue" phenomenon in Parkinson disease. *Neurology, 32*(5), 567–570.

McKinlay, A., Grace, R. C., Dalrymple-Alford, A. C., & Roger, D. (2010). Characteristics of executive function impairment in Parkinson's disease patients without dementia. *Journal of the International Neuropsychology Society, 16*(2), 268–277.

McMonagle, P., Blair, M., & Kertesz, A. (2006). Corticobasal degeneration and progressive aphasia. *Neurology, 67*(8), 1444–1451.

Menza, M. A., Cocchiola, J., & Golbe, L. I. (1995). Psychiatric symptoms in progressive supranuclear palsy. *Psychosomatics, 36*(6), 550–554.

Mimura, M., White, R. F., & Albert, M. L. (1997). Corticobasal degeneration: neuropsychological and clinical correlates. *Journal of Neuropsychiatry & Clinical Neuroscience, 9*(1), 94–98.

Monsch, A. U., Bondi, M. W., Salmon, D. P., Butter, N., Thal, L. J., Hansen, L. A., . . . Klauber, M.R.(1995). Clinical validity of the Mattis Dementia Rating Scale in detecting Dementia of the Alzheimer type. A double cross-validation and application to a community-dwelling sample. *Archives of Neurology, 52*(9), 899–904.

Mosimann, U. P., Mather, G., Wesnes, K. A., O'Brien, J. T., Burn, D. J., & McKeith, I. G. (2004). Visual perception in Parkinson disease dementia and dementia with Lewy bodies. *Neurology, 63*(11), 2091–2096.

Muslimovic, D., Post, B., Speelman, J. D., & Schmand, B. (2005). Cognitive profile of patients with newly diagnosed Parkinson disease. *Neurology, 65*(8), 1239–1245.

Muslimovic, D., Post, B., Speelman, J. D., De Haan, R. J., & Schmand, B.(2009). Cognitive decline in Parkinson's disease: a prospective longitudinal study. *Journal of the International Neuropsychology Society,* 15(3), 426–437.

Noe, E., Marder, K., Bell, K. L., Jacobs, D. M., Manly, J. J., & Stern, Y. (2004). Comparison of dementia with Lewy bodies to Alzheimer's disease and Parkinson's disease with dementia. *Movement Disorders, 19*(1), 60–67.

Pagonabarraga, J., Garcia-Sanchez, C., Llebaria, G., Pascual-Sedano, B., Gironell, A., & Kulisevsky, J. (2007). Controlled study of decision-making and cognitive impairment in Parkinson's disease. *Movement Disorders, 22*(10), 1430–1435.

Pagonabarraga, J., Kulisevsky, J., Llebaria, G., Garcia-Sanchez, C., Pascual-Sedano, B., & Gironell, A. (2008). Parkinson's disease-cognitive rating scale: a new cognitive scale specific for Parkinson's disease. *Movement Disorders, 23*(7), 998–1005.

Partiot, A., Verin, M., & Dubois, B. (1996). Delayed response tasks in basal ganglia lesions in man: further evidence for a striato-frontal cooperation in behavioural adaptation. *Neuropsychologia 34*(7), 709–721.

Paviour, D. C., Price, S. L., Johanshahi, M., Lees, A. J., & Fox, N.C. (2006). Longitudinal MRI in progressive supranuclear palsy and multiple system atrophy: rates and regions of atrophy. *Brain, 129*(Pt 4), 1040–1049.

Pillon, B., Blin, J., Vidailhet, M., Deweer, B., Sirgu, A., Dubois, B., & Agid, Y. (1995). The neuropsychological pattern of corticobasal degeneration: comparison with progressive supranuclear palsy and Alzheimer's disease. *Neurology, 45*(8), 1477–1483.

Poletti, M., Frosini, D., Lucetti, C., Dotto, P. D., Cervolo, R., & Bonuccelli, U. (2011). Impulsivity is associated with decision-making deficits in de-novo Parkinson's disease. *Journal of Neuropsychiatry & Clinical Neuroscience,* 23(3), E26.

Reginold, W., Armstrong, M. J., Duff-Canning, S., Lang, A., Tang-Wai, D., Fox, S., . . . Marras, C. (2012). The pill questionnaire in a nondemented Parkinson's disease population. *Movement Disorders, 27*(10), 1308–1311.

Riedel, O., Klotsche, J., Spottke, A., Deuschl, G., Förstl, H., Henn F., ... Wittchen, H. U. (2008). Cognitive impairment in 873 patients with idiopathic Parkinson's disease. Results from the German Study on Epidemiology of Parkinson's Disease with Dementia (GEPAD). *Journal of Neurology 255*(2), 255–264.

Rinne, J. O., Lee, M. S., Thompson, P. D., & Marsden, C. D. (1994). Corticobasal degeneration. A clinical study of 36 cases. *Brain, 117* (Pt 5), 1183–1196.

Robbins, T. W., James, M., Lange, K. W., Owen, A. M., Quinn, N. P., & Marsden, C. D. (1992). Cognitive performance in multiple system atrophy. *Brain, 115* (Pt 1), 271–291.

Robbins, T. W., James, M., Owen, A. M., Lange, K. W., Lees, A. J., Leigh, P. N., . . . Summers, B. A. (1994). Cognitive deficits in progressive supranuclear palsy, Parkinson's disease, and multiple system atrophy in tests sensitive to frontal lobe dysfunction. *Journal of Neurology, Neurosurgery and Psychiatry, 57*(1), 79–88.

Robert, G., Drapier, D., Verin, M., Millet, B., Azulay, J. P., & Blin, O. (2009). Cognitive impulsivity in Parkinson's disease patients: assessment and pathophysiology. *Movement Disorders, 24*(16), 2316–2327.

Rosenthal, E., Brennan, L., Xie, S., Hurtig, H., Milber, J., Weintraub, D., . . . Siderowf, A. (2010). Association between cognition and function in patients with Parkinson disease with and without dementia. *Movement Disorders, 25*(9), 1170–1176.

Roth, M., Tym, E., Mountjoy, C.Q., Huppert, F.A., Hendrie, H., Verma, S., & Goddard, R. (1986). CAMDEX. A standardised instrument for the diagnosis of mental disorder in the elderly with special reference to the early detection of dementia. *British Journal of Psychiatry, 149*, 698–709.

Sawle, G. V., Brooks, D. J., Marsden, C. D., & Frackowiak, R. S. (1991). Corticobasal degeneration. A unique pattern of regional cortical oxygen hypometabolism and striatal fluorodopa uptake demonstrated by positron emission tomography. *Brain 114* (Pt 1B), 541–556.

Schrag, A., Jahanshahi, M., & Quinn, N. (2000). What contributes to quality of life in patients with Parkinson's disease? *Journal of Neurology, Neurosurgery and Psychiatry, 69*(3), 308–312.

Shinotoh, H., Namba, H., Yamaguchi, M., Fukushi, K., Nagatsuka, S., Iyo, M., ..., Irie, T. (1999). Positron emission tomographic measurement of acetylcholinesterase activity reveals differential loss of ascending cholinergic systems in Parkinson's disease and progressive supranuclear palsy. *Annals of Neurology, 46*(1), 62–69.

Shulman, L. M., Gruber-Baldini, A. L., Anderson, K. E., Vaughan, C. G., Reich, S. G., Fish, P. S., & Weiner, W. J. (2008). The evolution of disability in Parkinson disease. *Movement Disorders, 23*(6), 790–796.

Soliveri, P., Monza, D., Paridi, D., Carella, F., Genitrini., S., Testa, D., & Girotti, F. (2000). Neuropsychological follow up in patients with Parkinson's disease, striatonigral degeneration-type multisystem atrophy, and progressive supranuclear palsy. *Journal of Neurology, Neurosurgery and Psychiatry, 69*(3), 313–318.

Soliveri, P., Monza, D., Paridi, D., Radice, D., Grisoli, M., Testa, D., . . . Girotti, F. (1999). Cognitive and magnetic resonance imaging aspects of corticobasal degeneration and progressive supranuclear palsy. *Neurology 53*(3), 502–507.

Soliveri, P., Piacentini, S., & Girotti, F. (2005). Limb apraxia in corticobasal degeneration and progressive supranuclear palsy. *Neurology 64*(3), 448–453.

Starkstein, S. E., Preziosi, T. J., Berthier, M. L., Bolduc, P. L., Mayberg, H. S., & Robinson, R. G. (1989). Depression and cognitive impairment in Parkinson's disease. *Brain, 112* (Pt 5), 1141–1153.

Starkstein, S. E., Sabe, L., Petracca, G., Chemerinski, E., Kuzis, G., Merello, M., & Leiguarda, R. (1996). Neuropsychological and psychiatric differences between Alzheimer's disease and Parkinson's disease with dementia. *Journal of Neurology, Neurosurgery and Psychiatry, 61*(4), 381–387.

Testa, D., Fetoni, V., Soliveri, P., Musicco, M., Palazzini, E., & Girotti, F. (1993). Cognitive and motor performance in multiple system atrophy and Parkinson's disease compared. *Neuropsychologia 31*(2), 207–210.

Troster, A. I., Paolo, A. M., Lyons, K. E., Glatt, S. L., Hubble, J. P., & Koller, W.C. (1995). The influence of depression on cognition in Parkinson's disease: a pattern of impairment distinguishable from Alzheimer's disease. *Neurology 45*(4), 672–676.

Troster, A. I., Woods, S. P., & Morgan, E. E. (2007). Assessing cognitive change in Parkinson's disease: development of practice effect-corrected reliable change indices. *Archives of Clinical Neuropsychology, 22*(6), 711–718.

Varanese, S., Perfetti, B., Ghilardi, M. F., & DiRocco, A. (2011). Apathy, but not depression, reflects inefficient cognitive strategies in Parkinson's disease. *PLoS One 6*(3), e17846.

Verbaan, D., Marinus, J., Visser, M. van Rooden S. M., Stiggelbout, A. M., Middelkoop, H. A. M., & van Hilten, J. J. (2007). Cognitive impairment in Parkinson's disease. *Journal of Neurology, Neurosurgery and Psychiatry, 78*(11), 1182–1187.

Wadia, P. M. & Lang, A. E. (2007). The many faces of corticobasal degeneration. *Parkinsonism & Related Disorders, 13*(Suppl 3), S336–340.

Weintraub, D., Moberg, P. J., Culbertson, W. C., Duda, J. E., & Stern, M. B. (2004). Evidence for impaired encoding and retrieval memory profiles in Parkinson disease. *Cognitive & Behavioral Neurology, 17*(4), 195–200.

Wenning, G. K., Litvan, I., Jankovic, J., Granata, R., Mangone, C. A., McKee, A., ... Pearce, R. K. (1998). Natural history and survival of 14 patients with corticobasal degeneration confirmed at postmortem examination. *Journal of Neurology, Neurosurgery and Psychiatry, 64*(2), 184–189.

Whittington, C. J., Podd, J., & Kan, M. M. (2000). Recognition memory impairment in Parkinson's disease: power and meta-analyses. *Neuropsychology, 14*(2), 233–246.

Whittington, C. J., Podd, J., & Stewart-Williams, S. (2006). Memory deficits in Parkinson's disease. *Journal of Clinical Experimental Neuropsychology, 28*(5), 738–754.

Williams-Gray, C. H., Evans, J. R., Goris, A., Foltynie, T., Ban, M., Robbins, T., W., . . . Barker, R. A. (2009). The distinct cognitive syndromes of Parkinson's disease: 5 year follow-up of the CamPaIGN cohort. *Brain, 132*(Pt 11), 2958–2969.

Zadikoff, C., Fox, S. H., Tang-Wai, D. F., Thomsen, T., de Bie, R. M., Wadia, P., . . . Marras, C. (2008). A comparison of the mini mental state exam to the Montreal cognitive assessment in identifying cognitive deficits in Parkinson's disease. *Movement Disorders, 23*(2), 297–299.

Zarranz, J. J., Alegre, J., Gómez-Esteban, J. C., Lezcano, E., Ros, R., Ampuero, I., . . . de Yebenes, J. G. (2004). The new mutation, E46K, of alpha-synuclein causes Parkinson and Lewy body dementia. *Annals of Neurology, 55*(2), 164–173.

3 A General Approach to Clinical Neuropsychological Assessment of Movement Disorders

Michele K. York and Adriana M. Strutt

INTRODUCTION

Neuropsychological assessments endeavor to provide an accurate and unbiased estimate of a patient's cognitive, psychological, and behavioral capacity. The task of the neuropsychologist is to dissect observed test performances to identify the individual's underlying cognitive strengths and weaknesses. For those patients who suffer from a movement disorder (MD), this task is further compounded for the neuropsychologist by the involuntary movements or variations in movements of the patient's condition, the psychological sequelae associated with or in reaction to the MD, and/or the behavioral tendencies that may interfere with the patient's task performance. Neuropsychological evaluations for individuals with MDs require unique considerations to elicit optimal performance and thus glean a reliable pattern of neurocognitive, emotional and behavioral functioning.

PURPOSE OF ASSESSMENT

In general, a neuropsychological examination seeks to provide a profile of the cognitive capacities of a patient to serve as an aid in differential diagnosis and as a guide to treatment management. Some specific indications for neuropsychological assessment in MDs are (a) to identify the presence and pattern of early or mild disturbances in cognitive function; (b) to aid in differential diagnosis of the type of movement disorder based on clinical history and neuropsychological profile (e.g., Parkinson's disease dementia versus Lewy body dementia); (c) to aid in the identification and differentiation of depression or other causes of behavioral impairment (e.g., impulse control, anxiety) from dementia and recommend appropriate psychological and behavioral interventions; (d) to elucidate the natural progression of cognitive changes or dementia through repeated administration of standardized tests; (e) to assist in treatment planning for cognitive rehabilitation strategies; (f) to evaluate the candidacy of individuals for deep brain stimulation (DBS) and to aid in the discussion of site of surgery (e.g., subthalamic nucleus (STN) versus internal globus pallidus (GPi)) based on the patient's cognitive profile and psychological status; (g) to evaluate the cognitive and behavioral side effect profile of surgical and nonsurgical treatments; and (h) to aid in making decisions regarding a person's ability to make his/her own health and financial decisions as well as future living planning.

PRACTICAL CLINICAL GUIDELINES

When examining individuals with MDs, there are practical issues that must also be considered and addressed, because these factors will impact an individual's test performance. In general, neuropsychological test batteries can take between 3 to 20 hours to administer depending on the level of neurologic impairment and the referral question, with the average clinical neuropsychological outpatient evaluation taking between 4 to 6 hours (Sweet, Peck, Abramowitz, & Etzweiler, 2002). For individuals with MDs, neuropsychological sessions may need to be limited to the evaluation of specific abilities due to known factors associated with MDs, such as variable attention/significant distractibility, limited physical and mental endurance, abrupt "on/off" medication periods, emotional lability, and disabling motor symptoms (e.g., dyskinesias, tremor, tics). Consequently, movement disorder evaluations are typically shorter in duration, and test selection and interpretation, considering the previously mentioned factors associated to MDs, become critical to answering the referral question.

Fixed versus flexible batteries. Test selection is dependent on a number of factors, including the goals of the evaluation or referral question, the need for serial assessments and alternate forms (e.g. pre- and postsurgery), reliability and validity of the available measures in comparison to the socio-demographics of the individual being assessed, and the individual's cognitive and physical functioning (Lezak, 2012). Test selection and strategies of neuropsychological assessment may be broadly categorized as utilizing a fixed battery (i.e., administration of a comprehensive, invariant series of tests) or a flexible or adjustive approach (selection of tests according to the reason for referral, pertinent clinical data, information obtained during an interview, the patient's ability to cooperate, and preliminary tests, which may suggest the presence of specific deficits). Although the use of ready-made batteries may attest to a lack of knowledge among inexperienced examiners (Sweet, Moberg, & Westergaard, 1996), these fixed batteries can be invaluable in research settings, especially in studies that will follow subjects longitudinally. Either strategy can provide a profile of abilities, and in practice, many examiners integrate complete test batteries or selected components with other procedures. Given the inefficiency of administering the same lengthy test battery to all patients and the lack of uniformity in a completely individualized approach, a practical compromise is to use a core battery consisting of carefully selected tests that require a few hours for administration and examine the major dimensions of cognition, mood, and behavior associated with the condition under investigation (Benton, 1992; Lezak, 2012). Depending on the specific referral question and the patient's pattern of performance on the core battery, specific impairments such as memory declines, visuospatial deficits or executive dysfunction can be explored in greater detail. Results of the core battery may be sufficient to answer the referral question in some cases, whereas, in other patients, an unequivocal diagnostic impression may elude the examiner despite detailed evaluation.

Environmental Conditions. Eliciting optimal performance is one of the primary responsibilities of the evaluator; consequently, numerous environmental factors should be considered when evaluating individuals with MDs. Several general modifications may need to be implemented due to poor vision (e.g., gaze palsy) or fine-motor deficiencies. It may be necessary to enlarge or to hold the stimuli closer to the individual to allow the patient a clear view of the material and large pencils or pencils with grips are recommended in assisting those patients with fine-motor deficiencies due to their MDs.

If the patient has a hyperkinetic condition, the testing environment many require modifications to aid the examiner in obtaining the best performance. It is recommended that patients with hyperkinetic movements be placed in a stationary chair with arms, which provides support for the patient to help control their movements. An adequate personal space surrounding the patient with a hyperkinetic disorder should be maintained, as sudden and violent involuntary movements can result in injury if the patient is too close to a wall or other hard surfaces. The evaluator may also consider restricting the movement of the stimuli and paper during visuospatial construction, motor and nonverbal memory testing. Additionally, it may be necessary for the evaluator to aid in the stabilization of the patient's movements during task performances (e.g., ensuring that their chair or table is stable as they work on a motor task).

Further, for patients who experience vocal or motor tics, the examiner may startle in reaction the examinee's nonrhythmic and unexpected vocalizations or motor behaviors. When this occurs, the experience can be awkward for both the examiner and the examinee, as many patients and clinicians are embarrassed due to their behaviors and reactions, respectively. The examiner should openly discuss this possibility with the patient, by informing them that due to their unexpected movement condition, the examiner may be caught off guard and react in response to the vocalizations and movements. Patients with Tourette's and other tic syndromes are usually understanding of their impact on those around them, and this introduction to the clinician's possible behavioral reactions allows for better communication and rapport building between examiner and examinee. Moreover, some patients with tic syndromes experience self-harming behaviors (i.e., slapping of the face, biting, head bumping, etc). The clinician should investigate the type of tics experienced by the patient and also openly discuss the alternatives for possible intervention should the behaviors be observed during the testing session. Although some patients are able to manage intrusive interventions (i.e., hand-holding with the examiner in an attempt to stop self-harm behaviors), others react in more intense self-harm actions when someone attempts to impede the tic. Therefore, it is vital that a discussion regarding possible clinician-focused interventions take place prior to attempting to stop such behavioral tendencies, because the examiner's response may unintentionally result in more harm than assistance.

For patients with hypokinetic movements, medication management during the evaluation should be a consideration. For example, individuals with Parkinson's disease are usually evaluated while "on" their movement disorder medication, so that they can be tested during the peak of their cognitive abilities. If the patient has an abrupt "off" medication time, the evaluation may need to be delayed until the medications are optimized again, particularly for timed measures or those requiring a written output. The timing of medication management should also be taken in to consideration during serial evaluations, with the neuropsychological testing scheduled for the same time of day for each evaluation. Patients with MDs often have a "best" time of day; therefore, when possible, patients' time preference should be considered when scheduling cognitive evaluations. Due to excessive daytime sleepiness, which is a prominent feature for several MDs, evaluations may also need to be divided in to several sessions in an attempt to ensure optimal effort across the testing battery. Some patients are prescribed stimulant medication to address their mental and physical fatigue. Given the possible side effects of pharmacological treatments, clinicians should be aware of the patient's medication regimen, as some stimulants can exacerbate the clinical symptoms evidenced by individuals with MDs (Hannay, Howieson, Loring, Fischer, & Lezak, 2012).

Cognitive and Psychological Sequelae. Due to a high prevalence of inattention/distractibility and frontal lobe mediated emotional and behavioral changes in MDs (e.g., apathy, disinhibition, perseveration), a distraction free testing environment is essential. Testing environments should be limited to only the examiner and the patient, and the testing table should be kept clear to reduce stimulus-bound behaviors (e.g., reaching for extraneous materials). Emotional lability and impulsive behavioral tendencies (e.g., crying, beginning the task before being instructed to do so, standing or walking around the testing room or attempting to exit the room) may be observed in individuals who suffer from MDs. Moreover, symptoms of psychosis (e.g., hallucinations and delusional thinking) can also interfere with standardized testing. For example, the patient may be quietly engaged in a hallucination while the unaware evaluator administers a test, or the patient may be experiencing paranoid ideations that impact the relationship between the evaluator and the examinee. The clinician is thus encouraged to inquire about past and current symptoms of psychosis as some patients may not openly discuss these symptoms. The clinician should also carefully observe and evaluate the psychological status and behavioral tendencies of the patient, control the testing environment (e.g., explanation of standardized procedure and expected behavior from both evaluator and patient) and implement breaks if decompensation in emotional status and/or behavioral tendencies is noted. Although these issues can be addressed in the clinician's behavioral observations, it is imperative that the administration of the tests be conducted as close to standardized procedures as possible to reduce the influence of confounding variables.

Computerized Neuropsychological Assessment. Application of computerized neuropsychological measures has expanded with technological advances and the widespread use of personal and laptop computers, tablets, and smart phones. Computerized testing offers some advantages over traditional cognitive testing, including more stringent standardization, easier scoring, more precise reaction-time measurement, randomization of test administration, and more convenient data storage. However, computerized cognitive testing has been criticized for neglecting the subtle behavioral nuances that are detected only with one-to-one contact during test administration. Although comprehensive computerized neuropsychological batteries (e.g., the Cambridge Neuropsychological Test Automated Battery (CANTAB) (Robbins et al., 1994)). Automated Neuropsychological Assessment Metrics (ANAM) (Kabat, Kane, Jefferson, & DiPino, 2001) have not yet gained widespread clinical use. Other computerized assessment batteries are used as cognitive screens (e.g., Neurotrax: Mindstreams, Computer Administered Neuropsychological Screen [CANS]; Hanna-Pladdy et al., 2010) to determine if a more standardized comprehensive neuropsychological assessment is recommended. Furthermore, individual computer administration of traditional neuropsychological measures has become more customary (e.g., Wisconsin Card Sorting Test (WCST) given technological advances (Lezak, 2012)). However, due to their heavy reliance on reaction time measurements as the primary measure of analysis, computerized neuropsychological assessments will likely result in a poor representation of the cognitive abilities in individuals who suffers from MDs. Additionally, most patients with MDs are older and lack experience with these new technologies, thus their lack of familiarity with the testing process may negatively impact their performance. Further, medical comorbidities, such as declines in vision, poor motor skills, and arthritis are usually evident in older patient populations, further confounding performance on these technological advancements. Therefore, computerized neuropsychological tasks should not be substituted for standardized pencil-and-paper tests administered by a human examiner. For patients with MDs, computerized tasks should be viewed as an adjunct to clinical evaluations.

Ethnic Minorities and Non-English Speaking Patients. When assessing minority patients, those who are bilingual, bicultural, and/or primarily non-English speaking, neuropsychologists must consider the influence of socio-demographic variables on neuropsychological test performance including culture, acculturation, language, education, years of residency in the primary culture, and socio-economic status (Strutt et al., 2012).

When the clinician shares linguistic similarities with the examinee but is unfamiliar with the patient's cultural and lifestyle practices, he/she is encouraged to learn about the patient's cultural social nuances, such as facial gestures, common expressions, and body language, to obtain a general understanding of the patient's cultural and lifestyle practices to better understand the observed behavioral observations of the patient. This may be an arduous task for the clinician and information gathered will unlikely be sufficient for a complete understanding of the interaction between examiner and examinee. However, this introductory information will afford the examiner the opportunity to ask the patient questions about his/her interaction style and behaviors prior to the evaluation, to assess for similarities and differences in comparison to the knowledge that has been acquired by the examiner.

Neuropsychologists who aim to conduct evaluations with non-English speakers are responsible for ensuring that they are adequately trained in conducting such evaluations (American Psychological Association, 2002). This training can include formal education, supervised experience, consultation, self-study, or professional experience. Ideally, neuropsychologists should receive formal training; however, currently, there are few and limited certification procedures to determine who is qualified to provide such supervision (Judd et al., 2009). As such, individual practitioners who are asked to provide services to non-English speaking minorities may find themselves inadequately prepared, yet may be disinclined to turn away referrals if they feel ethically responsible to provide services when a more appropriate provider is unavailable. A more concerning scenario involves the practitioner who lacks awareness regarding his/her limitations in providing such services.

Use of Interpreters. A survey conducted by Renteria and associates (2010) found that, 34.5% of the non-Spanish-speaking providers assessing primarily Spanish-speaking patients reported "always" using a Spanish-speaking interpreter, and 15.3% reported "always" referring out to a Spanish-speaking provider. Shockingly, 25.4% reported "never" referring out to Spanish-speaking providers, and 3.4% reported "always" conducting the Spanish testing themselves. Rivera-Mindt et al. (2008) suggest that professionally trained bilingual and socio-linguistically competent neuropsychologists and psychometrists should be utilized whenever possible to evaluate bilinguals. If such examiners are unavailable, then the bilingual client should be referred to such an examiner. When professionally trained bilingual examiners are unavailable, neuropsychologists should utilize trained, professional interpreters in order to provide services (Paradis, 2008), and it is the responsibility of neuropsychologist to educate the professional interpreter on the neuropsychological evaluation and expectations of translation (Judd et al., 2009).

The use of nonprofessional translators has potentially undesirable consequences, including possible secondary motivations to aid or hinder the client's performance (e.g., in the case of family), poor grasp of the language, and reticence to translate sensitive material (Paradis, 2008). Thus, whenever possible, neuropsychologists should avoid using family members, attorneys, and other persons known to the client as translators, unless circumstances dictate and permit such use (American Psychological Association, 2002). Despite the aforementioned concerns, many providers continue to use patients' family members or office staff as translators (15.3% of Renteria's English-speaking respondents reported "often" using patients' family or office staff, and 3.4% reported "always" using patients' family or office staff).

Moreover, research has documented a lack of test-wiseness in ethnic minority populations when Westernized neuropsychological measures are used (Manly, Byrd, Touradji, & Stern, 2004; Manly & Espino, 2004). Given the diversity that exists in socio-demographics across ethnic minorities, a clinician working with an individual from a minority group is encouraged to prepare the examinee for the testing process in order to ensure that the interpersonal exchange that will be observed during the standardized testing procedure is understood by the examinee and correctly interpreted by the examiner. For example, depending on cultural practices, ethnic minority patients may feel that the examiner is being dismissive or rude due to the lack of informal communication and interpersonal interaction between examiner and examinee during the standardized assessment procedure. Providing the patient with a basic explanation of the neuropsychological evaluation process will likely result in better rapport building between examiner and examinee, even when socio-demographic variables differ between the parties involved. Overall, it is imperative that, although the examiner is perceptive, he/she must also be considerate, compassionate, open-minded, and tolerant of the differences that may exist between him/her and the examinee.

COGNITIVE DOMAINS ASSESSED IN NEUROPSYCHOLOGICAL EVALUATIONS

Orientation and Basic Mental Status

Quantitative assessment of orientation is useful both in the detection of cerebral disease and in monitoring basic cognitive changes. Orientation is a basic cognitive capacity that is typically attained at the onset of a neurocognitive assessment. In response to the need for rapid cognitive screening, several measures and brief screening scales (5–30 minutes in length) have been designed to assess orientation and general mental status and/or to quickly examine the course of mental decline in dementing conditions. The Mini-Mental Status Exam (MMSE) (Folstein, Folstein, & McHugh, 1975) and the Montreal Cognitive Assessment (MoCA) (Nasreddine, Phillips, & Chertkow, 2012) are the two most widely used measures in both clinical and research settings when examining basic mental status and orientation. Research examining the psychometric qualities of these tools has shown that the MoCA is superior to the MMSE in detecting individuals at higher risk for of subcortical dementia (Dong et al., 2012; Kasten, Bruggemann, Schmidt, & Klein, 2010; Dalrymple-Alford et al., 2010, 2011). This is likely due to the inclusion of items that assess executive functioning and other abilities dependent upon intact subcortical functions. For individuals who suffer from MDs, the assessment of subcortical functioning is imperative; and, thus, the

MoCA provides a sample of the deficits, which may be found in individuals suffering from these conditions. One of the most widely used screening measures in the field of movement disorders is the Mattis Dementia Rating Scale-Second Edition (Jurica, Leitten, & Mattis, 2001), which is presently available in English and in Spanish (Strutt et al., 2012). This tool provides the examiner with a general understanding of an individual's abilities in attention, initiation/perseveration, construction, conceptualization, and memory and this tool is suitable for the screening of mild cognitive impairment and dementia (Matteau et al., 2011). When used for their stated purpose, namely, to identify cases that warrant more detailed study, these measures have proved to be fairly successful (Jurica, Leitten, & Mattis, 2001; Strutt et al., 2012). However, clinicians and researchers should be aware that subtle declines may not be revealed when using these tests due to the simplicity of the measures. Thus, it is critical to acknowledge that a negative performance (i.e., within normal limits results) does not rule out brain pathology, it only reveals which functions are considered to be reasonably intact (Lezak, Howieson, & Loring, 2004).

Premorbid Functioning and Intelligence

A basic impression of an individual's premorbid functioning is vital to understanding and interpreting the outcomes of a neuropsychological evaluation. This is a simple task when referring to functions with performance expectations. For example, adults who can no longer perform age-appropriate tasks (i.e., copy simple designs, speak fluently) evidence a clear functioning decline; however, obtaining a premorbid level can be a formidable task when the functions examined are normally distributed skills (i.e., breadth of vocabulary, which is known to be associated with education and social class). In this case, only an individual comparison provides a meaningful basis for assessing a possible deficit. A direct measurement of decline (i.e., the use of premorbid test scores or academic data), is recommended; however, clinicians rarely have the luxury of such information and patient self-report may be inaccurate. Hence, in most cases, the examiner must implement a nondirect method of deficit assessment from which individual comparison standards can be inferred (Lezak, 2012). The use of demographic equations (Krull, Sherer, & Adams, 1995; Axelrod, Vanderploeg, & Schinka, 1999), single-word reading tests of phonetically irregular and infrequently appearing words (Spreen & Strauss, 1998; Storandt, Stone, & LaBarge, 1995), and tests of mental ability (i.e., breadth of expressive vocabulary) (Krull, Scott, & Sherer, 1995) are the most common methods of calculating premorbid functioning and intellect estimates. However, these methods should be used with caution as there are many factors that may influence performance on these measures. Being aware of the quantity and quality of education, the individual's vocational history and other socio-demographic or cultural factors that are known to influence performance is critical for a neuropsychological evaluation (Strutt et al., 2012). Thus, equations combining socio-demographic variables with current test scores initially appeared to result in less overprediction of high scores and underprediction of low ones (Crawford et al., 1989). However, more recent research examining methods for estimating premorbid performance found that the phenomenon of regression to the mean affected all of the examined equations as scores at the extremes of the IQ spectrum were most vulnerable to estimation errors (Basso, Bornstein, Roper, & McCoy, 2000). Although these techniques for estimating premorbid functioning are available, all estimation techniques underscore the need for additional test data and historical information from both the patient and a collateral source.

Intelligence

Although a premorbid estimate of intelligence is helpful in determining the level of cognitive decline, a comprehensive evaluation of intelligence is usually not warranted for older patients who suffer from MDs. Due to the previously mentioned time constraints with individuals with MDs, time spent on the neuropsychological evaluation should be dedicated to the assessment of skills that are known to be disrupted by these neurological conditions and should not focus on a general assessment of intelligence. Examining discrete scores of subtests that are used to provide intellectual functioning scores (i.e., Weschler Adult Intelligence Scale-Fourth Edition (WAIS-IV): Block Design, Digit Span; 2012) will provide a better understanding of the neurocognitive strengths and weaknesses of the patient and how the neurological condition is affecting the individual's current abilities.

For those individuals who experience MDs at a younger age (i.e., early onset Parkinson's disease or Huntington's disease), a comprehensive evaluation of intelligence may be helpful in providing the patient with a general understanding of how their neurological illness has not only disrupted the cognitive skills associated with this condition (i.e., attention, working memory, information processing speed), but also how the declines associated with their neurological illness influences their general cognitive skills, including overall intellect. An examination of overall intelligence may also be used to assist the clinician in providing recommendations for the patient's educational and/or vocational future. Overall, the assessment of intelligence should be considered on a case by case basis and the decision to evaluate intellectual functioning should be dependent on several factors including patient age, stamina, referral question and need for recommendations.

Attention/Concentration

Attention is not a unitary concept. Several more or less independent types (e.g., simple, selective, divided, shifting) have been identified, referring to the different processes involved in how an individual becomes receptive to and how one processes or attends to internal and external stimuli. Research conceives attention as a hierarchical system in which processing occurs sequentially in a series of stages within different brains systems (Lezak, 2012). A salient characteristic of this system is its limited capacity (Lavie, 2001), as only a finite amount of processing can occur simultaneously and the complexity of the tasks involved will also impact these skills. Additionally, mood and both mental and physical fatigue can significantly impact an individual's level of attention/concentration (Zimmerman & Leclercq, 2002)

Impaired attention/concentration is among the most common neurocognitive difficulties associated with brain changes (Leclercq, Deloche, & Rousseaux, 2002; Lezak, 2012). The importance of attentional processes as a determinant of the level of diverse cognitive performances is widely recognized. It is clear that attentional deficits can be completely or partially responsible for observed impairments in learning, retention, perception, and problem solving, and overall cognitive productivity can suffer even when all other cognitive domains are intact (Stuss et al., 1989).

Individuals with MDs usually suffer from frontal and subcortical brain changes that impact reaction times, speed of encoding and sustained attention. Furthermore, individuals with MDs are impacted by external factors that may be simultaneously dividing their attention, including their involuntary movements (i.e., choreic movements in Huntington's disease; tremor in Parkinson's disease) or hypokinetic symptoms (i.e., rigidity and dyskinesias) leading to high levels of discomfort and distractibility. Many patients with MDs are also unable to quickly engage or complete the proposed tasks due to physical limitations. In light of the negative impact of inattention and distractibility on all other cognitive domains, the examiner evaluating individuals with MDs, especially when patients report a deficit in short-term memory, should carefully evaluate the role of sustained attention and information processing speed on encoding and recall.

Attentional processes are currently evaluated by a variety of examination procedures (e.g., simple auditory attention, visual attention and tracking, and simple and complex working memory exercises). Although many measures are available to test individuals with MDs, the examiner must be aware of the impact of abnormal movements and rigidity on the task at hand. Behavioral observations are a key element in detecting an patient's level of distractibility and difficulties with sustained attention. The examiner is encouraged to document attention lapses and how they affect an individual's performance throughout the testing session and within specific functional domains. Consequently, these lapses should be explored, when possible, to clarify the individual's ability to perform a particular type of task and to better understand how the variations or deficits in attention impact performance (Lezak, 2012; Lezak et al., 2004).

Processing Speed, Psychomotor Functioning, and Praxis

A salient mental effect of neurological disorders can be longer response latencies in initiating behavior and in responding to external stimuli. Research has shown that individuals diagnosed with MDs are likely to evidence slow reaction times and poor motor control due to rigidity or abnormal movements/tics, and, therefore, the interpretation of performance on neurocognitive measures assessing information processing speed must usually be interpreted with caveats in place. Given the physical limitations experienced by individuals diagnosed with MDs, an examination of written versus oral information processing speed is warranted. Understanding an individual's rate of processing is vital, as performance on all other assessed domains will be impacted by an individual's ability to understand, encode and recall the presented material. Clinicians should be aware that delayed response latencies are typical for patients suffering from MDs, and that patients usually benefit when provided with extended response time. Of course, this accommodation may not always be possible, depending on the task at hand; therefore, clinicians will, at times, have to test the individual's limits to ensure that incorrect responses were due to lack of knowledge or a deficit and not because of a delayed reaction or response.

Within a neuropsychological assessment, evaluation of fine and gross motor abilities is typically limited for individuals with MDs, as detailed motor testing is performed within the context of a comprehensive neurological evaluation. However, neuropsychologists may briefly evaluate motor functioning, using the Finger Tapping Test for motor speed and the Grooved Pegboard Test for fine motor control. Although apraxia is not a common clinical manifestation of the subcortical dementias typical of MDs, the presence of sequential orobuccal apraxia is characteristic of corticobasal degeneration (CBD) and should be screened for when attempting to provide a differential diagnosis of parkinsonian disorders (Lee, Williams, & Storey, 2012).

Memory

Disturbances of memory are such a frequent consequence of neurological illnesses that their assessment is usually considered to be the most important component of the neuropsychological examination. Distinctions are made between various contrasting forms of memory, each of which may be differentially impaired in patients with neurological conditions, including short versus long term memory, contextual versus noncontextual memory, free recall versus recognition memory, and verbal versus visual memory.

Short-Term and Long-Term Memory

Short-term memory (STM) operates within a time period of 45 seconds or less and with minimal opportunity for rehearsal; it also largely depends on attentional processes, processing speed, and the accurate perception of incoming information. STM is divided into *primary memory* or the ability to retain information in memory for a short time and *working memory* or the ability to maintain and manipulate the information held in primary memory. Although declines in working memory are often observed in patients diagnosed with MDs, age comparisons are imperative as declines in this domain are also known to be impacted by increases in age (Lezak, 2004), and, thus, what may appear as a decline in mental manipulation or subcortical functioning may reveal age-appropriate changes. Long-term memory (LTM), which involves the temporary or permanent storage of information, is itself divided into "recent memory" for events occurring hours or days before recall and "remote memory" for events that occurred further back in time.

For individuals with MDs, it is imperative for the clinician to understand the influence of attention/concentration and frontal lobe mediated functions when examining short- and long-term memory skills (e.g., organizing and planning during word-list learning, inability to encode contextual information due to impaired executive functioning). Despite the myriad of theoretical frameworks for memory functioning, for clinical purposes, a model of declarative memory provides the foundation for conceptualizing and understanding memory impairments: (1) registration or sensory memory; (2a) immediate memory—the first stage of STM; (2b) Rehearsal, (2c) STM—retention from one hour to several days, and (3) LTM—consolidation of information from several days to longer periods (Balota, Law, & Zevin, 2000; Lezak, 2012; Parkin, 2001).

Assessing Verbal Memory

Given the high prevalence of frontal lobe mediated dysfunction in individuals with MDs, the assessment of encoding and retrieval of both contextual and noncontextual/list-learning is recommended for this population. When using a list-learning task, the examiner can chose from nonsemantically related word lists that also present a distracter list or from less complex/shorter, semantically related lists without a distracter trial. These measures contain a recognition memory trial, which assists the examiner in identifying whether the patient's difficulties in STM are due to a primary encoding or retrieval deficit. Additionally, the recognition trial allows for a sample of the patient's ability to discriminate between relevant and nonrelevant stimuli (i.e., correct responses versus false positive errors). Further, the majority of these list-learning/noncontextual measures have alternate forms that can be used to assess an individual longitudinally.

STM should also be evaluated using contextual verbal memory measures, such as the encoding and recall of brief passages to clarify deficits in short-term verbal learning and retention. Some of these contextual verbal memory measures provide a rehearsal trial, where the story is repeated to the patient during the encoding phase of the test and a recognition trial is also usually included (Wechsler Memory Scale, 2012). These types of measures can assist the clinician in understanding whether the patient benefits from the repetition of information and whether the individual's level of attention/concentration is impacting their ability to encode the large amounts of presented material and if context aids the encoding and retention of information. Utilizing both contextual and noncontextual measures provides a clearer understanding of the patient's memory skills and whether the STM declines are due to encoding, retention and/or recognition deficits.

Assessing Visual Memory

Most measures used to assess visual memory include a visual motor component (i.e., drawing), which can be problematic when assessing patients diagnosed with MDs, since failure may arise from primary vision changes, constructional disability, impaired visual or spatial memory, or interaction between these variables and their abnormal movements (e.g., rigidity, chorea, dyskinesia; Lezak et al., 2004). Therefore, assessment of the patient's perception and visual acuity should precede the evaluation of visual memory skills, and the status of their MD should be noted during visual motor testing.

In regard to the assessment of this cognitive domain, visual reproduction (VR) from the Weschler series, the Brief Visual Memory Test-Revised (BVMT-R) and the Rey-Osterrieth Complex Figure Test (ROCFT) are some of the most widely used measures with individuals who suffer from MDs (Wechsler Memory Scale-IV, 2012; Meyers & Meyers, 1995; Benedict, 1997). The examiner should carefully weigh the benefits of repeated exposure (i.e., serial design paradigm of the BVMT-R) versus the longer exposure of less complex designs (i.e., WMS-VR) and the nontimed exposure of complex stimuli (i.e., ROCFT), along with the patient's motor abilities. Additionally, recognition memory testing is valuable when assessing visual memory skills as it overcomes the motor output limitations of patients with MDs, and allows the neuropsychologist to dissect the memory impairments into primary encoding or retrieval deficits.

Language

Although language impairments are commonly demonstrated in cortical conditions, such as Alzheimer's disease, language declines are also evident in MDs as these impairments arise from a primary subcortical pathology. Consequently, subcortical brain structures have also been incorporated into models of language providing more flexibility and a deeper understanding of the neural circuitry responsible for communication (Crosson, 1992; Geschwind, 1972). One distinction in language performance is made between receptive language (the awareness and comprehension of language) and expressive language (the formulation and production of appropriate language). Patients with MDs, at least earlier in the disease process, do not typically demonstrate receptive language impairments; however, they may develop expressive language difficulties, which are independent from the speech changes that are common in some MDs, including stuttering, dysarthria, and hypophonia (Crosson, 1992). Patients with MDs do not typically demonstrate deficiencies in vocabulary, grammar, syntax, comprehension of spoken material, or in their ability to follow sequential commands (Lezak, 2012). However, it should be noted that these abilities are influenced by gaps in attention/

concentration, which are prevalent in MD, which can necessitate evaluation of these language abilities. Word finding and retrieval disturbances are common in MDs (Brown & Marsden, 1988) with research demonstrating impairments in both phonemic and semantic fluency for patients with Parkinson's disease and progressive supranuclear palsy (Bayles, Trosset, Tomoeda, Montgomery, & Wilson, 1993; Cordato, Halliday, Caine, & Morris, 2006; Raskin, Sliwinski, & Borod, 1992). It is widely believed that lexical retrieval is impaired in disorders with a subcortical etiology, and that cueing can facilitate semantic retrieval (York, Levin, Grossman, Lai, & Krauss, 2003).

Standardized aphasia test batteries provide profiles of percentile scores for a variety of language functions, such as word association, repetition, naming, and receptive language ability (De Renzi & Vignolo, 1962; Orgass & Poeck, 1966). However, these comprehensive measures do not yield highly useful results in patients with MDs and can increase the length of a neuropsychological evaluation significantly. In practice, the examiner may select those subtests of an aphasia battery that are most relevant to the referral question, such as naming, verbal fluency, comprehension, and sequential commands. Assessment of naming ability, which is the most frequently impaired linguistic function in patients with brain disease, is assessed by procedures that require the naming of line drawings of objects to visual confrontation (e.g., The Boston Naming Test) (Kaplan, Goodglass, Weintraub, 1983). Phonemic fluency is the ability to generate words beginning with a specified letter, usually the letters F, A, and S are used for one minute per trial. Semantic fluency is the ability to generate exemplars of a specified category (e.g., animals, fruits and vegetables) within one minute. It should be noted that these fluency measures are timed; thus individuals with MDs may be at a disadvantage due to difficulties initiating responses and dysarthria. Phonemic fluency performance is not considered a pure language measure, but is thought to assess how well patients activate frontal-related strategies (Azuma et al., 2003; Henry & Crawford, 2004; Stuss et al., 1998; Troyer, Moscovitch, Winocur, Alexander, & Stuss, 1998). Consequently, phonemic fluency tasks will be discussed further in the executive function section.

Visuospatial Functioning

Visuospatial performance comprises a variety of abilities, such as visual and color discrimination, visuoperceptual organization, visual reasoning, construction, and visual neglect (Benton, Silvan, Hamsher, Varney, & Spreen, 1994; Dee, 1970; Lezak, 2012) Visuospatial functioning is often one of the more difficult cognitive domains to assess in MDs due to the heavy reliance of this skill on written output. Additionally, neuropsychological tasks used to assess visuospatial and visuoconstruction skills require a frontal lobe mediated resources (i.e., planning, organization, sequencing) and thus impairment in this domain may be difficult to identify and disentangle from general executive dysfunction.

Generally, the task of the neuropsychologist is to assess the patient's visuospatial performance by taking into account the patient's physical limitations due to their neurological condition. For example, is a poor visuoconstruction performance due to the patient's dystonic tremor or chorea interfering with their ability to hold the pencil and perform the task or due to a primary perceptual impairment? Several measures of visuospatial functioning do not require a written or motor output, including judgment of distance and direction, geographic orientation, facial recognition, or visuospatial reasoning; thus making these tasks attractive choices for use with individuals with MDs. Although the assessment of visuoconstruction abilities requires a motor output, it is the most commonly evaluated visuospatial ability in neuropsychological evaluations (e.g., Clock drawing, cube drawing) (Lezak, 2012). Other measures of visuospatial construction require the patient to integrate their visual abilities with their motor skills, and they also rely heavily on frontal lobe organizational abilities (e.g., The Rey-Osterrieth Complex Figure Test and RBANS Copy); thus, requiring the neuropsychologist to dissect these performances into their component abilities.

Executive Functions: Reasoning, Decision Making, and Problem Solving

In general, executive functions refer to "higher-level" cognitive processes (e.g., planning) involved in the control and regulation of "lower-level" cognitive processes (e.g., working memory, Spreen & Strauss, 1998). Reasoning, decision making, inhibition, judgment, planning, multitasking, cognitive flexibility, and problem solving are all considered executive functioning tasks. Research suggests that there are three component factors underlying executive functions: (1) inhibition and switching (Baldo, Shimamura, Delis, Kramer, & Kaplan, 2001; York et al., 2003); (2) working memory (Morris et al., 1988; Owen, 2004); and (3) sustained and selective attention (Manly & Robertson, 1997; Stuss, Floden, Alexander, Levine, & Katz, 2001). The dorsolateral prefrontal cortex has been linked to a variety of executive function tasks, including verbal and design fluency, response inhibition, working memory, organizational skills, maintaining and shifting set, planning, reasoning, problem solving, and abstract thinking (Barcelo, 2001). Frontostriatal functioning, which is often impaired in individuals with MDs, is vital for the execution of more complex tasks such as behavioral adaptation, everyday social interactions, management of occupational demands (e.g., switching from one task to another), safety, financial planning, and driving (Grafman & Litvan, 1999). Given the frontostriatal pathology implicated in MDs, executive functioning is a primary area for neuropsychologists to focus their cognitive evaluations (Bonelli & Cummings, 2007; Cummings, 1993; Grafman & Litvan, 1999).

Executive functions are assessed using a multitude of tasks, each which tap several aspects of cognitive processing or require integration of cognitive domains. The Delis–Kaplan Executive Function Scale (DKEFS) is a battery of stand-alone measures that can be used to assess verbal and nonverbal executive functions and include modifications of preexisting and novel tests (Delis, Kaplan, and Kramer, 2001). Determining through patient interview or caregiver rated questionnaires (e.g., Frontal Systems Behavioral Scale [FrsBE]; Grace & Mallow, 2011); Dysexecutive Questionnaire (DEX; Wilson, Alderman, Burgess, Emslie, & Evan, 1996) the patient's primary areas of impairment in this domain, may aid the examiner in choosing the most appropriate executive function measures to assess. Problem solving and reasoning are often assessed using measures of card sorting (e.g., Wisconsin Card Sorting Test, DKEFS Card sorting; Heaton, Chelune, Talley, & Kay, 1993), selection of relevant dimensions in response to stimuli (e.g., Booklet Category Test), judging the similarities or differences between items (e.g., WAIS-IV Similarities) or visual progressive matrices (e.g., WAIS-IV Matrix Reasoning) Set shifting, which is involved in multitasking and safety regulation, can be assessed with overlearned alternation tasks (e.g., Trail Making Test, Part B; DKEFS Alternating Fluency). Inhibition, which is the ability to stop a prepotent response, is often measured with the Stroop color naming paradigm (e.g., naming the color of the word "red" written in blue ink; Stroop, 1935) and behaviorally it is evaluated with self- or caregiver-reported measures (FrSBE, DEX). Phonemic fluency, which is a language task highly dependent on intact functioning of frontostriatal circuitry, has been an area of intense research focus in MDs (York et al., 2003). Phonemic fluency tasks require a timed response of word generation to specified letter, and several MDs have been shown to have early and definitive deficits on this measure, including Parkinson's disease, Tourette Syndrome, and Huntington disease (Dumas, van den Bogaard, Middelkoop, & Roos, 2013; Mahone, Koth, Cutting, Singer, & Denckla, 2001; Troyer Moscovitch, Winocur, Leach, & Freedman, 1998). Furthermore, impaired phonemic fluency performance is correlated with subsequent development of dementia in PD (Henry & Crawfod, 2005; Jacobs et al., 1995).

DIFFERENTIAL DIAGNOSIS

Individuals with MDs tend to demonstrate neurocognitive declines that localize to subcortical brain structures, including the basal ganglia (caudate, putamen and globus pallidus), subthalamic nucleus, substantia nigra, and their interconnections to each other and to the thalamic nuclei, are typical in movement conditions (Cummings, 1993). These declines include bradyphrenia (cognitive slowing), declines in attention/concentration, executive dysfunction including impaired concept manipulation and use of strategies, visuospatial abnormalities, and a memory decline characterized by difficulties with retrieval. In contrast to cortical dysfunction, a subcortical dementia does not include aphasia, agnosia, and apraxia as primary features. For example, progressive supranuclear palsy (PSP) is considered a prototypic subcortical dementia, with slowed processing speed, impaired memory retrieval, and cognitive inflexibility, whereas, in contrast, corticobasal degeneration (CBD) is considered to have a mixed cortical and subcortical pattern as patients often demonstrate aphasia and apraxia in addition to executive dysfunction (Goetz, Leurgans, Lang, & Litvan, 2003). Cortical versus subcortical classifications of dementia are generally utilized as a general characterization of cognitive, psychological, and behavioral symptoms, which are generally identifiable in the early stages of the disease process. However, as these conditions progress, both subcortical and cortical declines become evident and in later or final stages of dementia, the patterns are equivocal

Lee et al. (2012) quantified the effect sizes of cognitive abnormalities between parkinsonian disorders, such as PSP, CBD, multiple-systems atrophy (MSA) and PD, to assess the potential contribution of cognitive testing in differential diagnosis of parkinsonisms. They calculated Cohen's d and positive likelihood ratios for their critical review of 19 articles that directly compared at least 2 parkinsonism groups. This review found that fewer than half of the cognitive tests evaluated had sufficient effect sizes to provide clinically useful data. Specifically, cognitive testing was not found to be very useful in differentiating PD from MSA. In separating PSP from PD and MSA, phonemic and semantic fluency measures, Trail-Making Test Part B, and the Wisconsin Card Sorting Test were found to be moderately useful, and lower scores on the Frontal Assessment Battery differentiated PSP from PD. Cognitive tests alone were unable to differentiate CBD from other parkinsonisms; however, sequential orobuccal apraxia was associated with a diagnosis of CBD (Litvan et al., 2003). Overall, small effect sizes indicated that cognitive testing in isolation was not shown to be clinically useful in differentiating the parkinsonian disorders; however, the authors acknowledge that the utility of cognitive testing increases when other clinical characteristics (e.g., disease progression, medication response) are considered in conjunction with the testing pattern.

From this review, Lee and colleagues (2012) recommend a core battery of standard measures that are easy to administer and can be performed in a relatively short period of time to aid in the differential diagnosis of parkinsonian disorders. They recommend using verbal fluency tests, the Frontal Assessment Battery, Trail Making Test Parts A and B, and graded apraxia assessments. Although these measures were found to be very useful in differentiating some of the parkinsonian disorders, they do not constitute a comprehensive neuropsychological assessment and will not address other cognitive domains impacted by these and other MDs (i.e., short-term memory decline, lapses in attention). Therefore, to evaluate each of the cognitive domains in a comprehensive neuropsychological evaluation, taking into account the reported effect sizes, cognitive changes associated to these and other MDs, mood and behavioral symptomatology of these conditions, and additional influential factors (i.e., onset of illness, disease length, medical comorbidities) we recommend a battery of tests that neuropsychologists can chose from based on the patient's clinical presentation and referral question, stratified by cognitive domain (see Table 3-1).

MOOD AND BEHAVIORAL EVALUATIONS

In addition to the cognitive impairments associated with MDs, a comprehensive neuropsychological assessment should also examines the presence and

Table 3-1 Neuropsychological Tests by Cognitive Domain for the Assessment of MDs

Cognitive domain	*Test*
Orientation	Montreal Cognitive Assessment, Dementia Rating Scale-II
Premorbid	Wechsler Test of Adult Reading, Advanced Clinical Solutions premorbid
Verbal Memory	Hopkins Verbal Learning Test, Rey Adult Verbal Learning Test, California Verbal Learning Test, Wechsler Memory Scale-IV (WMS-IV) Logical Memory
Visual Memory	Brief Visual Memory Test-Revised, WMS-IV Visual Reproduction, Rey-Osterreith Complex Figure
Language	Semantic Fluency, Boston Naming Test, Token Test
Attention/Working Memory	Wechsler Adult Intelligence Scale-IV (WAIS-IV) Digit Span, Symbol Digit Modalities Test (oral and written conditions), Trail Making Test Part A
Visuospatial	Clock Drawing, Judgment of Line Orientation, Rey-Osterreith Complex Figure, WMS-IV Block Design
Motor	Finger Tapping, Grooved Pegboard, Praxis screening
Executive Function	Verbal Fluency, Alternating Fluency, Trail Making Test Part B, Frontal Assessment Battery, Wisconsin Card Sorting Test, Stroop Color Word Test
Mood/Behavior	Beck Depression Inventory-II, State Trait Anxiety Inventory, Questionnaire for Impulsive-Compulsive Disorders (QUIP), Columbia Suicide Severity Scale
Functional Status	Lawton's Physical Self-Maintenance Scale and Instrumental Activities of Daily Living Questionnaires

severity of neuropsychiatric symptoms, including depression, anxiety, apathy, impulse-control disorders and psychosis. These emotional or personality changes can either precede or follow a movement disorder diagnosis (Bonnet, Jutras, Czernecki, Corvol, & Vidailhet, 2012; Louis, Huey, Gerbin, & Viner, 2012; Reedeker et al., 2011) Although mood and behavioral symptoms are associated with specific brain pathologies (Lishman, 1997), individuals with MDs also demonstrate these symptoms in response to the life-style changes associated with their neurological illness. Few individuals will experience mood, personality, and behavioral changes that are simply either direct consequences of their neurological condition or secondary reactions to impairment and quality of life. For most, the observed declines are the product of extremely complex interactions involving the individual's premorbid behavioral patterns, current environmental demands, and their neurological symptomatology (Gainotti, 1993). All these factors can impact a neuropsychological assessment and should be considered when evaluating behavioral features of MDs.

DEPRESSION

Depression is a common behavioral manifestation of several MDs, with prevalence rates ranging from 30–50% in Parkinson's disease, 37% for dystonia, 34% for essential tremor patients, 2–9% in Tourette's syndrome (Kulisevsky et al., 2001), 20% for Progressive Supranuclear Palsy (Schrag et al., 2010). In MDs, the most commonly endorsed symptoms associated with depression are fatigability, difficulties with work, anhedonia, and sleep disturbances, whereas guilt, self-blame, and worthlessness were rarely endorsed by MD patients (Miller et al., 2007). For several MDs, depression is considered an antecedent symptom, occurring years prior to the first motor symptom (Shiba et al., 2000; Starkstein, Brockman, & Hayhow, 2012). To improve quality of life for patients with MDs, it is essential to evaluate for depression and make treatment recommendations. However, the assessment of depression in these populations is complicated by the large overlap between the physiological symptoms of depression and MDs (e.g., restlessness, changes in sleep or appetite, decreased energy) (Shulman, Taback, Rabinstein, & Weiner, 2002). A review of the scales used to assess patients with Parkinson's disease was undertaken by the Movement Disorders Society (MDS), with the Beck Depression Inventory-II and the Hamilton Depression Scale reported to be the best validated and widely used measures for this population (Schrag et al., 2007). However, evidence-based reviews of depression scales have not been carried out for other MDs.

ANXIETY

Anxiety encompasses feelings of worry, fear, or dread to specific events or stimuli or more generalized feelings. Anxiety disorders can be diagnosed as phobias, social anxiety, panic attacks, generalized anxiety, obsessive-compulsive disorder, and posttraumatic stress disorder. The literature regarding the prevalence and treatment of anxiety for MDs is limited to Parkinson's disease, with estimates ranging from 30% for panic disorders to 11% for generalized anxiety symptoms (Marsh, 2000; Menza & Dobkin, 2005). Anxiety has been related to increased motor symptoms, such as gait disturbances, dyskinesias, freezing, and on/off fluctuations and can negatively impact quality of life, if left untreated (Menza, Sage, Marshall, Cody, & Duvoisin, 1990). Significant overlap also exists with symptoms of anxiety and MDs (e.g., restlessness) confounding the assessment of this behavioral disorder for this population. The MDS also published a critical evidenced based review of anxiety for PD and was unable to recommend any scales for assessment due to the lack of validation studies (Leentjens et al., 2008).

APATHY

Apathy, defined as a multidimensional disorder of motivation that includes reduced goal-directed behavior, cognitive ability, and emotions has been observed in several MDs (Leentjens et al., 2008; Robert et al., 2009). For those who experience apathy, symptoms appear to progress over time and across disease stages and these symptoms appear to be intrinsic to the evolution and progression of certain MDs (Thompson et al., 2012). Apathy is conceptualized as a distinct construct from depression, although symptom overlap does exist (Lane-Brown & Tate, 2009), as research has documented the presence of apathy symptomatology in individuals who do not suffer from depression (Louis et al., 2012). Although research has shown a high prevalence of apathy in MDs, specifically, Parkinson's disease, studies have also indicated that the prevalence of apathy is significantly reduced once patients with concomitant depression and dementia are excluded (Starkstein, 2012). There is a higher prevalence of apathy in patients with hypokinetic MDs; whereas individuals diagnosed with hyperkinetic conditions exhibit significantly more agitation, irritability, anxiety, and euphoria (Kulisevsky et al., 2001). For some individuals with MDs, apathy has been shown to be associated to global and executive cognitive performance and severe depression (Weintraub & Hurtig, 2007; Reijnders et al., 2010; Reedeker et al., 2011). Although some research has shown that lower mental status baseline scores predict the onset of apathy (Reedeker et al., 2011), other research has found that apathy places individuals at higher risk for cognitive declines (Dujardin, Sockeed, Delliaux, Destee, & Defebvre, 2009).

Although a variety of rating scales have been developed, valid diagnostic interviews and standardized diagnostic criteria for apathy are still lacking (Starkstein et al., 2012). Research suggests that measures should be examined for reliability and validity and relevant confounders, such as depression, cognitive declines, and important contextual factors, are accounted for when evaluating for apathy (Starkstein, 2012). Clinicians should examine symptoms of apathy separately from depression and should be aware that patients with anosognosia associated with frontal dysfunction may under-report symptoms of apathy (Louis et al., 2012). Although apathy is a commonly observed condition in individuals with MDs, its mechanism remains poorly understood, and no effective treatments have been identified to date (Starkstein et al., 2012).

IMPULSE CONTROL DISORDERS IN MOVEMENT DISORDERS

Impulse control disorders (ICDs), such as compulsive gambling, excessive shopping, hypersexuality, excessive engagement in hobbies, and compulsive eating are recognized as serious complications of dopamine replacement therapy (Raja & Bentivoglio, 2012). Additionally, other behavioral tendencies, such as punding (stereotyped, repetitive, purposeless behaviors) and compulsive medication overuse (dopamine dysregulation syndrome-DDS) have been associated with dopaminergic medications, with a 2–3.5 times increased odds of having an ICD if individuals are taking these medications (Weintraub et al., 2010). While ICDs have been associated with high dosages of dopamine agonists, DDS is primarily associated with higher potency, shorter acting dopaminergic medications (Weintraub & Nirenberg, 2012; Raja & Bentivoglio, 2012).

Literature examining the prevalence and treatment of ICDs is exclusive to PD, with incidence documented to be as high as 14% (Raja & Bentivoglio, 2012; Weintraub et al., 2010). Although impulsive behavioral tendencies are evident in individuals who suffer from Tourette's disorder and Huntington's disease, these frontal lobe mediated behaviors, which can be an exacerbation of premorbid personality characteristics or are out-of-character behavioral tendencies are not considered ICDs but, rather, psychological changes associated with these neurological conditions (Stout, Rodawalt, & Siemers, 2001). The primary treatment for ICDs is the discontinuation of or significant reduction in dopamine agonists (Raja & Bentivoglio, 2012; Weintraub & Nirenberg, 2012). Although some research suggests the use of serotonin selective reuptake inhibitors, nalmefene, zonisamide, or low dose antidopaminergic drugs (quetuaoine or clozapine) can be effective (Raja & Bentivoglio, 2012), other research indicates that no empirical evidence supports the amelioration of ICDs in individuals who suffer from PD and take dopamine agonists (Weintraub & Nirenberg, 2012). It is recommended to inquire about ICDs in patients with PD to aid in the early identification and intervention of this condition as many patients are unlikely to report symptoms due to a myriad of factors, including lack of insight and embarrassment (Aarons, Peisah, & Wijeratne, 2012). Risk factors for ICDs include younger age of illness onset, younger age, a predisease history of impulse control problems or novelty-seeking personality traits, personal or family history of substance abuse, mental health comorbidities, and gambling problems (Weintraub & Nirenberg, 2012; Wu, Politis & Piccini, 2009).

PSYCHOSIS

Psychosis (visual hallucinations and delusional thinking, which in many cases includes pathological jealousy) in MDs is rare with the exception of PD, for which a prevalence rate of 20–40% has been documented (Weintraub & Hurtig, 2007). In 1973, Friedhoff and Alpert proposed a theory that suggested that an increase in dopaminergic activity or a decrease in cholinergic activity relieved symptoms of PD, but resulted in some cases in symptoms of psychosis. Since this discovery, dopaminergic medications have been recognized to induce hallucinations and/or delusional thinking by stimulating or inducing hypersensitivity of mesocorticolimbic dopamine receptors (Marsh, 2005).

However, given the complex interplay between dopamine, serotonin, acetylcholine, and noradrenalin systems, other neurotransmitter systems have also been implicated in the psychosis observed in patients with PD (Aarons, Peisah, & Wijeratne, 2012). Psychosis is associated with older age, older age at onset of illness, higher use of antiparkinsonian medication, presence of dementia, more severe Parkinsonism and comorbid depression, and the presence of rapid eye movement sleep behavior (Starkstein et al., 2012; Forsaa, Larsen, Wentzel-Larsen, & Alves, 2010). Symptoms of psychosis usually develop after patients have been on medication for longer periods of time. Patients who experience early-onset psychosis often either had an undisclosed premorbid mental health condition, or their PD symptoms had evolved into another neurodegenerative condition, such as dementia with Lewy bodies or Alzheimer's disease with extrapyramidal signs (Goetz, Vogel, Tanner, & Stebbins, 1998).

CONCLUSION

When approaching a neuropsychological evaluation for patients with MDs, a myriad of factors should be considered (i.e., referral question, mental and physical stamina, abnormal movements, mood, behavioral tendencies, and multicultural considerations) to provide an accurate impression of the individual's neurocognitive and psychological functioning and to aid in treatment planning and recommendations. The unique characteristics of this patient population, including their abnormal movements, their potential for executive dysfunction and subcortical dementia, and their distinctive behavioral changes, are manageable factors during a comprehensive evaluation. However, knowledge regarding these issues is vital in preplanning for the neurocognitive assessment of individuals who suffer from MDs.

REFERENCES

Aarons, S., Peisah, C., & Wijeratne, C. (2012). Neuropsychiatric effects of Parkinson's disease treatment. *Australasian Journal of Aging, 31*(3), 198–202.

American Psychological Association APA (2002). Guidelines on multicultural training research practice and organizational change for psychologists.

Axelrod, B. N., Vanderploeg, R. D., & Schinka, J. A. (1999). Comparing methods for estimating premorbid intellectual functioning. *Archives of Clinical Neuropsychology, 14*(4), 341–346.

Azuma, T., Cruz, R. F., Bayles, K. A., Tomoeda, C. K., & Montgomery, E. B., Jr. (2003). A longitudinal study of neuropsychological change in individuals with Parkinson's disease. *International Journal of Geriatric Psychiatry, 18*(12), 1115–1120.

Baldo, J. V., Shimamura, A. P., Delis, D. C., Kramer, J., & Kaplan, E. (2001). Verbal and design fluency in patients with frontal lobe lesions. *Journal of the International Neuropsychology Society, 7*(5), 586–596.

Balota, D. A., Law, M. B., & Zevin, J. D. (2000). The attentional control of lexical processing pathways: reversing the word frequency effect. *Memory and Cognition, 28*(7), 1081–1089.

Barcelo, F. (2001). Does the Wisconsin Card Sorting Test measure prefrontal function? *Spanish Journal of Psychology, 4*(1), 79–100.

Basso, M. R., Bornstein, R. A., Roper, B. L., & McCoy, V. L. (2000). Limited accuracy of premorbid intelligence estimators: a demonstration of regression to the mean. *Clinical Neuropsychology, 14*(3), 325–340.

Bayles, K. A., Trosset, M. W., Tomoeda, C. K., Montgomery, E. B., Jr., & Wilson, J. (1993). Generative naming in Parkinson disease patients. *Journal of Clinical Experimental Neuropsychology, 15*(4), 547–562. doi: 10.1080/01688639308402578

Benedict, R. H. B. (1997). *Brief visual memory test-revised.* Lutz, FL: Psychological Assessment Resources.

Benton, A. (1992). Clinical neuropsychology: 1960–1990. *Journal of Clinical Experimental Neuropsychology, 14*(3), 407–417. doi: 10.1080/01688639208407616

Benton, A. L., Sivan, A. B., Hamsher, K., Varney, N. R., & Spreen, O. (1994). *Contributions to neuropsychological assessment* (2nd ed.). New York, NY: Oxford University Press.

Bonelli, R., & Cummings, J. L. (2007). Frontal-subcortical circuitry and behavior. *Dialogues in Clinical Neuroscience, 9*, 141–151.

Bonnet, A. M., Jutras, M. F., Czernecki, V., Corvol, J. C., & Vidailhet, M. (2012). Nonmotor symptoms in Parkinson's disease in 2012: Relevant clinical aspects. *Parkinsons Disease, 2012*, 198316. doi: 10.1155/2012/198316

Brown, R. G., & Marsden, C. D. (1988). "Subcortical dementia": The neuropsychological evidence. [Review]. *Neuroscience, 25*(2), 363–387.

Cordato, N. J., Halliday, G. M., Caine, D., & Morris, J. G. (2006). Comparison of motor, cognitive, and behavioral features in progressive supranuclear palsy and Parkinson's disease. *Movement Disorders, 21*(5), 632–638. doi: 10.1002/mds.20779

Crawford, J. R., Stewart, L. E., Cochrane, R. H., Foulds, J. A., Besson, J. A., & Parker, D. M. (1989). Estimating premorbid IQ from demographic variables: regression equations derived from a UK sample. *British Journal of Clinical Psychology, 28*(Pt 3), 275–278.

Crosson, B. (1992). *Subcortical functions in language and memory*. New York, NY: Guilford Press.

Cummings, J. L. (1993). Frontal-subcortical circuits and human behavior. *Archives in Neurology, 50*(8), 873–880.

Cummings, J. L. (1988). The dementias of Parkinson's disease: Prevalence, characteristics, neurobiology, and comparison with dementia of the Alzheimer type. *European Neurology, 28*(Suppl 1),15–23.

Dalrymple-Alford, J. C., Livingston, L., MacAskill, M. R., Graham, C., Melzer, T. R., Porter, R. J., & Anderson, T. J. (2011). Characterizing mild cognitive impairment in Parkinson's disease. *Movement Disorders, 26*(4), 629–636. doi: 10.1002/mds.23592

Dalrymple-Alford, J. C., MacAskill, M. R., Nakas, C. T., Livingston, L., Graham, C., Crucian, G. P., . . . Anderson, T. J. (2010). The MoCA: well suited screen for cognitive impairment in Parkinson's disease. *Neurology, 75*, 1717–1725.

Dee, H. L. (1970). Visuoconstructive and visuoperceptive deficit in patients with unilateral cerebral lesions. *Neuropsychologia, 8*(3), 305–314.

Delis, D. C., Kaplan, E., & Kramer J. H. (2001). *Delis–Kaplan executive function system™ (D-KEFS™) manual*. San Antonio, TX: Pearson.

De Renzi, E., & Vignolo, L. A. (1962). The token test: A sensitive test to detect receptive disturbances in aphasics. *Brain, 85*, 665–678.

Dong, Y., Lee, W. Y., Basri, N. A., Collinson, S. L., Merchant, R. A., Venketasubramanian, N., & Chen, C. L. (2012). The Montreal cognitive assessment is superior to the mini-mental state examination in detecting patients at higher risk of dementia. *International Psychogeriatrics, 24*(11), 1749–1755. doi: 10.1017/S1041610212001068

Dujardin, K., Sockeed, P., Delliaux, M., Destee, A., & Defebvre, L. (2009). Apathy may herald cognitive decline and dementia in Parkinson's disease. *Movement Disorders, 24*(16), 2391–2397.

Dumas, E. M., van den Bogaard, S. J., Middelkoop, H. A., & Roos, R. A. (2013). A review of cognition in Huntington's disease. *Frontiers in Bioscience (Schol Ed), 5*, 1–18.

Folstein, M. F., Folstein, S. E., & McHugh, P. R. (1975). "Mini-mental state." A practical method for grading the cognitive state of patients for the clinician. *Journal of Psychiatric Research, 12*(3), 189–198.

Forsaa, E. B., Larsen, J. P., Wentzel-Larsen, T., & Alves, G. (2010). What predicts mortality in Parkinson's disease? A prospective population-based long-term study. *Neurology, 75*(14), 1270–1276.

Gainotti, G. (1993). The riddle of the right hemisphere's contribution to the recovery of language. *European Journal of Disorders of Communication, 28*(3), 227–246.

Geschwind, N. (1972). Language and the brain. *Scientific American, 226*(4), 76–83.

Goetz, C. G., Leurgans, S., Lang, A. E., & Litvan, I. (2003). Progression of gait, speech and swallowing deficits in progressive supranuclear palsy. *Neurology, 60*(6), 917–922.

Goetz, C. G., Vogel, C., Tanner, C. M., & Stebbins, G. T. (1998). Early dopaminergic drug-induced hallucinations in Parkinsonian patients. *Neurology 51*(3), 811–814.

Grace, J., & Mallow, P. F. (2011). *Frontal system behavior scale (FRSBE) manual.* Lutz, FL: Psychological Assessment Resources.

Grafman, J., & Litvan, I. (1999). Importance of deficits in executive functions. *Lancet, 354*(9194),1921–1923.

Hanna-Pladdy, B., Enslein, A., Fray, M., Gajewski, B. J., Pahwa, R., & Lyons, K. E. (2010). Utility of the NeuroTrax computerized battery for cognitive screening in Parkinson's disease: Comparison with the MMSE and the MoCA. *International Journal of Neuroscience, 120*(8), 538–543. doi: 10.3109/00207454.2010.496539

Hannay, J. H., Howieson, D. B., Loring, D. W., Fischer, J. S., & Lezak, M. D. (2012). *Neuropathology for Neuropsychologists* (4th ed.). New York, NY: Oxford University Press.

Heaton, R. K., Chelune, G. J., Talley, J. L., Kay, G. G., & Curtiss, G. (1993). *Wisconsin card sorting test manual: Revised and expanded.* Odessa, FL: Psychological Assessment Resources.

Henry, J. D., Crawford, J. R. (2004). Verbal fluency deficits in Parkinson's disease: A meta-analysis. *Journal of the International Neuropsychology Society, 10*(4), 608–622.

Jacobs, D. M., Marder, K., Cote, L. J., Sano, M., Stern, Y., & Mayeux, R. (1995). Neuropsychological characteristics of preclinical dementia in Parkinson's disease. *Neurology,45*(9, 1691–1696.

Judd, T., Capetillo, D., Carrion-Baralt, J., Marmol, L. M., Miguel-Montes, L. S., Navarrete, M. G., & Valdes, J. (2009). Professional considerations for improving the neuropsychological evaluation of Hispanics: A National Academy of Neuropsychology education paper. *Archives of Clinical Neuropsychology, 24*(2), 127–135. doi: 10.1093/arclin/acp016

Jurica, P. J., Leitten, C. L., & Mattis, S. (2001). *DRS-2: Dementia Rating Scale-2.* Lutz, Florida: Psychological Assessment Resources.

Kabat, M. H., Kane, R. L., Jefferson, A. L., & DiPino, R. K. (2001). Construct validity of selected Automated Neuropsychological Assessment Metrics (ANAM) battery measures. *Clinical Neuropsychology, 15*(4), 498–507. doi: 10.1076/clin.15.4.498.1882

Kaplan, E., Goodglass, H., & Weintraub, S. (1983). *The Boston naming test.* (2nd ed.). Philadelphia, PA: Lea & Febiger.

Kasten, M., Bruggemann, N., Schmidt, A., & Klein, C. (2010). Validity of the MoCA and MMSE in the detection of MCI and dementia in Parkinson disease. *Neurology, 75*(5), 478; author reply 478–479. doi: 10.1212/WNL.0b013e3181e7948a

Krull, K. R., Sherer, M., & Adams, R. L. (1995). A comparison of indices of premorbid intelligence in clinical populations. *Applied Neuropsychology, 2*(1), 35–38.

Kulisevsky, J., Litvan, I., Berthier, M. L., Pascual-Sedano, B., Paulsen, J. S., & Cummings, J. L. (2001). Neuropsychiatric assessment of Gilles de la Tourette patients: Comparative study with other hyperkinetic and hypokinetic movement disorders. *Movement Disorder, 16*(6), 1098–1104.

Lane-Brown, A. T., & Tate, R. L. (2009). Measuring apathy after traumatic brain injury: Psychometric properties of the Apathy Evaluation Scale and the Frontal Systems Behavior Scale. *Brain Injury, 23*(13–14), 999–1007.

Lavie, N. (2001). The role of capacity limits in selective attention: Behavioural evidence and implications for neural activity. In J. Braun & C. Koch (Eds.), *Visual Attention and Cortical Circuits* (pp. 49–68). Cambridge, MA: MIT Press.

Leclercq, M., Deloche, G., & Rousseaux, M. (2002). Attentional complaints evoked by traumatic brain-injured and stroke patients: Frequency and importance. In M. Leclerq & P. Zimmerman (Eds.), *Applied neuropsychology of attention: Theory, diagnosis, and rehabilitation* (pp. 89–109). London: Psychology Press.

Lee, W., Williams, D. R., & Storey, E. (2012). Cognitive testing in the diagnosis of parkinsonian disorders: a critical appraisal of the literature. *Movement Disorders, 27*(10), 1243–1254. doi: 10.1002/mds.25113

Leentjens, A. F., Dujardin, K., Marsh, L., Martinez-Martin, P., Richard, I. H., Starkstein, S. E.,... Goetz, C. G. (2008). Apathy and anhedonia rating scales in Parkinson's disease: critique and recommendations. *Movement Disorders, 23*(14), 2004–2014. doi: 10.1002/mds.22229

Lezak, M. D. (2012). *Neuropsychological assessment* (5th ed.). Oxford, England, and New York, NY: Oxford University Press.

Lezak, M. D., Howieson, D. B., & Loring, D. W. (2004). *Neuropsychological assessment* (4th ed.). New York, NY: Oxford University Press.

Litvan, I., Bhatia, K. P., Burn, D. J., Goetz, C. G., Lang, A. E., McKeith, I.,... Wenning, G. K. (2003). Movement Disorders Society Scientific Issues Committee report: SIC Task Force appraisal of clinical diagnostic criteria for Parkinsonian disorders. *Movement Disorders, 18*(5), 467–486. doi: 10.1002/mds.10459

Lishman, W. A. (1997). Organic psychiatry: The psychological consequences of cerebral disorders (3rd ed.). Boston, MA: Blackwell Scientific.

Louis, E. D., Huey, E. D., Gerbin, M., & Viner, A. S. (2012). Apathy in essential tremor, dystonia, and Parkinson's disease: a comparison with normal controls. *Movement Disorders, 27*(3), 432–434. doi: 10.1002/mds.24049

Mahone, E. M., Koth, C. W., Cutting, L., Singer, H. S., & Denckla, M. B. (2001). Executive function in fluency and recall measures among children with Tourette syndrome or ADHD. *Journal of the International Neuropsychology Society, 7*(1), 102–111.

Manly, J. J., Byrd, D. A., Touradji, P., & Stern, Y. (2004). Acculturation, reading level, and neuropsycholgical test performance among African American elders. *Applied Neuropsychology, 11*(1), 37–46.

Manly, J. J., & Espino, J. J. (2004). Cultural influences on dementia recognition and management. *Clinical Geriatric Medicine, 20*(1), 93–119.

Manly, T., & Robertson, I. (1997). Sustained attention and the frontal lobes. In P. Rabbitt (Ed.), *Methodology of frontal and executive function* (pp. 135–153). Hove, UK: Psychology Press.

Marsh, L. (2000). Anxiety disorders in Parkinson's disease. *International Review of Psychiatry, 12*, 307–318.

Marsh, L. (2005). Psychosis in Parkinson's disease. *Primary Psychiatry, 12*(7), 56–62.

Matteau, E., Dupré, N., Langlois, M., Jean, L., Thivierge, S., Provencher, P., & Simard, M. (2011). Mattis dementia rating scale 2: Screening for MCI and dementia. *American Journal of Alzheimers Disease & Other Dementias, 26*(5), 389–398. doi: 10.1177/1533317511412046

Menza, M., & Dobkin, R. D. (2005). Anxiety and Parkinson's disease. *Primary Psychiatry, 12*(7), 63–68.

Menza, M. A., Sage, J., Marshall, E., Cody, R., & Duvoisin, R. (1990). Mood changes and "on-off" phenomena in Parkinson's disease. *Movement Disorders, 5*(2), 148–151.

Meyers, J. E., & Meyers, K. R. (1995). *Rey complex figure test and recognition trial.* San Antonio, TX: The Psychological Corporation.

Miller, K. M., Okun, M. S., Fernandez, H. F., Jacobson, C. E. T., Rodriguez, R. L., & Bowers, D. (2007). Depression symptoms in movement disorders: comparing Parkinson's disease, dystonia, and essential tremor. *Movement Disorders, 22*(5), 666–672. doi: 10.1002/mds.21376

Moretti, R., Torre, P., Antonello, R. M., Rosin, M. V., Esposito, F., Furman, M. R., & Bellini, G. (2012). Apathy: A complex symptom specific to the clinical pattern of presentation of Parkinson's disease? *American Journal of Alzheimer's Disorders & Other Dementias, 27*(3), 196–201.

Morris, R. G., Downes, J. J., Sahakian, B. J., Evenden, J. L., Heald, A., & Robbins, T. W. (1988). Planning and spatial working memory in Parkinson's disease. *Journal of Neurology, Neurosurgery, & Psychiatry, 51*(6), 757–766.

Nasreddine, Z. S., Phillips, N., & Chertkow, H. (2012). Normative data for the Montreal Cognitive Assessment (MoCA) in a population-based sample. *Neurology, 78*(10), 765–766; author reply 766. doi: 10.1212/01.wnl.0000413072.54070.a3

Orgass, B., & Poeck, K. (1966). [A new aphasia-test for the diagnosis of speech comprehension disorders]. *Nervenarzt, 37*(3), 124–126.

Owen, A. M. (2004). Cognitive dysfunction in Parkinson's disease: The role of frontostriatal circuitry. *Neuroscientist, 10*(6), 525–537.

Owen, A. M., Roberts, A. C., Hodges, J. R., Summers, B. A., Polkey, C. E., & Robbins, T. W. (1993). Contrasting mechanisms of impaired attentional set-shifting in patients with frontal lobe damage or Parkinson's disease. *Brain, 116* (Pt 5), 1159–1175.

Paradis, M. (2008). Bilingualism and neuropsychiatric disorders. *Journal of Neurolinguistics, 21*, 199–230.

Parkin, A. J. (2001). The structure and mechanisms of memory. In B. Rapp (Ed.), *The handbook of cognitive neuropsychology: What deficits reveal about the human mind* (pp. 399–422). New York, NY: Psychology Press.

Raja, M., & Bentivoglio, A. R. (2012). Impulsive and compulsive behaviors during dopamine replacement treatment in Parkinson's disease and other disorders. *Current Drug Safety, 7*(1), 63–75.

Raskin, S. A., Sliwinski, M., & Borod, J. C. (1992). Clustering strategies on tasks of verbal fluency in Parkinson's disease. *Neuropsychologia, 30*(1), 95–99.

Reedeker, N., Bouwens, J. A., van Duijn, E., Giltay, E. J., Roos, R. A., & van der Mast, R. C. (2011). Incidence, course, and predictors of apathy in Huntington's disease: a two-year prospective study. *Journal of Neuropsychiatry & Clinical Neuroscience, 23*(4), 434–441. doi: 10.1176/appi.neuropsych.23.4.434

Reijnders, J. S., Scholtissen, B., Weber, W. E., Aalten, P., Verhey, F. R., & Leentjens, A. F. (2010). Neuroanatomical correlates of apathy in Parkinson's disease: A magnetic resonance imaging study using voxel-based morphometry. *Movement Disorders, 25*(14), 2318–2325. doi: 10.1002/mds.23268

Renteria, L., Li, S. T., & Pilskin, N. H. (2010). Reliability and validity of the Spanish language Wechsler Adult Intelligence Scare (3rd edition) in a sample of American, urban, Spanish-speaking Hispanics. *The Clinical Neuropsychologist, 22*(3), 455–470. doi: 10.1080/13854040701336428

Rivera-Mindt, M., Arentoft, A., Kubo, G. K., D'Aquila, E., Schneiner, D., Pizzirusso, M.,... Gollan, T. H. (2008). Neuropsychological, cognitive, and theoretical considerations for evaluation of biligual individuals. *Neuropsychological Review, 18*(3), 255–268. doi: 10.1007/s11065-008-9069-7

Robbins, T. W., James, M., Owen, A. M., Sahakian, B. J., McInnes, L., & Rabbitt, P. (1994). Cambridge Neuropsychological Test Automated Battery (CANTAB): A factor analytic study of a large sample of normal elderly volunteers. *Dementia, 5*(5), 266–281.

Robert, P., Onyike, C. U., Leentjens, A. F., Dujardin, K., Aalten, P., Starkstein, S., ... Byrne, J. (2009). Proposed diagnostic criteria for apathy in Alzheimer's disease and other neuropsychiatric disorders. *European Psychiatry, 24*(2), 98–104. doi: 10.1016/j.eurpsy.2008.09.001

Schrag, A., Barone, P., Brown, R. G., Leentjens, A. F., McDonald, W. M., Starkstein, S., ... Goetz, C. G. (2007). Depression rating scales in Parkinson's disease: critique and recommendations. *Movement Disorders, 22*(8), 1077–1092. doi: 10.1002/mds.21333

Schrag, A., Sheikh, S., Quinn, N. P., Lees, A. J., Selai, C., Mathias, C., ... Jahanshahi, M. (2010). A comparison of depression, anxiety, and health status in patients with progressive supranuclear palsy and multiple system atrophy. *Movement Disorders, 25*(8), 1077–1081. doi: 10.1002/mds.22794

Shiba, M., Bower, J. H., Maraganore, D. M., McDonnell, S. K., Peterson, B. J., Ahlskog, J. E.... Rocca, W. A. (2000). Anxiety disorders and depressive disorders preceding Parkinson's disease: a case-control study. *Movement Disorders, 15*(4), 669–677.

Shulman, L. M., Taback, R. L., Rabinstein, A. A., & Weiner, W. J. (2002). Nonrecognition of depression and other nonmotor symptoms in Parkinson's disease. *Parkinsonism & Related Disorders, 8*(3), 193–197.

Spreen, O., & Strauss, E. (1998). *A compendium of neuropsychological tests: Administration, norms, and commentary.* (2nd ed.). NY: Oxford University Press.

Starkstein, S. E. (2012). Apathy in Parkinson's disease: Diagnostic and etiological dilemmas. *Movement Disorders, 27*(2), 174–178.

Starkstein, S. E., Brockman, S., & Hayhow, B. D. (2012). Psychiatric syndromes in Parkinson's disease. *Current Opinions in Psychiatry, 25*, 468–472.

Storandt, M., Stone, K., & LaBarge, E. (1995). Deficits in reading performance in very mild dementia of the Alzheimer type. *Neuropsychology, 9*(2), 174–176.

Stout, J. C., Rodawalt, W. C., & Siemers, E. R. (2001). Risky decision making in Huntington's disease. *Journal of the International Neuropsychology Society, 7*(1), 92–101.

Stroop, J. R. (1935). Studies of interference in serial verbal reactions. *Journal of Experimental Psychology, 18* (6), 643–662.

Strutt, A. M., Ayanegui, I. G., Scott, B. M., Mahoney, M. L., York, M. K., & San Miguel Montes, L. E. (2012). Influence of socio-demographic characteristics on DRS-2 performance in Spanish-speaking older adults. *Archives of Clinical Neuropsychology, 27*(5), 545–556. doi: 10.1093/arclin/acs049

Stuss, D. T., Alexander, M. P., Hamer, L., Palumbo, C., Dempster, R., Binns, M., ... Izukawa, D. (1998). The effects of focal anterior and posterior brain lesions on verbal fluency. *Journal of the International Neuropsychology Society, 4*(3), 265–278.

Stuss, D. T., Floden, D., Alexander, M. P., Levine, B., & Katz, D. (2001). Stroop performance in focal lesion patients: dissociation of processes and frontal lobe lesion location. *Neuropsychologia, 39*(8), 771–786.

Stuss, D. T., Stethem, L. L., Hugenholtz, H., Picton, T., Pivik, J., & Richard, M. T. (1989). Reaction time after head injury: fatigue, divided and focused attention, and consistence of performance. *Journal of Neurology, Neurosurgery, & Psychiatry, 52*(6), 742–748.

Sweet, J. J., Moberg, P. J., & Westergaard, C. (1996). Five year follow-up survey of practices and beliefs of clinical neuropsychologists. *Clinical Neuropsychologist, 10*, 202–221.

Sweet, J. J., Peck, E. A., 3rd, Abramowitz, C., & Etzweiler, S. (2002). National Academy of Neuropsychology/Division 40 of the American Psychological Association practice survey of clinical neuropsychology in the United States, Part I: Practitioner and practice characteristics, professional activities, and time requirements. *Clinical Neuropsychology, 16*(2), 109–127. doi: 10.1076/clin.16.2.109.13237

Thompson, J. C., Harris, J., Sollom, A. C., Stopford, C. L., Howard, E., Snowden, J. S., & Craufurd, D. (2012). Longitudinal evaluation of neuropsychiatric symptoms in Huntington's disease. *Journal of Neuropsychiatry & Clinical Neuroscience, 24*(1), 53–60.

Troyer, A. K., Moscovitch, M., Winocur, G., Leach, L., & Freedman, M. (1998). Clustering and switching on verbal fluency tests in Alzheimer's and Parkinson's disease. *Journal of the International Neuropsychology Society, 4*(2), 137–143.

Troyer A. K., Moscovitch, M., Winocur, G., Alexander, M. P., & Stuss, D. (1998). Clustering and switching on verbal fluency: the effects of focal frontal—and temporal-lobe lesions. *Neuropsychologia, 36*(6), 499–504.

Wechsler Memory Scale fourth edition manual. (2012). San Antonio, TX: Pearson.

Weintraub, D., & Hurtig, H. I. (2007). Presentation and management of psychosis in Parkinson's disease and dementia with Lewy bodies. *American Journal of Psychiatry, 164*(10), 1491–1498.

Weintraub, D., Koester, J., Potenza, M. N., Siderowf, A. D., Stacy, M., Voon, V., . . . Lange, A. E. (2010). Impulse control disorders in Parkinson's disease: A cross-sectional study of 3090 patients. *Archives of Neurology, 67*(5), 589–595.

Weintraub, D. & Nirenberg, M. J. (2012). Impulse control and related disorders in Parkinson's disease. *Neurodegenerative Disorders., 11*(2), 63–71.

Wilson, B. A., Alderman, N., Burgess, P. W., Emslie, H., & Evan, J. (1996) *Behavioral assessment of the dysexecutive syndrome (BADS).* San Antonio, TX: Pearson.

Wu, K., Politis, M., & Piccini, P. (2009). Parkinson's disease and impulse control disorders: A review of clinical features, pathophysiology and management. *Postgraduate Medical Journal, 85*(1009), 590–596.

York, M. K., Levin, H. S., Grossman, R. G., Lai, E. C., & Krauss, J. K. (2003). Clustering and switching in phonemic fluency following pallidotomy for the treatment of Parkinson's disease. *Journal of Clinical Experimental Neuropsychology, 25*(1), 110–121. doi: 10.1076/jcen.25.1.110.13626

Zimmerman, P., & Leclercq, M. (2002). Neuropsychological aspects of attentional functions and disturbances. *Applied neuropsychology of attention: Theory, diagnosis, and rehabilitation* (pp.56–86). London: Psychology Press.

4 Movement Disorders and Their Impact on Quality of Life

Delia Lorenz and Günther Deuschl

INTRODUCTION

The World Health Organization defines "Quality of Life (QoL) as individuals' perception of their position in life in the context of culture and value systems in which they live and in relation to their goals, expectations, standards and concerns. It is affected in a complex way by the person's physical health, psychological state, level of independence, social relationships, personal beliefs and their relationship to salient features of their environment" (The WHOQOL Group, 1996). The definition of QoL can be further compartmentalized into five dimensions: (1) physical, (2) emotional, (3) social, (4) economic, and (5) spiritual. For the concept of QoL there is a considerable agreement that QoL is subjective and multidimensional. Because it is subjective, it is best measured from the patient's perspective. Because it is multidimensional, a broad range of life domains such as well-being in physical, economic, social, and emotional domains, and the development and activity must be included. Health-related QoL (HRQoL) is defined as a functional effect of a medical condition and/or its therapy upon a patient. So it provides a possibility to evaluate or measure the impact of the disease as a whole and the overall efficacy of specific treatment. We will use the term QoL here only for HRQoL. Quality of life assessment contributes to a better understanding of the disease's and treatment's impact on the patient, and thus helps in decision making. Quality-of-life evaluations reflect the point of view of patients (possibly conflicting with the clinical ratings). A systematic search of the Cochrane Controlled Trials register from 1980 to 1997 showed an increase in reporting on QoL from 0.63% to 4.2% for trials from all disciplines with drug therapy as the most common intervention (Sanders, Egger, Donovan, Tallon, & Frankel, 1998).

A more recent literature search using PubMed for the period 1970 to 2003 on QoL assessment and reporting in randomized controlled trials from all disciplines showed an increase from 0% (1970–1974) to 4.4% (2000–2003). However, QoL was defined only in a small percentage (15–32%) of the reported clinical trials (Naito, Nakayama, & Fukuhara, 2004). In addition, the use of a broad variety of different QoL profiles and indices complicates the validation and comparison of findings.

GENERIC QUALITY-OF-LIFE INSTRUMENTS

There are several generic QoL instruments available including the Nottingham Health Profile (Hagell, Whalley, McKenna, & Lindvall, 2003; Hunt et al., 1980),

Table 4-1 Generic quality of life instruments

	Number of items	*Number of domains*	*Time frame*	*Successful clinimetric testing*	*General population norms available*	*Multiple languages available*
Nottingham Health Profile (NHP)	38	6	At present time	+	+	+
Sickness Impact Profile (SIP)	136	12	Today	+	+	+
EuroQoL (EQ-5D)	5	5	Today	+	+	+
36-item Short-Form Health Survey (SF-36, SF-36v2)	36	8	Last 4 weeks	+	+	+
Schedule for the Evaluation of Individual QoL (SEIQoL)	46	5	At present time	+		
QoL Questionnaire 15 D (15D)	15	15	At present time	+		+
WHO QoL Assessment Short version (WHOQOL-BREF)	26	4	Last 4 weeks	+		+
Questions on Life Satisfaction-Movement Disorders (QLS-MD)	12	1	Last 4 weeks			(+)
Questions on Life Satisfaction-Deep Brain Stimulation (QLS-DBS)	5	1	Last 4 weeks			(+)

the Sickness Impact Profile (SIP) (Bergner, Bobbitt, Carter, & Gilson, 1981), the EuroQoL (EQ-5D) (EuroQol Group, 1990; Ware & Sherbourne, 1992) (http://www.sf-36.org/), the Schedule for the Evaluation of Individual Quality of Life (SEIQoL) (Browne, O'Boyle, McGee, McDonald, & Joyce, 1997), the Quality of Life Questionnaire 15D (15D) (Sintonen, 2001) (http://www.15d-instrument.net/15d), the World Health Organization Quality of Life Assessment Short Version (WHOQOL-BREF; Skevington, Lotfy, & O'Connell, 2004; http://www.who.int/substance_abuse/research_tools/whoqolbref/en/), the Questions on Life Satisfaction-Movement Disorders (QLS-MD) Module and the Questions on Life Satisfaction-Deep Brain Stimulation (QLS-DBS) Module (Kuehler et al., 2003) (Table 4-1).

PARKINSON'S DISEASE

Parkinson's disease (PD) is a chronic progressive illness that causes disability and impaired QoL. Motor, behavioral, and social functions, in addition to the effects of treatments, are significant contributors to QoL in patients with PD. A wide variety of outcome measures are used in PD research which range from disease staging scales such as the Hoehn and Yahr scale (Hoehn & Yahr, 1967), symptom-specific measures such as dyskinesia scales, disability scales such as the Schwab and England scale (Gillingham, 1969), disability/impairment scales such as the Unified Parkinson's Disease Rating Scale (UPDRS) (Fahn, Elton, & Members of the UPDRS Development Commitee, 1987) to QoL instruments. For decades, successful management of PD has been focusing on the control of motor symptoms using scales such as UPDRS. Recently, however, there is increasing recognition that not only the physical impairment of the disease is important, but also various nonmotor symptoms such as depression, cognitive impairment, sleep disturbances, the medical or surgical treatment, psychosocial well-being of the patient and their ability to perform their occupational and social roles contribute to the burden of the disease (Aarsland, Tandberg, Larsen, & Cummings, 1996; Lees, Blackburn, & Campbell, 1988; Tandberg, Larsen, Aarsland, & Cummings, 1996). The patient-perceived QoL does not simply reflect disease severity, but may include other factors such as neuropsychiatric complaints, cognitive impairment, and psychosocial factors. The health burden of PD can be assessed on several levels, each of which has a different perspective, symptom scales, generic QoL measures, and disease specific measures can all be used for this, either alone or in combination. It has been shown, that PD affects QoL and has an increasing impact on QoL along with the progression of the disease (Karlsen, Larsen, Tandberg, & Maeland, 1999).

QoL Tools in PD

There are several QoL instruments available for Patients with PD including the Parkinson's disease questionnaire 39 (PDQ-39) (Peto, Jenkinson, Fitzpatrick, &

Greenhall, 1995; Jenkinson, Fitzpatrick, Peto, Greenhall, & Hyman, 1997; http://www.publichealth.ox.ac.uk/research/hsru/PDQ/Intropdq), the Parkinson's disease questionnaire 8 (PDQ-8) (Jenkinson & Fitzpatrick, 2007). (http://www.publichealth.ox.ac.uk/research/hsru/PDQ/pdq8), the PD Quality of Life Scale (PDQUALIF; Welsh et al., 2003), the PD Quality of Life Questionnaire (PDQL; de Boer, Wijker, Speelman, & de Haes, 1996; Martinez-Martin, Serrano-Duenas, Forjaz, & Serrano, 2007), the Parkinson's Impact Scale (PIMS; Schulzer, Mak, & Calne, 2003), the Parkinson Quality of Life Questionnaire (PLQ;Van den Berg, 1998), the Scales for Outcomes in Parkinson's Disease Psychosocial (SCOPA-PS; Marinus, Visser, Martinez-Martin, van Hilten, & Stiggelbout, 2003), and the Parkinson's disease symptom inventory (PDSI; Hogan et al., 1999) (Table 4-2). In one comparison study of all PD QoL tools they showed an acceptable internal consistency. The content validity was adequate for the PDQ-39, PDQL, and PLQ but insufficient for the PIMS. Overall, the authors found the PDQ-39 to be the

Table 4-2 Health-related quality of life in Parkinson's disease

	Number of items	*Number of domains*	*Time frame*	*Successful clinimetric testing*	*Multiple languages available*
Parkinson's disease questionnaire 39 (PDQ-39)	39	8	Last month	+	+
Parkinson's disease questionnaire 8 (PDQ-8)	8	8	Last month	+	+
Parkinson's disease QoL Scale (PDQUALIF)	32	7	Flexible	+	(+)
Parkinson's disease QoL Questionnaire (PDQL)	37	4	Last 3 months	+	+
Parkinson's Impact Scale (PIMS)	10	4	At present time	+	(+)
Parkinson QoL Questionnaire (PLQ)	44	9	Past week		
Scales for Outcomes in Parkinson's Disease Psychosocial (SCOPA-PS)	11	1	Last month	+	(+)
Parkinson's disease symptom inventory (PDSI)	51			+	

most valuable QoL tool because of its validity, satisfactory clinimetric characteristics, and availability in multiple languages (Marinus, Ramaker, van Hilten, & Stiggelbout, 2002).

Factors Impacting QoL in PD

There are multiple factors impacting on QoL in PD and it is important to understand their particular weight on the overall disease perception. It has been demonstrated that QoL deteriorates with advancing disease, and later stages of illness are associated with poorer QoL (Schrag, Jahanshahi, & Quinn, 2000). Studies of QoL in PD have further confirmed that both the symptoms of PD and medication have a substantial impact on patients' QoL (Schrag et al., 2000). Overall, factors contributing to QoL in PD can mainly be divided to (a) physical/motor, (b) cognitive/psychiatric and (c) medication-related symptoms. For motor symptoms, there is an influence of specific PD symptoms tremor, rigidity, bradykinesia on QoL (Peto et al., 1995), but further physical symptoms such as difficulty in walking, start hesitation, shuffling gait, freezing, festination, propulsion, difficulty in turning, and difficulty in dressing also have a significant effect on QoL scores. Even though many of the motor symptoms significantly influence QoL, axial impairment including postural instability and gait difficulties seem to have the most meaningful impact on QoL in PD (Gomez-Esteban et al., 2007; Muslimovic, Post, Speelman, Schmand, & de Haan, 2008; Rahman, Griffin, Quinn, & Jahanshahi, 2008). Some of these motor symptoms cause a higher frequency of falls in PD patients. Falls have a strong influence on QoL in PD through injury and resulting in time in hospital. Also, the fear of falling can prevent PD patients from taking part in activities, further restricting their QoL (Bloem, Grimbergen, Cramer, Willemsen, & Zwinderman, 2001). Although severity of motor symptoms and their treatment are important factors influencing QoL in PD ("Factors Impacting on Quality of Life in Parkinson's Disease: Results from an International Survey," 2002), these factors only explain part of the variance of QoL scores.

Nonmotor symptoms in PD have gained relevance in recent years for their high prevalence in PD patients and their impact on patients' QoL (K. R. Chaudhuri, Healy, & Schapira, 2006). Psychiatric nonmotor symptoms, mainly anxiety and depression, represent the most common nonmotor symptoms in most of the studies (Barone et al., 2009). Frequencies of nonmotor symptoms in different studies were: psychiatric symptoms (66.8%), anxiety (40–48%), apathy (51%), depression (range 10–45%), attention/memory (42–44%), sleep disorders (64.1%), gastrointestinal symptoms (61%), urinary symptoms (57–59%), and pain (46–60%) (Barone et al., 2009; Martinez-Martin, Schapira, et al., 2007; Schrag et al., 2000). There is a strong impact of non-motor symptoms on the QoL showing a close association between number of nonmotor symptoms and worse QoL. This could be shown in studies evaluating the new Non-Motor Symptoms Scale (NMSS) (R. K. Chaudhuri et al., 2013). The NMSS showed a highly significant association with PDQ-39 SI and high to moderate correlation with all

PDQ-39 domains. As scores on the NMSS increased, QoL, measured by disease specific and generic scales became worse. Similarly QoL progressively declined as motor symptoms increased, although this association was weaker. High correlations between the PDQ-39 domains Mobility and ADL with the total NMSS score suggest an association between nonmotor symptoms and satisfaction with physical domains of QOL. Overall the correlation between nonmotor symptoms and the PDQ-39 summary index weights stronger than with motor symptoms. (K. R. Chaudhuri et al., 2007; Martinez-Martin, Rodriguez-Blazquez, Kurtis, & Chaudhuri, 2011). Nonmotor symptoms are present already at disease onset, and some, like psychiatric and sleep disorders, may even precede motor symptoms (Shiba et al., 2000). Nonmotor symptoms also contribute to institutionalization in advanced stages of Parkinson's disease.

Within the subgroup of cognitive/psychiatric symptoms depression is the factor with the most significant impact on QoL (Rahman et al., 2008), although it is still not clear if the association of depression with reduced QoL is causal. In a population-based study, depressive symptoms as measured by the MADRS accounted for 54% of the variance of QoL scores (Schrag et al., 2000). This is even more relevant since depression is common in PD (5.1% major depression, 45.5% milder depressive symptoms (Riedel et al., 2010)), and there is evidence of a high prevalence of depression already in the initial or even prodromal phase of the disease (Shiba et al., 2000). Anxiety also contributes to a poorer QoL in PD. Anxiety is poorly studied in PD, despite being present in up to 40% of PD patients. Anxiety can worsen the motor symptoms of PD, which can further increase anxiety (Rahman et al., 2008; Richard, 2005). Anxiety can manifest as "fear of falling," which has been reported by 46% of patients (Bloem et al., 2001), and can lead to avoidance of mobility, and hence, social isolation and poorer QoL. In one study, anxiety explained 29% of the variance in overall QoL in PD patients, whereas depression explained an additional 10% (Hanna & Cronin-Golomb, 2012). Moreover, cognitive impairment, confusion, and memory problems were found to significantly influence QoL (Rahman et al., 2008).

For the medication-related symptoms, unpredictable on/off states and dyskinesias have an important impact on QoL in PD. Increasing dyskinesia severity has also been associated with increased depression and higher health-care costs (Chapuis, Ouchchane, Metz, Gerbaud, & Durif, 2005). Hallucinations that are common in advanced PD stages with more drugs and higher drug dosages are associated with lower QoL, worse cognitive function, greater depression, and, with delusions, are associated with increased nursing home placement (Goetz & Stebbins, 1995; Holroyd, Currie, & Wooten, 2001). However, other studies did not find motor complications to be associated with lower levels of QoL (Schrag et al., 2000).

There are some further clinical factors that have been shown to be associated with poorer QoL in PD. These include sleep disorders/insomnia. Sleep disorders are frequent in PD patients. They include early and frequent awakening, cramps, pains, and nightmares. Sleep disorders have an impact on patients' QoL, and were, in one study, more predictive of distress than increased physical disability (Barone et al., 2009; Karlsen et al., 1999). A further factor contributing to poorer QoL in PD is fatique. Fatigue has been rated as among the most disabling symptoms of PD by a large percentage of patients. The prevalence of fatigue in PD ranged from 33 to 58% (Friedman & Friedman, 1993; Herlofson & Larsen, 2003). Autonomic symptoms such as urinary incontinence and constipation also have an influence on QoL. Urinary symptoms were most frequently reported (89.9%) at advanced disease stages. The high frequency of urinary symptoms may in part reflect the onset of a urinary disorder with increasing age (Barone et al., 2009). Further factors with an influence on QoL in PD patients are sweating (Swinn et al., 2003), and pain (Rahman et al., 2008). Treatment onset in PD has an impact on QoL. There was a significant deterioration in all eight domains of the PDQ-39 scale in PD patients who were left untreated at the first presentation. This pattern worsened if patients did not start treatment at the first review with further deterioration of QoL scores at the second review. This contrasts with untreated PD patients who were given specific anti-PD treatment at the first review. In these patients, the PDQ-39 scores remained stable and showed a trend toward improved QoL scores at the second follow-up, suggesting a beneficial effect of dopaminergic treatment on aspects of the PDQ-39 scale (Grosset et al., 2007). Another study identified the following management factors affecting QoL in PD: (a) Process of communicating the clinical diagnosis, (b) specialist clinicians' use of information and holistic therapies, (c) the ability of patients to gain the information on the disease, (d) patients' use of holistic therapies, (e) patients' emotional state (including depression), (f) patients' access to and use of a patient support group. It could be shown that depression (as assessed with the BDI), "satisfaction with the explanation of the condition at diagnosis," and "current feelings of optimism" had a statistically significant impact on QoL. In combination with disease severity and medication, these factors increased the ability to explain the variability of QoL in the PD population in this study to approximately 60% ("Factors Impacting on Quality of Life in Parkinson's Disease: Results from an International Survey," 2002).

Overall, the question if motor or nonmotor symptoms in PD have a higher or an equal impact on the patients' QoL is still open. Some studies found that physical mobility still is the most important single factor contributing to decline in QoL in PD, at least in a long-term perspective. More advanced disease severity and disability, predicted poorer outcome in the sections physical mobility and social isolation (Schrag et al., 2000). Other studies found nonmotor symptoms, especially depression and disability, as the major nonmotor determinants of QoL in PD (Gomez-Esteban et al., 2007). However, it seems evident that the use of a measure of motor function as the primary outcome measure in clinical trials is unlikely to determine the effect of one drug on the overall impact on QoL.

Predictors of QoL in PD

Longitudinal studies of QoL, particularly those following patients with PD prospectively over time, are few (Karlsen, Tandberg, Arsland, & Larsen, 2000; Marras, Lang, Krahn, Tomlinson, & Naglie, 2004; Reuther et al., 2007), and they are limited in their duration of follow-up. Only one of these studies is community based (Karlsen et al., 2000), hence, there is need for more information on predictors and changes of QoL derived from long-term investigations of unselected cohorts of patients with PD. So far, nearly all studies found that depression is as a strong predictor of QoL in PD. It has been shown that depressive symptoms as measured by the MADRS or BDI accounted for 41–54% of the variance of QoL scores (Schrag et al., 2000; Soh, Morris, & McGinley, 2011). Depression also was the strongest predictor of reduced QoL in patients with PD followed prospectively for 12 months (Reuther et al., 2007). A second important predictor is cognitive impairment (Karlsen et al., 1999; Schrag et al., 2000). Frequency and severity of nonmotor symptoms as a whole seem to be an important predictor of QoL in patients with PD as well (Martinez-Martin et al., 2011). It has been shown that measures of disease severity (e.g., as measured by the Hoehn and Yahr scale; Hoehn & Yahr, 1967) and disability (e.g., as measured by the Schwab and England scale; Gillingham, Donaldson, Schwab, & England, 1969) correlate with QoL scores, although there is some overlap in the content of QoL and disability scales. However, the motor part of the UPDRS (Fahn et al., 1987), although so far the primary outcome measure for most clinical trials with antiparkinsonian medication, does not contribute significantly to QoL in PD in one study (Rahman et al., 2008). Because postural instability, gait problems, and falls are core features of and thus define higher Hoehn and Yahr stages, although they are not similarly weighted in the UPDRS motor part, this observation may indicate that these symptoms are important predictors of poor QoL in PD. Indeed, axial symptoms and falls have been found to be associated with or predict lower levels of QoL in PD patients (Reuther et al., 2007; Schrag et al., 2000). Tremor and rigidity scores did not correlate with QoL scores, whereas gait problems and limb akinesia have been shown to be associated with worse QoL. Tremor dominant disease has usually been found to have a better prognosis than the akinetic rigid type. Findings of a better QoL in tremor-dominant PD further support this differentiation. The differences in study results regarding predictors of QoL may not only depend on the study population but also on the used QoL outcome scale. Hence, in one study with the PDQ-39 as the outcome QoL scale the factors age of PD onset, Hoehn and Yahr staging, Schwab and England disability ratings, and duration of illness cumulatively accounted for 42,9% of the variance in PDQ39-SI scores (Rahman et al., 2008), whereas another study using the NHP scale showed the highest predictive value for depression measured by MADRS, sleep disorders, and a low degree of independence (measured by the Schwab and England scale) (Karlsen et al., 1999). One study examined the relative importance of motor and nonmotor symptoms determining QoL in PD found that motor symptoms explained only 18.9% of the variance of total SF-36 score, whereas 61.7% of the variance of SF-36 score could be explained when nonmotor variables such as depression, sleep disorders, and fatigue were also included in the model (Qin et al., 2009).

In summary, the available studies found that the main factors to be depression, disability, disease severity (particularly related to axial features), and cognitive impairment.

Clinical Studies in Parkinson's Disease Using QoL as an Outcome Parameter

Studies of the last two decades found nonmotor symptoms important and maybe as the major determinant of QoL in PD. The sole use of a measure of motor function as the primary outcome measure in clinical trials is unlikely to determine the effect of one drug on all aspects of the disease or the overall impact on QoL. In this context, QoL becomes increasingly important as a crucial variable for clinical trials.

For levodopa (in combination with a dopa-decarboxylase inhibitor), the gold standard of therapy for PD, a short-term improvement of QoL could be demonstrated with the greatest improvement in physical-function domains. The gradual decline of the initial QoL improvements under therapy may reflect QoL impairment due to progressive increase in disease severity or may relate to the development of motor complications associated with long-term levodopa therapy (Noyes, Dick, & Holloway, 2006). For entacapone, an inhibitor of the catechol-O-methyl transferase (COMT) a review revealed 12 studies (9 open-label, 3 double-blind) of entacapone with QoL (generic or PD specific QoL measures) as an outcome measure (3 studies with QoL as primary endpoint; Gallagher & Schrag, 2008). Two double-blind, placebo-controlled trials showed no significant difference in the QoL scales on primary analysis, but improvements in QoL areas for patients treated with entacapone in the post-hoc analyses (Fenelon et al., 2003; Reichmann et al., 2005). A third double-blind, placebo-controlled trial of patients without motor fluctuations demonstrated a significant improvement for various areas of QoL (Olanow et al., 2004). For tolcapone, another COMT-inhibitor, four double-blind, placebo-controlled studies comparing adjunctive tolcapone to standard levodopa and placebo in advanced disease with motor fluctuations have used generic QoL measures as as secondary endpoint. Some of these studies showed an improvement in the SIP summary scores compared to placebo (M. D. Welsh, Dorflinger, Chernik, & Waters, 2000), whereas others showed no significant change (Adler et al., 1998). For rasagiline, a new generation monoamine oxidase inhibitor (MAO-B), two double-blind, placebo-controlled trials used the PDQUALIF as a secondary end point. One study showed a significant greater improvement versus placebo in total PDQUALIF score (Biglan et al., 2006), whereas the other study demonstrated no significant difference but only a trend for a greater improvement in the total score and significant improvement in some of the PDQUALIF subscores in the rasagiline arm ("A Randomized Placebo-Controlled Trial of Rasagiline in Levodopa-Treated Patients with Parkinson Disease and Motor Fluctuations: The PRESTO study," 2005). For continuous intraduodenal infusion of levodopa/carbidopa gel there are only data of three small open-label studies with an index of QoL as an outcome measure available. These revealed significant improvements in PDQ-39 total score and some of the subscores (Antonini et al., 2008). Within the group of dopamine receptor agonists there are studies with QoL as an endpoint available for rotigotine and pramipexole. For rotigotine two double-blind, placebo-controlled trials with QoL as a secondary outcome measure demonstrated significant improvement of QoL as measured with the EQ-5D and PDQ-39 compared with placebo (Jankovic, Watts, Martin, & Boroojerdi, 2007; Poewe et al., 2007). For pramipexole three double-blind studies with a QoL index as an outcome measure have been conducted. These showed that pramipexole had comparable efficacy to levodopa on QoL (Holloway et al., 2004; "Long-Term Effect of Initiating Pramipexole vs Levodopa in Early Parkinson Disease," 2009), that pramipexole as add-on therapy to levodopa showed significant greater improvement in PDQ-39 total score (Poewe et al., 2007) and subscores compared to placebo and a trend to greater improvement on PDQUALIF for pramipexole versus placebo ("Pramipexole in Levodopa-Treated Parkinson Disease Patients of African, Asian, and Hispanic Heritage," 2007). A large review of literature until 2009 on the efficacy of dopamine receptor agonists in improving QoL in PD patients found level I evidence demonstrating that pergolide, cabergoline, pramipexole, 24-hour extended-release ropinerole, and rotigotine is efficacious in improving QoL mostly in PD patients in advanced disease stages with wearing-off fluctuations (Martinez-Martin & Kurtis, 2009). One review is summarizing the effect of different interventions on QoL (Martinez-Martin & Deuschl, 2007).

DBS Trials for Parkinson's Disease Using QoL Measures as Outcome Parameter

Surgical therapy, such as ablative/lesioning procedures and deep brain stimulation (DBS), is an option for patients with an insufficient therapeutical effect under anti-Parkinsonian medication. Especially DBS has not only been demonstrated to improve the motor symptoms of PD but also QoL (Diamond & Jankovic, 2005). Evidence class 1 studies (evidence class 1 = randomized controlled trials) showed improvements of QoL for different surgical procedures. One study randomized to unilateral pallidotomy or bilateral STN-DBS and used the PDQL as a secondary outcome parameter. Both groups showed similar improvements in mean PDQL total scores at 3 months with a trend toward significance for a better improvement in the STN-DBS group (Esselink et al., 2004). Another study randomized 156 patients with advanced PD comparing STN-DBS with best medical treatment and defined QoL as the primary endpoint for the first time. Quality of life as measured by the PDQ-39 improved by 25% in the STN-DBS group and by 22% in the physical summary score of the SF-36, whereas there was practically no change in the medication group (Deuschl et al., 2006). Other studies showed an improvement of 58% using the SIP at 6 months in the bilateral STN-DBS group (Spottke et al., 2002); an improvement of 43% in total PDQL score in the bilateral STN-DBS group at 12 months (Lagrange et al., 2002); an improvement of 22.5% in the SF-36 global score that solely depended on significant improvements in the parts physical function and physical role (Drapier et al., 2005); significant improvements in NHP subscores assessing sleep, energy, emotional reaction, and social isolation (Erola et al., 2005); improvements of up to 62% using the PDQ-39 in different studies (Erola et al., 2005; Troster et al., 2003). There is evidence that improvement of QoL in PD following STN-DBS does not only depend on improvement of motor function but also correlate with improvements of levodopa induced motor complications and improvements in depression (Martinez-Martin et al., 2002; Troster et al., 2003). Other studies evaluated QoL in PD patients following different surgical procedures (uni- or bilateral pallidotomy, nucleus subthalamicus lesions, unilateral GPi-DBS, unilateral Vim-DBS, and STN-DBS) found significant improvements in the SIP physical score (Straits-Troster et al., 2000), for all dimensions of the SF-36 except role mental and mental health (Gray et al., 2002) and for parts of the PDQ-39 (Gray et al., 2002; Woods et al., 2001).

QUALITY OF LIFE IN ATYPICAL PARKINSONIAN DISORDERS

The term atypical parkinsonian disorders (APD) includes multiple system atrophy (MSA), dementia with Lewy bodies (DLB), progressive supranuclear palsy (PSP), and corticobasal degeneration (CBD). The clinical hallmarks of the APDs are a levodopa-unresponsive Parkinsonism and associated atypical features in the areas motor, autonomic, oculomotor, and cognitive / neurobehavioral. There is a heterogenous clinicopathological presentation of APDs leading to a classification according to protein aggregation type: (a) synucleinopathies (Parkinson's disease dementia (PDD), DLB, MSA), and (b) tauopathies (PSP, CBD) (Wenning, Litvan, & Tolosa, 2011). Multiple system atrophy (MSA) is a sporadic, chronic neurodegenerative disorder leading to progressive disability and decreased life expectancy. It is clinically characterized by combinations of Parkinsonian, autonomic, cerebellar, and pyramidal signs and thereby subdivided into the Parkinsonian variant (MSA-P) and the cerebellar variant (MSA-C) (Wenning, Geser, Stampfer-Kountchev, & Tison, 2003). Quality of life instruments were developed for idiopathic Parkinson's disease have been used in patients with MSA (Schrag, Geser, et al., 2006). These instruments do not address specific features important to patients with MSA such as severe autonomic dysfunction or bulbar involvement and, therefore, may lead to an underestimation of health problems in MSA. However, there is a disease-specific QoL questionnaire for MSA patients, the MSA health-related QoL scale (MSA-QoL). This is a scale with 3 subscales (14 motor items, 12 nonmotor items, 14 items for emotional/social functioning). The psychometric properties of the scale showed a good reliability, face and construct validity (Schrag et al., 2007). QoL is significantly impaired in MSA patients as measured with the SF-36 and EQ-5D and deteriorates with disease progression. QoL scores correlate with motor impairment as measured with the Unified MSA Rating Scale (UMSARS), with depression as measured by the Beck Depression Inventory (BDI) and with severity of autonomic dysfunction as measured with the Composite Autonomic Symptom Scale (COMPASS). Depression is a frequent accompanying symptom with up to 50% of the MSA patients having moderate to severe depression as measured with the BDI. However, although depression affects more than 40% of MSA patients, it seems not to be the main contributor to poor QoL as it is in PD patients, and other neuropsychiatric features appear uncommon (Kollensperger et al., 2010; Schrag, Geser, et al., 2006). A more important aspect determining QoL in MSA patients is the degree of dysautonomia. Patients with more symptoms of dysautonomia show an impaired QoL as measured with the SF-36 (Kollensperger et al., 2007), and autonomic dysfunction accounted for 22% of the variance in life satisfaction in one study (Benrud-Larson, Sandroni, Schrag, & Low, 2005). Activities of daily living as measured by the UMSARS and COMPASS scales were moderate to strong predictors for the SF-36 physical summary score and BDI and UMSARS motor scores were predictors for the SF-36 mental summary score (Schrag, Geser, et al., 2006).

The PSP is a common, sporadic atypical neurodegenerative Parkinsonian disorder with a mean onset in the mid-60s. Key features are early postural instability, vertical supranuclear gaze palsy, severe axial levodopa-unresponsive, akinetic-rigid syndrome, early pseudobulbar dysarthria and dysphagia, and early severe frontal dysfunction (Williams & Lees, 2009). So far, there is only one disease-specific QoL scale for PSP. The Progressive Supranuclear Palsy Quality of Life scale (PSP-QoL) has a physical subscale with 22 items and a mental subscale with 23 items. Psychometric properties showed a high reliability and a good validity (Schrag, Selai, et al., 2006). In comparison with PD patients, MSA and PSP patients report a worse health status. There are some qualitative differences in main areas of QoL impairment between the patient groups with more difficulties with self-care and more depressive symptoms in PSP patients and, greater pain / discomfort in MSA patients. The most important factors associated with health status in patients with atypical Parkinson syndromes were depressive symptoms followed by disease severity and anxiety in one study (Schrag et al., 2010).

Dementia with Lewy bodies (DLB) is a neurodegenerative dementia in elderly patients with a considerable overlap with Parkinson's disease dementia (PDD), a more common entity characterized by delayed-onset cognitive decline emerging at least 1 year after motor onset (McKeith et al., 2005). Corticobasal degeneration (CBD) is the least common neurodegenerative atypical parkinsonian disorder. CBD patients usually present with various clinical phenotypes (corticobasal syndrome, primary progressive nonfluent aphasia, and the behavioral variant of frontotemporal dementia) usually in the sixth or seventh decade. Symptoms of the corticobasal syndrome are a unilateral ideomotor or limb kinetic apraxia, dystonia, stimulus-sensitive myoclonus, parkinsonism unresponsive to dopaminergic therapy, and/or other lateralized cortical features (Ling et al., 2010). So far, there is only one clinical trial measuring the treatment effect of memantine with QoL as an outcome measure in DLB patients (V. Larsson et al., 2011), and there are no studies on QoL in CBD available.

QUALITY OF LIFE IN HUNTINGTON'S DISEASE

Huntington disease (HD) is a rare neurodegenerative disorder of the central nervous system with a variable onset. It is characterized by choreatic movements, behavioral and psychiatric disturbances and dementia. HD is autosomal dominant inherited, fully penetrant, and caused by an excess CAG repeat (36 repeats ore more) on the short arm of chromosome 4p16.3 in the Huntington gene. The clinical course is divided in the prodromal phase, the transition phase, and the clinical stage (Shoulson & Fahn, 1979). By progression of the disease, the patients experience a markedly decrease in independence and increase in the need for care (Roos, 2010). Huntington's disease has a profound impact on patients' physical and psychosocial well-being (Helder, Kaptein, van Kempen, van Houwelingen, & Roos, 2001). Patients within the different stages of the disease show differences of the areas of QoL, which are impaired. Studies examining reactions of asymptomatic gene carriers when informed about their positive test result suggest few long-term adverse consequences (Tibben, 2007), anxiety and depression increase temporarily for gene carriers, pessimism about the future and more suicidal ideation may occur (M. U. Larsson, Luszcz, Bui, & Wahlin, 2006). Patients in the prodromal phase report mostly concerns about occupational functioning and difficulties within the social and emotional area. Symptomatic HD patients report the main difficulties in the physical/functional area and cognition. In the late-stage HD physical impairment predominates whereas cognitive concerns are less important probably due to the increasing degree of cognitive impairment (Ho & Hocaoglu, 2011).

QoL Tools in Huntington's Disease

So far, there are 2 disease-specific QoL scales for HD patients. The Huntington's disease health-related Quality of Life questionnaire (HDQoL) is a 40-item questionnaire that includes 3 primary scales (physical/cognitive, primary emotions/self, primary services), and 6 specific scales (cognitive, hopes/worries, services, physical/functional, mood state, self/vitality), which can be added to get a summary score. The HDQoL showed good test-retest reliability, construct validity, and scale acceptability (Hocaoglu, Gaffan, & Ho, 2012).

The Huntington Quality of life instrument (H-QoL-I that) consists of 11 items, which are divided into three dimensions: motor functioning (four items), psychology (four items) and socializing (three items). The H-QoL-I showed an acceptable reliability and validity in patients with HD (Clay et al., 2012).

Factors Impacting QoL in Huntington's Disease

Factors associated with impaired QoL are total motor score, cognitive decline as measured with the Mini-Mental State test, and the duration of the disease (Helder et al., 2001). Another study found a significant association of impaired QoL with higher levels of depressive mood and lower functional capacity, whereas motor symptoms and cognitive function influenced QoL to a lesser extent (Ho, Gilbert, Mason, Goodman, & Barker, 2009). Behavioral, psychiatric, and cognitive symptoms are frequent and often precede motor symptoms in HD. Affective symptoms are most common, followed by apathy and irritability. Further neuropsychiatric / behavioral symptoms include agitation, disinhibition, irritability, anxiety, psychotic symptoms, and aberrant motor behavior. The neuropsychiatric symptoms are hardly associated with cognitive or motor measures indicating that behavioral aspects of basal ganglia diseases are often independent of cognitive and motor symptoms (Paulsen, Ready, Hamilton, Mega, & Cummings, 2001). Although the positive motor features, particularly chorea and dystonia, are the most obvious features of HD, they are not the best predictors for the level of disability. Rather, disability correlates better with negative motor features such as poverty of movement, including bradykinesia, apraxia, and cognitive impairment (Mahant, McCusker, Byth, & Graham, 2003). So, rating HD primarily on the severity of chorea or dystonia will not necessarily relate to the level of function. The severity of functional impairment in patients with HD is also related to the behavioral abnormalities that occur in the disease. Apathy is a common and probably the most significant behavioral abnormality. One study found that symptoms of apathy/executive dysfunction are strongly associated with decline in activities of daily living even after controlling for the effects of motor and cognitive deficits. So behavioral dysfunction not only contributes to functional decline in HD patients but may also impair the patients' ability to utilize remaining motor or cognitive skills (Hamilton et al., 2003). Furthermore, behavioral and cognitive symptoms change the patient's perspective and perception of QoL so that the interpretation of QoL scales/questionnaires may be limited. For patients with mental disorders, it could be shown that factors such as affective state, reality distortion, and poor cognition lead to a distortion of responses within the QoL areas of social roles and material and social living conditions. The patients' judgments differ from their spouses'/caregivers' mainly for social and occupational aspects of QoL (Katschnig, 2006). For patients with dementia cognitive limitations and lack of insight can be barriers to self-reporting QoL since communication, attention, memory, and judgment are necessary skills to answer survey questions. There is evidence that mild to moderately cognitively impaired individuals can still articulate feelings, concerns, and wishes, and thereby provide evaluations of their QoL For severe dementia, common QoL tools are not sufficient. Proxy-interviews of QoL in demented patients consistently showed lower QoL rates in contrast to the patients' rating so that proxies are only a poor substitute for obtaining the patient's perspective of his / her health status (Logsdon, Gibbons, McCurry, & Teri, 2002).

The patients' perceived QoL is also influenced by the illness perception of spouses and caregivers. Studies revealed that the spouses' role problems, their unsupportive behavior, and the marital relationship itself are factors influencing patients' QoL (Manne, Pape, Taylor, & Dougherty, 1999). In HD, similar factors influence both patient and caregiver QoL; these are functional capacity and cognitive scores (Ready, Mathews, Leserman, & Paulsen, 2008). However, studies examining the effect of partners' perceptions in HD revealed only an influence for the area of physical functioning, but not for other areas of QoL or total QoL perception (Kaptein et al., 2007).

Predictors of QoL in Huntington's Disease

Predictors of physical aspects of QoL in HD are motor score, cognitive decline, and the duration of the disease. These factors predicted 42% of the variance of the physical dimension in contrast to only 11% of the psychosocial dimension of the SIP. Other studies found that depression is a strong predictor of QoL in HD, followed by motor impairment, independent functioning, and cognitive impairment (Helder et al., 2001). However, one study found no association of an overall index of neuropsychiatric symptoms with patient or caregiver QoL (Ready et al., 2008).

Studies on the effect of genetic testing in HD have shown that perceived low social support, the expectation of an unfavorable genetic test result before the testing procedure, and being childless are predictors for low mental health in gene carriers (Tibben, 2007).

Clinical Studies in Huntington's Disease Using QoL as an Outcome Parameter

In HD, current drug therapy has no effect on the progression of the disability but is a therapy of specific symptoms such as hyperkinesias and psychiatric symptoms. Clinical trials in HD have usually defined motor function (mostly chorea) as their primary outcome measure and not QoL measures as end points. However "classical" HD scales such as the Unified Huntington's Disease Rating Scale (UHDRS) (Huntington Disease Group, 1996) comprise important areas of QoL. Components of the UHDRS are motor, cognitive, and behavioral assessment, independence scale, functional assessment, and the total functional capacity. The total functional capacity subscale includes the areas of occupation, financial affairs, domestic responsibilities, activities of daily living, and independent living. The independence scale is rated from 0 to 100 with higher scores on the function scales indication better functioning.

Overall, there is poor evidence in the management of HD today, not only for the treatment of motor symptoms such as chorea but also for other neurologic symptoms, psychiatric disturbances, and dementia, mainly due to a lack of randomized controlled trials. Anti-choreatic agents include conventional dopamine-blocking antipsychotics, tetrabenazine, atypical antipsychotic drugs, amantadine, and riluzole. For the treatment of psychiatric and behavioral symptoms, antidepressants and conventional and atypical antipsychotic drugs are used. For dementia, unsaturated fatty acids, riluzole, and minocycline have shown to provide mild cognitive benefits in open-label trials. Possible neuroprotective agents include coenzyme Q10, minocycline and unsaturated fatty acids (Bonelli & Hofmann, 2007).

QUALITY OF LIFE IN DYSTONIA

Dystonia is a heterogeneous group of hyperkinetic movement disorders characterized by involuntary sustained muscle contractions that lead to abnormal postures and repetitive movements (S. Fahn, Marsden, C.D., Calne, D.B., 1987). Classification of dystonia is based on etiology (idiopathic: familial and sporadic; secondary: heredodegenerative and environmental) and bodily distribution (focal, segmental, and generalized). Dystonia is a disabling disorder that can affect many aspects of patients' daily living such as walking, sitting, and eating. Due to the awkward postures dystonia is also a disfiguring disorder that can lead to embarrassment, social avoidance, and isolation. Health related QoL is significantly worse for different forms of dystonia compared to the general population (Page, Butler, & Jahanshahi, 2007). Even though dystonia is typically considered a movement disorder characterized by motor symptoms, there is now emerging evidence for the presence and importance of nonmotor symptoms in primary and other genetic forms of dystonia, although it is unclear if these symptoms are secondary to motor manifestations and subsequent psychosocial impairment or if they are a primary feature of the disease. Nonmotor symptoms include affective and other psychiatric disorders, cognition, sleep and energy, pain, autonomic symptoms, abnormalities in sensory and perceptual functions as well as low self-esteem, embarrassment, and limited social interaction (Kuyper, Parra, Aerts, Okun, & Kluger, 2011; Stamelou, Edwards, Hallett, & Bhatia, 2011). It has been shown that physical and emotional factors are associated with a lower perceived QoL. The main impairment of QoL in dystonia, however, lies in the domains of social and physical functioning, pain, anxiety, and depression (Page et al., 2007).

QoL Tools for Dystonia

The craniocervical dystonia questionnaire (CDQ-24) is a 24-item instrument for patients with CD and BSP and is based on five subscales: stigma, emotional well-being, pain, activities of daily living, and social/family life. Reliability was satisfactory for all subscales. The CDQ-24 subscales showed moderate to high correlations with those SF-36 subscales measuring similar aspects and were sensitive to change in de novo patients over a defined period of time (Muller et al., 2004).

The Cervical Dystonia Impact Profile (CDIP-58) is a patient-based 58-item rating scale measuring the health impact of CD in 8 areas (head and neck symptoms, pain and discomfort, upper-limb activities, walking, sleep, annoyance, mood, and psychosocial functioning). It has shown good reliability and validity (Cano et al., 2004).

The Oromandibular Dystonia Questionnaire (OMDQ-25) is a 25-item questionnaire with good reliability and validity and sensitive to change after Botulinum Toxin A treatment (Merz, Deakin, & Hawthorne, 2010).

Factors Impacting QoL in Dystonia

Factors influencing the magnitude of impact on QoL in dystonic patients are the extent of dystonia, disability, deformity, pain, age, employment status, living situation, and lifestyle changes of the patients. Most of the studies have been evaluating patients with focal dystonia with CD as the most common form. Health-related QoL was reduced in patients with focal dystonia compared with that in controls (Ben-Shlomo, Camfield, & Warner, 2002; Muller et al., 2002). The QoL impairment as measured by the SF-36 was thereby comparable to patients with other severe neurologic disorders such as Parkinson's disease, multiple sclerosis or stroke (Pekmezovic et al., 2009). Patients with focal dystonia do not only show impaired QoL for aspects of physical function but also strikingly for aspects of mental health (Muller et al., 2002). This effect on mental well-being may reflect a stigmatizing effect of living with such a visible and disfiguring disorder. There are differences for QoL between the different types of focal dystonia. Patients with CD seem to be more severely impaired by pain and depression than patients with BSP and writer's cramp (Pekmezovic et al., 2009). For BSP, there was a gender difference with women having a worse QoL and more depressive symptoms than males, whereas patients with CD showed no gender differences but pain as the main determinant for depression and impaired QoL in one study (Muller et al., 2002). Another study showed a stronger impairment of physical and social functioning and a lower perception of general health in patients with BSP in contrast to CD. Overall the patients with BSP seemed to experience a higher degree of disability related to an impaired QoL (Hilker, Schischniaschvili, Ghaemi, Jacobs, & Rudolf, 2001). Different types of dystonia (focal, segmental, and generalized) showed an impairment of HRQL for all age groups irrespective of gender. Patients with generalized dystonia had a poorer QoL than those with focal dystonia particularly in the domains of physical and social functioning. Irrespective of type of dystonia, poorer QoL was also found in separated/divorced and younger patients (Page et al., 2007). A higher activity level, more social engagement, and more work-related responsibilities in contrast to older people may cause the greater interference of dystonic symptoms with everyday life in younger patients.

Motor symptoms in dystonia obviously influence QoL since they result in awkward positions, disfigurement and pain. The postural abnormalities in combination with excessive muscle contractions are the main factor for psychosocial adjustment for all forms of dystonia. The physical appearance/attractiveness influences interpersonal interaction and social perception so that disfigurement in dystonia leads to a worse self-perception and a poorer QoL (Page et al., 2007).

Nonmotor symptoms are common in dystonia and are increasingly considered as important factors regarding patient's perception of health status and QoL. The most frequent nonmotor symptoms are depression and anxiety with a prevalence of 25–50% over the course of a lifetime (Fabbrini et al., 2010). There are different prevalence rates of depression for different types of dystonia, for example, 47% depression as measured by the BDI in patients with CD in contrast to 37% in patients with BSP (Muller et al., 2002). Depression and anxiety have a profound impact on both physical and mental aspects of the QoL, and thus are the most important determinants of worse QoL (Ben-Shlomo et al., 2002). For patients with CD, it has been shown that body concept and disfigurement are the main factors determining the psychosocial adjustment of the patients and that self-rated disfigurement was the most important predictor of depression in this patient group (Page et al., 2007). Further associated psychiatric disorders are obsessive-compulsive disorders with a frequency up to nearly 20% in patients with idiopathic focal dystonia (Voon et al., 2010) and social phobia (Gundel et al., 2003). Alcohol abuse and dependence have mainly been reported for patients with the DYT11 mutation. Given the typical sensitivity of myoclonus to alcohol in this patient group, the alcohol dependence may be due to the alcohol's symptomatic effects rather than a real associated comorbidity (Saunders-Pullman et al., 2002). Results of the so far few studies addressing sleep in patients with dystonia suggest an impairment of either sleep structure or quality, whereas they showed mixed evidence if dystonia leads to sleepiness. Depressive symptoms may be a confounding factor for impaired sleep quality in dystonia (Avanzino et al., 2010). One study found the strongest correlation for tired subscore of the Visual Analogue Mood Scale with overall QoL (Soeder et al., 2009). Pain is one of the most common and disabling complaints in many patients with dystonia. For patients with CD, prevalence rates for pain up to 75% are described (Chan, Brin, & Fahn, 1991). Reasons for this high frequency and impact of pain in dystonic patients may be alterations in the threshold for experiencing pain, in pain processing, or in the somatosensory system (Abbruzzese & Berardelli, 2003; Lobbezoo, Tanguay, Thon, & Lavigne, 1996). Depression again, may be a confounding factor for symptoms of pain in patients with dystonia. For patients with CD, it has been shown that neck pain had a significant impact on all SF-36 domains and represented the main determinant of depression in this patient group (Muller et al., 2002). Factors positively influencing QoL in this patient group are level of physical activity and satisfaction with treatment (Zetterberg, Aquilonius, & Lindmark, 2009).

Predictors of QoL in Dystonia

Similar to other movement disorders, depression, dysfunctional mood, and anxiety are predictors of QoL in patients with dystonia. Depression has also been one of the major predictors of QoL in mixed samples of patients with focal, segmental, hemi-, and generalized dystonia so that this factor is independent of the type of dystonia (Page et al., 2007; Pekmezovic et al., 2009). Other predictors for QoL of patients with dystonia include milestones of the disease such as disease severity, longer disease duration, extent of dystonia, higher age, pain, and functional disability, social factors such as living alone, poor financial situation, being unemployed or retired status but also psychological factors such as body concept, sense of disfigurement, social participation, perceptions of stigma, acceptance of illness and intrinsic personality features such as self-esteem and self-deprecation. These intrinsic personality features are also important factors for QoL since they seem to modify the patients' ability to cope with the disease. Higher age and longer disease duration are associated with better coping with the disease, which may be due to the development of successful coping strategies (Ben-Shlomo et al., 2002; Muller et al., 2002). So there is an important effect of psychological variables in dystonia that can mediate or modify the effect of disease severity on QoL. This has already been shown for QoL in patient groups with other neurological diseases (Schrag et al., 2000; Suurmeijer, Reuvekamp, & Aldenkamp, 2001).

Clinical Trials in Dystonia Using QoL as an Outcome Parameter

In most cases of dystonia, treatment is merely symptomatic, designed to improve posture and function and to relieve associated pain. Treatment options in focal dystonia have substantially improved especially after the introduction of botulinum toxin type A (BtxA) as a neuromuscular paralytic agent. Placebo controlled studies showed an efficient reduction of the increased muscle tone in dystonia after BtxA treatment and a long-term clinical efficacy of the injections, so that this therapy is now considered as the first line treatment in cranial and cervical dystonia (Albanese et al., 2011; Jankovic & Brin, 1991). The magnitude of the effect of BTX on health-related quality of life is unclear and studies differ on this point, which may be due to different types of dystonia and short follow-up in some of the studies. Studies showed an improvement of QoL by botulinum toxin treatment and a reduced intensity of depressive symptoms (Hilker et al., 2001). Botulinum toxin B (BtxB) is also effective and safe for treating focal dystonia. However data for long-term efficacy and safety as well as relative indications for BtxA, BtxB, and other treatments such as deep brain stimulation are still insufficient (Costa, Borges, et al., 2009; Costa, Espírito-Santo, et al.,2009b).

Patients with focal dystonia improve significantly with BTX treatment when symptoms are measured with dystonia-specific scoring instruments (Costa, Espírito-Santo, et al., 2009a). Quality of life improved for several QoL dimensions under BtxA therapy and QoL improvement persists after long-term Btx therapy. Pain as an important aspect especially in CD patients (Chan et al., 1991) showed a significant amelioration following BtxA injections, but also aspects of psychological well-being such as mental health, social functioning, and vitality improved under BtxA therapy in patients with focal dystonia (Hilker et al., 2001; Snaith & Wade, 2011). Treatment of the motor symptoms of dystonia may or may not lead to improvement in depression and health-related QOL (Muller et al., 2002), but some studies showed that successful treatment of CD with BtxA injections was also accompanied with improvement in depression and disability, whereas negative body concept and low self-esteem as aspects of psychological function did not change significantly with symptomatic improvement of dystonia maybe because of the only temporary effect of BtxA (Jahanshahi & Marsden, 1992). An improvement of QoL following Btx treatment could also be demonstrated for patients with jaw-opening oromandibular dystonia and laryngeal focal dystonia/spasmodic dysphonia (Charous, Comella, & Fan, 2011; Hogikyan, Wodchis, Spak, & Kileny, 2001). The magnitude of benefit is largely independent of the time course of therapy (Bhattacharyya & Tarsy, 2001). On the contrary, it has been shown that improvement of clinical symptoms in focal dystonia following BtxA therapy is often not accompanied by significant improvements for QoL (Hilker et al., 2001). This mismatch may indicate that measures of functional health status such as QoL measures reflect the therapeutic efficacy of BtxA treatment better than clinical outcome scores.

Information on the clinical effectiveness and impact on QoL of other drugs used for dystonia treatment is quite rare. Besides Btx, Trihexyphenidyl, an anticholinergic drug, is the most commonly used drug, for the treatment of focal dystonia. Anticholinergic therapy shows moderate to marked effects in focal dystonia (Lang, 1986). So far, there is only one trial comparing this drug to BtxA in patients with CD. Trihexyphenidyl was worse tolerated and significantly less effective compared to BTX in improving symptoms on clinical scales for dystonia (Tsui, TWSTRS) (Costa et al., 2005). Reviews of literature found no systematic review or randomized clinical trials evaluating other drugs for the treatment of focal dystonia, such as antipsychotics, dopamine (ant-)agonists or serotonin (ant-)agonists (Snaith & Wade, 2011).

For generalized dystonia, drug therapy in general is not very effective. Anticholinergics, especially in high dosage are the only substance class for which controlled studies are available showing that trihexyphenidyl is effective for generalized dystonia (Burke, Fahn, & Marsden, 1986). Other substances, which may or may not be effective, include levodopa, benzodiazepines, pimozid, or tetrabenzin. Baclofen can be administered orally or intrathecally. Orally administered baclofen has been shown to be effective in children and adolescents with idiopathic dystonia. The response to baclofen of adults with focal dystonia has been less dramatic. Patients who responded to baclofen did have a significantly shorter duration of symptoms before therapy (Greene, 1992). Intrathecal administration of baclofen is now considered a safe and effective treatment for severe dystonia of different etiologies in some studies. Significant benefit has not only been demonstrated for motor symptoms in dystonia, but is also reflected in improvement of QoL, activities of daily living, and level of function (Walker et al., 2000). Botulinum toxin injections may be a useful therapy for selected muscle groups in generalized dystonia (Jankovic, 2004).

DBS Trials for Dystonia Using QoL as an Outcome Parameter

The treatment of patients with generalized dystonia, previously restricted to only a few oral medications with often-intolerable side effects, has been radically changed and improved with the therapeutic option of DBS of the globus pallidus internus (GPi). Deep brain stimulation should be considered as a treatment option for patients with severe, medically refractory dystonia (Krauss, 2010). There are differences for the degree of possible improvement by DBS dependent on type (primary / secondary) and topography (cranial / axial / limb) of dystonia (Lubarr & Bressman, 2011). Treatment with GPi-DBS has been effective in patients with primary generalized dystonia (Kupsch et al., 2006), segmental dystonia (Kupsch et al., 2006), cervical dystonia (Skogseid et al., 2012), blepharospasm-oromandibular cranial dystonia (Reese et al., 2011), myoclonus dystonia (Trottenberg et al., 2001), and tardive dystonia (Trottenberg et al., 2005). Besides efficacy for motor symptoms, QoL also improves by DBS in dystonia. One large randomized, sham-stimulation controlled trial on GPi-DBS in primary segmental or generalized dystonia (Kupsch et al., 2006) with QoL as an outcome endpoint found significant improvements of QoL in the GPi-DBS group for all dimensions of the SF-36 as well as for depression scores as measured by the BDI (Mueller et al., 2008). Another large trial showed improvements only for two of the physical SF-36 domains (general health, physical function) (Vidailhet et al., 2005). One smaller study found an improvement of QoL of 37% as measured with a modified version of the PDQ-39 in patients with primary and tardive dystonia (Halbig et al., 2005). For focal dystonia, improvements in clinical scores, in disability and pain scores, as well as for physical aspects of the SF-36 and depression scores have been demonstrated in patients with CD (Skogseid et al., 2012), and Meige-Syndrome (Reese et al., 2011). Quality of life parameters, mainly physical aspects, were also improved in patients with tardive dystonia following GPi-DBS (Gruber et al., 2009).

QUALITY OF LIFE IN ESSENTIAL TREMOR

Essential tremor (ET) is the most common pathological tremor in humans. The defining feature in patients with ET is a 4–12 Hz kinetic tremor of the hands and arms, but tremor of the head, voice or other parts of the body often occurs. Overall, the tremor phenomenology is heterogeneous. Not only kinetic and postural tremor, but also intention tremor, and tremor at rest may occur. The etiologies of ET are still unclear and are likely to be diverse and many, including genetic and environmental factors (Elble & Deuschl, 2009; Lorenz & Deuschl, 2007). For a long time, ET has been considered a pure tremor disorder and has often been termed a benign condition. The clinical dimensions of ET must be expanded to include non-motor manifestations of the disease (Tan et al., 2005). Furthermore a high frequency of distinct physical and psychological handicaps in ET patients has been uncovered (Lorenz, Schwieger, Moises, & Deuschl, 2006). In ET, the inability to eat or drink due to tremor may increase stress and embarrassment leading to social isolation, which leads to worsening QoL (Jankovic, 2002). So, clinical experience suggests that patients do not only suffer from tremor symptoms but that the impact of tremor on the patient's life is rather defined by social handicap, disability, and impaired QoL. So far, there are only few data available on QoL (Lorenz et al., 2006; Troster, Pahwa, Fields, Tanner, & Lyons, 2005) and specific aspects of psychosocial functioning and mediating factors in ET patients that may influence the perception of and coping with the disease (Lorenz, Poremba, Papengut, Schreiber, & Deuschl, 2011).

QoL Tools in ET

So far, there is only one disease-specific QoL instrument available for ET. The Quality of life in Essential Tremor (QUEST) scale is 30-item ET-specific QoL scale including five subscales (physical, psychosocial, communication, hobbies/leisure, and work/finance). The psychometric properties are good to satisfactory (Martinez-Martin et al., 2010; Troster et al., 2005).

Factors Impacting QoL in ET

Essential tremor leads to decreased QoL and has a profound negative impact on patients' lives. Different dimensions of QoL are impaired in ET patients; however studies showed that the impairment is more due to mental rather than physical domains in this disorder commonly classified as a pure movement disorder. In comparison to other movement disorders such as PD and dystonia, ET patients showed less impairment in physical domains but similar decreased QoL for the mental domains (Lorenz et al., 2006). Studies have demonstrated that a relevant psychosocial impairment in professional and everyday life, disabilities in daily activities with a resulting avoidance of these activities, and a subjectively felt need for tremor concealment are very frequent. Patients matched for tremor severity showed significant differences, particularly for psychological aspects. These included higher scores for clinically relevant psychological symptoms as measured by the Brief Symptom Inventory indicating a higher level and intensity of psychiatric symptoms, significant differences for distinct personality traits, a higher frequency of depressive episodes, and a more pronounced impairment in different aspects of professional and everyday life (Lorenz et al., 2011). Age and gender are general factors that may influence QoL and perceived health status in ET. It has been demonstrated that age, independent of tremor severity, is associated with poorer functional outcomes (Louis et al., 2001). Essential tremor is defined by its' motor symptoms, namely the postural and kinetic tremor of the hands and arms but also other body parts (Deuschl, Bain, & Brin, 1998). However, it has been shown that tremor severity does not correlate well with tremor related disability (Bain, 1998). One study has demonstrated that for postural tremor without load neither power nor amplitude was significantly correlated with disability measures, whereas postural tremor with load correlated well with tremor-related disability measures such as the tremor disability questionnaire. Kinetic tremor that occurs during voluntary movements is more disabling than the postural tremor and interferes with many different activities of daily living such as writing, pouring, eating, and dressing. It has been shown that kinetic tremor is strongly associated with tremor-related disability measures (Norman, D'Amboise, Pari, & Heroux, 2011), so evaluation of kinetic tremor in a clinical setting may provide more valuable information for treatment decisions in ET patients. Intention tremor as a special type of kinetic tremor is a tremor during target-directed movements with increase of tremor amplitude at the termination of the movement. The patients with intention tremor have a higher degree of disability; maybe it is even the most important reason for disability in ET (Deuschl, Wenzelburger, Loffler, Raethjen, & Stolze, 2000). It has been shown that tremor severity is logarithmically related to disability, for example, a unit increase in disability is associated with exponential increase in severity. This would imply that a treatment must produce an exponential reduction in severity in order to be associated with a clinically relevant reduction in disability (Elble et al., 2006). Aside from the tremor phenomenology, other motor features have been described in ET. Gait difficulties, which are not uncommon in patients with ET, are the most important complaints in this group.

In several studies, postural instability and mild to moderate ataxic gait, beyond that seen in normal aging, have been demonstrated in patients with ET, and especially those patients with other cerebellar signs (e.g., intention tremor) (Stolze, Petersen, Raethjen, Wenzelburger, & Deuschl, 2001).

The physical disability caused by the tremor of ET has traditionally been regarded as the most important feature of the disease that causes distress, and it has received the most attention for the management of patients. This point of view has now changed since ET is increasingly recognized to have several nonmotor manifestations. Patients with ET have higher prevalence and higher mean scores of depression, anxiety, fatigue, sleep disturbances, and pain, as well as distinct personality traits (Tan et al., 2005). Psychological factors such as anxiety and depression do also have functional consequences in patients with ET. These factors may partly explain the phenomenon that only a minority of ET patients seeks medical attention for their tremor. Possible differences between individuals seeking medical attention or not, have hardly been studied so far. It has been shown that those who seek medical treatment for ET are more functionally impaired than those who do not. So, patients with psychological comorbidities do not only perceive that they are more disabled, but also, their execution of tasks is objectively more impaired (Louis et al., 2001). The reason why individuals with ET with similar disease severity do or do not seek medical help is unclear and depression or other so-far-undetermined individual factors may account for this. Another explanation for the difference in disease perception may be the use of different coping strategies for the disease. However, different groups of ET patients (outpatients versus community-based sample) showed similar coping strategies with active problem-orientated coping as the main coping strategy in one study (Lorenz et al., 2011).

Psychiatric features of ET have been studied in more detail recently. Possible psychiatric symptoms / comorbidities include depression, anxiety, embarrassment, and apathy. One study showed that ET patients reported more nonmotor symptoms than healthy controls, and that they scored significantly higher for the subscales anxiety, phobic anxiety, and psychoticism in a questionnaire for psychiatric symptoms (SCL-90R) (Tan et al., 2005). Depressive symptoms occur in a considerable number of patients and are significantly associated with QoL, so patients with severe depressive symptoms show the lowest QoL as measured with the QUEST (Louis, Huey, Gerbin, & Viner, 2012b). Another study showed that depression was even the only nonmotor feature that affected the patient's QOL (Chandran et al., 2012). The question of whether depression in ET is either a psychiatric response to disabling tremor, a mood disorder as part of the underlying disease, a confounding factor, a maladaptative coping mode, or an expression of an insufficient psychosocial adaptation is still unsolved. One study showed that depressive symptoms seemed to precede the onset of the motor manifestations in prospective analyses, so that a mood disorder may be part of the underlying disease process rather than a response to the tremor (Louis, Benito-Leon, & Bermejo-Pareja, 2007). Embarrassment, defined as an experience of having an unacceptable condition witnessed by others, has been demonstrated to be common in ET patients, to contribute to lower QoL, and to correlate with depressive symptoms (Louis & Rios, 2009). Anxiety is a common symptom in ET with prevalence rates up to 66%. Anxiety scores of ET patients were significantly higher compared to controls in different studies and correlated with tremor severity (Tan et al., 2005). Social phobia as another disorder within the anxiety spectrum does occur in ET patients with a prevalence of 32% for primary and secondary social phobia, whereas cases with secondary social phobia reported a later age at onset, a greater fear and avoidance of fine motor tasks in public, and demonstrated more severe tremor and tremor-related disability (Schneier, Barnes, Albert, & Louis, 2001). Patients with ET showed lower vigor and elevated apathy scores compared to controls (Louis, Huey, Gerbin, & Viner, 2012a). Apathy occurs in ET as in other movement disorders as a function of depression, but one study could demonstrate that some patients do have features of apathy without depression (Louis et al., 2012a). Besides the neuropsychiatric symptoms in ET, distinct personality traits and cognitive changes have been described. Studies on personality in ET showed higher harm avoidance and a trend toward social introversion. So far, it is not clear whether the ET personality profile is premorbid or is a co-morbid feature of the illness; however, one study found that the personality profile was not entirely related to tremor severity and tremor-related disability, so that it may be a primary disease feature (Chatterjee, Jurewicz, Applegate, & Louis, 2004; Lorenz et al., 2006). Cognitive changes have been reported in several studies including mostly clinically subtle, mild attentional, and executive dysfunction accompanying the disorder, such as deficits on tests of verbal fluency, naming, mental set-shifting, verbal and working memory, complex auditory attention, visual attention, and response inhibition (Benito-Leon, Louis, & Bermejo-Pareja, 2006b). These neuropsychological changes can be attributed to a functional disturbance of frontal areas due to a remote effect within the cerebellothalamo-cortical circuits as a consequence of cerebellar pathology loops and / or can be influenced by confounding factors such as anxiety, chronic motor dysfunction, and depression (Sahin et al., 2006; Troster et al., 2002). So far, 2 population-based studies and 1 prospective follow-up study described an association of elderly onset essential tremor with dementia and a nearly twofold increased risk for developing dementia (Benito-Leon, Louis, & Bermejo-Pareja, 2006a; Bermejo-Pareja, Louis, & Benito-Leon, 2007; Thawani, Schupf, & Louis, 2009). The significance of these results, however, remains unclear, since age associated brain pathology in older patients must be considered and very large patient populations would be required to decipher the potential confounds: depression, anxiety, education, comorbidities, medications, and sampling bias (Deuschl & Elble, 2009).

Overall, besides tremor severity, several nonmotor symptoms, especially depression, anxiety, and psychosocial factors contribute to lower QoL in ET. Nonmotor aspects of ET play significant roles in determining the QoL and may even outweigh the impact of impaired activities of daily living due to motor symptoms (Lorenz et al., 2011).

Predictors of QoL in ET

Comparable to other movement disorders, studies in ET patients have demonstrated that not only occurrence and severity of the motor symptoms, but mainly nonmotor symptoms predict a lower perceived health status and a QoL. Depression, dysfunctional mood, and anxiety, as well as cognitive impairment are predictors of QoL in ET patients (Louis et al., 2012b). Depressive symptoms have been found to be a strong predictor of tremor-related QoL in several studies. It could be demonstrated that depression, as measured by the BDI, was the only predictive factor for QoL summary scores, that depressive symptoms were a stronger predictor of QoL than was the main motor feature of ET itself, and that increased symptoms of depression were associated with lower psychosocial health status (Lorenz et al., 2011; Louis et al., 2012b). Cognitive impairment was another important factor associated with lower perceived health status in ET. Deficits in executive functions and lower vigor were independently predictive of poorer physical health status after considering the effects of ET disease severity (Woods, Scott, Fields, Poquette, & Troster, 2008). Similar results were shown in a study on functional correlates of lower cognitive tests in ET. Cognitive test scores were a better predictor of functional disability than was the tremor severity (Louis, 2010).

Clinical Studies of Essential Tremor Using QoL as an Outcome Parameter

The pharmacological treatment of ET is not optimal since there are still only two first-line medications, primidone and propranolol, and since the efficacy of medication is often insufficient. Only 30–50% of the ET patients respond to medication, medications rarely reduce the tremor to asymptomatic levels, and troublesome side effects can occur and lead to a discontinuation of the therapy (Koller & Vetere-Overfield, 1989; Louis, Rios, & Henchcliffe, 2010).

Propranolol (Cleeves & Findley, 1988; Winkler & Young, 1974), a nonselective beta-adrenergic receptor antagonist, and primidone (Findley, Cleeves, & Calzetti, 1985; Sasso, Perucca, Fava, & Calzetti, 1991) have been shown to reduce the amplitude of both postural and kinetic tremor, so that handwriting, drinking, and eating improved under therapy. However, the patients' embarrassment remained unchanged in one study (W. Koller, Biary, & Cone, 1986). There are no studies on efficacy of propranolol and primidone in ET with QoL or health status as endpoints, probably due to the fact that most studies on this topic were published before 2000. Further drugs that are used in ET include gabapentin, pregabalin, topiramate, other selective beta-1-adreonreceptor antagonists such as atenolol and sotalol, benzodiazepines, clozapine, and injections of botulinum toxin more for head than for hand tremor (Deuschl, Raethjen, Hellriegel, & Elble, 2011; Ferreira et al., 2013).

Gabapentin, an anticonvulsant with a structure similar to gamma-aminobutyric acid (GABA), has been shown to reduce tremor severity significantly (W. Ondo, Hunter, Vuong, Schwartz, & Jankovic, 2000). Another trial showed no significant difference for total tremor score, as well as no difference for QoL as measured with the SIP between placebo and gabapentin (Pahwa et al., 1998).

Topiramate is an anticonvulsant that blocks sodium channels and potentiates GABA activity. Studies have demonstrated a tremor improvement using clinical rating scales and demonstrated reduced functional disability in the treatment group compared to placebo (Connor, Edwards, & Tarsy, 2008; W. G. Ondo et al., 2006). For Pregabalin, an anticonvulsant drug, two double-blind, placebo controlled trials showed inconsistent results with a significant reduction in tremor amplitude compared with placebo in one study (Zesiewicz et al., 2007), but no improvement for tremor severity, as well as a statistically significant worsening of QoL as measured with QUEST in the Pregabalin group (Ferrara et al., 2009).

Carisbamate, an investigational neuromodulator currently in development for epilepsy, and placebo treatment did not differ in their effects on the tremor severity or on measures of affect, mood, or quality of life (Elble, Biondi, Ascher, Wiegand, & Hulihan, 2010).

DBS Trials for Essential Tremor Using QoL as an Outcome Parameter

Stereotactic surgery is an option for patients with disabling hand tremor that is not suppressed adequately by drug treatment. Previous reviews have suggested that DBS of the nucleus ventrointermedius (Vim) of the thalamus and Vim thalamotomy were highly efficacious treatments for upper limb tremor in patients with ET but gave these procedures only a limited recommendation, because results from double-blind placebo-controlled trials of these procedures were not available (Zesiewicz et al., 2005). Recent reviews of DBS trials in ET have found that the quality of available evidence was still limited, so that case series and case reports have to be used to evaluate safety and effectiveness of DBS. Quality of life outcomes for patients receiving DBS were also just recently made available considering these studies of lower evidence, so that the impact of DBS on the patient cannot be definitely estimated so far (Deuschl et al., 2011). Studies with a shorter follow-up of up to 12 months following DBS demonstrated improvement only in the patients' emotional constraint after surgery as measured by the NHP I and a positive impact on home maintenance, social life, and interests/hobbies as measured by the NHP II (Hariz, Lindberg, & Bergenheim, 2002), improvements in anxiety and QoL with respect to activities of daily living, stigma, emotional well-being, and communication as measured by a modified version of the PDQ-39 (Troster et al., 1999), and improvements for the domain's activities of daily living, emotional well-being, and perceived stigma as measured by a modified version of the PDQ-39 (Fields et al., 2003). Furthermore, several studies demonstrated, that ET patients have a marked improvement in daily functioning with thalamic DBS (Lyons et al., 1998), and an improvement from preoperative ADL scores to last follow-up (Pahwa et al., 1999). Long-term effects of DBS in ET have been evaluated by two studies so far. One study found a significant improvement of tremor severity, activities of daily living, and QoL as measured by a modified PDQ-39 for the dimensions of emotional well-being, stigma, and for total scores up to 7 years after surgery compared with presurgical scores. However, at the longest follow-up (up to 12 years), only the PDQ-39 stigma score was significantly improved (Nazzaro, Pahwa, & Lyons, 2012). In another series of patients followed for 7 years, the initial improvement in ADL at 1 year was no longer sustained at long term, except for the ability to eat, whereas social life remained improved (Hariz, Blomstedt, & Koskinen, 2008). Two studies evaluated QoL following DBS in the caudal zona incerta and found statistically significant improvements in the psychosocial and activities of daily living subscores of the QUEST, but not in any of the SF-36 domains or total score (Plaha et al., 2011; Sandvik, Koskinen, Lundquist, & Blomstedt, 2012).

QUALITY OF LIFE IN RESTLESS LEGS SYNDROME

Restless legs syndrome (RLS) is possibly the most common neurological movement disorder. Reported prevalence rates range from 1.9% to 15%, depending on case definition (Ohayon, O'Hara, & Vitiello, 2011). Approximately 2.5% of adults with RLS are having symptoms severe enough to require medical intervention (Yeh, Walters, & Tsuang, 2011). Clinical symptoms of RLS include a distressing urge to move the lower limbs at rest periods and especially at nighttime rest. This urge is frequently accompanied by an unpleasant sensation felt deep inside the affected limb. The symptoms appear during rest periods and are relieved by movement. The RLS can be classified as a primary disease or as a secondary condition to iron deficiency or renal failure, for example. It is known, that some medications can worsen or trigger RLS (Leschziner & Gringras, 2012). An association of RLS with PD and diabetes mellitus is discussed controversially (Innes, Selfe, & Agarwal, 2012; Moller, Unger, Stiasny-Kolster, & Oertel, 2010). Age at onset of RLS symptoms is variable. About 25% of adults with RLS report onset of symptoms between ages of 10 and 20 years (Picchietti et al., 2011). In patients with an older age at onset (>50y) RLS symptoms are often more intense (Allen et al., 2003). The RLS seems to be a hereditary disease with 9 out of 10 patients reporting a family history of RLS (Winkelmann & Ferini-Strambi, 2006). Results of genetic studies in RLS show a genetic heterogeneity of the disease. Gender is also a risk factor for RLS with women about twice as often affected by RLS as males (Leschziner & Gringras, 2012). Other risk factors for RLS include low iron levels, lower socioeconomic status, poor health, older age, and comorbidity with psychiatric disorders (Yeh et al., 2011). Furthermore, there is evidence that RLS is associated with metabolic dysregulation, autonomic dysfunction, and risk of cardiovascular disease (Innes, Selfe, & Agarwal, 2011).

Diagnostic criteria of RLS include 4 essential criteria (1. an urge to move the legs, usually accompanied or caused by uncomfortable and unpleasant sensations in the legs, 2. the urge to move or unpleasant sensations begin or worsen during periods of rest or inactivity such as lying down or sitting, 3. the urge to move or unpleasant sensations are partially or totally relieved by movement, at least as long as the activity continues, 4. the urge to move or unpleasant sensations are worse in the evening or at night than during the day, or only occur in the evening or night (Allen et al., 2003)). However, studies could demonstrate that not the essential RLS symptoms, but the negative effect of these RLS symptoms on sleep, daytime functional status, and cognitive function probably has the main impact on patients' perception of health, well-being, and QoL (Abetz et al., 2004). RLS remains largely undiagnosed, even though it is a common, and often a clinically significant medical condition (Allen, Stillman, & Myers, 2010). Sleep disturbance is the primary reason for patients with RLS to seek treatment (Allen et al., 2010; Hening et al., 2004). Although the condition is not life-threatening, it could be demonstrated that RLS produces an economic burden for society and patient. All RLS-related costs increased with RLS symptom severity, with increasingly significant decrements in health status, sleep disturbance, and work productivity, so that RLS carries a significant personal and social burden (Allen, Bharmal, & Calloway, 2011). Restless legs-syndrome patients showed an impaired QoL in comparison to the normative general population and to other patient samples (e.g., those with cardiovascular conditions or diabetes; Abetz et al., 2004). The negative impact of RLS symptoms on the patients' QoL is thereby comparable with other serious diseases such as type 2 diabetes mellitus and depression (Allen et al., 2005). Assessing the disease burden and the impact of RLS on QoL is also critical for evaluating treatment benefits.

QoL Tools in Restless Legs Syndrome

The RLS Quality of Life questionnaire (RLSQoL) is a validated questionnaire consisting of 18 items, 13 of which are scored on a 5-point scale (0 = not at all, to 4 = all the time/a lot), the remainder being recorded as either a numerical value or a dichotomous response. Ten of the items contribute to a single summary score, the overall-life-impact score, whereas the remaining 8 items concern employment (1 question), sexual interest (2 questions), and work (5 questions), and are summarized individually. Higher scores on the RLSQoL overall-life-impact score indicate a better QoL. The RLSQoL has been found to be reliable, valid, and responsive to change (Abetz et al., 2006).

The Restless Legs Syndrome Quality of Life Questionnaire (QoL-RLS) is a 12-item questionnaire including a global rating of QoL as well as items related to sleep, activities of daily living, mood, social interactions, to the consequences of disturbed sleep on everyday life and tiredness during the day and on mood, to consequences of pain and side effects of treatments on daily activities, and to coping behavior. Psychometric properties were good in one study as well as in a reanalysis with the data of a large-scale clinical-trial population (Kohnen et al., 2007).

The Restless Legs Quality of Life Instrument (RLS-QLI) comprises 17 items to be rated on a five point scale that could be allocated to factors: daily function, social function, sleep quality, emotional well-being. The psychometric quality of this instrument was good with high reliability scores and validity (Atkinson et al., 2004). So far, the RLS-QLI has not been used in published clinical trials.

The Restless Legs Syndrome-Next Day Impact (RLS-NDI) questionnaire is a 14-item self-reported outcome measure to assess the impact of disturbed sleep due to RLS on next day functioning as measured by the domains activities of daily living, cognitive functioning, emotional functioning, physical functioning, energy, daytime sleepiness, and social functioning. In one study, the RLS-NDI demonstrated content validity (Lasch et al., 2011).

Factors Impacting QoL in Restless Legs Syndrome

The RLS has profound negative effects on QoL (Allen et al., 2010). Studies showed lower mean SF-36 scores compared with U.S. population norms, and similar SF-36 scores as patients with other medical conditions, such as type 2 diabetes mellitus or depression (C. Kushida et al., 2007). Quality of life is reduced in both physical and mental domains among patients with RLS (C. Kushida et al., 2007; Winkelman et al., 2009). Quality of life in RLS is also affected by special domains such as cognitive deficits (Pearson et al., 2006) or daytime tiredness (Moller et al., 2006), so that QoL instruments should address these domains as well.

The RLS is described as a sensorimotor neurological disorder without sleep-related symptoms in the diagnostic criteria (Allen et al., 2003). However, RLS symptoms have a marked impact on sleep. Sleep disturbance, rather than the primary symptoms of RLS (urge to move, etc.) mediates the effects of RLS symptoms on primary outcomes, including QoL, emotional distress, daytime alertness, cognitive dysfunction, and psychiatric morbidity (C. A. Kushida, Allen, & Atkinson, 2004). Sleep disturbance is reported by up to 88% of RLS patients and include impaired sleep latency, shorter total sleep time, lower sleep efficiency, higher arousal index, more stage shifts, longer REM latency and abnormalities in the percentages of the different sleep stages (Allen et al., 2005; Winkelman et al., 2009). Many RLS sufferers reported performance-related effects, presumably resulting from RLS-related sleep disruption, such as daytime sleepiness and difficulty in concentrating the following day. In a large survey of the general populations of six countries, 85% of RLS patients reported a negative impact of the RLS symptoms on their daytime functioning, including a negative influence on their mood, a lack of energy, a disturbance of daily activities and social life, distraction from doing their job, and disturbance of their personal relationships. Therefore, a primary treatment goal should be the reduction of the sleep disturbance of RLS, both to decrease the RLS-related nocturnal distress and to improve daytime functioning (C. A. Kushida et al., 2004).

The serious adverse effects on sleep due to RLS symptoms leave patients with daytime fatigue and decreased motivation, which, in some cases, can lead to depression and anxiety (Allen & Earley, 2001). Increased symptom severity is furthermore associated with serious psychological impairment in multiple psychological domains such as psychological distress. One study showed a higher psychological distress and higher scores in the subscales compulsivity, depression, anxiety, hostility, phobic anxiety, and paranoid ideation by using the

Symptom Checklist 90-R questionnaire (Scholz, Benes, et al., 2011). Results of studies suggest a strong association between RLS and major depressive disorder and / or panic disorder. The lifetime prevalence of comorbid depression and anxiety disorders is elevated by odds ratio of 2.1 to 5.3 in RLS compared to the community (Lee et al., 2008; Winkelmann et al., 2005). These results suggest that RLS patients are at increased risk of having specific anxiety and depressive disorders. However, a considerable proportion of these co-morbidities may be due to the RLS symptomatology.

Clinical Trials in Restless Legs Syndrome Using QoL as an Outcome Parameter

In the past years, evidence-based guidelines have been published by taskforces for the Movement Disorders Society (Trenkwalder et al., 2008), the European Federation of Neurological Sciences (Vignatelli et al., 2006), and the European Restless Legs Syndrome Study Group (EURLSSG) (Garcia-Borreguero et al., 2011). There is a wide array of treatment options for RLS including pharmacological and nonpharmacologic interventions. In the pharmacological pathway, a number of agents are used for the treatment of patients with RLS (Garcia-Borreguero et al., 2012; Trenkwalder et al., 2008). The treatment varies according to symptom severity and frequency, and the presence or absence of painful symptoms. Treatments may relieve some or all of the symptoms of RLS, but they can also be associated with side effects, including increased symptom severity (augmentation = defined as the worsening of RLS symptoms including earlier onset and higher intensity) in the long term (Trenkwalder et al., 2004). So, not only the disorder, but also its treatment, may have an impact on patients' QoL.

Dopaminergic therapy is the first-line treatment in RLS. For Levodopa a recent review has shown that Levodopa therapy is efficacious for the short-term treatment of RLS, whereas augmentation, as the clinically most-relevant adverse event, was not investigated sufficiently in most studies (Scholz, Trenkwalder, et al., 2011b). RLS symptom severity was more reduced with levodopa than placebo, and QoL as measured by Visual Analogue Scales improved significantly compared to placebo (Benes et al., 1999; Trenkwalder et al., 1995). One controlled trial showed smaller effects with levodopa than with cabergoline for QoL (Trenkwalder et al., 2007). For the group of dopamine agonists, a recent review showed that they were superior to placebo in randomized controlled trials with up to seven months' follow-up (Scholz, Trenkwalder, et al., 2011a), and a further meta-analysis of 35 trials showed moderate improvements in symptom severity, self-rated sleep quality, and disease specific quality of life (Hornyak, Trenkwalder, Kohnen, & Scholz, 2012). On the other hand treatment with has agonists can also induce side effects. These agents can be associated with augmentation (Allen, Ondo, et al., 2011) and they can induce impulse control disorders. In RLS, impulse control disorders may affect as many as one in five patients with RLS who are taking dopamine agonists (Voon et al., 2011).

CONCLUSIONS

Quality-of-life measurements have become an important tool to assess the real-life-burden of a disease and to measure efficacy of drug or surgical treatment in the field of movement disorders. Although movement disorders are defined by their motor symptoms, studies of the last two decades could demonstrate that often the nonmotor symptoms, especially depression, anxiety, and cognitive impairment, have the main impact on patients' and are also predictors of QoL. The number of clinical trials using QoL measurements as outcome parameters has accelerated in the last years profoundly. However, the variety of different QoL instruments on one side and the lack of disease-specific QoL measurements on the other side require a detailed assessment of available tools for each specific clinical trial.

REFERENCES

Aarsland, D., Tandberg, E., Larsen, J. P., & Cummings, J. L. (1996). Frequency of dementia in Parkinson disease. *Archives of Neurology, 53*(6), 538–542.

Abbruzzese, G., & Berardelli, A. (2003). Sensorimotor integration in movement disorders. *Movement Disorders, 18*(3), 231–240.

Abetz, L., Allen, R., Follet, A., Washburn, T., Earley, C., Kirsch, J., & Knight, H. (2004). Evaluating the quality of life of patients with restless legs syndrome. *Clinical Therapy, 26*(6), 925–935.

Abetz, L., Arbuckle, R., Allen, R. P., Garcia-Borreguero, D., Hening, W., Walters, A. S.,…Kirsch, J. M. (2006). The reliability, validity and responsiveness of the International Restless Legs Syndrome Study Group rating scale and subscales in a clinical-trial setting. *Sleep Medicine, 7*(4), 340–349.

Adler, C. H., Singer, C., O'Brien, C., Hauser, R. A., Lew, M. F., Marek, K. L.,…Yoo, K. (1998). Randomized, placebo-controlled study of tolcapone in patients with fluctuating Parkinson disease treated with levodopa-carbidopa. Tolcapone Fluctuator Study Group III. *Archives in Neurology, 55*(8), 1089–1095.

Albanese, A., Asmus, F., Bhatia, K. P., Elia, A. E., Elibol, B., Filippini, G.,…Valls-Sole, J. (2011). EFNS guidelines on diagnosis and treatment of primary dystonias. *European Journal of Neurology, 18*(1), 5–18.

Allen, R. P., Bharmal, M., & Calloway, M. (2011). Prevalence and disease burden of primary restless legs syndrome: results of a general population survey in the United States. *Movement Disorders, 26*(1), 114–120.

Allen, R. P., & Earley, C. J. (2001). Validation of the Johns Hopkins restless legs severity scale. *Sleep Medicine, 2*(3), 239–242.

Allen, R. P., Ondo, W. G., Ball, E., Calloway, M. O., Manjunath, R., Higbie, R. L.,… Nisbet, P. A. (2011). Restless legs syndrome (RLS) augmentation associated with dopamine agonist and levodopa usage in a community sample. *Sleep Medicine, 12*(5), 431–439.

Allen, R. P., Picchietti, D., Hening, W. A., Trenkwalder, C., Walters, A. S., & Montplaisi, J. (2003). Restless legs syndrome: diagnostic criteria, special considerations, and epidemiology. A report from the restless legs syndrome diagnosis and epidemiology workshop at the National Institutes of Health. *Sleep Medicine, 4*(2), 101–119.

Allen, R. P., Stillman, P., & Myers, A. J. (2010). Physician-diagnosed restless legs syndrome in a large sample of primary medical care patients in western Europe: Prevalence and characteristics. *Sleep Medicine, 11*(1), 31–37.

Allen, R. P., Walters, A. S., Montplaisir, J., Hening, W., Myers, A., Bell, T. J., & Ferini-Strambi, L. (2005). Restless legs syndrome prevalence and impact: REST general population study. *Archives of Internal Medicine, 165*(11), 1286–1292.

Antonini, A., Mancini, F., Canesi, M., Zangaglia, R., Isaias, I. U., Manfredi, L., ... Pezzoli, G. (2008). Duodenal levodopa infusion improves quality of life in advanced Parkinson's disease. *Neurodegenerative Diseases, 5*(3-4), 244–246.

Atkinson, M. J., Allen, R. P., DuChane, J., Murray, C., Kushida, C., & Roth, T. (2004). Validation of the restless legs syndrome quality of life instrument (RLS-QLI): Findings of a consortium of national experts and the RLS Foundation. *Quality of Life Research, 13*(3), 679–693.

Avanzino, L., Martino, D., Marchese, R., Aniello, M. S., Minafra, B., Superbo, M., ... Abbruzzese, G. (2010). Quality of sleep in primary focal dystonia: a case-control study. *European Journal of Neurology, 17*(4), 576–581.

Bain, P. G. (1998). Clinical measurement of tremor. *Movement Disorders, 13*(Suppl 3), 77–80.

Barone, P., Antonini, A., Colosimo, C., Marconi, R., Morgante, L., Avarello, T. P., ... Dotto, P. D. (2009). The PRIAMO study: A multicenter assessment of nonmotor symptoms and their impact on quality of life in Parkinson's disease. *Movement Disorders, 24*(11), 1641–1649.

Benes, H., Kurella, B., Kummer, J., Kazenwadel, J., Selzer, R., & Kohnen, R. (1999). Rapid onset of action of levodopa in restless legs syndrome: a double-blind, randomized, multicenter, crossover trial. *Sleep, 22*(8), 1073–1081.

Benito-Leon, J., Louis, E. D., & Bermejo-Pareja, F. (2006a). Elderly-onset essential tremor is associated with dementia. *Neurology, 66*(10), 1500–1505.

Benito-Leon, J., Louis, E. D., & Bermejo-Pareja, F. (2006b). Population-based case-control study of cognitive function in essential tremor. *Neurology, 66*(1), 69–74.

Benrud-Larson, L. M., Sandroni, P., Schrag, A., & Low, P. A. (2005). Depressive symptoms and life satisfaction in patients with multiple system atrophy. *Movement Disorders, 20*(8), 951–957.

Ben-Shlomo, Y., Camfield, L., & Warner, T. (2002). What are the determinants of quality of life in people with cervical dystonia? *Journal of Neurology, Neurosurgery and Psychiatry, 72*(5), 608–614.

Bergner, M., Bobbitt, R. A., Carter, W. B., & Gilson, B. S. (1981). The sickness impact profile: Development and final revision of a health status measure. *Medical Care, 19*(8), 787–805.

Bermejo-Pareja, F., Louis, E. D., & Benito-Leon, J. (2007). Risk of incident dementia in essential tremor: A population-based study. *Movement Disorders, 22*(11), 1573–1580.

Bhattacharyya, N., & Tarsy, D. (2001). Impact on quality of life of botulinum toxin treatments for spasmodic dysphonia and oromandibular dystonia. *Archives of Otolaryngology & Head Neck Surgery, 127*(4), 389–392.

Biglan, K. M., Schwid, S., Eberly, S., Blindauer, K., Fahn, S., Goren, T., ... Shoulson, I. (2006). Rasagiline improves quality of life in patients with early Parkinson's disease. *Movement Disorders, 21*(5), 616–623.

Bloem, B. R., Grimbergen, Y. A., Cramer, M., Willemsen, M., & Zwinderman, A. H. (2001). Prospective assessment of falls in Parkinson's disease. *Journal of Neurology, 248*(11), 950–958.

Bonelli, R. M., & Hofmann, P. (2007). A systematic review of the treatment studies in Huntington's disease since 1990. *Expert Opinions in Pharmacotherapy, 8*(2), 141–153.

Browne, J. P., O'Boyle, C. A., McGee, H. M., McDonald, N. J., & Joyce, C. R. (1997). Development of a direct weighting procedure for quality of life domains. *Quality of Life Research, 6*(4), 301–309.

Burke, R. E., Fahn, S., & Marsden, C. D. (1986). Torsion dystonia: a double-blind, prospective trial of high-dosage trihexyphenidyl. *Neurology, 36*(2), 160–164.

Cano, S. J., Warner, T. T., Linacre, J. M., Bhatia, K. P., Thompson, A. J., Fitzpatrick, R., & Hobart, J. C. (2004). Capturing the true burden of dystonia on patients: the Cervical Dystonia Impact Profile (CDIP-58). *Neurology, 63*(9), 1629–1633.

Chan, J., Brin, M. F., & Fahn, S. (1991). Idiopathic cervical dystonia: clinical characteristics. *Movement Disorders, 6*(2), 119–126.

Chandran, V., Pal, P. K., Reddy, J. Y., Thennarasu, K., Yadav, R., & Shivashankar, N. (2012). Non-motor features in essential tremor. *Acta Neurologica Scandinavica, 125*(5), 332–337.

Chapuis, S., Ouchchane, L., Metz, O., Gerbaud, L., & Durif, F. (2005). Impact of the motor complications of Parkinson's disease on the quality of life. *Movement Disorders, 20*(2), 224–230.

Charous, S. J., Comella, C. L., & Fan, W. (2011). Jaw-opening dystonia: Quality of life after botulinum toxin injections. *Ear Nose Throat Journal, 90*(2), E9.

Chatterjee, A., Jurewicz, E. C., Applegate, L. M., & Louis, E. D. (2004). Personality in essential tremor: further evidence of non-motor manifestations of the disease. *Journal of Neurology, Neurosurgery and Psychiatry, 75*(7), 958–961.

Chaudhuri, K. R., Healy, D. G., & Schapira, A. H. (2006). Non-motor symptoms of Parkinson's disease: diagnosis and management. *Lancet Neurology, 5*(3), 235–245.

Chaudhuri, K. R., Martinez-Martin, P., Brown, R. G., Sethi, K., Stocchi, F., Odin, P., . . . Schapira, A. H. (2007). The metric properties of a novel non-motor symptoms scale for Parkinson's disease: Results from an international pilot study. *Movement Disorders, 22*(13), 1901–1911.

Chaudhuri, R. K., Rojo, J. M., Schapira, A. H., Brooks, D. J., Stocchi, F., Odin, P., Antonini, A., Brown, R. J., Martinez-Martin, P. (2013). A proposal for a comprehensive grading of Parkinson's disease severity combining motor and non-motor assessments: Meeting an unmet need. *PLoS One, 8*(2)(e57221.).

Clay, E., De Nicola, A., Dorey, J., Squitieri, F., Aballea, S., Martino, T., . . . Toumi, M. (2012). Validation of the first quality-of-life measurement for patients with Huntington's disease: The Huntington quality of life instrument. *International Clinical Psychopharmacology, 27*(4), 208–214.

Cleeves, L., & Findley, L. J. (1988). Propranolol and propranolol-LA in essential tremor: a double blind comparative study. *Journal of Neurology, Neurosurgery and Psychiatry, 51*(3), 379–384.

Connor, G. S., Edwards, K., & Tarsy, D. (2008). Topiramate in essential tremor: findings from double-blind, placebo-controlled, crossover trials. *Clinical Neuropharmacology, 31*(2), 97–103.

Costa, J., Borges, A.A., Espírito-Santo, C.C., Ferreira, J., Coelho, M.M., Moore, P., Sampaio, C. (2009). Botulinum toxin type A versus botulinum toxin type B for cervical dystonia. *Cochrane Database Systematic Review*(1).

Costa, J., Espirito-Santo, C., Borges, A., Ferreira, J. J., Coelho, M., & Sampaio, C. (2005). Botulinum toxin type A versus anticholinergics for cervical dystonia. *Cochrane Database Systematic Review*(1), CD004312.

Costa, J., Espírito-Santo, C. C., Borges, A. A., Ferreira, J., Coelho, M. M., Moore, P., Sampaio, C. (2009a). Botulinum toxin type A therapy for cervical dystonia. *Cochrane Database Systematic Review* (1).

Costa, J., Espírito-Santo, C. C., Borges, A. A., Ferreira, J., Coelho, M. M., Moore, P., Sampaio, C. (2009b). Botulinum toxin type B for cervical dystonia. *Cochrane Database Systematic Review* (1).

de Boer, A. G., Wijker, W., Speelman, J. D., & de Haes, J. C. (1996). Quality of life in patients with Parkinson's disease: development of a questionnaire. *Journal of Neurology, Neurosurgery and Psychiatry, 61*(1), 70–74.

Deuschl, G., Bain, P., & Brin, M. (1998). Consensus statement of the Movement Disorder Society on Tremor. Ad Hoc Scientific Committee. *Movement Disorders, 13 Suppl 3*, 2–23.

Deuschl, G., & Elble, R. (2009). Essential tremor--neurodegenerative or nondegenerative disease towards a working definition of ET. *Movement Disorders, 24*(14), 2033–2041.

Deuschl, G., Raethjen, J., Hellriegel, H., & Elble, R. (2011). Treatment of patients with essential tremor. *Lancet Neurology, 10*(2), 148–161.

Deuschl, G., Schade-Brittinger, C., Krack, P., Volkmann, J., Schafer, H., Botzel, K.,... Voges, J. (2006). A randomized trial of deep-brain stimulation for Parkinson's disease. *New England Journal of Medicine, 355*(9), 896–908.

Deuschl, G., Wenzelburger, R., Loffler, K., Raethjen, J., & Stolze, H. (2000). Essential tremor and cerebellar dysfunction clinical and kinematic analysis of intention tremor. *Brain, 123 (Pt 8)*, 1568–1580.

Diamond, A., & Jankovic, J. (2005). The effect of deep brain stimulation on quality of life in movement disorders. *Journal of Neurology, Neurosurgery and Psychiatry, 76*(9), 1188–1193.

Drapier, S., Raoul, S., Drapier, D., Leray, E., Lallement, F., Rivier, I.,... Verin, M. (2005). Only physical aspects of quality of life are significantly improved by bilateral subthalamic stimulation in Parkinson's disease. *Journal of Neurology, 252*(5), 583–588.

Elble, R. J., Biondi, D. M., Ascher, S., Wiegand, F., & Hulihan, J. (2010). Carisbamate in essential tremor: brief report of a proof of concept study. *Movement Disorders, 25*(5), 634–638.

Elble, R. J., & Deuschl, G. (2009). An update on essential tremor. *Current Neurology & Neuroscience Report, 9*(4), 273–277.

Elble, R. J., Pullman, S. L., Matsumoto, J. Y., Raethjen, J., Deuschl, G., & Tintner, R. (2006). Tremor amplitude is logarithmically related to 4- and 5-point tremor rating scales. *Brain, 129*(Pt 10), 2660–2666.

Erola, T., Karinen, P., Heikkinen, E., Tuominen, J., Haapaniemi, T., Koivukangas, J., & Myllyla, V. (2005). Bilateral subthalamic nucleus stimulation improves health-related quality of life in Parkinsonian patients. *Parkinsonism & Related Disorders, 11*(2), 89–94.

Esselink, R. A., de Bie, R. M., de Haan, R. J., Lenders, M. W., Nijssen, P. C., Staal, M. J.,... Speelman, J. D. (2004). Unilateral pallidotomy versus bilateral subthalamic nucleus stimulation in PD: a randomized trial. *Neurology, 62*(2), 201–207.

The EuroQol Group. (1990). EuroQol—A new facility for the measurement of health-related quality of life. *Health Policy, 16*(3), 199–208.

Fabbrini, G., Berardelli, I., Moretti, G., Pasquini, M., Bloise, M., Colosimo, C.,... Berardelli, A. (2010). Psychiatric disorders in adult-onset focal dystonia: a case-control study. *Movement Disorders, 25*(4), 459–465.

Factors impacting on quality of life in Parkinson's disease: results from an international survey. (2002). *Movement Disorders, 17*(1), 60–67.

Fahn, S., Elton, R., & Members of the UPDRS Development Commitee. (1987). The Unified Parkinson's Disease Rating Scale. In S. Fahn, C. D. Marsden, D. B. Calne, & M. Goldstein (Eds.), *Recent Developments in Parkinson's Disease* (Vol. 2, pp. 153–163, 293–304). Florham Park, NJ: Macmillan Healthcare Information.

Fahn, S., Marsden, C.D., Calne, D.B.. (1987). Classification and investigation of dystonia. In C. D. Marsden and S. Fahn (Eds.), *Movement disorders 2* (pp. 332–358). London, England: Butterworth.

Fenelon, G., Gimenez-Roldan, S., Montastruc, J. L., Bermejo, F., Durif, F., Bourdeix, I.,... Schadrack, J. (2003). Efficacy and tolerability of entacapone in patients with Parkinson's disease treated with levodopa plus a dopamine agonist and experiencing wearing-off motor fluctuations. A randomized, double-blind, multicentre study. *Journal of Neural Transmission, 110*(3), 239–251.

Ferrara, J. M., Kenney, C., Davidson, A. L., Shinawi, L., Kissel, A. M., & Jankovic, J. (2009). Efficacy and tolerability of pregabalin in essential tremor: a randomized, double-blind, placebo-controlled, crossover trial. *Journal of Neurological Science, 285*(1-2), 195–197.

Ferreira, J. J., Katzenschlager, R., Bloem, B. R., Bonuccelli, U., Burn, D., Deuschl, G.,... Oertel, W. H. (2013). Summary of the recommendations of the EFNS/MDS-ES review on therapeutic management of Parkinson's disease. *European Journal of Neurology, 20*(1), 5–15. doi: 10.1111/j.1468-1331.2012.03866.x

Fields, J. A., Troster, A. I., Woods, S. P., Higginson, C. I., Wilkinson, S. B., Lyons, K. E.,... Pahwa, R. (2003). Neuropsychological and quality of life outcomes 12 months after unilateral thalamic stimulation for essential tremor. *Journal of Neurology, Neurosurgery and Psychiatry, 74*(3), 305–311.

Findley, L. J., Cleeves, L., & Calzetti, S. (1985). Primidone in essential tremor of the hands and head: a double blind controlled clinical study. *Journal of Neurology, Neurosurgery and Psychiatry, 48*(9), 911–915.

Friedman, J., & Friedman, H. (1993). Fatigue in Parkinson's disease. *Neurology, 43*(10), 2016–2018.

Gallagher, D. A., & Schrag, A. (2008). Impact of newer pharmacological treatments on quality of life in patients with Parkinson's disease. *Central Nervous System Drugs, 22*(7), 563–586.

Garcia-Borreguero, D., Ferini-Strambi, L., Kohnen, R., O'Keeffe, S., Trenkwalder, C., Hogl, B.,... Williams, A. M. (2012). European guidelines on management of restless legs syndrome: report of a joint task force by the European Federation of Neurological Societies, the European Neurological Society and the European Sleep Research Society. *European Journal of Neurology, 19*(11), 1385–1396.

Garcia-Borreguero, D., Stillman, P., Benes, H., Buschmann, H., Chaudhuri, K. R., Gonzalez Rodriguez, V. M.,... Zucconi, M. (2011). Algorithms for the diagnosis and treatment of restless legs syndrome in primary care. *BMC Neurology, 11*, 28.

Gillingham, F. J., Donaldson, I. M. L., Schwab, R. S., England, A. C. (1969). Projection technique for evaluating surgery in Parkinson's disease. In F. J. Gillingham, and I. M. L. Donaldson (Eds.), *Third symposium on surgery in Parkinson's disease* (pp. 152–157). Edinburgh, Scotland: Livingstone.

Goetz, C. G., & Stebbins, G. T. (1995). Mortality and hallucinations in nursing home patients with advanced Parkinson's disease. *Neurology, 45*(4), 669–671.

Gomez-Esteban, J. C., Zarranz, J. J., Lezcano, E., Tijero, B., Luna, A., Velasco, F.,... Garamendi, I. (2007). Influence of motor symptoms upon the quality of life of patients with Parkinson's disease. *European Neurology, 57*(3), 161–165.

Gray, A., McNamara, I., Aziz, T., Gregory, R., Bain, P., Wilson, J., & Scott, R. (2002). Quality of life outcomes following surgical treatment of Parkinson's disease. *Movement Disorders, 17*(1), 68–75.

Greene, P. (1992). Baclofen in the treatment of dystonia. *Clinical Neuropharmacology, 15*(4), 276–288.

Grosset, D., Taurah, L., Burn, D. J., MacMahon, D., Forbes, A., Turner, K., ... Chaudhuri, K. R. (2007). A multicentre longitudinal observational study of changes in self reported health status in people with Parkinson's disease left untreated at diagnosis. *Journal of Neurology, Neurosurgery and Psychiatry, 78*(5), 465–469.

Gruber, D., Trottenberg, T., Kivi, A., Schoenecker, T., Kopp, U. A., Hoffmann, K. T., ... Kupsch, A. (2009). Long-term effects of pallidal deep brain stimulation in tardive dystonia. *Neurology, 73*(1), 53–58.

Gundel, H., Wolf, A., Xidara, V., Busch, R., Ladwig, K. H., Jacobi, F., ... Ceballos-Baumann, A. O. (2003). High psychiatric comorbidity in spasmodic torticollis: a controlled study. *Journal of Nervous & Mental Disease, 191*(7), 465–473.

Hagell, P., Whalley, D., McKenna, S. P., & Lindvall, O. (2003). Health status measurement in Parkinson's disease: validity of the PDQ-39 and Nottingham Health Profile. *Movement Disorders, 18*(7), 773–783.

Halbig, T. D., Gruber, D., Kopp, U. A., Schneider, G. H., Trottenberg, T., & Kupsch, A. (2005). Pallidal stimulation in dystonia: effects on cognition, mood, and quality of life. *Journal of Neurology, Neurosurgery and Psychiatry, 76*(12), 1713–1716.

Hamilton, J. M., Salmon, D. P., Corey-Bloom, J., Gamst, A., Paulsen, J. S., Jerkins, S., ... Peavy, G. (2003). Behavioural abnormalities contribute to functional decline in Huntington's disease. *Journal of Neurology, Neurosurgery and Psychiatry, 74*(1), 120–122.

Hanna, K. K., & Cronin-Golomb, A. (2012). Impact of anxiety on quality of life in Parkinson's disease. *Parkinson's Disease, 2012*, 640707.

Hariz, G. M., Blomstedt, P., & Koskinen, L. O. (2008). Long-term effect of deep brain stimulation for essential tremor on activities of daily living and health-related quality of life. *Acta Neurologica Scandinavica, 118*(6), 387–394.

Hariz, G. M., Lindberg, M., & Bergenheim, A. T. (2002). Impact of thalamic deep brain stimulation on disability and health-related quality of life in patients with essential tremor. *Journal of Neurology, Neurosurgery and Psychiatry, 72*(1), 47–52.

Helder, D. I., Kaptein, A. A., van Kempen, G. M., van Houwelingen, J. C., & Roos, R. A. (2001). Impact of Huntington's disease on quality of life. *Movement Disorders, 16*(2), 325–330.

Hening, W., Walters, A. S., Allen, R. P., Montplaisir, J., Myers, A., & Ferini-Strambi, L. (2004). Impact, diagnosis and treatment of restless legs syndrome (RLS) in a primary care population: the REST (RLS epidemiology, symptoms, and treatment) primary care study. *Sleep Medicine, 5*(3), 237–246.

Herlofson, K., & Larsen, J. P. (2003). The influence of fatigue on health-related quality of life in patients with Parkinson's disease. *Acta Neurologica Scandinavica, 107*(1), 1–6.

Hilker, R., Schischniaschvili, M., Ghaemi, M., Jacobs, A., & Rudolf, J. (2001). Health related quality of life is improved by botulinum neurotoxin type A in long term treated patients with focal dystonia. *Journal of Neurology, Neurosurgery and Psychiatry, 71*(2), 193–199.

Ho, A. K., Gilbert, A. S., Mason, S. L., Goodman, A. O., & Barker, R. A. (2009). Health-related quality of life in Huntington's disease: Which factors matter most? *Movement Disorders, 24*(4), 574–578.

Ho, A. K., & Hocaoglu, M. B. (2011). Impact of Huntington's across the entire disease spectrum: the phases and stages of disease from the patient perspective. *Clinical Genetics, 80*(3), 235–239.

Hocaoglu, M. B., Gaffan, E. A., & Ho, A. K. (2012). The Huntington's Disease health-related Quality of Life questionnaire (HDQoL): a disease-specific measure of health-related quality of life. *Clinical Genetics, 81*(2), 117–122.

Hoehn, M. M., & Yahr, M. D. (1967). Parkinsonism: onset, progression and mortality. *Neurology, 17*(5), 427–442.

Hogan, T., Grimaldi, R., Dingemanse, J., Martin, M., Lyons, K., & Koller, W. (1999). The Parkinson's disease symptom inventory (PDSI): a comprehensive and sensitive instrument to measure disease symptoms and treatment side-effects. *Parkinsonism & Related Disorders, 5*(3), 93–98.

Hogikyan, N. D., Wodchis, W. P., Spak, C., & Kileny, P. R. (2001). Longitudinal effects of botulinum toxin injections on voice-related quality of life (V-RQOL) for patients with adductory spasmodic dysphonia. *Journal of Voice, 15*(4), 576–586.

Holloway, R. G., Shoulson, I., Fahn, S., Kieburtz, K., Lang, A., Marek, K., ... Watts, A. (2004). Pramipexole vs levodopa as initial treatment for Parkinson disease: a 4-year randomized controlled trial. *Archives of Neurology, 61*(7), 1044–1053.

Holroyd, S., Currie, L., & Wooten, G. F. (2001). Prospective study of hallucinations and delusions in Parkinson's disease. *Journal of Neurology, Neurosurgery and Psychiatry, 70*(6), 734–738.

Hornyak, M., Trenkwalder, C., Kohnen, R., & Scholz, H. (2012). Efficacy and safety of dopamine agonists in restless legs syndrome. *Sleep Medicine, 13*(3), 228–236.

Hunt, S. M., McKenna, S. P., McEwen, J., Backett, E. M., Williams, J., & Papp, E. (1980). A quantitative approach to perceived health status: a validation study. *Journal of Epidemiology & Community Health, 34*(4), 281–286.

Huntington Study Group. Unified Huntington's disease rating scale: reliability and consistency. (1996). *Movement Disorders, 11*(2), 136–142.

Innes, K. E., Selfe, T. K., & Agarwal, P. (2011). Prevalence of restless legs syndrome in North American and Western European populations: a systematic review. *Sleep Medicine, 12*(7), 623–634.

Innes, K. E., Selfe, T. K., & Agarwal, P. (2012). Restless legs syndrome and conditions associated with metabolic dysregulation, sympathoadrenal dysfunction, and cardiovascular disease risk: A systematic review. *Sleep Medicine Review, 16*(4), 309–339.

Jahanshahi, M., & Marsden, C. D. (1992). Psychological functioning before and after treatment of torticollis with botulinum toxin. *Journal of Neurology, Neurosurgery and Psychiatry, 55*(3), 229–231.

Jankovic, J. (2002). Essential tremor: a heterogenous disorder. *Movement Disorders, 17*(4), 638–644.

Jankovic, J. (2004). Dystonia: medical therapy and botulinum toxin. *Advances in Neurology, 94*, 275–286.

Jankovic, J., & Brin, M. F. (1991). Therapeutic uses of botulinum toxin. *New England Journal of Medicine, 324*(17), 1186–1194.

Jankovic, J., Watts, R. L., Martin, W., & Boroojerdi, B. (2007). Transdermal rotigotine: double-blind, placebo-controlled trial in Parkinson disease. *Archives of Neurology, 64*(5), 676–682.

Jenkinson, C., & Fitzpatrick, R. (2007). Cross-cultural evaluation of the short form 8-item Parkinson's Disease Questionnaire (PDQ-8): results from America, Canada, Japan, Italy and Spain. *Parkinsonism & Related Disorders, 13*(1), 22–28.

Jenkinson, C., Fitzpatrick, R., Peto, V., Greenhall, R., & Hyman, N. (1997). The Parkinson's Disease Questionnaire (PDQ-39): development and validation of a Parkinson's disease summary index score. *Age & Ageing, 26*(5), 353–357.

Kaptein, A. A., Scharloo, M., Helder, D. I., Snoei, L., van Kempen, G. M., Weinman, J.,...Roos, R. A. (2007). Quality of life in couples living with Huntington's disease: the role of patients' and partners' illness perceptions. *Quality of Life Research, 16*(5), 793–801.

Karlsen, K. H., Larsen, J. P., Tandberg, E., & Maeland, J. G. (1999). Influence of clinical and demographic variables on quality of life in patients with Parkinson's disease. *Journal of Neurology, Neurosurgery and Psychiatry, 66*(4), 431–435.

Karlsen, K. H., Tandberg, E., Arsland, D., & Larsen, J. P. (2000). Health related quality of life in Parkinson's disease: a prospective longitudinal study. *Journal of Neurology, Neurosurgery and Psychiatry, 69*(5), 584–589.

Katschnig, H. (2006). Quality of life in mental disorders: challenges for research and clinical practice. *World Psychiatry, 5*(3), 139–145.

Kohnen, R., Allen, R. P., Benes, H., Garcia-Borreguero, D., Hening, W. A., Stiasny-Kolster, K., & Zucconi, M. (2007). Assessment of restless legs syndrome--methodological approaches for use in practice and clinical trials. *Movement Disorders, 22*(Suppl 18), S485–494.

Kollensperger, M., Geser, F., Ndayisaba, J. P., Boesch, S., Seppi, K., Ostergaard, K.,...Wenning, G. K. (2010). Presentation, diagnosis, and management of multiple system atrophy in Europe: final analysis of the European multiple system atrophy registry. *Movement Disorders, 25*(15), 2604–2612.

Kollensperger, M., Stampfer-Kountchev, M., Seppi, K., Geser, F., Frick, C., Del Sorbo, F.,...Wenning, G. K. (2007). Progression of dysautonomia in multiple system atrophy: a prospective study of self-perceived impairment. *European Journal of Neurology, 14*(1), 66–72.

Koller, W., Biary, N., & Cone, S. (1986). Disability in essential tremor: effect of treatment. *Neurology, 36*(7), 1001–1004.

Koller, W. C., & Vetere-Overfield, B. (1989). Acute and chronic effects of propranolol and primidone in essential tremor. *Neurology, 39*(12), 1587–1588.

Krauss, J. K. (2010). Surgical treatment of dystonia. *European Journal of Neurology, 17 Suppl 1*, 97–101.

Kuehler, A., Henrich, G., Schroeder, U., Conrad, B., Herschbach, P., & Ceballos-Baumann, A. (2003). A novel quality of life instrument for deep brain stimulation in movement disorders. *Journal of Neurology, Neurosurgery and Psychiatry, 74*(8), 1023–1030.

Kupsch, A., Benecke, R., Muller, J., Trottenberg, T., Schneider, G. H., Poewe, W.,...Volkmann, J. (2006). Pallidal deep-brain stimulation in primary generalized or segmental dystonia. *New England Journal of Medicine, 355*(19), 1978–1990.

Kushida, C., Martin, M., Nikam, P., Blaisdell, B., Wallenstein, G., Ferini-Strambi, L., & Ware, J. E., Jr. (2007). Burden of restless legs syndrome on health-related quality of life. *Quality of Life Research, 16*(4), 617–624.

Kushida, C. A., Allen, R. P., & Atkinson, M. J. (2004). Modeling the causal relationships between symptoms associated with restless legs syndrome and the patient-reported impact of RLS. *Sleep Medicine, 5*(5), 485–488.

Kuyper, D. J., Parra, V., Aerts, S., Okun, M. S., & Kluger, B. M. (2011). Nonmotor manifestations of dystonia: a systematic review. *Movement Disorders, 26*(7), 1206–1217.

Lagrange, E., Krack, P., Moro, E., Ardouin, C., Van Blercom, N., Chabardes, S.,... Pollak, P. (2002). Bilateral subthalamic nucleus stimulation improves health-related quality of life in PD. *Neurology, 59*(12), 1976–1978.

Lang, A. E. (1986). High dose anticholinergic therapy in adult dystonia. *Canadian Journal of Neurological Science, 13*(1), 42–46.

Larsson, M. U., Luszcz, M. A., Bui, T. H., & Wahlin, T. B. (2006). Depression and suicidal ideation after predictive testing for Huntington's disease: a two-year follow-up study. *Journal of Genetics Counseling, 15*(5), 361–374.

Larsson, V., Engedal, K., Aarsland, D., Wattmo, C., Minthon, L., & Londos, E. (2011). Quality of life and the effect of memantine in dementia with lewy bodies and Parkinson's disease dementia. *Dementia & Geriatric Cognitive Disorders, 32*(4), 227–234.

Lasch, K. E., Abraham, L., Patrick, J., Piault, E. C., Tully, S. E., & Treglia, M. (2011). Development of a next day functioning measure to assess the impact of sleep disturbance due to restless legs syndrome: the restless legs syndrome-next day impact questionnaire. *Sleep Medicine, 12*(8), 754–761.

Lee, H. B., Hening, W. A., Allen, R. P., Kalaydjian, A. E., Earley, C. J., Eaton, W. W., & Lyketsos, C. G. (2008). Restless legs syndrome is associated with DSM-IV major depressive disorder and panic disorder in the community. *Journal of Neuropsychiatry & Clinical Neuroscience, 20*(1), 101–105.

Lees, A. J., Blackburn, N. A., & Campbell, V. L. (1988). The nighttime problems of Parkinson's disease. *Clinical Neuropharmacology, 11*(6), 512–519.

Leschziner, G., & Gringras, P. (2012). Restless legs syndrome. *British Medical Journal, 344*, e3056.

Ling, H., O'Sullivan, S. S., Holton, J. L., Revesz, T., Massey, L. A., Williams, D. R.,... Lees, A. J. (2010). Does corticobasal degeneration exist? A clinicopathological re-evaluation. *Brain, 133*(Pt 7), 2045–2057.

Lobbezoo, F., Tanguay, R., Thon, M. T., & Lavigne, G. J. (1996). Pain perception in idiopathic cervical dystonia (spasmodic torticollis). *Pain, 67*(2-3), 483–491.

Logsdon, R. G., Gibbons, L. E., McCurry, S. M., & Teri, L. (2002). Assessing quality of life in older adults with cognitive impairment. *Psychosomatic Medicine, 64*(3), 510–519.

Long-term effect of initiating pramipexole vs levodopa in early Parkinson disease. (2009). *Archives of Neurology, 66*(5), 563–570.

Lorenz, D., & Deuschl, G. (2007). Update on pathogenesis and treatment of essential tremor. *Current Opinions in Neurology, 20*(4), 447–452.

Lorenz, D., Poremba, C., Papengut, F., Schreiber, S., & Deuschl, G. (2011). The psychosocial burden of essential tremor in an outpatient- and a community-based cohort. *European Journal of Neurology, 18*(7), 972–979.

Lorenz, D., Schwieger, D., Moises, H., & Deuschl, G. (2006). Quality of life and personality in essential tremor patients. *Movement Disorders, 21*(8), 1114–1118.

Louis, E. D. (2010). Functional correlates of lower cognitive test scores in essential tremor. *Movement Disorders, 25*(4), 481–485.

Louis, E. D., Barnes, L., Albert, S. M., Cote, L., Schneier, F. R., Pullman, S. L., & Yu, Q. (2001). Correlates of functional disability in essential tremor. *Movement Disorders, 16*(5), 914–920.

Louis, E. D., Benito-Leon, J., & Bermejo-Pareja, F. (2007). Self-reported depression and anti-depressant medication use in essential tremor: cross-sectional and prospective analyses in a population-based study. *European Journal of Neurology, 14*(10), 1138–1146.

Louis, E. D., Huey, E. D., Gerbin, M., & Viner, A. S. (2012a). Apathy in essential tremor, dystonia, and Parkinson's disease: a comparison with normal controls. *Movement Disorders, 27*(3), 432–434.

Louis, E. D., Huey, E. D., Gerbin, M., & Viner, A. S. (2012b). Depressive traits in essential tremor: impact on disability, quality of life, and medication adherence. *European Journal of Neurology, 19*(10), 1349–1354.

Louis, E. D., & Rios, E. (2009). Embarrassment in essential tremor: prevalence, clinical correlates and therapeutic implications. *Parkinsonism & Related Disorders, 15*(7), 535–538.

Louis, E. D., Rios, E., & Henchcliffe, C. (2010). How are we doing with the treatment of essential tremor (ET)?: Persistence of patients with ET on medication: data from 528 patients in three settings. *European Journal of Neurology, 17*(6), 882–884.

Lubarr, N., & Bressman, S. (2011). Treatment of generalized dystonia. *Current Treatment Options in Neurology, 13*(3), 274–289.

Lyons, K. E., Pahwa, R., Busenbark, K. L., Troster, A. I., Wilkinson, S., & Koller, W. C. (1998). Improvements in daily functioning after deep brain stimulation of the thalamus for intractable tremor. *Movement Disorders, 13*(4), 690–692.

Mahant, N., McCusker, E. A., Byth, K., & Graham, S. (2003). Huntington's disease: clinical correlates of disability and progression. *Neurology, 61*(8), 1085–1092.

Manne, S. L., Pape, S. J., Taylor, K. L., & Dougherty, J. (1999). Spouse support, coping, and mood among individuals with cancer. *Annals of Behavioral Medicine, 21*(2), 111–121.

Marinus, J., Ramaker, C., van Hilten, J. J., & Stiggelbout, A. M. (2002). Health related quality of life in Parkinson's disease: a systematic review of disease specific instruments. *Journal of Neurology, Neurosurgery and Psychiatry, 72*(2), 241–248.

Marinus, J., Visser, M., Martinez-Martin, P., van Hilten, J. J., & Stiggelbout, A. M. (2003). A short psychosocial questionnaire for patients with Parkinson's disease: the SCOPA-PS. *Journal of Clinical Epidemiology, 56*(1), 61–67.

Marras, C., Lang, A., Krahn, M., Tomlinson, G., & Naglie, G. (2004). Quality of life in early Parkinson's disease: impact of dyskinesias and motor fluctuations. *Movement Disorders, 19*(1), 22–28.

Martinez-Martin, P., & Deuschl, G. (2007). Effect of medical and surgical interventions on health-related quality of life in Parkinson's disease. *Movement Disorders, 22*(6), 757–765.

Martinez-Martin, P., Jimenez-Jimenez, F. J., Carroza Garcia, E., Alonso-Navarro, H., Rubio, L., Calleja, P., . . . Benito-Leon, J. (2010). Most of the Quality of Life in Essential Tremor Questionnaire (QUEST) psychometric properties resulted in satisfactory values. *Journal of Clinical Epidemiology, 63*(7), 767–773.

Martinez-Martin, P., & Kurtis, M. M. (2009). Systematic review of the effect of dopamine receptor agonists on patient health-related quality of life. *Parkinsonism & Related Disorders, 15*(Suppl 4), S58–64.

Martinez-Martin, P., Rodriguez-Blazquez, C., Kurtis, M. M., & Chaudhuri, K. R. (2011). The impact of non-motor symptoms on health-related quality of life of patients with Parkinson's disease. *Movement Disorders, 26*(3), 399–406.

Martinez-Martin, P., Schapira, A. H., Stocchi, F., Sethi, K., Odin, P., MacPhee, G., . . . Chaudhuri, K. R. (2007). Prevalence of nonmotor symptoms in Parkinson's disease in an international setting; study using nonmotor symptoms questionnaire in 545 patients. *Movement Disorders, 22*(11), 1623–1629.

Martinez-Martin, P., Serrano-Duenas, M., Forjaz, M. J., & Serrano, M. S. (2007). Two questionnaires for Parkinson's disease: are the PDQ-39 and PDQL equivalent? *Quality of Life Research, 16*(7), 1221–1230.

Martinez-Martin, P., Valldeoriola, F., Tolosa, E., Pilleri, M., Molinuevo, J. L., Rumia, J., & Ferrer, E. (2002). Bilateral subthalamic nucleus stimulation and quality of life in advanced Parkinson's disease. *Movement Disorders, 17*(2), 372–377.

McKeith, I. G., Dickson, D. W., Lowe, J., Emre, M., O'Brien, J. T., Feldman, H., ... Yamada, M. (2005). Diagnosis and management of dementia with Lewy bodies: third report of the DLB Consortium. *Neurology, 65*(12), 1863–1872.

Merz, R. I., Deakin, J., & Hawthorne, M. R. (2010). Oromandibular dystonia questionnaire (OMDQ-25): a valid and reliable instrument for measuring health-related quality of life. *Clinical Otolaryngology, 35*(5), 390–396.

Moller, J. C., Korner, Y., Cassel, W., Meindorfner, C., Kruger, H. P., Oertel, W. H., & Stiasny-Kolster, K. (2006). Sudden onset of sleep and dopaminergic therapy in patients with restless legs syndrome. *Sleep Medicine, 7*(4), 333–339.

Moller, J. C., Unger, M., Stiasny-Kolster, K., & Oertel, W. H. (2010). Restless Legs Syndrome (RLS) and Parkinson's disease (PD)-related disorders or different entities? *Journal of Neurological Science, 289*(1-2), 135–137.

Mueller, J., Skogseid, I. M., Benecke, R., Kupsch, A., Trottenberg, T., Poewe, W., ... Volkmann, J. (2008). Pallidal deep brain stimulation improves quality of life in segmental and generalized dystonia: results from a prospective, randomized sham-controlled trial. *Movement Disorders, 23*(1), 131–134.

Muller, J., Kemmler, G., Wissel, J., Schneider, A., Voller, B., Grossmann, J., ... Poewe, W. (2002). The impact of blepharospasm and cervical dystonia on health-related quality of life and depression. *Journal of Neurology, 249*(7), 842–846.

Muller, J., Wissel, J., Kemmler, G., Voller, B., Bodner, T., Schneider, A., ... Poewe, W. (2004). Craniocervical dystonia questionnaire (CDQ-24): development and validation of a disease-specific quality of life instrument. *Journal of Neurology, Neurosurgery and Psychiatry, 75*(5), 749–753.

Muslimovic, D., Post, B., Speelman, J. D., Schmand, B., & de Haan, R. J. (2008). Determinants of disability and quality of life in mild to moderate Parkinson disease. *Neurology, 70*(23), 2241–2247.

Naito, M., Nakayama, T., & Fukuhara, S. (2004). Quality of life assessment and reporting in randomized controlled trials: a study of literature published from Japan. *Health & Quality of Life Outcomes, 2*, 31.

Nazzaro, J. M., Pahwa, R., & Lyons, K. E. (2012). Long-term benefits in quality of life after unilateral thalamic deep brain stimulation for essential tremor. *Journal of Neurosurgery, 117*(1), 156–161.

Norman, K. E., D'Amboise, S. N., Pari, G., & Heroux, M. E. (2011). Tremor during movement correlates well with disability in people with essential tremor. *Movement Disorders, 26*(11), 2088–2094.

Noyes, K., Dick, A. W., & Holloway, R. G. (2006). Pramipexole versus levodopa in patients with early Parkinson's disease: effect on generic and disease-specific quality of life. *Value Health, 9*(1), 28–38.

Ohayon, M. M., O'Hara, R., & Vitiello, M. V. (2011). Epidemiology of restless legs syndrome: a synthesis of the literature. *Sleep Medicine Review, 16*(4), 283–295.

Olanow, C. W., Kieburtz, K., Stern, M., Watts, R., Langston, J. W., Guarnieri, M., & Hubble, J. (2004). Double-blind, placebo-controlled study of entacapone in levodopa-treated patients with stable Parkinson disease. *Archives of Neurology, 61*(10), 1563–1568.

Ondo, W., Hunter, C., Vuong, K. D., Schwartz, K., & Jankovic, J. (2000). Gabapentin for essential tremor: a multiple-dose, double-blind, placebo-controlled trial. *Movement Disorders, 15*(4), 678–682.

Ondo, W. G., Jankovic, J., Connor, G. S., Pahwa, R., Elble, R., Stacy, M. A.,... Hulihan, J. F. (2006). Topiramate in essential tremor: a double-blind, placebo-controlled trial. *Neurology, 66*(5), 672–677.

Page, D., Butler, A., & Jahanshahi, M. (2007). Quality of life in focal, segmental, and generalized dystonia. *Movement Disorders, 22*(3), 341–347.

Pahwa, R., Lyons, K., Hubble, J. P., Busenbark, K., Rienerth, J. D., Pahwa, A., & Koller, W. C. (1998). Double-blind controlled trial of gabapentin in essential tremor. *Movement Disorders, 13*(3), 465–467.

Pahwa, R., Lyons, K. L., Wilkinson, S. B., Carpenter, M. A., Troster, A. I., Searl, J. P.,... Koller, W. C. (1999). Bilateral thalamic stimulation for the treatment of essential tremor. *Neurology, 53*(7), 1447–1450.

Paulsen, J. S., Ready, R. E., Hamilton, J. M., Mega, M. S., & Cummings, J. L. (2001). Neuropsychiatric aspects of Huntington's disease. *Journal of Neurology, Neurosurgery and Psychiatry, 71*(3), 310–314.

Pearson, V. E., Allen, R. P., Dean, T., Gamaldo, C. E., Lesage, S. R., & Earley, C. J. (2006). Cognitive deficits associated with restless legs syndrome (RLS). *Sleep Medicine, 7*(1), 25–30.

Pekmezovic, T., Svetel, M., Ivanovic, N., Dragasevic, N., Petrovic, I., Tepavcevic, D. K., & Kostic, V. S. (2009). Quality of life in patients with focal dystonia. *Clinical Neurology & Neurosurgery, 111*(2), 161–164.

Peto, V., Jenkinson, C., Fitzpatrick, R., & Greenhall, R. (1995). The development and validation of a short measure of functioning and well being for individuals with Parkinson's disease. *Quality of Life Research, 4*(3), 241–248.

Picchietti, D. L., Arbuckle, R. A., Abetz, L., Durmer, J. S., Ivanenko, A., Owens, J. A.,... Walters, A. S. (2011). Pediatric restless legs syndrome: analysis of symptom descriptions and drawings. *Journal of Child Neurology, 26*(11), 1365–1376.

Plaha, P., Javed, S., Agombar, D., G, O. F., Khan, S., Whone, A., & Gill, S. (2011). Bilateral caudal zona incerta nucleus stimulation for essential tremor: outcome and quality of life. *Journal of Neurology, Neurosurgery and Psychiatry, 82*(8), 899–904.

Poewe, W. H., Rascol, O., Quinn, N., Tolosa, E., Oertel, W. H., Martignoni, E.,... Boroojerdi, B. (2007). Efficacy of pramipexole and transdermal rotigotine in advanced Parkinson's disease: a double-blind, double-dummy, randomised controlled trial. *Lancet Neurology, 6*(6), 513–520.

Pramipexole in levodopa-treated Parkinson disease patients of African, Asian, and Hispanic heritage. (2007). *Clinical Neuropharmacology, 30*(2), 72–85.

Qin, Z., Zhang, L., Sun, F., Fang, X., Meng, C., Tanner, C., & Chan, P. (2009). Health related quality of life in early Parkinson's disease: impact of motor and non-motor symptoms, results from Chinese levodopa exposed cohort. *Parkinsonism & Related Disorders, 15*(10), 767–771.

Rahman, S., Griffin, H. J., Quinn, N. P., & Jahanshahi, M. (2008). Quality of life in Parkinson's disease: the relative importance of the symptoms. *Movement Disorders, 23*(10), 1428–1434.

A randomized placebo-controlled trial of rasagiline in levodopa-treated patients with Parkinson disease and motor fluctuations: The PRESTO study. (2005). *Archives of Neurology, 62*(2), 241–248.

Ready, R. E., Mathews, M., Leserman, A., & Paulsen, J. S. (2008). Patient and caregiver quality of life in Huntington's disease. *Movement Disorders, 23*(5), 721–726.

Reese, R., Gruber, D., Schoenecker, T., Bazner, H., Blahak, C., Capelle, H. H.,... Krauss, J. K. (2011). Long-term clinical outcome in meige syndrome treated with internal pallidum deep brain stimulation. *Movement Disorders, 26*(4), 691–698.

Reichmann, H., Boas, J., Macmahon, D., Myllyla, V., Hakala, A., & Reinikainen, K. (2005). Efficacy of combining levodopa with entacapone on quality of life and activities of daily living in patients experiencing wearing-off type fluctuations. *Acta Neurologica Scandinavica, 111*(1), 21–28.

Reuther, M., Spottke, E. A., Klotsche, J., Riedel, O., Peter, H., Berger, K., . . . Dodel, R. C. (2007). Assessing health-related quality of life in patients with Parkinson's disease in a prospective longitudinal study. *Parkinsonism & Related Disorders, 13*(2), 108–114.

Richard, I. H. (2005). Anxiety disorders in Parkinson's disease. *Advances in Neurology, 96*, 42–55.

Riedel, O., Klotsche, J., Spottke, A., Deuschl, G., Forstl, H., Henn, F., . . . Wittchen, H. U. (2010). Frequency of dementia, depression, and other neuropsychiatric symptoms in 1,449 outpatients with Parkinson's disease. *Journal of Neurology, 257*(7), 1073–1082.

Roos, R. A. (2010). Huntington's disease: a clinical review. *Orphanet Journal of Rare Diseases, 5*(1), 40.

Sahin, H. A., Terzi, M., Ucak, S., Yapici, O., Basoglu, T., & Onar, M. (2006). Frontal functions in young patients with essential tremor: a case comparison study. *Journal of Neuropsychiatry & Clinical Neuroscience, 18*(1), 64–72.

Sanders, C., Egger, M., Donovan, J., Tallon, D., & Frankel, S. (1998). Reporting on quality of life in randomised controlled trials: bibliographic study. *British Medical Journal, 317*(7167), 1191–1194.

Sandvik, U., Koskinen, L. O., Lundquist, A., & Blomstedt, P. (2012). Thalamic and subthalamic deep brain stimulation for essential tremor: where is the optimal target? *Neurosurgery, 70*(4), 840–845; discussion 845–846.

Sasso, E., Perucca, E., Fava, R., & Calzetti, S. (1991). Quantitative comparison of barbiturates in essential hand and head tremor. *Movement Disorders, 6*(1), 65–68.

Saunders-Pullman, R., Shriberg, J., Heiman, G., Raymond, D., Wendt, K., Kramer, P., . . . Bressman, S. B. (2002). Myoclonus dystonia: possible association with obsessive-compulsive disorder and alcohol dependence. *Neurology, 58*(2), 242–245.

Schneier, F. R., Barnes, L. F., Albert, S. M., & Louis, E. D. (2001). Characteristics of social phobia among persons with essential tremor. *Journal of Clinical Psychiatry, 62*(5), 367–372.

Scholz, H., Benes, H., Happe, S., Bengel, J., Kohnen, R., & Hornyak, M. (2011). Psychological distress of patients suffering from restless legs syndrome: a cross-sectional study. *Health & Quality of Life Outcomes, 9*, 73.

Scholz, H., Trenkwalder, C., Kohnen, R., Riemann, D., Kriston, L., & Hornyak, M. (2011a). Dopamine agonists for restless legs syndrome. *Cochrane Database Systematic Review* (3), CD006009.

Scholz, H., Trenkwalder, C., Kohnen, R., Riemann, D., Kriston, L., & Hornyak, M. (2011b). Levodopa for restless legs syndrome. *Cochrane Database Systematic Review* (2), CD005504.

Schrag, A., Geser, F., Stampfer-Kountchev, M., Seppi, K., Sawires, M., Kollensperger, M., . . . Wenning, G. K. (2006). Health-related quality of life in multiple system atrophy. *Movement Disorders, 21*(6), 809–815.

Schrag, A., Jahanshahi, M., & Quinn, N. (2000). What contributes to quality of life in patients with Parkinson's disease? *Journal of Neurology, Neurosurgery and Psychiatry, 69*(3), 308–312.

Schrag, A., Jahanshahi, M., & Quinn, N. P. (2001). What contributes to depression in Parkinson's disease? *Psychology & Medicine, 31*(1), 65–73.

Schrag, A., Selai, C., Mathias, C., Low, P., Hobart, J., Brady, N., & Quinn, N. P. (2007). Measuring health-related quality of life in MSA: the MSA-QoL. *Movement Disorders, 22*(16), 2332–2338.

Schrag, A., Selai, C., Quinn, N., Lees, A., Litvan, I., Lang, A.,... Hobart, J. (2006). Measuring quality of life in PSP: the PSP-QoL. *Neurology, 67*(1), 39–44.

Schrag, A., Sheikh, S., Quinn, N. P., Lees, A. J., Selai, C., Mathias, C.,...Jahanshahi, M. (2010). A comparison of depression, anxiety, and health status in patients with progressive supranuclear palsy and multiple system atrophy. *Movement Disorders, 25*(8), 1077–1081.

Schulzer, M., Mak, E., & Calne, S. M. (2003). The psychometric properties of the Parkinson's Impact Scale (PIMS) as a measure of quality of life in Parkinson's disease. *Parkinsonism & Related Disorders, 9*(5), 291–294.

Shiba, M., Bower, J. H., Maraganore, D. M., McDonnell, S. K., Peterson, B. J., Ahlskog, J. E.,... Rocca, W. A. (2000). Anxiety disorders and depressive disorders preceding Parkinson's disease: a case-control study. *Movement Disorders, 15*(4), 669–677.

Shoulson, I., & Fahn, S. (1979). Huntington disease: clinical care and evaluation. *Neurology, 29*(1), 1–3.

Sintonen, H. (2001). The 15D instrument of health-related quality of life: properties and applications. *Annals of Medicine, 33*(5), 328–336.

Skevington, S. M., Lotfy, M., & O'Connell, K. A. (2004). The World Health Organization's WHOQOL-BREF quality of life assessment: psychometric properties and results of the international field trial. A report from the WHOQOL group. *Quality of Life Research, 13*(2), 299–310.

Skogseid, I. M., Ramm-Pettersen, J., Volkmann, J., Kerty, E., Dietrichs, E., & Roste, G. K. (2012). Good long-term efficacy of pallidal stimulation in cervical dystonia: a prospective, observer-blinded study. *European Journal of Neurology, 19*(4), 610–615.

Snaith, A., & Wade, D. (2011). Dystonia. *Clinical Evidence (Online), 2011.*

Soeder, A., Kluger, B. M., Okun, M. S., Garvan, C. W., Soeder, T., Jacobson, C. E.,... Fernandez, H. H. (2009). Mood and energy determinants of quality of life in dystonia. *Journal of Neurology, 256*(6), 996–1001.

Soh, S. E., Morris, M. E., & McGinley, J. L. (2011). Determinants of health-related quality of life in Parkinson's disease: a systematic review. *Parkinsonism & Related Disorders, 17*(1), 1–9.

Spottke, E. A., Volkmann, J., Lorenz, D., Krack, P., Smala, A. M., Sturm, V.,... Dodel, R. C. (2002). Evaluation of healthcare utilization and health status of patients with Parkinson's disease treated with deep brain stimulation of the subthalamic nucleus. *Journal of Neurology, 249*(6), 759–766.

Stamelou, M., Edwards, M. J., Hallett, M., & Bhatia, K. P. (2011). The non-motor syndrome of primary dystonia: clinical and pathophysiological implications. *Brain,* 135(Pt 6), 1668–1681.

Stolze, H., Petersen, G., Raethjen, J., Wenzelburger, R., & Deuschl, G. (2001). The gait disorder of advanced essential tremor. *Brain, 124*(Pt 11), 2278–2286.

Straits-Troster, K., Fields, J. A., Wilkinson, S. B., Pahwa, R., Lyons, K. E., Koller, W. C., & Troster, A. I. (2000). Health-related quality of life in Parkinson's disease after pallidotomy and deep brain stimulation. *Brain & Cognition, 42*(3), 399–416.

Suurmeijer, T. P., Reuvekamp, M. F., & Aldenkamp, B. P. (2001). Social functioning, psychological functioning, and quality of life in epilepsy. *Epilepsia, 42*(9), 1160–1168.

Swinn, L., Schrag, A., Viswanathan, R., Bloem, B. R., Lees, A., & Quinn, N. (2003). Sweating dysfunction in Parkinson's disease. *Movement Disorders, 18*(12), 1459–1463.

Tan, E. K., Fook-Chong, S., Lum, S. Y., Gabriel, C., Koh, K. K., Prakash, K. M., & Louis, E. D. (2005). Non-motor manifestations in essential tremor: Use of a validated instrument to evaluate a wide spectrum of symptoms. *Parkinsonism & Related Disorders, 11*(6), 375–380.

Tandberg, E., Larsen, J. P., Aarsland, D., & Cummings, J. L. (1996). The occurrence of depression in Parkinson's disease. A community-based study. *Archives of Neurology, 53*(2), 175–179.

Thawani, S. P., Schupf, N., & Louis, E. D. (2009). Essential tremor is associated with dementia: prospective population-based study in New York. *Neurology, 73*(8), 621–625.

Tibben, A. (2007). Predictive testing for Huntington's disease. *Brain Research Bulletin, 72*(2-3), 165–171.

Trenkwalder, C., Benes, H., Grote, L., Happe, S., Hogl, B., Mathis, J.,... Kohnen, R. (2007). Cabergoline compared to levodopa in the treatment of patients with severe restless legs syndrome: results from a multi-center, randomized, active controlled trial. *Movement Disorders, 22*(5), 696–703.

Trenkwalder, C., Garcia-Borreguero, D., Montagna, P., Lainey, E., de Weerd, A. W., Tidswell, P.,... Ferini-Strambi, L. (2004). Ropinirole in the treatment of restless legs syndrome: results from the TREAT RLS 1 study, a 12 week, randomised, placebo controlled study in 10 European countries. *Journal of Neurology, Neurosurgery and Psychiatry, 75*(1), 92–97.

Trenkwalder, C., Hening, W. A., Montagna, P., Oertel, W. H., Allen, R. P., Walters, A. S.,... Sampaio, C. (2008). Treatment of restless legs syndrome: an evidence-based review and implications for clinical practice. *Movement Disorders, 23*(16), 2267–2302.

Trenkwalder, C., Stiasny, K., Pollmacher, T., Wetter, T., Schwarz, J., Kohnen, R.,... et al. (1995). L-dopa therapy of uremic and idiopathic restless legs syndrome: a double-blind, crossover trial. *Sleep, 18*(8), 681–688.

Troster, A. I., Fields, J. A., Pahwa, R., Wilkinson, S. B., Strait-Troster, K. A., Lyons, K.,... Koller, W. C. (1999). Neuropsychological and quality of life outcome after thalamic stimulation for essential tremor. *Neurology, 53*(8), 1774–1780.

Troster, A. I., Fields, J. A., Wilkinson, S., Pahwa, R., Koller, W. C., & Lyons, K. E. (2003). Effect of motor improvement on quality of life following subthalamic stimulation is mediated by changes in depressive symptomatology. *Stereotactic & Functional Neurosurgery, 80*(1-4), 43–47.

Troster, A. I., Pahwa, R., Fields, J. A., Tanner, C. M., & Lyons, K. E. (2005). Quality of life in Essential Tremor Questionnaire (QUEST): development and initial validation. *Parkinsonism & Related Disorders, 11*(6), 367–373.

Troster, A. I., Woods, S. P., Fields, J. A., Lyons, K. E., Pahwa, R., Higginson, C. I., & Koller, W. C. (2002). Neuropsychological deficits in essential tremor: an expression of cerebello-thalamo-cortical pathophysiology? *European Journal of Neurology, 9*(2), 143–151.

Trottenberg, T., Meissner, W., Kabus, C., Arnold, G., Funk, T., Einhaupl, K. M., & Kupsch, A. (2001). Neurostimulation of the ventral intermediate thalamic nucleus in inherited myoclonus-dystonia syndrome. *Movement Disorders, 16*(4), 769–771.

Trottenberg, T., Volkmann, J., Deuschl, G., Kuhn, A. A., Schneider, G. H., Muller, J.,... Kupsch, A. (2005). Treatment of severe tardive dystonia with pallidal deep brain stimulation. *Neurology, 64*(2), 344–346.

Van den Berg, M. (1998). Leben mit Parkinson: Entwicklung und psychometrische Testung des Fragenbogens PLQ. *Neurological Rehabilitation, 4*, 221–226.

Vidailhet, M., Vercueil, L., Houeto, J. L., Krystkowiak, P., Benabid, A. L., Cornu, P.,... Pollak, P. (2005). Bilateral deep-brain stimulation of the globus pallidus in primary generalized dystonia. *New England Journal of Medicine, 352*(5), 459–467.

Vignatelli, L., Billiard, M., Clarenbach, P., Garcia-Borreguero, D., Kaynak, D., Liesiene, V.,... Montagna, P. (2006). EFNS guidelines on management of restless legs syndrome and periodic limb movement disorder in sleep. *European Journal of Neurology, 13*(10), 1049–1065.

Voon, V., Butler, T. R., Ekanayake, V., Gallea, C., Ameli, R., Murphy, D. L., & Hallett, M. (2010). Psychiatric symptoms associated with focal hand dystonia. *Movement Disorders, 25*(13), 2249–2252.

Voon, V., Schoerling, A., Wenzel, S., Ekanayake, V., Reiff, J., Trenkwalder, C., & Sixel-Doring, F. (2011). Frequency of impulse control behaviours associated with dopaminergic therapy in restless legs syndrome. *BMC Neurology, 11*, 117.

Walker, R. H., Danisi, F. O., Swope, D. M., Goodman, R. R., Germano, I. M., & Brin, M. F. (2000). Intrathecal baclofen for dystonia: benefits and complications during six years of experience. *Movement Disorders, 15*(6), 1242–1247.

Ware, J. E., Jr., & Sherbourne, C. D. (1992). The MOS 36-item short-form health survey (SF-36). I. Conceptual framework and item selection. *Medical Care, 30*(6), 473–483.

Welsh, M., McDermott, M. P., Holloway, R. G., Plumb, S., Pfeiffer, R., & Hubble, J. (2003). Development and testing of the Parkinson's disease quality of life scale. *Movement Disorders, 18*(6), 637–645.

Welsh, M. D., Dorflinger, E., Chernik, D., & Waters, C. (2000). Illness impact and adjustment to Parkinson's disease: before and after treatment with tolcapone. *Movement Disorders, 15*(3), 497–502.

Wenning, G. K., Geser, F., Stampfer-Kountchev, M., & Tison, F. (2003). Multiple system atrophy: an update. *Movement Disorders, 18 Suppl 6*, S34–42.

Wenning, G. K., Litvan, I., & Tolosa, E. (2011). Milestones in atypical and secondary Parkinsonisms. *Movement Disorders, 26*(6), 1083–1095.

WHOQOL Group. (1996). *What Quality of Life?* Paper presented at the World Health Forum, Geneva.

Williams, D. R., & Lees, A. J. (2009). Progressive supranuclear palsy: clinicopathological concepts and diagnostic challenges. *Lancet Neurology, 8*(3), 270–279.

Winkelman, J. W., Redline, S., Baldwin, C. M., Resnick, H. E., Newman, A. B., & Gottlieb, D. J. (2009). Polysomnographic and health-related quality of life correlates of restless legs syndrome in the Sleep Heart Health Study. *Sleep, 32*(6), 772–778.

Winkelmann, J., Czamara, D., Schormair, B., Knauf, F., Schulte, E. C., Trenkwalder, C., ... Meitinger, T. (2012). Genome-wide association study identifies novel restless legs syndrome susceptibility loci on 2p14 and 16q12.1. *PLoS Genet, 7*(7), e1002171.

Winkelmann, J., & Ferini-Strambi, L. (2006). Genetics of restless legs syndrome. *Sleep Medicine Review, 10*(3), 179–183.

Winkelmann, J., Prager, M., Lieb, R., Pfister, H., Spiegel, B., Wittchen, H. U., ... Strohle, A. (2005). "Anxietas tibiarum". Depression and anxiety disorders in patients with restless legs syndrome. *Journal of Neurology, 252*(1), 67–71.

Winkler, G. F., & Young, R. R. (1974). Efficacy of chronic propranolol therapy in action tremors of the familial, senile or essential varieties. *New England Journal of Medicine, 290*(18), 984–988.

Woods, S. P., Fields, J. A., Lyons, K. E., Koller, W. C., Wilkinson, S. B., Pahwa, R., & Troster, A. I. (2001). Neuropsychological and quality of life changes following unilateral thalamic deep brain stimulation in Parkinson's disease: a one-year follow-up. *Acta Neurochirurgica (Wien), 143*(12), 1273–1277; discussion 1278.

Woods, S. P., Scott, J. C., Fields, J. A., Poquette, A., & Troster, A. I. (2008). Executive dysfunction and neuropsychiatric symptoms predict lower health status in essential tremor. *Cognitive & Behavioral Neurology, 21*(1), 28–33.

Yeh, P., Walters, A. S., & Tsuang, J. W. (2011). Restless legs syndrome: A comprehensive overview on its epidemiology, risk factors, and treatment. *Sleep Breath, 16*(4), 987–1007.

Zesiewicz, T. A., Elble, R., Louis, E. D., Hauser, R. A., Sullivan, K. L., Dewey, R. B., Jr., ... Weiner, W. J. (2005). Practice parameter: therapies for essential tremor: report of the Quality Standards Subcommittee of the American Academy of Neurology. *Neurology, 64*(12), 2008–2020.

Zesiewicz, T. A., Ward, C. L., Hauser, R. A., Salemi, J. L., Siraj, S., Wilson, M. C., & Sullivan, K. L. (2007). A pilot, double-blind, placebo-controlled trial of pregabalin (Lyrica) in the treatment of essential tremor. *Movement Disorders, 22*(11), 1660–1663.

Zetterberg, L., Aquilonius, S. M., & Lindmark, B. (2009). Impact of dystonia on quality of life and health in a Swedish population. *Acta Neurologica Scandinavica, 119*(6), 376–382.

PART TWO

PARKINSON'S DISEASE AND PARKINSON'S DISEASE WITH DEMENTIA

5 Neuropathology, Biomarkers, and Cognition in Parkinson's Disease

Eiron Cudaback, Brenna A. Cholerton, Kathleen S. Montine, and Thomas J. Montine

INTRODUCTION

The British physician Dr. James Parkinson first described the now eponymous idiopathic malady of aged individuals almost two hundred years ago in his treatise of observations titled "An Essay on the Shaking Palsy" (reprinted in Parkinson, 2002). Figure 5-1 shows a classic illustration of Parkinson's disease (PD) from 1866. In particular, Parkinson noted the profound impact that disease-associated discordant movements imposed on the daily activities of affected individuals. Although Parkinson definitively stated that the minds of the six subjects he observed remained "uninjured" by their disorder (Parkinson, 2002), it is now widely accepted that non-motor symptoms, especially those constituting diminished cognitive capacity, contribute significantly to the overall burden suffered by patients with PD during all phases of disease progression.

Although nondemented PD patients commonly present with a vast heterogeneity of cognitive impairments, especially marked are those deficits associated with executive function. Included in this cognitive domain are the various goal-driven behaviors underlying the purposeful planning, execution, monitoring, and switching of tasks, as well as the general awareness of intent and appropriateness, particularly in the context of psychosocial settings. In addition to the resultant spectrum of dysexecutive symptoms, PD patients frequently report diminished visuospatial and working memory capacities, attention deficits, and depression-independent

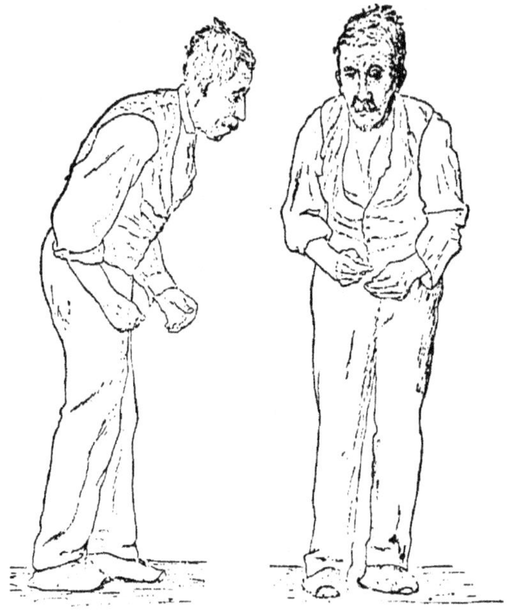

FIGURE 5-1
Illustration of Parkinson's disease by William Richard Gowers. First published in *A Manual of Diseases of the Nervous System (1866).*

emotional blunting including apathy and anhedonia. However, significant controversy persists among behavioral investigators over whether these additional neuropsychological sequelae comprise discrete impairments beyond the influence of the circumscribed executive suite. Nonetheless, current estimates forecast a greater than fivefold risk of dementia in PD patients compared to the general population, underscoring the importance of characterizing neuropathologic correlates of PD-associated cognitive impairment. Indeed, the early cognitive impairment seen in PD patients prior to motor symptom presentation is highly predictive of the dementia frequently observed during later disease stages.

NEUROPATHOLOGIC LESIONS OF PARKINSON'S DISEASE

Gross examination of the PD brain rarely illuminates disease, and not until nearly a full century after Parkinson's initial observations did the German-born neurologist Fritz Heinrich Lewy first describe the microscopic neuronal inclusions that are now considered the neuropathologic hallmark of the disorder. These inclusions, known as Lewy bodies (Figure 5-2), were originally identified by staining with the acidic dye eosin, likewise being insoluble in various organic solvents, suggesting a highly ordered protein composition. Although inextricably associated with PD, Lewy bodies can be distributed throughout the diseased brain, confounding efforts to determine the anatomic origin and progression of the disease.

Within decades of Lewy's findings, and in addition to the reported widespread characteristic Lewy body pathology, a significant loss of pigment was noted in the substantia nigra of PD subjects, eventually leading to speculation that neuron loss from this brain stem region was causal for PD-related motor symptoms. Indeed, postmortem analyses of PD brains confirm marked depigmentation (Figure 5-3) due to extensive loss of dopaminergic (substantia nigra) and noradrenergic (locus coeruleus) projections from brain stem, a finding thought to parallel in time the onset of PD motor symptoms, and possibly even the observed cognitive deficits (discussed below). Nevertheless, the correlation between initial motor symptoms and brainstem pathology led many to hypothesize that PD neuropathology begins in the substantia nigra pars compacta, subsequently radiating to eventually affect more distal cortical structures. Braak and Braak (Braak et al., 2003) attempted to characterize more precisely the spatial aspects of disease progression, and ultimately developed a neuropathologic staging paradigm for PD in which disease appears to originate in the dorsal motor nucleus of the vagus nerve, to advance rostrally through the pons and basal forebrain, and eventually to involve neocortical structures. However, in light of sporadic PD cases to the contrary, as well as documented early neuropsychological changes, such presumptions have been revisited with some favoring a more ubiquitous etiology over the assumed diaspora out of the brain stem and midbrain. Lending further neuropathologic support to the clinical observation of PD-associated cognitive impairment, extranigral Lewy body disease also has been confirmed in the basal forebrain, limbic structures, and various cerebral cortical regions. Yet even with

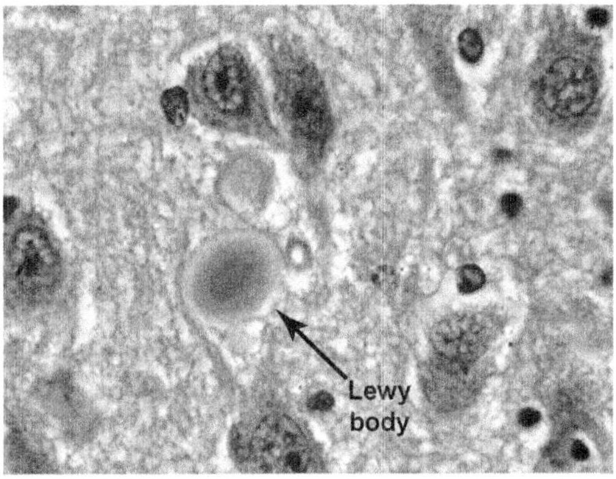

FIGURE 5-2
Lewy body (Kondi Wong, Armed Forces Institute of Pathology; www.genome.gov).

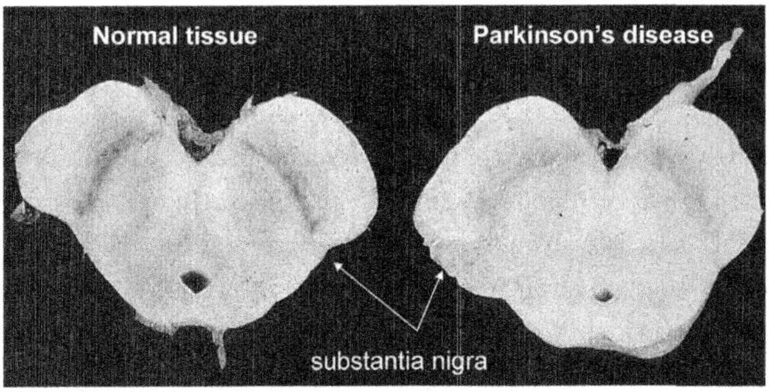

FIGURE 5-3
Depigmentation of the substantia nigra in Parkinson's disease (note the pallor in the right compared to left image).

nearly two centuries of intense investigation, the clinical diagnosis of PD, like many other neurodegenerative diseases, has continued to represent a significant challenge, even to highly trained specialists.

The 19th century French neurologist Charcot originally enumerated four cardinal symptoms of PD: bradykinesia, rigidity, resting tremor, and postural instability. As a testament to the significant relationship between these classic motor deficits and the underlying disease, Charcot's original observations still form the basis for clinical diagnosis of PD. However, while reasonably objective indicators of specific neuropathologic changes, these classical presentations are more indicative of established disease, and, therefore, offer somewhat limited utility for early detection, prognosis, and effective prevention. Furthermore, confirmation of diagnostic accuracy is still mostly substantiated after postmortem pathologic findings are correlated with antemortem clinical observations. Therefore, identification of molecular determinants specific to PD pathologic changes, as well as relevant nonmotor prodromes, especially cognitive impairment, would be of particular clinical importance.

Not until the 1990s and a sweeping scientific revolution in human genetics were the unique molecular determinants underlying PD neuropathologic changes revealed. Of particular interest, missense mutations detected in the alpha synuclein gene (*SNCA*) were found to correlate with the inheritance of more severe autosomal-dominant forms of PD (Kruger et al., 1998; Michell et al., 2005; Polymeropoulos et al., 1997; Zarranz et al., 2004). In addition to mutations, *SNCA* duplications (Ahn et al., 2008; Chartier-Harlin et al., 2004; Elia et al., 2003; Fuchs et al., 2007; Nishioka et al., 2009) also are associated with earlier onset and more rapid progression of PD symptoms, including cognitive impairment and dementia. More recently, a link between discreet nucleotide variations in *SNCA* and sporadic cases of PD have been confirmed in large genome-wide association studies (Nalls et al., 2011). However, while genetics can enlighten disease risk and prognosis, the mechanistic relationship between the *SNCA* product, alpha synuclein, and PD pathogenesis remains to be clarified fully.

Nearly a decade before *SNCA* was unequivocally implicated in the inheritance of familial PD, it was cloned from electric eel and rodent CNS (Maroteaux, Campanelli & Scheller,1988). Alpha-synuclein is a 140 amino acid cytoplasmic protein that is predominantly found associated with vesicle membranes in presynaptic neuron terminals, with marked expression seen in the substantia nigra, hippocampus, and neocortex. Although the physiological function of alpha-synuclein remains unclear, animal studies strongly suggest an essential role in neurotransmission. Furthermore, although principally cytoplasmic, alpha-synuclein has been detected in various biological fluids, including cerebral spinal fluid (CSF), plasma, urine, and saliva, strongly suggesting that it may be actively secreted from neurons. Of particular significance to PD, a major protein constituent of Lewy body inclusions was identified as an aggregated form of alpha-synuclein, directly implicating abnormal alpha-synuclein function in PD etiology and disease progression. Although additional aggregated proteins have been identified as components of Lewy body inclusions, including but not limited to neurofilament and ubiquitin, significant emphasis has been placed on the potential pleiotropy that alpha-synuclein exerts on PD pathogenesis.

BIOMARKERS

Biomarkers represent uniformly objective measures or laboratory tests used for the identification of molecular and structural signatures of normal physiology or disease. Because significant strides have been made toward the identification of clinically relevant biomarkers in Alzheimer's disease (AD) pathogenesis, it is hoped that PD is poised for similar success. Indeed, few current diagnostic laboratory tests exist for the definitive assessment and prognosis of neurodegenerative diseases, and, in the case of PD, clinical diagnosis wholly relies on the identification of classical motor symptoms in affected individuals. Interestingly, motor deficits have been observed to be coincident with widespread neuropathologic changes, including marked reductions in dopaminergic projections from the substantia nigra, suggesting that significant pathologic changes likely precede these clinically defining motor disturbances. Associated nonmotor prodromes are highly variable in both presentation and onset, and are presumed to derive in part from the more expansive disease pattern. However, the neuropsychological and neuropsychiatric changes frequently observed in preclinical PD tend to be nonspecific in nature, making it difficult to differentiate stochastic or PD-independent alterations in cognition and behavior from those deficits linked to PD, and so complicate the underlying clinical utility of their assessment. In addition, although evaluation of such early-stage clinical determinants for PD may provide significant diagnostic and prognostic utility, cognitive prodromes can be especially subtle so as not to register on the more subjective psychometric analyses frequently employed. Thus the development of reproducibly sensitive metrics for detection and assessment of early-stage PD-associated changes in cognition would provide an opportunity for more reliable risk assessment, early diagnosis, and disease stage, in addition to widening the therapeutic window for effective intervention strategies.

Biomarkers derived from biological fluids, including cerebral spinal fluid (CSF), blood, urine, and saliva, offer the greatest clinical utility for PD assessment given the relative ease with which practitioners are able to procure samples for analysis. Particularly promising is the fact that alpha-synuclein is detectable in these fluids, and appears to be associated with Lewy body accumulation, and therefore with PD. Unfortunately, specificity for PD has been questioned since significant overlap appears to exist with multiple system atrophy (Shi et al., 2011; Tateno et al., 2012), in addition to more recently inconsistent findings in CSF (Constantinescu & Mondello, 2012). Genetics studies have likewise implicated the *PARK7* gene in familial PD pathogenesis, therefore drawing interest toward the resulting gene product as a potential biomarker candidate in sporadic PD. Indeed, *PARK7* encodes DJ-1, a protein of unknown but critical function found in a variety of body fluids (Lin et al., 2012). There is also significant interest in the PD translation of established AD biomarkers, such as amyloid beta ($A\beta_{42}$) and tau protein, due to the overlapping clinical relationship with disease-associated cognitive deficits. As with α-synuclein, PD-associated CSF levels of DJ-1 (Hong et al., 2010; Shi et al., 2011), $A\beta_{42}$ (Leverenz et al/, 2011; Mollenhauer et al., 2006), and total tau (Mollenhauer et al., 2011; Shi et al., 2011) have all been investigated as potential markers for preclinical PD. As with alpha-synuclein, conflicting data exists as to the particular association, and disease selectivity remains a legitimate concern (Constantinescu & Mondello, 2012; Gonzalez-Cuyar et al., 2011). Taken together, however, one could imagine that measurement inconsistency and a lack of disease specificity suggest the need to pursue a more multi-faceted approach, including several relevant biomarkers instead of a single measurement.

In an attempt to assess the efficacy of putative PD biomarkers, we have previously suggested (Gonzalez-Cuyar et al., 2011; Sonnen, Montine, Quinn, Breitner, & Montine, 2010) the following multilevel ranking for biomarker development (a) initial observation—disease association with expert diagnosis, which may include postmortem classification of disease; (b) confirmation—replication of the initial observation in independent sample that includes multiple related diseases; (c) validation— multisite replication in independent samples; (d) clinical research—standardization of bioassay and use as disease endpoint in clinical research; and (e) primary care— adopted as part of the standard care in primary clinical settings. Currently, PD biomarker discovery and development is in the early stages between initial observation and confirmation. In the next section, we focus on neuropathologic changes of cognitive dysfunction in PD and the current evidence for proposed biomarkers.

COGNITIVE DYSFUNCTION AND NEUROPATHOLOGY IN PD

Cognitive impairment is increasingly recognized as a pervasive and debilitating component of Parkinson's disease (PD). Although historically associated primarily with dopamine depletion in the substantia nigra, recent findings that relate extranigral and cortical dysfunction to the development and progression of cognitive impairment in PD challenge the long-held assertion that cognitive dysfunction in PD is purely "subcortical" in nature. Indeed, numerous neuropathologic processes working both in conjunction with and independently from one another have been related to cognitive function in PD, including accumulation of Lewy body inclusions, disruptions to multiple neurotransmitter systems, and other disease processes such as Alzheimer disease pathologic changes and vascular brain injury. Cognitive changes in patients with PD are heterogeneous in presentation and progression, and thus likely reflect the multiple neuropathologic processes.

Lewy Body Inclusions and Alpha-Synuclein

Characterization of alpha-synuclein now allows for more accurate Lewy body identification using immunostaining, especially extranigral pathologic changes.

Recent results reported by large, community-based autopsy cohort studies provide support for an association between Lewy body accumualtion and cognitive test performance in the general population. In the combined community-based Rush Religious Orders/Memory and Aging cohorts, neocortical (but not limbic or striatal) Lewy bodies were associated with faster global cognitive decline and increased dementia risk, while limbic Lewy bodies were independently associated with worse performance on visuospatial tasks (Schneider et al., 2012). In contrast, findings from the Adult Changes in Thought cohort demonstrated that Lewy body formation in the cortex and striatum were strongly associated with a simple visuo-contruction task, and, to a lesser extent, performance on language-related measures, but not to global cognition (Cholerton et al., 2013). However, although community-based autopsy studies support an association between Lewy body neuropathology and cognition, extensive Lewy body accumulation in the cortex may not always confer significant cognitive decline and dementia in PD patients. Although a number of PD-specific clinicopathologic studies have demonstrated correlations between Braak staging of Lewy body formation and dementia, global cognition, and episodic memory (Aarsland, Brown, Larsen, & Ballard, 2005; Irwin et al., 2012; Mattila, Rhinne, Helenius, Dickson, & Roytta, 2000), others suggest that the presence of substantial Lewy bodies alone does not necessarily lead to clinical symptoms of cognitive decline (Braak, Ryb, Jansen Steur, Del Tredici, & de Vos, 2005; Colosimo, Hughes, Kilford, & Lees, 2003; Parkkinen, Pirttila, Tervahauta, & Alafuzoff, 2005).

Routine identification of brain stem Lewy body pathology, especially in medulla, pons, and midbrain, can be accomplished effectively using standard histologic techniques. However, progressive extranigral pathologic changes associated with amygdala, cingulate gyrus, and neocortex, proves a more significant challenge for detection. In addition to fostering increased understanding of the molecular basis for PD pathogenesis, characterization of alpha-synuclein also has allowed for the development of more accurate and sensitive immunohistochemical approaches to Lewy body detection in brain regions most likely associated with early- as well as late-stage cognitive impairment. Therefore, similarly powerful analytic methodologies provide an opportunity to delineate clearly the associations between key neuropathologic changes and cognitive deficits in PD subjects.

Autopsy studies may obscure the relationship between alpha-synuclein accumulation and cognitive test performance or dementia status prior to death given that, by the time of autopsy, Lewy body accumulation is likely to be extensive in the brains of PD patients. Very few studies to date, however, have examined the relationship between CSF alpha-synuclein and cognition. PD patients have lower levels of CSF alpha-synuclein than patients with other neurological disorders and controls (Mollenhauer et al., 2011); however, correlations between alpha-synuclein and global cognitive test performance have been shown in dementia with Lewy bodies (DLB), Alzheimer's disease (AD), and mild cognitive impairment, but not necessarily PD (Korff, Liu, Ginghina, Shi, & Zhang, 2013; Reesink et al., 2010). Further studies are thus needed to determine whether early accumulation of alpha-synuclein correlates with specific measures of cognitive decline.

Disruption to Neurotransmitter Systems

Dopaminergic Loss and Damage to the Fronto-Striatal Pathways

Recent neuroimaging studies confirm previous postmortem observations relating cognitive impairment in nondemented PD subjects to striatal hypofunction, reduced radiotracer uptake by caudate and putamen specifically (Cropley et al., 2008; Jokinen, Bruck, Aalto, Forsback, Parkkola, & Rinne, 2009) and subsequent disruption of projecting fronto-striatal pathways. The earliest cognitive alterations reported in PD, namely subtle dys-executive symptoms consisting of mild impairments in attention, working memory, and processing speed, seem to parallel the initial loss of dopamine in the substantia nigra and subsequent impact on the fronto-striatal pathways that support executive function. Dopamine is associated with reward-related learning, cognitive flexibility, action planning, working memory, set shifting, and other executive processes (Kulisevsky, 2000). Reductions in dopamine transporter (DAT) density in the caudate nucleus are associated with impaired memory and executive function, and predict later executive, visuospatial, language, and verbal memory decline. Of note, however, more specific predictive ability was found when DAT findings were combined with other measures (e.g., DAT and perfusion on SPECT imaging in posterior cortical regions areas predicted language and verbal memory decline) (Arnaldi et al., 2012). Thus, although initial brain stem reductions in dopamine may predict later cognitive dysfunction, neuropathologic changes occurring elsewhere in the brain likely serve to increase the variability in cognitive performance seen in PD patients.

Loss of dopamine in the substantia nigra leading to insufficient dopamine in the nonmotor frontostriatal pathways is perhaps the most strongly implicated neuropathologic feature underpinning the pervasive executive dysfunction seen in early PD. These pathways, including the dorsolateral prefrontal, anterior cingulate, and orbitofrontal circuits have all been implicated, to varying degrees, in performance on multiple measures of executive functioning in PD (Nobili et al., 2010; Zgaljardic et al., 2006). Working memory, a primary neuropsychological function subserved by the frontostriatal pathways, correlated with reduced signal on fMRI in cognitively impaired PD subjects as compared to those without cognitive impairments (Lewis, Dove, Robbins, Barker, & Owen, 2003). In nondemented drug naïve patients with early PD, impaired verbal fluency impairment correlated not only with reduced dopamine in the caudate nucleus, but also with metabolism in the dorsolateral prefrontal and anterior cingulate circuits (Polito et al., 2012). Further, Niethammer and colleagues (Niethammer et al., 2013) demonstrated that a loss of dopamine in the frontostriatal circuits correlated with the expression of a validated PD "cognition related metabolic pattern." Overall, defects in the frontostriatal pathways, resulting primarily from dopamine loss in the brainstem, are often seen as the primary causative factor in early cognitive deficits associated with PD.

Although initial cognitive deficits in PD are most likely related to striatal dopamine loss, dopamine levels and dopamine receptor expression in the prefrontal cortex may also play a modulatory role in cognition. Cortical dopamine levels are not consistently reduced early in PD, although as the disease progresses dopamine receptor expression and overall levels in the cortex are altered (Sawamoto et al., 2008). Dopamine D1 receptors are found abundantly in the prefrontal cortex, and recent human imaging studies suggest that too little or too much activation of the D1 receptors in the prefrontal cortex can lead to impairment on the Wisconsin Card Sorting task (Takahashi, Yamada, & Suhara, 2012), a finding that has implications for individual management of PD symptoms with currently available treatments. D2 and D3 receptors are also associated with various executive cognitive functions, including memory, attention, learning, processing speed, task-switching, response inhibition, social recognition, and others (Stelzel, Fiebach, Cools, Tafazoli, & D'Esposito, 2013; van Holstein et al., 2011). Blockade of D3 receptors improves cognition, thus possibly providing one explanation for why impaired cognition can occur with certain dopamine agonists (Nakajima et al., 2013).

Cholinergic Degeneration in the Basal Forebrain

Alpha-synuclein accumulation in the cholinergic neurons in the basal forebrain occurs early in the course of PD (Nobili et al., 2011). Ascending projections from the basal forebrain distribute acetycholine widely throughout the brain; disruptions in this system can lead to notable cognitive impairments, particularly in attention, learning, and memory, and these changes may occur in conjunction with and independently from striatal dopamine depletion (Pavese, Rivero-Bosch, Lewis, Whone, & Brooks, 2011). Recent animal models suggest that mice over-expressing alpha-synuclein show altered extracellular dopamine release and decreased cortical acetylcholine even prior to striatal dopamine loss, with concomitant changes in learning and recognition (Magen et al., 2012). In mice, simultaneous depletion of dopamine and acetylcholine led to greater impairments in attention and object recognition than either alone (Zurkovsky et al., 2013). Although cholinergic deficits are primarily associated with attention and learning, they may also provide another substrate for understanding the visual disruption that can occur in PD. Projections to the occipital visual cortex show early and substantial reductions in acetylcholine, and may provide a neuropathologic basis for the onset of visual hallucinations and other visuoperceptual impairments in PD (Kuhl et al., 1996). Of note, both visuospatial changes and acetylcholine degeneration are associated with later onset of dementia, providing further support for a role of cholinergic deficits in the development of dementia in PD (Bohnen & Albini, 2011). Notably, initial studies examining the effects of treatment with cholinesterase inhibitors on cognition in PD patients demonstrated that treated patients show greater improvements primarily in executive abilities (Dubois et al., 2012).

Norepinephrine

Beyond the cognitive deficits produced by the pathological hallmark of dopamine loss, it is important to note that disruptions to other monoaminergic systems occurring in PD either alongside, or as a result of, dopamine depletion, can have negative repercussions for cognition. Loss of locus coeruleus noradrenergic neurons also occurs early in the course of PD (possibly even years prior to the onset of motor symptoms), and may provide another substrate for the impairments in executive function seen in PD. In particular, impairments in the noradrenergic system have been implicated in cognitive inflexibility in both animal PD models and human studies (Kehagia, Murray, & Robbins, 2010; Vazey & Aston-Jones, 2012). Higher CSF norepinephrine levels also are associated with poorer performance on tests requiring attention, processing speed, and working memory in cognitively normal adults, lending support to the assertion that there is an optimal range of norepinephrine necessary to enhance working memory, whereas too much serves an inhibitory effect (Wang et al., 2013; Zhang, Cordeiro Matos, Jego, Admantidis, & Seguela, 2013).

Serotonin

Serotonin depletion also occurs in PD and may play a significant role in the psychiatric symptoms associated with PD; however, its effects on cognition are controversial and not well understood. Further, the serotonergic system may not be affected in early PD, and thus may not substantially impact initial changes in cognition (Scholtissen, Verhey, Steinbusch, & Leentjens, 2006). Given the potential impact of serotonergic disruptions on psychiatric syndromes, however, including mood disturbance, sleep-related impairments, and anxiety, indirect effects on executive and attentional processes may be associated with serotonin depletion.

Other Disease

AD Neuropathologic Changes

It has been hypothesized that AD-related abnormalities may interact with alpha-synuclein as a cause of dementia in some PD patients. This is supported by autopsy studies that demonstrate substantial overlap between AD and PD neuropathologic changes (Compta et al., 2011; Sabbagh et al., 2009), as well as experimental models that demonstrate increased cognitive decline in mice with abnormal Aβ, tau, and alpha-synuclein (Clinton, Blurton-Jones, Myczek, Trojanowski, & LaFerla, 2010). In addition, in a magnetic resonance imaging study, PD patients with a baseline pattern of atrophy consistent with an AD profile showed long-term global decline compared to those without this pattern (Weintraub et al., 2012). Genetic studies provide further support for this relationship: APOE ε4 genotype has been independently associated with cognitive decline and dementia in PD patients (Morley et al., 2012). Indeed, it has been suggested that although early changes in executive impairment in PD patients is primarily associated with prefrontal dysfunction, progression to dementia requires additional involvement of temporal-lobe structures (Pagonabarraga et al., 2012).

Other biomarker studies are less clear; however. There appears to be at least a subgroup of PD dementia patients with an AD-like cerebrospinal fluid (CSF) pattern of high tau and low Aβ (Buongiorno, Compta, & Marti, 2011; Montine et al., 2010). However, unlike AD, CSF total tau and phosphorylated tau181 were lower in patients with PD compared to controls in several large-scale studies (Alves et al., 2010; Montine et al., 2010; Shi et al., 2011). The relationship between CSF biomarkers and performance on specific cognitive tests is likewise mixed: $A\beta_{42}$ and the $A\beta_{42}$/t-tau ratio have been related to executive functions, memory, semantic fluency, and global cognitive decline (Alves et al., 2010; Leverenz et al., 2011; Siderowf et al., 2010). Tau-related CSF measures have been less typically associated with cognition (Alves et al., 2010; Siderowf et al., 2010), although some studies have shown a relationship between increased tau and global functioning, memory, naming, and executive functions (Compta et al., 2009; Leverenz et al., 2011).

Reports that evaluate brain amyloid imaging techniques in PD patients similarly show that only a subgroup of patients appears to have elevations in Pittsburgh compound B (PiB) that mirror AD (Petrou et al., 2012), although PiB uptake is higher in PD patients with dementia as compared to nondemented patients (Edison et al., 2008; Gomperts et al., 2008). Interestingly, PiB retention over time correlated with worse performance in executive function over time but not motor impairment (Gomperts et al., 2013). Taken together, research conducted to date suggests that AD pathophysiologic processes are related to and increase the risk for cognitive dysfunction in a subgroup of PD patients. Small sample size, stage of disease, cognitive measures incorporated, and included covariates may all contribute to the seemingly incongruent results presented to date, and additional prospective, longitudinal studies will help to elucidate the relationship between AD-related biomarkers and cognition in PD patients.

Vascular Neuropathology

Vascular brain injury is commonly comorbid in patients with idiopathic PD, and thus represents another potential source of variance in the cognitive profile of PD patients. The presence of microvascular lesions is increasingly indicated in overall dementia risk (Inaba et al., 2011), and population-based studies demonstrate associations between executive processes, memory, language, and visuospatial construction and the presence of cortical and subcortical lesions (Cholerton et al., 2013; Launer, Hughes, & White, 2011). White matter lesions may increase dementia risk specifically in PD patients, and have been associated with lower performance on tests of global cognition, executive functions, attention, learning, and memory (Marshall, Shchelchkov, Kaufer, Ivanco, & Bohnen, 2006; Melzer et al., 2013). Not all studies have found an association between vascular injury and cognition in PD, however; thus, the impact of such lesions on specific cognitive functions is likely influenced by their location and severity.

Other Cerebral Cortical Changes

Global cerebral cortical atrophy may be a marker for later dementia, and is associated with decline on global cognitive measures. Even in nondemented PD patients, cortical thinning is observed in frontal, temporal, parietal, and occipital lobes, and increases in those with cognitive impairment (Nishio et al., 2010). Localized imaging has shown that hippocampal atrophy occurs in PD, and is associated with reduced verbal memory performance in nondemented patients (Ibarretxe-Bilbao et al., 2008). Further, many patients with PD-related dementia exhibit hippocampal atrophy, thus suggesting that impairments in learning and memory might be expected later in the disease. Although several studies using advanced perfusion imaging techniques have identified regional hypoperfusion of brain regions especially critical for executive functions in cognitively impaired nondemented PD subjects, it remains unclear whether reduced local blood flow results from underlying PD-specific neuropathology or vice versa (Hattori et al., 2013).

Reduced cortical metabolism has been demonstrated in moderate to advanced PD patients in FDG PET studies, and recently these findings have been extended to include patients with early-stage disease (Borghammer, 2012). In PD patients with mild cognitive impairment, hypometabolism in frontal, parietal, and occipital regions in comparison with cognitively normal PD patients has been demonstrated (Pappata et al., 2011). Reductions in metabolism in both the frontal lobes and more posterior regions have been associated with impaired executive function, whereas visuospatial deficits are more specifically related to hypometabolism in occipitoparietal and temporal regions, memory with temporal and parietal regions, and language (naming and fluency) with frontal regions (Garcia-Garcia et al., 2012). It has been suggested by many that, although frontostriatal cognitive deficits are ubiquitous in PD, impairments related to more posterior areas (semantic fluency, memory, and visuospatial abilities) are more likely to herald the onset of dementia. Thus, imaging studies such as these may provide insight into those patients most likely to benefit from cognitive therapeutic interventions as such treatments become available.

CONCLUSION

Although discrete motor dysfunction has remained the clinical cornerstone of PD diagnosis for the better part of two centuries, mounting evidence strongly supports the existence of significant nonmotor symptoms throughout the disease course. Of particular interest, prodromal PD symptoms, especially cognitive impairment, may be reproducibly assessed for effective diagnostic utility. However, development of such clinical tools requires a thorough understanding of the molecular determinants that underlie PD and the specific role that each plays in disease progression. For this reason, the identification of conspicuous neuropathologic correlates for distinct changes in cognition and behavior associated with PD is critical for the development of early-stage detection strategies.

Indeed, successful biomarker discovery and development will continue to rely heavily on expanding neuropathologic approaches for PD and other neurodegenerative diseases.

FUTURE DIRECTIONS

Advanced age represents the greatest overall risk factor for the development of dementia-associated neurodegenerative diseases, including PD (Montine & Larsen, 2009). The rapidly advancing age of world populations underscores a therapeutic imperative, one reinforced by the current focus of significant scientific resource on cognitive impairment and dementia in PD. Yet, as revealed in this chapter, many questions remain.

- Can neuropathologic techniques or approaches advance and improve for the benefit of more informative PD diagnosis? Neuropathologic evaluation will continue to contribute to our understanding of disease in humans. Limitations inherent in postmortem examination can be addressed by coupling with animal model and clinical investigations that use biomarkers or imaging. Evolving quantitative molecularly specific approaches in neuropathology, especially in combination with genetic association studies, also will deepen our understanding of the relevant molecular mechanisms of disease (Postupna et al., 2012).
- Can PD-specific biomarkers achieve the same efficacy as their AD counterparts? The success achieved so far in the development of biomarkers for AD has clearly promoted confidence that similar goals can likely be realized in the PD arena. As with AD, however, significant resources will need to be made available if even reasonable objectives are to be met. Indeed, significant public and private support are evidenced by the promotion of a PD Biomarkers Identification Network (National Institute of Health) and the Parkinson's Progression Markers Initiative (Michael J. Fox Foundation).
- Will neuropathologic correlates of PD-associated cognitive impairment eventually lead to the development of highly predictive biomarkers? As presented in this chapter, the evidence for specific neuropathologic signatures of prodromal cognitive impairment in PD is accumulating, and by extension, relevant biomarker development is within our grasp. Intelligent strategy, resources, and persistence are the ingredients necessary for success.

REFERENCES

Aarsland, D., Perry, R., Brown, A., Larsen, J. P., & Ballard, C. (2005). Neuropathology of dementia in Parkinson's disease: a prospective, community-based study. *Annals of Neurology, 58*, 773–776.

Ahn, T. B., Kim, S. Y., Kim, J. Y., Park, S. S., Lee, D. S., Min, H. J.,...Jeon, B. S. (2008). alpha-Synuclein gene duplication is present in sporadic Parkinson disease. *Neurology, 70*, 43–49.

Alves, G., Bronnick, K., Aarsland, D., Blennow, K., Zetterberg, H., Ballard, C., ... Mulugeta, E. (2010). CSF amyloid-beta and tau proteins, and cognitive performance, in early and untreated Parkinson's disease: the Norwegian ParkWest study. *Journal Of Neurology Neurosurgery and Psychiatry, 81*, 1080–1086.

Arnaldi, D., Campus, C., Ferrara, M., Fama, F., Picco, A., De Carli, F., ... Nobili, F. (2012). What predicts cognitive decline in de novo Parkinson's disease? *Neurobiology of Aging, 33*, e11–20.

Bohnen, N. I., & Albin, R. L. (2011). The cholinergic system and Parkinson disease. *Behavioural Brain Research, 221*, 564–573.

Borghammer, P. (2012). Perfusion and metabolism imaging studies in Parkinson's disease. *Danish Medical Journal, 59*, B4466.

Braak, H., Del Tredici, K., Rub, U., de Vos, R. A., Jansen Steur, E. N., & Braak, E. (2003). Staging of brain pathology related to sporadic Parkinson's disease. *Neurobiology of Aging, 24*, 197–211.

Braak, H., Rub, U., Jansen Steur, E. N., Del Tredici, K., & de Vos, R. A. (2005). Cognitive status correlates with neuropathologic stage in Parkinson disease. *Neurology, 64*, 1404–1410.

Buongiorno, M., Compta, Y., & Marti, M. J. (2011). Amyloid-beta and tau biomarkers in Parkinson's disease-dementia. *Journal of the Neurological Sciences, 310*, 25–30.

Chartier-Harlin, M. C., Kachergus, J., Roumier, C., Mouroux, V., Douay, X., Lincoln, S., ... Destee A. (2004). Alpha-synuclein locus duplication as a cause of familial Parkinson's disease. *Lancet, 364*, 1167–1169.

Cholerton, B., Larson, E. B., Baker, L. D., Craft, S., Crane, P. K., Millard, S. P., ... Montine, T, J. (2013). Neuropathologic correlates of cognition in a population-based sample. *Journal of Alzheimer's Disease, 36*, 699–709.

Clinton, L. K., Blurton-Jones, M., Myczek, K., Trojanowski, J. Q., & LaFerla, F. M. (2010). Synergistic Interactions between Abeta, tau, and alpha-synuclein: acceleration of neuropathology and cognitive decline. *Journal of the Neurological Sciences, 30*, 7281–7289.

Colosimo, C., Hughes, A. J., Kilford, L., & Lees, A. J. (2003). Lewy body cortical involvement may not always predict dementia in Parkinson's disease. *Journal of Neurology Neurosurgery and Psychiatry, 74*, 852–856.

Compta, Y., Marti, M. J., Ibarretxe-Bilbao, N., Junque, C., Valldeoriola, F., Munoz, E., ... Tolosa, E. (2009). Cerebrospinal tau, phospho-tau, and beta-amyloid and neuropsychological functions in Parkinson's disease. *Movement Disorders, 24*, 2203–2210.

Compta, Y., Parkkinen, L., O'Sullivan, S. S., Vandrovcova, J., Holton, J. L., Collins, C., ... Revesz, T. (2011). Lewy- and Alzheimer-type pathologies in Parkinson's disease dementia: Which is more important? *Brain, 134*, 1493–1505.

Constantinescu, R., & Mondello, S. (2012). Cerebrospinal fluid biomarker candidates for parkinsonian disorders. *Frontiers in Neurology, 3*, 187.

Cropley, V. L., Fujita, M., Bara-Jimenez, W., Brown, A. K., Zhang, X. Y., Sangare, J., ... Innis, R. B. (2008). Pre- and post-synaptic dopamine imaging and its relation with frontostriatal cognitive function in Parkinson disease: PET studies with [11C]NNC 112 and [18F]FDOPA. *Psychiatry Research, 163*, 171–182.

Dubois, B., Tolosa, E., Katzenschlager, R., Emre, M., Lees, A. J., Schumann, G., ... Moline, M. L. (2012). Donepezil in Parkinson's disease dementia: A randomized, double-blind efficacy and safety study. *Movement Disorders, 27*, 1230–1238.

Edison, P., Rowe, C. C., Rinne, J. O., Ng, S., Ahmed, I., Kemppainen, N.,... Brooks, D. J. (2008). Amyloid load in Parkinson's disease dementia and Lewy body dementia measured with [11C]PIB positron emission tomography. *Journal Of Neurology Neurosurgery and Psychiatry, 79*, 1331–1338.

Elia, A. E., Petrucci, S., Fasano, A., Guidi, M., Valbonesi, S., Bernardini, L.,... Valente, E. M. (2013). Alpha-synuclein gene duplication: Marked intrafamilial variability in two novel pedigrees. *Movement Disorders, 28*, 813–817.

Fuchs, J., Nilsson, C., Kachergus, J., Munz, M., Larsson, E. M., Schule, B.,... Farrer, M. J. (2007). Phenotypic variation in a large Swedish pedigree due to SNCA duplication and triplication. *Neurology, 68*, 916–922.

Garcia-Garcia, D., Clavero, P., Gasca Salas, C., Lamet, I., Arbizu, J., Gonzalez-Redondo, R.,... Rodriguez-Oroz, M. C. (2012). Posterior parietooccipital hypometabolism may differentiate mild cognitive impairment from dementia in Parkinson's disease. *European Journal of Nuclear Medicine and Molecular Imaging, 39*, 1767–1777.

Gomperts, S. N., Rentz, D. M., Moran, E., Becker, J. A., Locascio, J. J., Klunk, W. E.,... Johnson, K. A. (2008). Imaging amyloid deposition in Lewy body diseases. *Neurology, 71*, 903–910.

Gomperts, S. N., Locascio, J. J., Rentz, D., Santarlasci, A., Marquie, M., Johnson, K.A., & Growdon, J. H. (2013). Amyloid is linked to cognitive decline in patients with Parkinson disease without dementia. *Neurology, 80*, 85–91.

Gonzalez-Cuyar, L. F., Sonnen, J. A., Montine, K. S., Keene, C. D., & Montine, T. J. (2011). Role of cerebrospinal fluid and plasma biomarkers in the diagnosis of neurodegenerative disorders and mild cognitive impairment. *Current Neurology and Neuroscience Reports, 11*, 455–463.

Hattori, N., Yabe, I., Hirata, K., Shiga, T., Sakushima, K., Tsuji-Akimoto, S.,... Tamaki, N. (2013). Brain regions associated with cognitive impairment in patients with Parkinson disease: quantitative analysis of cerebral blood flow using 123I iodoamphetamine SPECT. *Clinical Nuclear Medicine, 38*, 315–320.

Hong, Z., Shi, M., Chung, K. A., Quinn, J. F., Peskind, E. R., Galasko, D.,... Zhang, J. (2010). DJ-1 and alpha-synuclein in human cerebrospinal fluid as biomarkers of Parkinson's disease. *Brain, 133*, 713–726.

Ibarretxe-Bilbao, N., Ramirez-Ruiz, B., Tolosa, E., Marti, M. J., Valldeoriola, F., Bargello, N., & Dunque, C. (2008). Hippocampal head atrophy predominance in Parkinson's disease with hallucinations and with dementia. *Journal of Neurology, 255*, 1324–1331.

Inaba, M., White, L., Bell, C., Chen, R., Petrovitch, H., Launer, L.,... Masaki, K. (2011). White matter lesions on brain magnetic resonance imaging scan and 5-year cognitive decline: The Honolulu-Asia aging study. *Journal of the American Geriatrics Society, 59*, 1484–1489.

Irwin, D. J., White, M. T., Toledo, J. B., Xie, S. X., Robinson, J. L., Van Deerlin, V.,... Trojanowski, J. Q. (2012). Neuropathologic substrates of Parkinson disease dementia. *Annals of Neurology, 72*, 587–598.

Jokinen, P., Bruck, A., Aalto, S., Forsback, S., Parkkola, R., & Rinne, J. O. (2009). Impaired cognitive performance in Parkinson's disease is related to caudate dopaminergic hypofunction and hippocampal atrophy. *Parkinsonism and Related Disorders, 15*, 88–93.

Kehagia, A. A., Murray, G. K., Robbins, T. W. (2010). Learning and cognitive flexibility: frontostriatal function and monoaminergic modulation. *Current Opinion in Neurobiology, 20*, 199–204.

Korff, A., Liu, C., Ginghina, C., Shi, M., & Zhang, J. (2013). Alpha-synuclein in cerebrospinal fluid of Alzheimer's disease and mild cognitive impairment. *Journal of Alzheimer's Disease, 36*, 679–688.

Kruger, R., Kuhn, W., Muller, T., Woitalla, D., Graeber, M., Kosel, S., . . . Riess, O. (1998). Ala30Pro mutation in the gene encoding alpha-synuclein in Parkinson's disease. *Nature Genetics, 18*, 106–108.

Kuhl, D. E., Minoshima, S., Fessler, J. A., Frey, K. A., Foster, N. L., Ficaro, E.P., . . . Koeppe, R. A. (1996). In vivo mapping of cholinergic terminals in normal aging, Alzheimer's disease, and Parkinson's disease. *Annals of Neurology, 40*, 399–410.

Kulisevsky, J. (2000). Role of dopamine in learning and memory: Implications for the treatment of cognitive dysfunction in patients with Parkinson's disease. *Drugs & Aging, 16*, 365–379.

Launer, L. J., Hughes, T. M., & White, L. R. (2011). Microinfarcts, brain atrophy, and cognitive function: The Honolulu Asia Aging Study Autopsy Study. *Annals of Neurology, 70*, 774–780.

Leverenz, J. B., Watson, G. S., Shofer, J., Zabetian, C. P., Zhang, J., & Montine, T. J. (2011). Cerebrospinal fluid biomarkers and cognitive performance in nondemented patients with Parkinson's disease. *Parkinsonism and Related Disorders, 17*, 61–64.

Lewis, S. J., Dove, A., Robbins, T. W., Barker, R. A., & Owen, A. M. (2003). Cognitive impairments in early Parkinson's disease are accompanied by reductions in activity in frontostriatal neural circuitry. *Journal of the Neurological Sciences, 23*, 6351–6356.

Lin, X., Cook, T. J., Zabetian, C. P., Leverenz, J. B., Peskind, E. R., Hu, S. C., . . . Zhang, J. (2012). DJ-1 isoforms in whole blood as potential biomarkers of Parkinson disease. *Scientific Reports, 2*, 954.

Magen, I., Fleming, S. M., Zhu, C., Garcia, E. C., Cardiff, K. M., Dinh, D., . . . Chesselet, M. F. (2012). Cognitive deficits in a mouse model of pre-manifest Parkinson's disease. *European Journal of Neuroscience, 35*, 870–882.

Maroteaux, L., Campanelli, J. T., & Scheller, R. H. (1988). Synuclein: a neuron-specific protein localized to the nucleus and presynaptic nerve terminal. *Journal of the Neurological Sciences, 8*, 2804–2815.

Marshall, G. A., Shchelchkov, E., Kaufer, D. I., Ivanco, L. S., Bohnen, N. I. (2006). White matter hyperintensities and cortical acetylcholinesterase activity in parkinsonian dementia. *Acta Neurologica Scandinavica, 113*, 87–91.

Mattila, P. M., Rinne, J. O., Helenius, H., Dickson, D. W., & Rotta. M. (2000). Alpha-synuclein-immunoreactive cortical Lewy bodies are associated with cognitive impairment in Parkinson's disease. *Acta Neuropathologica, 100*, 285–290.

Melzer, T. R., Watts, R., MacAskill, M. R., Pitcher, T. L., Livingston, L., Keenan R. J., . . . Anderson T. J. (2013). White matter microstructure deteriorates across cognitive stages in Parkinson disease. *Neurology, 80*, 1841–1849.

Michell, A. W., Barker, R. A., Raha, S. K., & Raha-Chowdhury, R. (2005). A case of late onset sporadic Parkinson's disease with an A53T mutation in alpha-synuclein. *Journal of Neurology Neurosurgery and Psychiatry, 76*, 596–597.

Mollenhauer, B., Trenkwalder, C., von Ahsen, N., Bibl, M., Steinacker, P., Brechlin, P., . . . Otto, M. (2006). Beta-amlyoid 1–42 and tau-protein in cerebrospinal fluid of patients with Parkinson's disease dementia. *Dementia and Geriatric Cognitive Disorders, 22*, 200–208.

Mollenhauer, B., Locascio, J. J., Schulz-Schaeffer, W., Sixel-Doring, F., Trenkwalder, C., Schlossmacher, M. G. (2011). alpha-Synuclein and tau concentrations in cerebrospinal fluid of patients presenting with parkinsonism: A cohort study. *Lancet Neurology, 10*, 230–240.

Montine, T. J., & Larson, E. B. (2009). Late-life dementias: does this unyielding global challenge require a broader view? *JAMA, 302*, 2593–2594.

Montine, T. J., Shi, M., Quinn, J. F., Peskind, E. R., Craft, S., Ginghina, C., . . . Zhang, J. (2010). CSF Abeta(42) and tau in Parkinson's disease with cognitive impairment. *Movement Disorders, 25*, 2682–2685.

Morley, J. F., Xie, S. X., Hurtig, H. I., Stern, M. B., Colcher, A., Horn, S., . . . Siderowf, A. (2012). Genetic influences on cognitive decline in Parkinson's disease. *Movement Disorders, 27*, 512–518.

Nakajima, S., Gerretsen, P., Takeuchi, H., Caravaggio, F., Chow, T., Le Foll, B., . . . Graff-Guerrero, A. (2013). The potential role of dopamine D receptor neurotransmission in cognition. *European Neuropsychopharmacology, 3*, 799–813.

Nalls, M. A., Plagnol, V., Hernandez, D. G., Sharma, M., Sheerin, U. M., Saad, M., . . . Wood, N. W. (2011). Imputation of sequence variants for identification of genetic risks for Parkinson's disease: a meta-analysis of genome-wide association studies. *Lancet, 377*, 641–649.

Niethammer, M., Tang, C. C., Ma, Y., Mattis, P. J., Ko, J. H., Dhawan, V., Eidelberg, D. (2013). Parkinson's disease cognitive network correlates with caudate dopamine. *Neuroimage, 78*, 204–209.

Nishio, Y., Hirayama, K., Takeda, A., Hosokai, Y., Ishioka, T., Suzuki, K., . . . Mori, E. (2010). Corticolimbic gray matter loss in Parkinson's disease without dementia. *European Journal of Neurology, 17*, 1090–1097.

Nishioka, K., Ross, O. A., Ishii, K., Kachergus, J. M., Ishiwata, K., Kitagawa, M., . . . Hattori, N. (2009). Expanding the clinical phenotype of SNCA duplication carriers. *Movement Disorders, 24*, 1811–1819.

Nobili, F., Campus, C., Araldi, D., De Carli, F., Cabassi, G., Brugnolo, A., . . . Rodriguez, G. (2010). Cognitive-nigrostriatal relationships in de novo, drug-naive Parkinson's disease patients: a [I-123]FP-CIT SPECT study. *Movement Disorders, 25*, 35–43.

Nobili, F., Araldi, D., Campus, C., Ferrara, M., De Carli, F., Brugnolo, A., . . . Rodriguez, G. (2011). Brain perfusion correlates of cognitive and nigrostriatal functions in de novo Parkinson's disease. *European Journal of Nuclear Medicine and Molecular Imaging, 38*, 2209–2218.

Pagonabarraga. J., Gomez-Anson. B., Rotger, R., Llebaria, G., Garcia-Sanchez, C., Pascual-Sedano, B., . . . Kulisevsky, J. (2012). Spectroscopic changes associated with mild cognitive impairment and dementia in Parkinson's disease. *Dementia and Geriatric Cognitive Disorders, 34*, 312–318.

Pappata, S., Santangelo, G., Aarsland, D., Vicidomini, C., Longo, K., Bronnick, K., . . . Barone, P. (2011). Mild cognitive impairment in drug-naive patients with PD is associated with cerebral hypometabolism. *Neurology, 77*, 1357–1362.

Parkinson, J. (2002). An essay on the shaking palsy. [originally published in 1817]. *Journal of Neuropsychiatry and Clinical Neurosciences, 14*, 223–236; discussion 222.

Parkkinen, L., Pirttila, T., Tervahauta, M., & Alafuzoff, I. (2005). Widespread and abundant alpha-synuclein pathology in a neurologically unimpaired subject. *Neuropathology, 25*, 304–314.

Pavese, N., Rivero-Bosch, M., Lewis, S. J., Whone, A. L., Brooks, D. J. (2011). Progression of monoaminergic dysfunction in Parkinson's disease: a longitudinal 18F-dopa PET study. *Neuroimage, 56*, 1463–1468.

Petrou, M., Bohnen, N. I., Muller, M. L., Koeppe, R. A., Albin, R. L., Frey, K. A. (2012). Abeta-amyloid deposition in patients with Parkinson disease at risk for development of dementia. *Neurology, 79,* 1161–1167.

Polito, C., Berti, V., Ramat, S., Vanzi, E., De Cristofaro, M. T., Pellicano, G.,... Pupi, A. (2012). Interaction of caudate dopamine depletion and brain metabolic changes with cognitive dysfunction in early Parkinson's disease. *Neurobiology of Aging, 33,* 206 e229–239.

Polymeropoulos, M. H., Lavedan, C., Leroy, E., Ide, S. E., Dehejia, A., Dutra, A.,... Nussbaum, R. L. (1997). Mutation in the alpha-synuclein gene identified in families with Parkinson's disease. *Science, 276,* 2045–2047.

Postupna, N., Rose, S. E., Bird, T. D., Gonzalez-Cuyar, L. F., Sonnen, J. A., Larson, E. B.,... Montine, T. J. (2012). Novel antibody capture assay for paraffin-embedded tissue detects wide-ranging amyloid beta and paired helical filament-tau accumulation in cognitively normal older adults. *Brain Pathology, 22,* 472–484.

Reesink, F. E., Lemstra, A. W., van Dijk, K. D., Berendse, H. W., van de Berg, W. D., Klein, M.,... van der Flier, W. M. (2010). CSF alpha-synuclein does not discriminate dementia with Lewy bodies from Alzheimer's disease. *Journal of Alzheimer's Disease, 22,* 87–95.

Sabbagh, M. N., Adler, C. H., Lahti, T. J., Connor, D. J., Vedders, L., Peterson, L. K.,... Beach, T. G. (2009). Parkinson disease with dementia: Comparing patients with and without Alzheimer pathology. *Alzheimer Disease & Associated Disorders, 23,* 295–297.

Sawamoto, N., Piccini, P., Hotton, G., Pavese, N., Thielemans, K., & Brooks, D. J. (2008). Cognitive deficits and striato-frontal dopamine release in Parkinson's disease. *Brain, 131,* 1294–1302.

Schneider, J. A., Arvanitakis, Z., Yu, L., Boyle, P. A., Leurgans, S. E., & Bennett, D. A. (2012). Cognitive impairment, decline and fluctuations in older community-dwelling subjects with Lewy bodies. *Brain, 135,* 3005–3014.

Scholtissen, B., Verhey, F. R., Steinbusch, H. W., & Leentjens, A. F. (2006). Serotonergic mechanisms in Parkinson's disease: opposing results from preclinical and clinical data. *Journal of Neural Transmission, 113,* 59–73.

Shi, M., Bradner, J., Hancock, A. M., Chung, K. A., Quinn, J. F., Peskind, E. R.,... Zhang, J. (2011). Cerebrospinal fluid biomarkers for Parkinson disease diagnosis and progression. *Annals of Neurology, 69,* 570–580.

Siderowf, A., Xie, S. X., Hurtig, H., Weintraub, D., Duda, J., Chen-Plotkin, A.,... Clark, C. (2010). CSF amyloid beta 1-42 predicts cognitive decline in Parkinson disease. *Neurology, 75,* 1055–1061.

Sonnen, J. A., Montine, K. S., Quinn, J. F., Breitner, J. C., & Montine, T. J. (2010). Cerebrospinal fluid biomarkers in mild cognitive impairment and dementia. *Journal of Alzheimers Disease, 19,* 301–309.

Stelzel, C., Fiebach, C. J., Cools, R., Tafazoli, S., & D'Esposito, M. (2013). Dissociable fronto-striatal effects of dopamine D2 receptor stimulation on cognitive versus motor flexibility. *Cortex, 49,* 2799–2811.

Takahashi, H., Yamada, M., & Suhara, T. (2012). Functional significance of central D1 receptors in cognition: beyond working memory. *Journal of Cerebral Blood Flow and Metabolism, 32,* 1248–1258.

Tateno, F., Sakakibara, R., Kawai, T., Kishi, M., & Murano, T. (2012). Alpha-synuclein in the cerebrospinal fluid differentiates synucleinopathies (Parkinson Disease, dementia with Lewy bodies, multiple system atrophy) from Alzheimer disease. *Alzheimer Disease & Associated Disorders, 26*, 213–216.

van Holstein, M., Aarts, E., van der Schaaf, M. E., Geurts, D. E., Verkes, R. J., Franke, B.,... Cools, R. (2011). Human cognitive flexibility depends on dopamine D2 receptor signaling. *Psychopharmacology (Berlin), 218*, 567–578.

Vazey, E. M., & Aston-Jones, G. (2012). The emerging role of norepinephrine in cognitive dysfunctions of Parkinson's disease. *Frontiers in Behavioral Neuroscience, 6*, 48.

Wang, L. Y., Murphy, R. R., Hanscom, B., Li, G., Millard, S. P., Petrie, E. C., Galasko, D. R.,... Peskind, E. R. (2013). Cerebrospinal fluid norepinephrine and cognition in subjects across the adult age span. *Neurobiology of Aging, 34*, 2287–2292.

Weintraub, D., Dietz, N., Duda, J. E., Wolk, D. A., Doshi, J., Xie, S. X.,... Siderowf, A. (2012). Alzheimer's disease pattern of brain atrophy predicts cognitive decline in Parkinson's disease. *Brain, 135*, 170–180.

Zarranz, J. J., Alegre, J., Gomez-Esteban, J. C., Lezcano, E., Ros, R., Ampuero, I.,... de Yebenes, J. G. (2004). The new mutation, E46K, of alpha-synuclein causes Parkinson and Lewy body dementia. *Annals of Neurology, 55*, 164–173.

Zgaljardic, D. J., Borod, J. C., Foldi, N. S., Mattis, P. J., Gordon, M. F., Feigin, A., & Eidelberg, D. (2006). An examination of executive dysfunction associated with frontostriatal circuitry in Parkinson's disease. *Journal of Clinical and Experimental Neuropsychology, 28*, 1127–1144.

Zhang, Z., Cordeiro Matos, S., Jego, S., Adamantidis, A., & Seguela, P. (2013). Norepinephrine Drives Persistent Activity in Prefrontal Cortex via Synergistic alpha1 and alpha2 Adrenoceptors. *PLoS One, 8*, e66122.

Zurkovsky, L., Bychkov, E., Tsakem, E. L., Siedlecki, C., Blakely, R. D, & Gurevich, E. V. (2013). Cognitive effects of dopamine depletion in the context of diminished acetylcholine signaling capacity in mice. *Dis Models & Mechanisms, 6*, 171–183.

6 Structural and Functional Neuroimaging of Cognition and Emotion in Parkinson's Disease

Carme Junque

INTRODUCTION

The origin and evolution of cognitive impairment in PD is still a matter of debate (Emre 2003; Owen 2004; Caballoll, Marti, &Tolosa 2007; Rodriguez-Oroz et al., 2009). In the 1980s and 1990s, evidence from neuroimaging studies using single photon emission computed tomography (SPECT) suggested that dopaminergic dysfunction was a major cause of cognitive deficits in PD. However, sophisticated magnetic resonance imaging (MRI) techniques with a high power for identifying early gray matter alterations and their correlations with neuropsychological impairment have clearly demonstrated that there are several regional gray matter changes in the limbic and neocortical regions that are involved in the cognitive deficits.

The evidence of neuropathological changes in limbic structures (the hippocampus, amygdala and medial temporal lobe) at the time of PD diagnosis and their correlation with memory and emotional changes seriously challenged the earlier models that had attempted to explain the neuropsychological dysfunctions on a neurochemical basis alone. There is increasing evidence that cognitive dysfunction in PD is due to brain structural changes. This is not surprising, since, at the time of PD diagnosis, neural degeneration has advanced to affect structures subserving several cognitive functions. Specifically, according to Braak et al. (2003) staging, when motor symptoms emerge, patients present degenerative changes in the amygdala, hippocampus, and cingulate cortex in addition to midbrain atrophy. These degenerative changes can explain apathy, impaired emotional perception, and memory disturbances.

In this chapter we review the current evidence provided by structural and functional neuroimaging data that seek to explain the neuropsychological deficits observed in newly diagnosed PD patients and the progressive evolution of the disease to dementia.

STRUCTURAL MRI STUDIES

Magnetic resonance imaging analysis allows *in vivo* detection and quantification of global and regional cerebral atrophy. The methods used to study the correlations between structure and functions include visual inspection performed by expert neuroradiologists, quantification of the volumes of cerebral structures, voxel-based morphometry (VBM) analyses, measures of cortical thickness, and diffusion tensor imaging (DTI) (see Table 6-1).

The classical volumetric analysis of regions of interest (ROI) involves manual tracking of the surfaces of a selected structure, followed by automatic calculation of the volumes. To demonstrate selectivity in brain atrophy, the volume of a specific structure (e.g., the caudate nucleus or hippocampus) must be corrected by the whole brain volume; this is to avoid the effect of interindividual variability due to gender and the degree of general atrophy produced by aging and by the degenerative process itself. The whole brain volume can be obtained from the sum of partial volumes of gray matter, white matter, and cerebrospinal fluid extracted from the segmentation of the native MR scans prior to spatial normalization. Manual volumetric analysis is labor-intensive and time-consuming, and is also affected by inter-rater variability; it requires two different operators in order to obtain the inter-rater correlation, or alternatively two measures must be made by the same operator to obtain the intra-rater reliability coefficient.

Currently available software includes semi-automated measures to calculate the volume of the cerebral structures. MRICro, for instance, is a semi-automated program that was used in the pioneer studies designed to quantify brain atrophy in PD *in vivo*. Another more accurate semi-automated method for obtaining volumetric measures of structures like the hippocampus is the stereological analysis provided by the ANALYZE program. Today, one of the most frequently used

Table 6-1 Structural neuroimaging methods used to detect in vivo brain changes associated with cognitive deficits

Rating scales from visual inspection
Manual volumetry
Semiautomated volumetry
Voxel-based morphometry (VBM) whole brain analyses
Voxel-based morphometry region of interest (ROI) analyses
Cortical thickness (CTh)
Diffusion tensor imaging (DTI)

programs is the FreeSurfer software (http://surfer.nmr.mgh.harvard.edu), which allows automatic volumetric measures.

Degrees of Atrophy and Semiautomatic and Automatic Volumetry

Using a visual rating scale of MRI atrophy on coronal slices, Bruck et al. (2004) reported a correlation between bilateral atrophy of the hippocampus and verbal memory functions in PD. The correlation appeared to be selective, because sustained attention was found to be related to prefrontal but not to hippocampal atrophy. A similar procedure was used recently by Jokinen et al. (2009), who also found the degree of hippocampal atrophy to be correlated with declarative memory measures but not with prefrontal scores. Using quantitative volumetric measures of the hippocampus, Riekkinen et al. (1998) showed that patients with memory impairment had greater hippocampal volume reductions than patients with normal memory performance, and that the hippocampal volumes correlated with declarative memory but not with working memory or set-shifting measures. These results suggest that failure of verbal/visual memory in PD may be due to hippocampal atrophy. By contrast, impairment in spatial working memory and attentional set shifting seems to depend on a dysfunction in the "fronto-striatal" systems.

Not all studies have shown selectivity or dissociations in the correlation analyses. Some authors have reported similar correlations between declarative memory functions and hippocampus and amygdala (Bouchard et al., 2008; Junque et al., 2005). This finding is to be expected, since both cerebral structures form part of the limbic system and degenerate at a similar neuropathological stage of the disease according to the Braak and Braak classification (Braak et al., 2003). Moreover, hippocampal volume has also been found to be correlated with global scores on the Mini Mental State Examination (MMSE) (Apostolova et al., 2012; Camicioli et al., 2003; Junque et al., 2005), probably reflecting the coexistence of a general cognitive decline in patients with more severe memory dysfunction. Despite these considerations, different teams of researchers using a variety of methodologies have consistently reported the association between declarative memory impairment and hippocampal degeneration. Combining manual and automatic volumetry and also shape analysis of the hippocampus, Apostolova et al. (2012) recently found that even patients without mild cognitive impairment (MCI) have hippocampal degeneration, and Beyer et al. (2013) reported that verbal memory is associated with structural hippocampal changes in newly diagnosed Parkinson's disease.

Following the model of fronto-striatal impairment as a putative cause of cognitive deficits in PD (see Owen, 2004 for a review) the caudate nucleus has been selected as a region of interest (ROI) in several volumetric studies. Studying samples of PD, PD plus diffuse Lewy bodies, and Alzheimer's disease, Almeida et al. (2003) did not find significant differences in caudate volume between PD patients without dementia and controls. The correlation analyses were also negative; these authors found no significant correlation between caudate volume and either global cognitive function, executive performance, or processing speed in any of the subsamples. The authors concluded that caudate atrophy assessed *in vivo* did not appear to contribute to the cognitive impairment observed in PD patients. Negative results for caudate atrophy in nondemented PD were also reported by Apostolova et al. (2010); using sophisticated 3D statistical maps of the caudate, these authors demonstrated significant atrophy in selective regions such as the left medial and lateral and right medial regions, but only in demented PD patients. Tinaz, Courtney, and Stern (2011) also found negative results for caudate atrophy in nondemented PD; in patients at early stages of the disease, they found volumetric reduction in the putamen and a trend toward a reduction in the nucleus accumbens, but not in the caudate nuclei. Nor did patients with MCI have evidence of caudate atrophy. Other recent results recorded in large samples and analyzing the whole brain also suggest a lack of caudate degeneration in early PD. As part of the population-based multicenter Norwegian ParkWest study, Dalaker et al. (2010) selected a sample of 87 subjects with newly diagnosed PD in order to investigate the degree of subcortical brain atrophy in patients with mild cognitive impairment (MCI PD) and without (non-MCI PD). In this study, only the left inferior lateral ventricle, third ventricle, and fourth ventricle sizes achieved statistical significance in the group comparison. Patients with MCI differed in these ventricular measures from cognitively preserved patients and also from controls. However, the results for the volumetric analyses of subcortical gray matter structures were unrevealing. This study suggests that ventricular enlargement, but not basal ganglia degeneration is associated with early cognitive impairment in PD, and that ventricular enlargement is probably due to neocortical gray matter atrophy. In the same cohort, Apostolova et al. (2012) reported that volume and shape of the ventricular system seem to be related to cognitive impairment: the patterns of ventricular atrophy were able to differentiate between PD patients with and without MCI and controls. The investigators found that PD patients with MCI showed significant enlargement of all portions of the lateral ventricles relative to normal controls and significantly greater bilateral expansion of the temporal and occipital and left frontal lateral ventricles than PD patients with normal cognitive performance. Interestingly, nonamnestic PD patients with MCI had significant enlargement in all parts of the lateral ventricle, whereas those with amnestic MCI showed changes localized to the left occipital horn, suggesting medial temporal lobe atrophy. In agreement with these findings, Camicioli et al. (2011) found that ventricular volume correlated with MMSE scores and also concluded that ventricular enlargement is a good measure of progressive brain atrophy in both demented and nondemented PD patients.

Voxel-Based Morphometry

Voxel-based morphometry (VBM) involves an automated image analysis of T1-weighted magnetic resonance imaging (MRI) scans that allows the study of regional atrophy. The standard procedure is relatively unbiased because it allows examination of the differences throughout the whole brain and does not require any a priori assumptions concerning the structures to be assessed (Ashburner & Friston, 2009). VBM analysis involves a complex semiautomatic process of segmentation, normalization, and smoothing. Early studies were performed examining density or concentration (unmodulated images) or volume (modulated images) (Mechelli, Price, Friston & Ashburner, 2005). Although VBM processes are automatic, there are several steps that require raters to take decisions, and this may affect the final results (Ridgway et al., 2008). Errors in segmentation due to the threshold selected are common in the case of degenerative illness. Another issue is that the kernel selected in the smoothing procedure may affect the potential to detect changes in relatively small structures such as the hippocampus. For example, in whole brain analysis a 12 mm kernel is commonly used, whereas, for the detection of hippocampal changes, the optimal kernel size is between 4 and 8 mm (Honea, Crow, Passingham, & Mackay, 2005). The cut-off criteria for statistical significance are also relevant: in VBM studies performed with PD samples, the criteria range from the liberal uncorrected $p<0.01$ to the restrictive family-wise-error (FWE) corrected. Another methodological discrepancy between VBM studies is the choice of the software, which may use either parametric or nonparametric statistical analyses. The version of a specific program used for the analysis and the confounding covariates entered in the analyses (i.e., whole intracranial brain volume, whole gray matter volume, age, gender, illness severity, motor impairment) should also be taken in account in the interpretation of the published data. Discrepancies between studies may also be due to the selection of either a standard template or a specific template created with the subjects and controls from the study itself. Focusing on the difficulties in comparing VBM studies and in performing meta-analyses of the studies, Ridgway et al. (2008) published "Ten Simple Rules for Reporting Voxel-Based Morphometry Studies."

The first studies using VBM in PD to assess cognitive impairment tried to identify patterns of gray matter atrophy in demented and nondemented patients. In comparison with nondemented PD, demented PD patients have more pronounced gray matter loss in the posterior cerebral regions (temporo-parietal and occipital areas), but nondemented PD also have gray matter decreases in limbic and paralimbic regions compared to controls (Burton, McKeith, Burn, Williams & O'Brien, 2004; Summerfield et al., 2005). Another early approach was to differentiate between cognitively normal PD and subjects classified as having MCI. Beyer, Janvin, Larsen, and Aarsland (2007) found that PD patients with MCI had decreased volumes of the left middle frontal, precentral, left superior temporal, and right inferior temporal gyri compared with noncognitively impaired PD patients. The same group of researchers reported the relevance of time of dementia onset on the differential patterns of gray matter reductions (Beyer & Aarsland, 2008). Following the evidence suggesting that early cognitive impairment was a predictor of dementia, Nishio et al. (2010) aimed to define the structural neuroimaging features of patients with PD with a high dementia risk. Using criteria based on the Clinical Dementia Rating Scale, they divided nondemented patients with PD into those with and those without impaired cognition. They found that gray matter loss occurred in limited parts of the cerebral cortex in patients without apparent cognitive impairment, but it extended into widespread cortical and limbic regions in cognitively impaired, nondemented patients. The gray matter reductions in PD described in this study are clearly more extensive than those previously reported in similar samples. The authors attributed these discrepancies to differences in methodological approach, arguing that whereas previous studies had used the optimized VBM procedure, they used a more recent unified segmentation-normalization algorithm. In a sample of 42 newly diagnosed PD (11 with MCI), Dalaker et al. (2011) failed to find regional differences between patients and controls or between patients with and without MCI; however, they reported a significant correlation between neuropsychological performance and gray matter volume. Specifically, attention-executive tests correlated with medial and inferior frontal gyri and the right middle temporal gyrus. However, no volumetric correlations were found for memory or visuospatial functions.

The relationship between the regional progression of atrophy and cognitive decline has also been investigated using VBM. With a mean follow-up period of 25 months, PD patients without dementia showed gray matter volume decreases in limbic, paralimbic, and neocortical associative temporo-occipital regions. Over the same follow-up period, neuropsychological assessment showed decreases only in digits-span-forward task (Ramirez-Ruiz et al., 2005). Visual hallucinations have been proposed as a marker for evolution to dementia in idiopathic PD and are among the main indicators of the presence of diffuse cortical Lewy bodies. Cross-sectional studies showed that PD patients with visual hallucinations are more cognitively impaired than patients of the same age without hallucinations. The profile of cognitive impairment comprises several visuoperceptual memory deficits suggestive of greater atrophy in the visual associative regions (Ramirez-Ruiz, Junque, Marti, Valldeoriola, & Tolosa, 2006). VBM studies of patients with hallucinations demonstrated greater atrophy in the parietal and temporal pathways in visual associative regions than in a group of patients without hallucinations matched by age, motor impairment, and disease duration (Ramirez-Ruiz, Marti, et al., 2007). Thus, there was a strong correspondence between structural findings and neuropsychological results. In the follow-up of this sample over two and a half years, patients with visual hallucinations suffered from clearly greater declines than patients without hallucinations in memory, visuoperceptual, executive and language functions, and this deterioration was accompanied by widespread gray matter changes involving limbic, paralimbic, and neocortical associative regions. Moreover, the percentage of changes in the scores of cognitive tests correlated with gray matter reductions: for instance, verbal learning correlated positively with hippocampal gray matter, and semantic fluency decline with left thalamic reductions. Interestingly, patients without visual hallucinations had stable memory functions and presented gray matter decreases only in the cerebellum and cortical motor regions (Ibarretxe-Bilbao et al., 2010).

VBM data have demonstrated that cortical atrophy in PD presents regional patterns that are, in turn, related to specific neuropsychological deficits. Global brain atrophy or white matter intensities did not predict cognitive performance in PD, but regional gray or white matter atrophy assessed by VBM was able to explain specific cognitive deficits (Dalaker, Larsen, Bergsland, et al., 2009; Dalaker, Larsen, Dwyer, et al., 2009). The relationship between reductions in regional cerebral structures and cognitive dysfunctions in PD has been investigated using two statistical designs: group comparison and correlation analyses. Several studies have focused on the gray matter substrates of the impairment of specific cognitive functions such as memory, executive, and perceptual functions.

Besides whole brain analyses, VBM using SPM software also enables researchers to focus automatically on regions of interest by means of the FW Pickatlas tool (Maldjian, Laurienti, Kraf, & Burdette, 2003). Using an ROI analysis of the hippocampus, verbal learning has been found to be correlated with the hippocampal head volume (Ibarretxe-Bilbao et al., 2008). This correlation was seen for the whole sample of PD patients, and also for a subsample with visual hallucinations. The same relationship was observed in group comparison analyses. Patients with hippocampal gray matter reduction in the individual analyses performed significantly worse on verbal learning tasks than patients without this reduction. Another research group observed correlations between the hippocampal head volume and memory in aged subjects (Bouchard et al., 2008). Atrophy in demented PD patients involves the entire hippocampus, but the medial part is relatively preserved (Ibarretxe-Bilbao et al., 2008). As one longitudinal study reported, the atrophy of the hippocampal head in Parkinson's disease with hallucinations progresses toward generalized atrophy but is accompanied by an extensive gray matter loss in the limbic, paralimbic, and neocortical areas (Ibarretxe-Bilbao et al., 2010). However, for memory functions, whole brain VBM analyses have demonstrated that other regions in addition to the hippocampus may be related to memory impairment. Camicioli et al. (2009) assessed nondemented PD patients using the California Verbal Learning Test (CVLT) and a composite of index of executive function (EF): Stroop Interference, Trail Making Test Part B, and digit ordering. Poor memory was associated with gray matter (GM) atrophy in the left (uncus, middle temporal and fusiform gyri) and right temporal lobes and left putamen. Impairment in executive functions was also associated with GM atrophy in the middle temporal gyri, the left precuneus and cerebellum. Notably, executive functions did not correlate with frontal lobe atrophy.

Impairment in verbal fluency is one of the most frequently observed cognitive changes in Parkinson's disease and is seen even at early stages of the disease. It has usually been assumed to reflect executive dysfunctions. Deficits in phonemic and semantic fluencies were attributed to frontal lobe dysfunctions because both types of fluency were impaired in patients with structural frontal lesions, but semantic fluency was more closely related to temporal damage than phonemic fluency (Henry, 2004). In a sample of nondemented PD patients, correlations between semantic fluency and gray matter in temporal, frontal, and cerebellar areas were observed, suggesting that semantic fluency impairment may reflect structural gray matter changes in regions involved in language. In contrast, no cortical gray matter regions were found to be associated with phonemic fluency tests (Pereira, Junque, Marti, Ramirez-Ruiz, Bargallo, et al., 2009). The Trail

Making Test is also commonly used to assess prefrontal functions. Using the time to complete Trail Making Test B minus the time to complete Trail Making Test A as a measure of working memory or shifting ability in PD, Biundo et al. (2011) found correlations with the anterior and posterior cingulate regions as well as the supplementary motor area and the middle frontal gyrus.

The model of dopaminergic depletion causing dysfunction in the fronto-striatal circuitry cannot be satisfactorily explain visuoperceptual deficits in PD. VBM procedures have facilitated research into the neuroanatomical substrates of these deficits and the possible dissociation between dorsal and ventral stream processing of complex visual information. In the visual cortex, the occipito-temporal pathway (the ventral stream) is essential for perceiving the identity of faces, whereas the occipito-parietal pathway (the dorsal stream) is involved in spatial relationships between objects. In agreement with the "what/where" dissociation in relation to ventral versus dorsal stream structures, facial recognition impairment correlated with gray matter reduction in medial temporal lobe regions, whereas Benton's Visual-Form discrimination, which involves more spatial reasoning, correlated with the superior parietal regions (Pereira, Junque, Marti, Ramirez-Ruiz, Bartres-Faz, et al., 2009). Nagano-Saito et al. (2005) found that the raven-colored progressive matrices scores correlated with (among other cerebral regions) the left fusiform gyrus a region involved in visuoperceptual functions.

Recognition of facial expressions of emotions and odor identification are other perceptual functions that are often impaired in PD. Ekman's test, which assesses the ability to ascribe emotions to facial expressions, is found to be altered even at early stages of the disease. Total scores on Ekman's test have been reported to be correlated with bilateral regions of the orbitofrontal cortex. This result indicates that impairment in the recognition of emotions is explained by atrophy of the associative regions (Ibarretxe-Bilbao et al., 2009). Moreover, there is some specificity for the pattern of correlations within the limbic system and the type of emotion. For example, sadness correlates with the right amygdala and right orbitofrontal cortex, anger correlates with the bilateral nucleus accumbens, and disgust with the anterior cingulate cortex (Baggio et al., 2012).

Olfactory dysfunctions—that is, odor threshold, odor identification, and odor recognition— can be seen in several degenerative diseases. In 1998, the results of a meta-analysis were published examining the impairment in these olfactory domains in Alzheimer's (AD) and Parkinson's disease. A quantitative analysis of 43 studies of odor identification, recognition, and memory in AD and PD revealed extremely large effects across all domains; olfactory dysfunctions can, therefore, be considered perceptual cognitive deficits, because they are not explained solely by sensory impairment (Mesholam, Moberg, Mahr, & Doty, 1998). In a VBM study, early PD patients showed a significant correlation between gray matter volume and olfaction in the right piriform cortex. Patients at moderately advanced disease stages exhibited correlation between olfaction and the right amygdaloid complex, a region corresponding to secondary olfactory projection areas (Wattendorf et al., 2009).

Cortical Thickness

Surface-based cortical thickness (Cth) analysis performs better than VBM for the detection of cerebral cortical changes. VBM gray matter analysis includes both local cortical surface and cortical folding, and it depends on the overall brain size; therefore, its estimation of gray matter is less accurate. Cortical thickness analysis offers subvoxel precision because thickness values are assigned to individual vertices rather than voxels, and it is less susceptible to positional variance than VBM, given that the extraction of the cortex follows the gray matter surface despite local variations in its position (Hutton, Draganski, Ashburne & Weiskopf, 2009; Kim et al., 2005). In a multimodal study with the same sample, VBM identified only reduction in the left superior temporal region, whereas cortical thickness showed bilateral decreases in occipital and parietal regions in addition to temporal and frontal thinning of areas in the left hemisphere (Pereira et al., 2012) (see Figure 6-1). As for cognitive functions, the study by Pereira et al. found that CTh of PD patients correlated with age and Hoehn and Yahr stage, but not with global measures of cognitive functions.

In mild PD, Lyoo, Ryu, and Lee (2010) found widespread cortical thinning in the inferior parietal, rostral frontal, and orbitofrontal cortices, with predominance in the temporal cortex. The greater extent of CTh observed compared to Pereira et al.'s study is probably due to the use of a statistical significance cut-off of $p < 0.001$ uncorrected for multiple comparisons. Interestingly, despite this extensive cortical thinning, the authors did not observe changes in prefrontal regions. In early PD, Jubault et al. (2011) reported no differences in global cortical thickness between patients and controls, but observed two clusters exhibiting thinning: the left medial supramarginal area and the right dorsal pre-supramarginal area. Disease duration correlated with the thickness of left temporal pole, the bilateral occipital cortex, and Broca's area. The authors

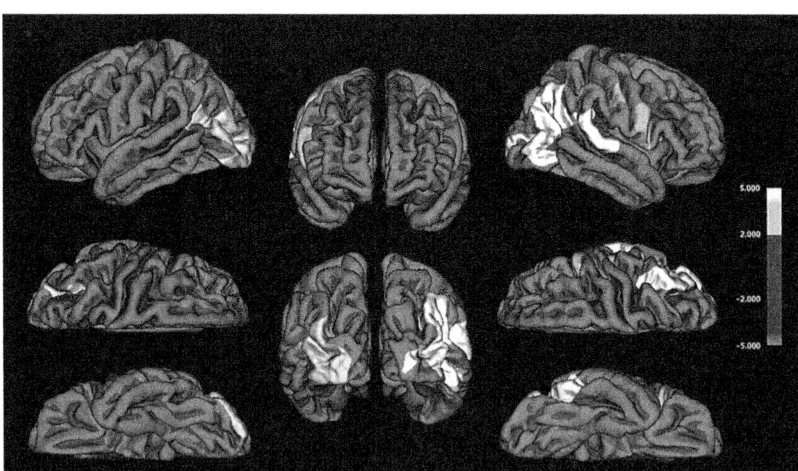

FIGURE 6-1

Results of the cortical thickness analysis showing cortical thinning in Parkinson's disease patients compared to healthy elderly controls. From Pereira et al. (2012).

suggested that correlation between disease duration and thickness in the occipital cortex may indicate the increase in PD-related visuospatial deficits, and the emergence of hallucinations. Similar results were published by Tinaz, Courtney, and Stern (2011) in a sample of 15 patients at early stages of the disease. These authors did not find global thinning of the cortex, but whole brain maps identified thinning in several regions of the left hemisphere (inferior frontal gyrus, pars triangularis, middle and inferior occipital gyrus, lingual and fusiform gyri, and cuneus/calcarine sulcus) and also in the right hemisphere (inferior frontal gyrus, pars orbitalis extending to the *pars triangularis*, and orbital gyrus). The ROI analysis confirmed thinning in the left triangular and right orbital parts of the inferior frontal gyri, the banks of the left parietal sulcus intermedius primus, and the banks of the left posterior collateral transverse. The authors did not find significant correlations with the composite z scores of psychomotor speed (digit-symbol and symbol search scores), executive function (digit span total, trails A-B, and FAS scores), and emotional status (STAI-S and STAI-T scores). In summary, Cth has been shown to be a useful tool for detecting early gray matter changes in PD, and the regions described are known to be involved in complex cognitive functions, but correlation analyses failed to yield findings of statistical significance, perhaps because only linear relationships have been explored.

Diffusion Tensor Imaging

Diffusion tensor imaging (DTI) is an MRI technique that can indirectly evaluate the integrity of white matter tracts by measuring water diffusion and its directionality in three dimensions. The magnitude (diffusivity) and directionality (anisotropy) of water molecular displacement by diffusion in the brain can be quantified by mean diffusivity (MD) and fractional anisotropy (FA). To analyze DTI for group comparison or correlation purposes, several procedures are available: voxel-based whole brain analysis, voxel-based ROI analyses, whole Tract-Based Spatial Statistics (TBSS), quantification of FA and MD of specific fibers, and tractography. An advantage of quantitative fiber tracking over other methods of DTI quantification is its ability to measure the diffusion properties of isolated fiber tracts along their full extent. A number of methods are now available for fiber identification and tracking quantification (for review, see Chanraud, Zahr, Sullivan, & Pfefferbaum, 2010).

DTI has been found to be more sensitive than VBM in detecting structural changes in patients at early stages of the disease (Karagulle Kendi, Lehericy, Luciana, Ugurbil, & Tuite, 2008). As expected, FA values in the substantia nigra and its projections were lower in PD compared with healthy controls (Chan et al., 2007) and in de novo PD patients (Vaillancourt, et al., 2009), and FA values correlated inversely with disease severity (Chan et al., 2007). Combining substantia nigra volumetry and its connectivity with the thalamus, the classification sensitivity of PD versus controls reached 100% and its specificity reached 80% (Menke et al., 2009). The combination of FA and MD values from DTI in addition to tractography has also been found to be useful to differentiate PD from atypical parkinsonian disorders such as multiple system atrophy (MSA) and progressive supranuclear palsy (PSP) (Nilsson et al., 2007).

In demented patients, one study reported lower FA values in patients compared with controls in bilateral frontal, left temporal and left parietal white matter (Lee et al., 2010). PD patients with dementia have FA reductions in bilateral posterior cingulate bundles compared to nondemented PD patients. Moreover, FA values in the left posterior cingulate bundle showed significant correlations with many cognitive parameters: the Dementia Rating Scale, the Mattis Dementia Rating Scale, Mini-Mental State Examination, and the revised version of Hasegawa's dementia scale. Thus, posterior cingulate areas may play an important role in the dementia process in PDD (Matsui, Nishinaka, Oda, Niikawa, Kubori, et al., 2007). The same researchers reported that PD patients with cognitive deficits, specifically executive dysfunctions, showed reduced FA in the right frontal and left parietal white matter (Matsui, Nishinaka, Oda, Niikawa, Komatsu, et al., 2007).

In nondemented PD, odor impairment has been found to be correlated with FA values in the cerebellum (Zhang et al., 2011) and with white matter surrounding the gyrus rectus (Ibarretxe-Bilbao et al., 2010). FA values in the olfactory regions may be of clinical interest because they clearly distinguished Parkinson's subjects from controls, suggesting they have a role in the preclinical identification of PD (Rolheiser et al., 2011).

FUNCTIONAL NEUROIMAGING STUDIES

There is strong evidence that neurochemical changes contribute to cognitive dysfunction in PD. Neuroimaging studies such as single photon emission tomography (SPECT), positron emission tomography (PET), and functional magnetic resonance imaging (fMRI), as well as transcranial magnetic stimulation (TMS), pre- and postsurgical treatments and direct brain stimulation of the brain have all provided strong evidence of the role of the dysfunctions in the frontostriatal circuitry in cognitive deficits in PD, specifically, executive functions and procedural and implicit learning (Carbon & Eidelberg, 2006; MacDonald & Monchi 2011; MacDonald et al., 2011; Monchi, Ko, & Strafella 2006; Owen et al., 1997; 1998)

SPECT and PET Studies

Since the pathological hallmark of PD is the degeneration of ascending projections of the midbrain dopamine neurons, it seems possible that cognitive deficits may be attributable to frontal lobe dysfunction as a direct consequence of impaired meso-frontal dopaminergic transmission or as a secondary consequence of impaired nigro-striatal dopaminergic function. An alternative hypothesis is that the cognitive deficits reflect a functional disturbance of the frontal cortex itself caused by locally impaired dopaminergic transmission. Both these hypotheses have been investigated using SPECT and PET.

Cerebral blood flow can be assessed by SPECT using 99mTC-HMPAO and by PET using H2 15O/PET. In addition, PET can measure the glucose metabolism using 18F-fluorodeoxyglucose (FDG). Dopaminergic function can be investigated by PET using the radiotracer (18F)-fluorodopa (FDOPA) and by SPECT by means of dopamine transporter (DAT) density (see Table 6-2).

Classifying PD patients according to their degree of cognitive impairment and using 99mTC-HMPAO SPECT, it has been reported that patients without cognitive impairment have no regional reductions in cerebral blood flow, that patients with mild cognitive impairment show blood-flow reductions mainly in posterior cerebral regions, but that reductions in patients with dementia are extensive and bilaterally symmetrical, involving both anterior and posterior brain regions. These findings suggest a widespread cortical, mainly posterior, type of dysfunction and a relationship between the degree of cognitive impairment and the magnitude of blood flow reductions (Wallin et al., 2007). Similarly, global cognitive impairment assessed by means of MMSE has been found to be correlated with a ratio reflecting the pattern of cortical metabolism from FDG-PET. This ratio is less associated with motor functions or with psychiatric symptoms (Liepelt et al., 2009).

Another topic that has been investigated is the relationship between disease progression, metabolic changes, and neuropsychological impairment. Paschali et al. (2010) studied a sample of nondemented PD patients by two single-photon-emission-computed- tomography (SPECT) studies (perfusion and dopamine transporter binding) and neuropsychological evaluation. Patients were divided into four groups according to the Hoehn and Yahr (H&Y) staging system. In the first stage of the disease, there were perfusion decreases in 55% of the patients bilaterally in the prefrontal lobes and in 22% in the right motor and

Table 6-2 Functional neuroimaging methods used to detect in vivo brain changes associated with cognitive deficits

Single Photon Emission Computed Tomography (SPECT),
99mTC-HMPAO. Blood Flow
Dopamine transporter (DAT)
N-isopropyl-p-[123I]iodoamphetamine (123I -IMP)
Positron emission tomography (PET)
18F-fluorodeoxyglucose (FDG). Glucose metabolism
18F-fluorodopa (FDOPA). Dopaminergic function
D2-receptor availability 11C-raclopride (RAC) PET
Pittsburgh compound B (PiB) PET imaging.
Functional magnetic resonance imaging (fMRI)
Task related
Study of segregated regions involved in a function (regional activation or deactivation)
Study of brain connectivity between regions (networks)
Resting state networks

supplementary motor cortex area. These percentages increased in stage 2 of the disease to 70% and 50%, respectively. These results are in agreement with observations that suggest that the cerebral cortex and, particularly, the frontal cortex are affected at relatively early stages of the disease. At stage 3 of the disease, all patients showed hypoperfusion in the prefrontal lobes and 73% bilaterally in the parietal lobes. By the late stages of the disease (4 and 5) most of the patients showed hypoperfusion in all cortical areas. Regarding neuropsychological performance, patients in the early stages of the disease differed significantly from controls both on semantic and phonological fluency and on visuospatial functions. Patients in later stages differed significantly from controls in all tests (semantic and phonological fluency, verbal and visual delayed recall, and visuospatial functions). They found cognitive deficits especially in the late PD stages compared to the early stages and associations between cognitive decrements and diminished cortical perfusion in the frontal and posterior cortical areas, but not in the basal ganglia.

One of the main clinical interests in functional neuroimaging relates to its possible power to predict dementia. Bohnen et al. (2011) evaluated subcortical and cortical metabolic changes in PD subjects who developed dementia after two years of follow-up. FDG PET was obtained for each subject at entry to the study and during follow-up. The findings indicate that incident dementia in idiopathic PD is heralded by metabolic changes within visual association and posterior cingulate cortices. Progression to dementia was associated with prominent hypometabolism of the cuneus and precuneus, but widespread cortical changes were also observed involving the mesiofrontal lobes. These results suggest that visual association and posterior cingulate cortex metabolic changes may be a useful biomarker for use in studies of the evolution of dementia in PD.

It is widely accepted that motor and cognitive impairments in PD have different neural substrates, but neuroimaging studies have only recently described these correlates. Using resting FDG and high-resolution positron emission tomography (PET), Lozza et al. (2004) carried out a network analysis of regional metabolic data to identify specific covariation patterns associated with motor and executive dysfunctions. They detected two independent patterns relating to each of the two clinical abnormalities. The first pattern was characterized by a relative increase in activity in the striatum and the mediodorsal thalamus associated with a relative decrease in the prefrontal and cingulate regions. This pattern explained the motor impairment. The second pattern, called the "PET cognitive pattern," was characterized by ventromedial frontal, hippocampal, and striatal hypometabolism and correlated with the conditional associative learning and the Brown Peterson tests. Huang et al. (2007) reported a similar dissociation and detected a covariance pattern that correlated significantly with performance on memory and executive functioning tests. This PD-related cognitive pattern was characterized by metabolic reductions in frontal and parietal association areas and relative increases in the cerebellar vermis and dentate nuclei. The degree of activation of the cognitive pattern predicted memory performance, visuospatial function, and perceptual motor speed. In addition, advancing disease in early PD was associated with declining metabolism in the prefrontal orbital (BA 9 and 10) and inferior parietal regions.

Besides the dissociation between cognitive and motor functions, differential patterns of metabolic abnormalities for cognitive and mood dysfunctions have been identified. Using FDOPA-PET, two independent topographic patterns have been described: pattern 1, including the parieto-occipito-temporal and medial temporal brain regions, and pattern 2, including the lateral frontal and anterior limbic cortex. Patterns 1 and 2 exhibited a double dissociation in their behavioral correlates, whereas pattern 1 correlated with visuospatial and memory functions but not dysphoria, and pattern 2 correlated with dysphoria but not cognitive measures (Mentis et al., 2002).

Metabolic correlates of specific cognitive dysfunctions in PD have focused on executive and memory functions and to a lesser degree on visuospatial functions. Following literature reports that impairment of frontal lobe functions is the earliest cognitive deficit in PD (Owen, 2004), several studies selected executive function tests and correlated performance with basal ganglia nuclei or the prefrontal cortex or both using ROI analyses. However, the conclusions of some of these studies should be treated with caution because the metabolism of the whole brain or the posterior cortex was not always assessed, and in several studies, the correlations of cognitive functions other than executive functions were not investigated.

The differential contributions of caudate and putamen metabolic deficits to cognitive deficits was investigated by van Beilen et al. (2008) in a sample of advanced PD patients. The neuropsychological tests included measures of memory, executive functioning, and fluency. Memory was tested with the memory scale of the Mattis Dementia Rating Scale and the 15 Words Test (learning score and recall score). Executive functioning was evaluated with the Odd Man Out test, the Stroop Interference Index, and time taken on Trail Making B divided by time taken on the Trail Making A. Fluency was measured with two category tests (animals and professions, 1 min each), and three letter-fluency tests. The authors found that three composite scores of memory, executive functioning, and fluency correlated with both caudate and putamen metabolic indices. In our view, these results probably reflect disease severity rather than specific contributions of the basal ganglia to the cognitive dysfunctions in PD. The authors did not assess other cerebral regions that are probably involved in the cognitive deficits of these patients.

Using FDOPA-PET uptake values in PD patients, Rinne et al. (2000) found that the dysfunction of the dopamine system in the caudate, but not in the putamen, is related to certain characteristics of cognitive impairment. Specifically, they reported that dopaminergic function in the caudate nucleus was negatively associated with performance on the attention-demanding Stroop interference task. In turn, dopaminergic function in the frontal cortex was positively correlated with performance on digit span backwards, verbal fluency, and verbal immediate recall tests. These results indicate that dopaminergic dysfunctions of the basal ganglia and prefrontal cortex explain different executive dysfunctions. In a small sample of nonmedicated PD patients, Bruck et al. (2001) investigated correlations of L-Dopa metabolism in the caudate and putamen with two classical frontal lobe function tests (the Stroop test and the WCST). They reported that decreased FDOPA uptake in the right caudate was related to slow processing time. In contrast, they did not find functional correlates of putaminal dopamine metabolism or neural correlates of WCST performance. A later study (Bruck et al., 2005) focused on neural correlates of specific Stroop task measures. They found that reaction time on the vigilance test correlated positively with FDOPA uptake in the right dorsolateral prefrontal cortex, and that reaction time on the Stroop test correlated negatively with FDOPA uptake in an area including the medial frontal cortex and the anterior cingulate. Thus, different components of the same test of executive functions had different basal ganglia and prefrontal correlates.

Relationships between the dopamine transporter (DAT) density in the basal ganglia and cognitive functions seem to be nonspecific. The DAT metabolism of both the head of the caudate and the putamen correlated with two tests of executive functions: the digit ordering test and perseverations on a modified card-sorting test. However, caudate head dopaminergic metabolism also correlated with memory measures and global cognitive scores (Müller, Wächter, Barthel, Reuter & von Cramon, 2000). Thus, it seems that the degree of caudate dopaminergic dysfunction probably reflects disease evolution, which, in turn, involves global cognitive dysfunctions.

Correlations between task performance and concurrent neural changes allow stronger causal inference than correlations between metabolic and cognitive data recorded separately. Sawamoto et al. (2008) investigated whether the executive deficits in early PD patients were associated with impaired dopaminergic transmission in the striatum, frontal cortex, or both. They monitored changes in regional synaptic dopamine levels using 11C-raclopride (RAC-PET) as a marker of D2-receptor availability. During RAC-PET, patients with PD and age-matched healthy controls were administered a spatial working memory (SWM) and a visuomotor control task (VMT). In controls, RAC binding was reduced in the dorsal caudate during performance of the SWT compared with the VMT, a finding compatible with increased levels of endogenous dopamine release due to the executive process. In PD patients, this RAC binding reduction was not observed. In contrast, a comparable level reduced RAC binding in the anterior cingulate cortex within the medial prefrontal cortex during the spatial working memory task in both controls and PD patients. These data suggest that executive deficits in patients with early-stage PD are associated with impaired nigrostriatal dopaminergic function resulting in abnormal processing in the cortico-basal ganglia circuits, but the mesocortical dopaminergic transmission appears well preserved at this stage of the illness.

The effects of L-dopa on executive functions can also be examined by performing neuroimaging tests in on-off L-dopa conditions. Testing the whole brain, in an $H_2{}^{15}O$ PET study and using an on-off design while performing the Tower of London and a working memory task, levodopa decreased blood flow in the right dorsolateral prefrontal cortex and increased blood flow in the right occipital lobe during both tasks (Cools, Stefanova, Barker, Robbins & Owen, 2002). Also using

PET, Nagano-Saito, Liu, Doyon and Dagher (2009) found that after administration of a dopamine agonist, PD patients showed an inverse correlation between activation of the ventro-medial prefrontal cortex and the problem complexity of the Tower of London task.

Regarding memory functions, Holthoff-Detto et al. (1997) reported that patients at an advanced stage of disease showed a significant correlation between reduced caudate uptake of FDOPA and impairment in delayed recall performance. With a more extensive neuropsychological battery, Jokinen et al. (2009) reported that the impaired dopaminergic function of the caudate nucleus is related to the impairments in verbal memory, visual memory and delayed recall in nondemented PD patients. However, it should be noted that these memory scores also correlated with hippocampal atrophy measured by structural MRI.

Implicit and explicit motor-learning tasks have been increasingly used to investigate the neural basis of motor-skill or procedural-learning impairment in PD. This learning depends on fronto-striatal integrity. Functional imaging studies in normal subjects have revealed that this cognitive process is associated with a distinct activation pattern involving prefrontal, premotor, and posterior parietal cortical regions, as well as the basal ganglia. In early stage PD, it has been reported that, for explicit motor sequence learning, patients recruited additional cortical regions compensating for abnormalities in basal ganglia function (Nakamura et al., 2001). Similar results were observed in mildly affected PD patients who demonstrated only modest impairment of learning during the first 30 seconds of the task and performed similarly to controls thereafter. However, the mechanism by which they achieved similar performance involved greater activation of the regions subserving motor learning and recruitment of contralateral cortical regions (Mentis et al., 2003). Within the basal ganglia, DAT binding shows more impairment of the putamen than of the caudate; however, motor learning correlates with dopamine reductions in the caudate but not in the putamen (Carbon et al., 2004). However, a longitudinal study by the same authors found that changes in sequence-learning-related activity demonstrate progressive changes in the neural responses that mediate sequence learning during the early clinical course of PD. Learning-related activation declined in dorsolateral prefontal cortex and parietal associative cortex; by contrast, increased activation over time was noted in the anterior cingulate cortex. An increase in hippocampal activation was also found, suggesting a compensatory mechanism of this structure, probably supporting the main role of the striatum in motor learning (Carbon, Reetz, Ghilardi, Dhawan & Eidelberg, 2010).

The substrate of the impairment in perceptual functions in PET and SPECT studies was investigated for two visuoperceptual tasks without a motor component: Raven's colored progressive matrices (RCPM) and a Poppelreuter-like task. In a SPECT study using N-isopropyl-p-[^{123}I]iodoamphetamine (^{123}I-IMP), PD patients without dementia showed significantly reduced rCBF bilaterally in occipital and posterior parietal cortices and there was a strong positive correlation between the RCPM score and the rCBF in the right visual association area (Abe et al., 2003). The misidentifications of figures in the Poppelreuter-like task by patients were correlated with hypometabolism in the associative visual cortices, including the right inferior temporal gyrus and the bilateral temporo-parieto-occipital junction (Ishioka et al., 2011).

PET studies also permit estimation of cholinergic activity. It has been reported that odor identification test scores correlated positively with acetylcholinesterase activity in the hippocampal formation, amygdala and neocortex, and with the monoaminergic activity in the striatum. However, multiple regression analysis demonstrated a significant effect only for limbic acetylcholinesterase activity. These results indicate that cholinergic denervation of the limbic archicortex is a more robust determinant of hyposmia than nigrostriatal dopaminergic denervation (Bohnen et al., 2010).

Recently, PET scans have allowed the measurement of the amyloid burden *in vivo* using Pittsburgh compound B (PiB) PET imaging. Although PiB is mainly used in Alzheimer's research, recently it has also been used to assess the possible comorbidity of PD with AD. The amyloid burden in PD with dementia (a Lewy body dementia) is debated but it is increased in dementia with Lewy bodies (DLB). The regional amyloid burden in the parietal (lateral and precuneus)/posterior cingulate region, but not in the occipital region, has been found to be related with deficits in the Benton visual form discrimination test in PD and DLB groups but not in AD or controls. Memory and frontal lobe functions did not correlate with PiB measures in either PD or DLB (Gomperts et al., 2008).

Functional Magnetic Resonance Imaging (fMRI)

Functional MRI provides an *in vivo* method for investigating the neural underpinnings of cognitive functions by measuring regional hemodynamic changes presumably related to underlying cellular activity. The most widely used functional MRI technique to identify cerebral activation is based on imaging of the endogenous blood-oxygen-level-dependent (BOLD) contrast. BOLD fMRI is considered to reflect the integrated synaptic activity of neurons via MRI signal changes due to changes in blood flow, blood volume, and the blood oxyhemoglobin/deoxyhemoglobin ratio (Logothetis, Pauls, Augath, Trinath, & Oelterman, 2001). In addition to the increases observed in the BOLD signal in activated brain areas, negative BOLD responses or "deactivations," which are thought to represent decreases in neuronal activity below baseline levels of activity, may also be critical responses within large-scale networks (Shmuel, Augath, Oeltermann, & Logothetis, 2006).

Early fMRI experiments compared the MR signal during one cognitive condition to a control task or to a passive baseline condition (e.g., visual fixation). This can be done using "block designs," in which stimuli of each cognitive condition are grouped together in blocks lasting 20–40 seconds, or in "event-related" paradigms, in which single stimuli from several different conditions are interspersed. The peak hemodynamic response is typically observed 4–6 seconds after the stimulus onset. The cognitive task induces positive and negative BOLD responses (task-related responses), which are reported as activations (increased BOLD) or deactivations (decreased BOLD). More recent studies have been based on the functional connectivity between nodes of cerebral networks.

Among functional neuroimaging techniques, fMRI has many potential advantages in studying patients with neurodegenerative disorders. For instance, fMRI sessions can be repeated many times over the course of a longitudinal study, because it is a noninvasive imaging technique that does not require injection of a contrast agent, and is thus well suited as a measure in clinical drug trials. However, disease-related alterations in brain structure may make it difficult to interpret the source of abnormalities in functional data. For example, hypoactivation may reflect atrophy in a specific cerebral region. In addition, fMRI measures may also be affected by transient brain and body states at the time of imaging, such as arousal, attention, sleep deprivation, sensory processing of irrelevant stimuli, or the effects of pharmacologic treatment (Sperling et al., 2010).

In addition to functional task-related activation studies, there has recently been considerable interest in studying the intrinsic connectivity of brain networks during the resting state using BOLD fMRI techniques, often referred to as functional connectivity or fc-MRI. Functional connectivity is defined as the temporal dependence of neuronal activity patterns of anatomically separate brain regions (van den Heuvel & Hulshoff Pol, 2010). fc-MRI techniques examine the correlation between the intrinsic oscillations or time courses of activity in brain regions, and have identified a number of brain networks that demonstrate significant consistency in the spontaneous activity of distributed nodes.

Based on findings from neuroimaging studies, Raichle et al. (2001) drew attention to synchronized resting state networks (RSN) and especially to spatially coherent spontaneous BOLD fluctuations. The RSN model postulates that the brain is spontaneously active in the absence of a task. The term *brain at rest* refers to the examination of conditions during which the subject has his or her eyes closed but is not sleeping. The hallmark characteristic of these RSNs is their synchronicity, which reflects not a genuine activation within the observed network, but rather the consistent collaboration and functional interconnectedness of the cortical regions involved (Wermke, Sorg, Wohlschlager, & Drzezga, 2008). In part, RSNs reflect structural connectivity. The correlation between cerebral regions (*functional connections*) in resting-state networks tends to be strongly related to structural white matter connections, suggesting the existence of an underlying structural core of functional connectivity networks (van den Heuvel & Hulshoff Pol, 2010). Damoiseaux and Greicius (2009) concluded in a review of studies that directly investigated the relationship between functional connectivity during the default mode and structural connectivity measured by DTI, that although the studies used slightly different approaches (whole brain versus ROI, mean FA versus number of tracts (fiber count), etc.) their results were largely convergent. All studies show that the strength of resting state functional connectivity correlates positively with structural connectivity strength.

The most consistently reported resting-state networks across studies include the primary sensorimotor network; the primary visual and extra-striate visual network; a network consisting of bilateral temporal/insular and anterior cingulate cortex regions; left and right lateralized networks consisting of superior parietal and superior frontal regions; and the default mode network (DMN) consisting of the precuneus, medial frontal, inferior parietal cortical regions, and medial temporal lobe (van den Heuvel & Hulshoff Pol, 2010). Thus, the default mode network is one of several RSNs; its regions are active during rest and deactivated or attenuated during goal-directed tasks (Wermke et al., 2008).

As was the case in SPECT and PET studies, fMRI has mainly been used to reveal abnormalities during the performance of executive functions. Lewis, Dove, Robbins, Barker & Owen (2003) demonstrated, for the first time, that fMRI can be used to identify the neural locus of the selective executive deficit in a subgroup of patients with early PD. This team studied the neural basis of cognitive heterogeneity in PD using a working memory task with an event-related functional magnetic resonance brain imaging (fMRI) design applied to patients at early stages of the disease. Two groups of patients were matched on a range of clinical and neuropsychological measures, but differed in their performance on the Tower of London test. The fMRI analysis was performed with ROI, and memory retrieval and manipulation processes during the executive task were contrasted separately with a motor control period. The authors observed a significant bilateral underactivation of the caudate nuclei during retrieval in the patient subgroup with executive impairment compared with the patient subgroup without cognitive impairment. The hypoactivation of the bilateral caudate was also observed during manipulation, but during this condition significantly lower activation was also found in the dorsolateral ventrolateral prefrontal cortex (Lewis et al., 2003).

The prefrontal cortex plays an important role in modulating action by attentional control, known as "attention to action." In normal controls, attention to action increases the connectivity between prefrontal cortex and premotor and supplementary frontal cortex, but in patients with PD this effect is not seen, suggesting a functional disconnection between these cerebral regions (Rowe et al., 2002). Using an on-off medication design during an attentional task, it has been reported that dopaminergic treatments have a clear differential effect for motor functions, reward, and attention (Rowe et al., 2008).

Using an event-related paradigm, Monchi et al. (2004) demonstrated that both hyper and hypoactivations are seen in PD patients compared to controls during the performance of an adapted version of the Wisconsin card sorting test. Decreased activation was observed in the PD group in the ventrolateral PFC when receiving negative feedback and in the posterior PFC when matching after negative feedback. In contrast, greater activation was found in the PD group compared with the matched control group in prefrontal regions, such as the posterior and the dorsolateral PFC when receiving positive or negative feedback. The same group of researchers (Monchi, Petrides, Mejia-Constain & Strafella, 2007) reported that patients presented increased cortical activation compared with controls in the condition that did not specifically require the caudate nucleus, but decreased cortical activation in the condition that did significantly involve this region. Thus, this study showed a pattern of cortical activation in PD characterized by either reduced or increased activation, depending on whether the caudate nucleus was involved in the task. The authors believe that these observations provide further support for the hypothesis that both the nigrostriatal and the mesocortical dopaminergic substrate may play a significant role in cognitive deficits in PD.

Simultaneous or dual tasks are clearly impaired in PD and it has been hypothesized that this impairment is due to the increased competition between fronto-striatal circuitry as a consequence of dopaminergic depletion. The cerebral dysfunctions responsible for such impairments were investigated by Wu and Hallet (2008). During dual tasks, patients had greater activity in the cerebellum, premotor area, parietal cortex, precuneus and prefrontal cortex compared with normal subjects, suggesting a compensatory activation.

Sequencing has been considered to be a component of executive functions. Tinaz, Schendan, Schon, and Stern (2006) designed a semantic-event sequencing task, which is a variant of the Picture Arrangement subtest of the Wechsler Adult Intelligence Scale-III for use in fMRI studies The task required subjects to examine four pictures of meaningful events, determine their correct temporal relationship, and, finally, re-order the pictures into a coherent sequence. Contrasted with a visuoperceptual task, this task mainly activates several frontal lobe regions. Using ROI analyses, the authors found that, in patients with PD, distinct areas of the prefrontal cortex showed both hypoactivation and hyperactivation, and that left caudate hyperactivation was also observed. The authors concluded that the hyperactivation seems to be compensatory but does not indicate more efficiency.

Following this line of investigation on the role of dopaminergic activation in executive processes, early fMRI studies in PD aimed to investigate the modulatory effects of dopaminergic therapy on neural systems subserving working memory and motor functions. In a study using a medication on-off design, cortical motor regions activated during the motor task showed greater activation during the dopamine-replete state, whereas the cortical regions subserving working memory functions displayed greater activation during the hypodopaminergic state. Interestingly, the increase in cortical activation during the working memory task in the hypodopaminergic state correlated positively with errors in task performance, and the increased activation in the cortical motor regions during the dopamine-replete state correlated positively with improvement in motor function. These results suggest that dopamine modulates the cortical networks subserving working memory and motor functions via two distinct mechanisms: nigrostriatal projections facilitate the motor function indirectly via thalamic projections to motor cortices, whereas the mesocortical dopaminergic system facilitates working memory function via direct inputs to the prefrontal cortex (Mattay et al., 2002).

Farid et al. (2009) compared the BOLD response during a go/no-go task in medication on and off conditions in the same patients, and reported different patterns of brain activation depending on the dopaminergic status. In the drug-off state, brain activation was widely distributed, mainly in the bilateral caudate. Levodopa induced changes in the pattern of cingulate cortex activity, which was more pronounced in the rostral part in the drug-off state and in the caudal part after levodopa intake. The complex effects of dopaminergic modulation were also seen on performance on the Stroop test. Fera et al. (2007) found that after a prolonged off medication state, patients showed activations during the Stroop test in anterior cingulate and presupplementary motor areas, which are hypothesized to operate at a higher level of basal dopaminergic modulation. Levodopa administration attenuated these responses and enhanced the prefrontal cortex response, which was correlated with improved task accuracy. The results of this experiment demonstrate the interference effect is significantly reduced after the administration of levodopa.

Impaired recognition of facial emotions could be explained as a perceptual or a theory-of-mind deficit in PD. In an fMRI study using angry and fearful facial expressions, PD patients had lower activations of the amygdala and fusiform gyrus compared to controls in both on and off states. After levodopa administration, both regions increased activation during the task, thus neurochemical dysfunction in regions related to perception of faces as well as regions related to emotions seems to contribute to the impairment in the judgment of facial emotions in PD (Tessitore et al., 2002).

Odor identification is seen in early stages of PD. Moessnang et al. (2011) found that PD patients have a pattern of hyperactivation during perception of common odors such as banana, pineapple, and lavender oil. Specifically, significant hyperactivation in patients was seen in the piriform cortex, the main part of the primary olfactory cortex, and in the orbitofrontal area. The authors interpreted the increased activation as a compensatory mechanism due to neurodegeneration caused by the loss of signal transmission.

The default mode network (DMN) can be observed as a component of fMRI acquired during resting state or as a network that is deactivated during a complex cognitive task. In PD, the DMN has recently been used to identify network dysfunctions. For the successful performance of cognitive tasks, it has been reported that the integrity of a network showing task-related deactivations may be particularly relevant. According to these hypotheses, deactivation of the prefrontal components of the default mode network could signal a reduction in inhibitory processes (disinhibition) but also the ability to redirect attentional processes from self-reflection to goal-directed behavior (i.e., internal to external reference). Since PD is marked by a loss of dopaminergic neurons projecting to the striatum, it is widely accepted that this leads to a relative functional disconnection of the striato-thalamo-frontal loop, ultimately resulting in impaired modulation of frontal activity. Van Eimeren, Monchi, Ballanger, and Strafella (2009) hypothesized that dopamine depletion in the ventromedial NC might lead to a functional disconnection of the DMN, consequently resulting in a failure to appropriately modulate DMN activity when performing an executive task. They used the Montreal card-sorting task in an fMRI study comparing unmedicated PD and matched controls. The results did not show the expected changes in prefrontal regions: both groups showed comparable deactivation of the medial prefrontal cortex but different degrees of deactivation in the posterior cingulate cortex and the precuneus. Compared with controls, patients with PD not only showed less deactivation of the posterior cingulate cortex and the precuneus, but even demonstrated a reversed pattern of activation and deactivation. Connectivity analysis showed that, in contrast to healthy individuals, the medial prefrontal cortex and the rostral ventromedial caudate nucleus were functionally disconnected, in patients, probably explaining the executive dysfunctions.

The effects of L-Dopa on the ventromedial prefrontal cortex region of the DMN in a procedural learning-related deactivation were described in a PET study (Argyelan et al., 2008). Using fMRI, Wu et al. (2009) also showed that patients in the medication off state had abnormal patterns of functional connectivity that were reversible after levodopa administration. Delaveau et al. (2010) evaluated the effect of levodopa on DMN deactivation in nondemented, nondepressed PD patients who received acute doses of either levodopa or placebo in two fMRI sessions. Brain deactivation was evaluated during a facial emotion recognition task. Although the control subjects showed the classical brain deactivation pattern during the emotion task, the PD patients taking placebo deactivated only the ventral medial prefrontal cortex and failed to deactivate the posterior midline and lateral parts of the DMN network. After levodopa administration, this network was restored in PD patients and was accompanied by an increased attentional resource to external stimuli.

Recognition memory is of high clinical interest because it is relatively preserved in nondemented PD patients and is clearly impaired in demented ones. It is, therefore, useful as an early marker for evolution toward dementia. Using independent component analyses of the BOLD signal in an fMRI study, it was demonstrated that the cerebral networks involved in recognition of words are impaired before the patients presented deficits in this function. During the recognition task of 35 previously seen words, patients performed normally in terms of correct responses and reaction time. However, compared to controls, patients failed to adequately deactivate areas of the DMN such as the precuneus, supramarginal gyrus and temporo-occipital cortex (Ibarretxe el al., 2011) (see Figure 6-2). The DMN has been related to memory functions in normal and pathological conditions, and its deactivation has been found to correlate with recognition-memory performance (Segura et al., 2013). Impaired DMN function could, therefore, be an early marker of declarative memory dysfunctions and can be used to investigate the progression of degenerative processes in nondemented PD.

CONCLUSIONS

Structural MRI studies have shown that PD patients with dementia have widespread cortical atrophy, involving almost all neocortical regions. PD patients without dementia also have reduced gray matter, and this reduction is observed especially those persons with visual hallucinations or mild cognitive impairment. Neocortical abnormalities are seen even at the early stages of the disease. In the prefrontal cortex, gray matter loss is more frequent in the orbital than in the dorsolateral region. Volumetric analyses have demonstrated that the hippocampus is more susceptible to early degeneration than the caudate nucleus, and its atrophy is

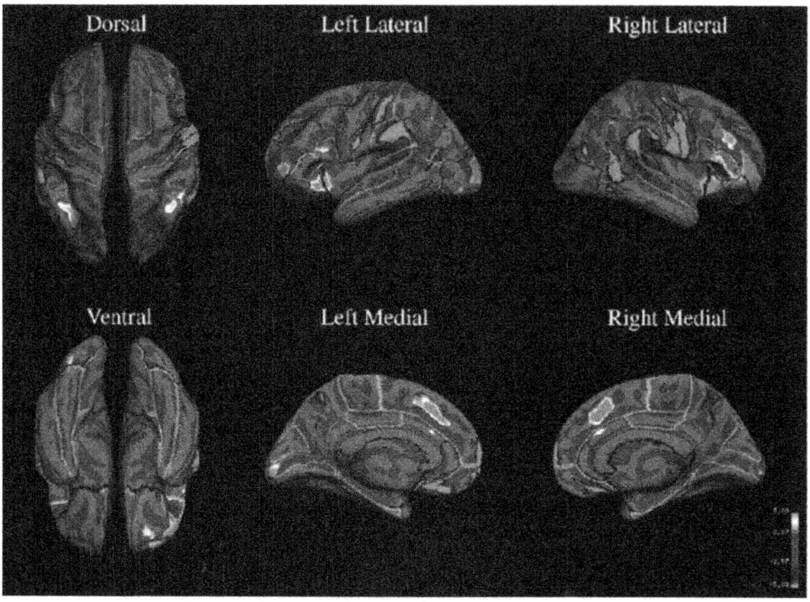

FIGURE 6-2
Regions that showed decreased activations and deactivations in PD patients compared to controls during a recognition memory task. From Ibarretxe-Bilbao et al. (2011).

correlated with declarative memory deficits. Different, albeit nonspecific, neural correlates have been identified for visuospatial, visuoperceptual, and memory and executive functions. Orbitofrontal gray matter reductions have been found to be associated with impaired perception of facial emotions.

Early PET and SPECT studies performed with ROI analyses suggested a major role of the basal ganglia in PD cognitive dysfunctions, especially executive and memory dysfunctions. Later studies assessing the prefrontal cortex also found correlations between prefrontal metabolism and neuropsychological impairment. Finally, whole brain studies highlighted the role of the posterior regions in the evolution of PD dementia.

Functional magnetic resonance imaging studies during task performance have demonstrated patterns of hypo- and hyperactivation in several brain regions. The patterns of brain hypoactivation may reflect dopaminergic failure or underlying cerebral degeneration, whereas patterns of hyperactivation at early stages of the disease may reflect compensatory mechanisms. Independent component analysis has identified changes in PD patients in the activation of specific cerebral networks and in the strength of brain connectivity between the nodes of these networks. The changes in the activation and deactivation patterns associated with a cognitive task may precede clinical evidence of impaired task performance. The resting state and, in particular, the default node network have shown their potential for detecting the effects of levodopa on cerebral networks subserving cognitive functions.

The most remarkable limitation of neuroimaging studies is the correlational nature of almost all the studies that do not allow us to determine the causality of cognitive dysfunctions in PD. Structural and functional studies often seems to be contradictory but probably are complementary. In the future, the multimodal PET/MRI studies in the same samples, as well as longitudinal studies in large cohorts of patients, could clarify the origin and evolution of cognitive and emotional deficits in PD.

REFERENCES

Abe, Y., Kachi, T., Kato, T., Arahata, Y., Yamada, T., Washimi, Y.,...Sobue, G. (2003). Occipital hypoperfusion in Parkinson's disease without dementia: Correlation to impaired cortical visual processing. *Journal of Neurology, Neurosurgery and Psychiatry, 74*(4), 419–422.

Almeida, O. P., Burton, E. J., McKeith, I., Gholkar, A., Burn, D., & O'Brien, J. T. (2003). MRI study of caudate nucleus volume in Parkinson's disease with and without dementia with Lewy bodies and Alzheimer's disease. *Dementia and Geriatric Cognitive Disorders, 16*(2), 57–63.

Apostolova, L. G., Beyer, M., Green, A. E., Hwang, K. S., Morra, J. H., Chou, Y.,...Thompson, P. M. (2010). Hippocampal, caudate, and ventricular changes in Parkinson's disease with and without dementia. *Movement Disorders, 25*(6), 687–695.

Apostolova, L., Alves, G., Hwang, K. S., Babakchanian, S., Bronnick, K. S., Larsen, J. P.,...Beyer, M. K. (2012). Hippocampal and ventricular changes in Parkinson's disease mild cognitive impairment. *Neurobiology of Aging* 33(9):2113–24.

Argyelan, M., Carbon, M., Ghilardi, M. F., Feigin, A., Mattis, P., Tang, C.,...Eidelberg, D. (2008). Dopaminergic suppression of brain deactivation responses during sequence learning. *Journal of Neuroscience, 28*(42), 10687–10695.

Ashburner, J., & Friston, K. J. (2009). Computing average shaped tissue probability templates. *NeuroImage, 45*(2), 333–341.

Baggio, H. C., Segura, B., Ibarretxe-Bilbao, N., Valldeoriola, F., Marti, M. J., Compta, Y.,...Junqué, C. (2012) Structural correlates of facial emotion recognition deficits in Parkinson's disease patients. *Neuropsychologia, 50*(8), 2121–2128.

Beyer, M. K., & Aarsland, D. (2008). Grey matter atrophy in early versus late dementia in Parkinson's disease. *Parkinsonism & Related Disorders, 14*(8), 620–625.

Beyer, M. K., Janvin, C. C., Larsen, J. P., & Aarsland, D. (2007). A magnetic resonance imaging study of patients with Parkinson's disease with mild cognitive impairment and dementia using voxel-based morphometry. *Journal of Neurology, Neurosurgery and Psychiatry, 78*(3), 254–259.

Beyer, M. K., Bronnick, K. S., Hwang, K. S., Bergsland, N., Tysnes, O. B., Larsen, J. P.,...Apostolova, L. G. (2013). Verbal memory is associated with structural hippocampal changes in newly diagnosed Parkinson's disease. *Journal of Neurology, Neurosurgery and Psychiatry, 84*(1), 23–28.

Biundo, R., Formento-Dojot, P., Facchini, S., Vallelunga, A., Ghezzo, L., Foscolo, L.,...Antonini, A. (2011). Brain volume changes in Parkinson's disease and their relationship with cognitive and behavioural abnormalities. *Journal of the Neurological Sciences, 310*(1-2), 64–69.

Bohnen, N. I., Müller, M. L., Kotagal, V., Koeppe, R. A., Kilbourn, M. A., Albin, R. L., & Frey, K. A. (2010) Olfactory dysfunction, central cholinergic integrity and cognitive impairment in Parkinson's disease. *Brain,* 133, 1747–54.

Bohnen, N. I., Koeppe, R. A., Minoshima, S., Giordani, B., Albin, R. L., Frey, K. A.,... Kuhl, D. E. (2011). Cerebral glucose metabolic features of Parkinson disease and incident dementia: Longitudinal study. *Journal of Nuclear Medicine 52*(6), 848–855.

Bouchard, T. P., Malykhin, N., Martin, W. R., Hanstock, C. C., Emery, D. J., Fisher, N. J.,... Camicioli, R. M. (2008). Age and dementia-associated atrophy predominates in the hippocampal head and amygdala in Parkinson's disease. *Neurobiology of Aging, 29*(7), 1027–1039.

Braak, H., Del Tredici, K., Rub, U., de Vos, R. A., Jansen Steur, E. N., & Braak, E. (2003). Staging of brain pathology related to sporadic Parkinson's disease. *Neurobiology of Aging, 24*(2), 197–211.

Bruck, A., Aalto, S., Nurmi, E., Bergman, J., & Rinne, J. O. (2005). Cortical 6-[18F] fluoro-L-dopa uptake and frontal cognitive functions in early Parkinson's disease. *Neurobiology of Aging, 26*(6), 891–898.

Bruck, A., Kurki, T., Kaasinen, V., Vahlberg, T., & Rinne, J. O. (2004). Hippocampal and prefrontal atrophy in patients with early non-demented Parkinson's disease is related to cognitive impairment. *Journal of Neurology, Neurosurgery and Psychiatry, 75*(10), 1467–1469.

Bruck, A., Portin, R., Lindell, A., Laihinen, A., Bergman, J., Haaparanta, M.,... Rinne, J. O. (2001). Positron emission tomography shows that impaired frontal lobe functioning in Parkinson's disease is related to dopaminergic hypofunction in the caudate nucleus. *Neuroscience Letters, 311*(2), 81–84.

Burton, E. J., McKeith, I. G., Burn, D. J., Williams, E. D., & O'Brien, J. T. (2004). Cerebral atrophy in Parkinson's disease with and without dementia: A comparison with Alzheimer's disease, dementia with Lewy bodies and controls. *Brain, 127*, 791–800.

Caballol, N., Marti, M. J., & Tolosa, E. (2007). Cognitive dysfunction and dementia in Parkinson disease. *Movement Disorders, 22*(Suppl 17), S358–S366.

Camicioli, R., Moore, M. M., Kinney, A., Corbridge, E., Glassberg, K., & Kaye, J. A. (2003). Parkinson's disease is associated with hippocampal atrophy. *Movement Disorders, 18*(7), 784–790.

Camicioli, R., Gee, M., Bouchard, T. P., Fisher, N. J., Hanstock, C. C., Emery, D. J.,... Martin, W. R. (2009). Voxel-based morphometry reveals extra-nigral atrophy patterns associated with dopamine refractory cognitive and motor impairment in parkinsonism. *Parkinsonism & Related Disorders, 15*(3), 187–195.

Camicioli, R., Sabino, J., Gee, M., Bouchard, T., Fisher, N., Hanstock, C.,... Martin, W. R. (2011). Ventricular dilatation and brain atrophy in patients with Parkinson's disease with incipient dementia. *Movement Disorders, 26*(8), 1443–1450.

Carbon, M., & Eidelberg, D. (2006). Functional imaging of sequence learning in Parkinson's disease. *Journal of the Neurological Sciences, 248*(1-2), 72–77.

Carbon, M., Ma, Y., Barnes, A., Dhawan, V., Chaly, T., Ghilardi, M. F.,... Eidelberg, D. (2004). Caudate nucleus: Influence of dopaminergic input on sequence learning and brain activation in parkinsonism. *NeuroImage, 21*(4), 1497–1507.

Carbon, M., Reetz, K., Ghilardi, M. F., Dhawan, V., & Eidelberg, D. (2010). Early Parkinson's disease: Longitudinal changes in brain activity during sequence learning. *Neurobiology of Disease, 37*(2), 455–460.

Chan, L. L., Rumpel, H., Yap, K., Lee, E., Loo, H. V., Ho, G. L.,... Tan, E. K. (2007). Case control study of diffusion tensor imaging in Parkinson's disease. *Journal of Neurology, Neurosurgery and Psychiatry, 78*(12), 1383–1386.

Chanraud, S., Zahr, N., Sullivan, E. V., & Pfefferbaum, A. (2010). MR diffusion tensor imaging: A window into white matter integrity of the working brain. *Neuropsychology Review, 20*(2), 209–225.

Cools, R., Stefanova, E., Barker, R. A., Robbins, T. W., & Owen, A. M. (2002). Dopaminergic modulation of high-level cognition in Parkinson's disease: The role of the prefrontal cortex revealed by PET. *Brain, 125*, 584–594.

Dalaker, T. O., Larsen, J. P., Bergsland, N., Beyer, M. K., Alves, G., Dwyer, M. G.,...Zivadinov, R. (2009). Brain atrophy and white matter hyperintensities in early Parkinson's disease(a). *Movement Disorders, 24*(15), 2233–2241.

Dalaker, T. O., Larsen, J. P., Dwyer, M. G., Aarsland, D., Beyer, M. K., Alves, G., & Zivadinov, R. (2009). White matter hyperintensities do not impact cognitive function in patients with newly diagnosed Parkinson's disease. *NeuroImage, 47*(4), 2083–2089.

Dalaker, T. O., Zivadinov, R., Larsen, J. P., Beyer, M. K., Cox, J. L., Alves, G.,...Aarsland, D. (2010). Gray matter correlations of cognition in incident Parkinson's disease. *Movement Disorders, 25*(5), 629–633.

Dalaker, T. O., Zivadinov, R., Ramasamy, D. P., Beyer, M. K., Alves, G., Bronnick, K. S.,...Larsen, J. P. (2011). Ventricular enlargement and mild cognitive impairment in early Parkinson's disease. *Movement Disorders, 26*(2), 297–301.

Damoiseaux, J. S., & Greicius, M. D. (2009). Greater than the sum of its parts: a review of studies combining structural connectivity and resting-state functional connectivity. *Brain Structure & Function,* 213(6), 525–33.

Delaveau, P., Salgado-Pineda, P., Fossati, P., Witjas, T., Azulay, J. P., & Blin, O. (2010). Dopaminergic modulation of the default mode network in Parkinson's disease. *European Neuropsychopharmacology, 20*(11), 784–792.

Emre, M. (2003). What causes mental dysfunction in Parkinson's disease? *Movement Disorders, 18*(Suppl 6), S63–71.

Farid, K., Sibon, I., Guehl, D., Cuny, E., Burbaud, P., & Allard, M. (2009). Brain dopaminergic modulation associated with executive function in Parkinson's disease. *Movement Disorders 24*(13), 1962–1969.

Fera, F., Nicoletti, G., Cerasa, A., Romeo, N., Gallo, O., Gioia, M. C.,...Quattrone, A. (2007). Dopaminergic modulation of cognitive interference after pharmacological washout in Parkinson's disease. *Brain Research Bulletin, 74*(1-3), 75–83.

Gomperts, S. N., Rentz, D. M., Moran, E., Becker, J. A., Locascio, J. J., Klunk, W. E., & Jhonson, K. A. (2008). Imaging amyloid deposition in Lewy body diseases. *Neurology, 71*(12), 903–910.

Henry, J. D., & Crawford, J. R. (2004). Verbal fluency deficits in Parkinson's disease: A meta-analysis. *Journal of the International Neuropsychological Society: JINS, 10*(4), 608–622.

Holthoff-Detto, V. A., Kessler, J., Herholz, K., Bonner, H., Pietrzyk, U., Wurker, M.,...Heiss W. D. (1997). Functional effects of striatal dysfunction in Parkinson disease. *Archives of Neurology, 54*(2), 145–150.

Honea, R., Crow, T. J., Passingham, D., & Mackay, C. E. (2005). Regional deficits in brain volume in schizophrenia: A meta-analysis of voxel-based morphometry studies. *The American Journal of Psychiatry, 162*(12), 2233–2245.

Huang, C., Mattis, P., Tang, C., Perrine, K., Carbon, M., & Eidelberg, D. (2007). Metabolic brain networks associated with cognitive function in Parkinson's disease. *NeuroImage, 34*(2), 714–723.

Hutton, C., Draganski, B., Ashburner, J., & Weiskopf, N. (2009). A comparison between voxel-based cortical thickness and voxel-based morphometry in normal aging. *NeuroImage, 48*(2), 371–380.

Ibarretxe-Bilbao, N., Ramirez-Ruiz, B., Tolosa, E., Marti, M. J., Valldeoriola, F., Bargallo, N.,...Junqué, C. (2008). Hippocampal head atrophy predominance in

Parkinson's disease with hallucinations and with dementia. *Journal of Neurology, 255*(9), 1324–1331.

Ibarretxe-Bilbao, N., Junque, C., Tolosa, E., Marti, M. J., Valldeoriola, F., Bargallo, N.,...Zarei, M. (2009). Neuroanatomical correlates of impaired decision-making and facial emotion recognition in early Parkinson's disease. *European Journal of Neuroscience, 30*(6), 1162–1171.

Ibarretxe-Bilbao, N., Junque, C., Marti, M. J., Valldeoriola, F., Vendrell, P., Bargallo, N.,...Tolosa, E. (2010). Olfactory impairment in Parkinson's disease and white matter abnormalities in central olfactory areas: A voxel-based diffusion tensor imaging study. *Movement Disorders, 25*(12), 1888–1894.

Ibarretxe-Bilbao, N., Ramirez-Ruiz, B., Junque, C., Marti, M. J., Valldeoriola, F., Bargallo, N.,...Tolosa, E. (2010). Differential progression of brain atrophy in Parkinson's disease with and without visual hallucinations. *Journal of Neurology, Neurosurgery and Psychiatry, 81*(6), 650–657.

Ibarretxe-Bilbao, N., Zarei, M., Junque, C., Marti, M. J., Segura, B., Vendrell, P.,...Tolosa, E. (2011). Dysfunctions of cerebral networks precede recognition memory deficits in early Parkinson's disease. *NeuroImage, 57*(2), 589–597.

Ishioka, T., Hirayama, K., Hosokai, Y., Takeda, A., Suzuki, K., Nishio, Y.,...Mori, E. (2011). Illusory misidentifications and cortical hypometabolism in Parkinson's disease. *Movement Disorders, 26*(5), 837–843.

Jokinen, P., Bruck, A., Aalto, S., Forsback, S., Parkkola, R., & Rinne, J. O. (2009). Impaired cognitive performance in Parkinson's disease is related to caudate dopaminergic hypofunction and hippocampal atrophy. *Parkinsonism & Related Disorders, 15*(2), 88–93.

Jubault, T., Gagnon, J. F., Karama, S., Ptito, A., Lafontaine, A. L., Evans, A. C.,...Monchi, O. (2011). Patterns of cortical thickness and surface area in early Parkinson's disease. *NeuroImage, 55*(2), 462–467.

Junque, C., Ramirez-Ruiz, B., Tolosa, E., Summerfield, C., Marti, M. J., Pastor, P.,... Mercader, J. M. (2005). Amygdalar and hippocampal MRI volumetric reductions in Parkinson's disease with dementia. *Movement Disorders, 20*(5), 540–544.

Karagulle Kendi, A. T., Lehericy, S., Luciana, M., Ugurbil, K., & Tuite, P. (2008). Altered diffusion in the frontal lobe in Parkinson disease. *American Journal of Neuroradiology, 29*(3), 501–505.

Kim, J. S., Singh, V., Lee, J. K., Lerch, J., Ad-Dab'bagh, Y., MacDonald, D.,...Evans, A. C. (2005). Automated 3-D extraction and evaluation of the inner and outer cortical surfaces using a laplacian map and partial volume effect classification. *NeuroImage, 27*(1), 210–221.

Lee, J. E., Park, H. J., Park, B., Song, S. K., Sohn, Y. H., Lee, J. D.,...Lee, P. H. (2010). A comparative analysis of cognitive profiles and white-matter alterations using voxel-based diffusion tensor imaging between patients with Parkinson's disease dementia and dementia with Lewy bodies. *Journal of Neurology, Neurosurgery and Psychiatry, 81*(3), 320–326.

Lewis, S. J., Cools, R., Robbins, T. W., Dove, A., Barker, R. A., & Owen, A. M. (2003). Using executive heterogeneity to explore the nature of working memory deficits in Parkinson's disease. *Neuropsychologia, 41*(6), 645–654.

Lewis, S. J., Dove, A., Robbins, T. W., Barker, R. A., & Owen, A. M. (2003). Cognitive impairments in early Parkinson's disease are accompanied by reductions in activity in frontostriatal neural circuitry. *The Journal of Neuroscience 23*(15), 6351–6356.

Liepelt, I., Reimold, M., Maetzler, W., Godau, J., Reischl, G., Gaenslen, A.,...Berg, D. (2009). Cortical hypometabolism assessed by a metabolic ratio in Parkinson's disease primarily reflects cognitive deterioration-[18F]FDG-PET. *Movement Disorders 24*(10), 1504–1511.

Logothetis, N. K., Pauls, J., Augath, M., Trinath, T., & Oeltermann, A. (2001). Neurophysiological investigation of the basis of the fMRI signal. *Nature, 412*(6843), 150–157.

Lozza, C., Baron, J. C., Eidelberg, D., Mentis, M. J., Carbon, M., & Marie, R. M. (2004). Executive processes in Parkinson's disease: FDG-PET and network analysis. *Human Brain Mapping, 22*(3), 236–245.

Lyoo, C. H., Ryu, Y. H., & Lee, M. S. (2010). Topographical distribution of cerebral cortical thinning in patients with mild Parkinson's disease without dementia. *Movement Disorders, 25*(4), 496–499.

MacDonald, P. A., MacDonald, A. A., Seergobin, K. N., Tamjeedi, R., Ganjavi, H., & Provost, J. S. (2011). The effect of dopamine therapy on ventral and dorsal striatum-mediated cognition in Parkinson's disease: Support from functional MRI. *Brain, 134*, 1447–1463.

Macdonald, P. A., & Monchi, O. (2011). Differential effects of dopaminergic therapies on dorsal and ventral striatum in Parkinson's disease: Implications for cognitive function. *Parkinson's Disease, 2011*.

Maldjian, J. A., Laurienti, P. J., Kraft, R. A., & Burdette, J. H. (2003). An automated method for neuroanatomic and cytoarchitectonic atlas-based interrogation of fMRI data sets. *NeuroImage, 19*(3), 1233–1239.

Matsui, H., Nishinaka, K., Oda, M., Niikawa, H., Kubori, T., & Udaka, F. (2007). Dementia in Parkinson's disease: Diffusion tensor imaging. *Acta Neurologica Scandinavica, 116*(3), 177–181.

Matsui, H., Nishinaka, K., Oda, M., Niikawa, H., Komatsu, K., Kubori, T.,...Udaka, F. (2007). Wisconsin card sorting test in Parkinson's disease: Diffusion tensor imaging. *Acta Neurologica Scandinavica, 116*(2), 108–112.

Mattay, V. S., Tessitore, A., Callicott, J. H., Bertolino, A., Goldberg, T. E., Chase, T. N.,...Weinberger, D. R. (2002). Dopaminergic modulation of cortical function in patients with Parkinson's disease. *Annals of Neurology, 51*(2), 156–164.

Menke, R. A., Scholz, J., Miller, K. L., Deoni, S., Jbabdi, S., Matthews, P. M., & Zarei, M. (2009). MRI characteristics of the substantia nigra in Parkinson's disease: A combined quantitative T1 and DTI study. *NeuroImage, 47*(2), 435–441.

Mentis, M. J., Dhawan, V., Nakamura, T., Ghilardi, M. F., Feigin, A., Edwards, C.,... Eidelberg, D. (2003). Enhancement of brain activation during trial-and-error sequence learning in early PD. *Neurology, 60*(4), 612–619.

Mentis, M. J., McIntosh, A. R., Perrine, K., Dhawan, V., Berlin, B., Feigin, A.,...Eidelberg, D. (2002). Relationships among the metabolic patterns that correlate with mnemonic, visuospatial, and mood symptoms in Parkinson's disease. *American Journal of Psychiatry, 159*(5), 746–754.

Mesholam, R. I., Moberg, P. J., Mahr, R. N., & Doty, R. L. (1998). Olfaction in neurodegenerative disease: A meta-analysis of olfactory functioning in Alzheimer's and Parkinson's diseases. *Archives of Neurology, 55*(1), 84–90.

Mechelli, A., Price, C. J., Friston, K. J., Ashburner, J. T1 Voxel-based morphometry of the human brain: methods and applications. *Current Medical Imaging Review 1*, 105–113, 2005.

Moessnang, C., Frank, G., Bogdahn, U., Winkler, J., Greenlee, M. W., & Klucken, J. (2011). Altered activation patterns within the olfactory network in Parkinson's disease. *Cerebral Cortex, 21*(6), 1246–1253.

Monchi, O., Ko, J. H., & Strafella, A. P. (2006). Striatal dopamine release during performance of executive functions: A [(11)C] raclopride PET study. *NeuroImage, 33*(3), 907–912.

Monchi, O., Petrides, M., Doyon, J., Postuma, R. B., Worsley, K., & Dagher, A. (2004). Neural bases of set-shifting deficits in Parkinson's disease. *Journal of Neuroscience, 24*(3), 702–710.

Monchi, O., Petrides, M., Mejia-Constain, B., & Strafella, A. P. (2007). Cortical activity in Parkinson's disease during executive processing depends on striatal involvement. *Brain, 130*, 233–244.

Muller, U., Wachter, T., Barthel, H., Reuter, M., & von Cramon, D. Y. (2000). Striatal [123I]beta-CIT SPECT and prefrontal cognitive functions in Parkinson's disease. *Journal of Neural Transmission 107*(3), 303–319.

Nagano-Saito, A., Washimi, Y., Arahata, Y., Kachi, T., Lerch, J. P., Evans, A. C., . . . Ito, K. (2005). Cerebral atrophy and its relation to cognitive impairment in Parkinson disease. *Neurology, 64*(2), 224–229.

Nagano-Saito, A., Liu, J., Doyon, J., & Dagher, A. (2009). Dopamine modulates default mode network deactivation in elderly individuals during the tower of London task. *Neuroscience Letters, 458*(1), 1–5.

Nakamura, T., Ghilardi, M. F., Mentis, M., Dhawan, V., Fukuda, M., Hacking, A., . . . Eidelberg, D. (2001). Functional networks in motor sequence learning: Abnormal topographies in Parkinson's disease. *Human Brain Mapping, 12*(1), 42–60.

Nilsson, C., Markenroth Bloch, K., Brockstedt, S., Latt, J., Widner, H., & Larsson, E. M. (2007). Tracking the neurodegeneration of parkinsonian disorders—a pilot study. *Neuroradiology, 49*(2), 111–119.

Nishio, Y., Hirayama, K., Takeda, A., Hosokai, Y., Ishioka, T., Suzuki, K., . . . Mori, E. (2010). Corticolimbic gray matter loss in Parkinson's disease without dementia. *European Journal of Neurology 17*(8), 1090–1097.

Owen, A. M. (2004). Cognitive dysfunction in Parkinson's disease: The role of frontostriatal circuitry. *The Neuroscientist,10*(6), 525–537.

Owen, A. M., Iddon, J. L., Hodges, J. R., Summers, B. A., & Robbins, T. W. (1997). Spatial and non-spatial working memory at different stages of Parkinson's disease. *Neuropsychologia, 35*(4), 519–532.

Owen, A. M., Doyon, J., Dagher, A., Sadikot, A., & Evans, A. C. (1998). Abnormal basal ganglia outflow in Parkinson's disease identified with PET. Implications for higher cortical functions. *Brain, 121*, 949–965.

Paschali, A., Messinis, L., Kargiotis, O., Lakiotis, V., Kefalopoulou, Z., Constantoyannis, C., . . . Vassilakos, P. (2010). SPECT neuroimaging and neuropsychological functions in different stages of Parkinson's disease. *European Journal of Nuclear Medicine and Molecular Imaging, 37*(6), 1128–1140.

Pereira, J. B., Junque, C., Marti, M. J., Ramirez-Ruiz, B., Bargallo, N., & Tolosa, E. (2009). Neuroanatomical substrate of visuospatial and visuoperceptual impairment in Parkinson's disease. *Movement Disorders, 24*(8), 1193–1199.

Pereira, J. B., Junque, C., Marti, M. J., Ramirez-Ruiz, B., Bartres-Faz, D., & Tolosa, E. (2009). Structural brain correlates of verbal fluency in Parkinson's disease. *Neuroreport, 20*(8), 741–744

Pereira, J. B., Ibarretxe-Bilbao, N., Marti, M. J., Compta, Y., Junque, C., Bargallo, N., . . . Tolosa, E. (2012). Assessment of cortical degeneration in patients with Parkinson's disease by voxel-based morphometry, cortical folding, and cortical thickness. *Human Brain Mapping* 33(11), 2521–34.

Raichle, M. E., MacLeod, A. M., Snyder, A. Z., Powers, W. J., Gusnard, D. A., & Shulman, G. L. (2001). A default mode of brain function. *Proceedings of the National Academy of Sciences of the United States of America, 98*(2), 676–682.

Ramirez-Ruiz, B., Marti, M. J., Tolosa, E., Bartres-Faz, D., Summerfield, C., Salgado-Pineda, P.,... Junqué, C. (2005). Longitudinal evaluation of cerebral morphological changes in Parkinson's disease with and without dementia. *Journal of Neurology, 252*(11), 1345–1352.

Ramirez-Ruiz, B., Junque, C., Marti, M. J., Valldeoriola, F., & Tolosa, E. (2006). Neuropsychological deficits in Parkinson's disease patients with visual hallucinations. *Movement Disorders, 21*(9), 1483–1487.

Ramirez-Ruiz, B., Junque, C., Marti, M. J., Valldeoriola, F., & Tolosa, E. (2007). Cognitive changes in Parkinson's disease patients with visual hallucinations. *Dementia and Geriatric Cognitive Disorders, 23*(5), 281–288.

Ramirez-Ruiz, B; Marti, M. J., Tolosa, E., Gimenez, M., Bargallo N., Valldeoriola, F.,... Junqué, C. (2007). Cerebral atrophy in Parkinson's disease patients with visual hallucinations. *European Journal of Neurology, 14*(7),750–756.

Ridgway, G. R., Henley, S. M., Rohrer, J. D., Scahill, R. I., Warren, J. D., & Fox, N. C. (2008). Ten simple rules for reporting voxel-based morphometry studies. *NeuroImage, 40*(4), 1429–1435.

Riekkinen, P., Jr, Kejonen, K., Laakso, M. P., Soininen, H., Partanen, K., & Riekkinen, M. (1998). Hippocampal atrophy is related to impaired memory, but not frontal functions in non-demented Parkinson's disease patients. *Neuroreport, 9*(7), 1507–1511.

Rinne, J. O., Portin, R., Ruottinen, H., Nurmi, E., Bergman, J., Haaparanta, M.,... Solin, O. (2000). Cognitive impairment and the brain dopaminergic system in Parkinson disease: [18F]fluorodopa positron emission tomographic study. *Archives of Neurology, 57*(4), 470–475.

Rodriguez-Oroz, M. C., Jahanshahi, M., Krack, P., Litvan, I., Macias, R., Bezard, E.,... (2009). Initial clinical manifestations of Parkinson's disease: Features and pathophysiological mechanisms. *Lancet Neurology, 8*(12), 1128–1139.

Rolheiser, T. M., Fulton, H. G., Good, K. P., Fisk, J. D., McKelvey, J. R., Scherfler, C.,... Robertson, H. A. (2011). Diffusion tensor imaging and olfactory identification testing in early-stage Parkinson's disease. *Journal of Neurology, 258*(7), 1254–1260.

Rowe, J., Stephan, K. E., Friston, K., Frackowiak, R., Lees, A., & Passingham, R. (2002). Attention to action in Parkinson's disease: Impaired effective connectivity among frontal cortical regions. *Brain, 125*, 276–289.

Rowe, J. B., Hughes, L. E., Barker, R. A., & Owen, A. M. (2010). Dynamic causal modelling of effective connectivity from fMRI: Are results reproducible and sensitive to Parkinson's disease and its treatment? *NeuroImage, 52*(3), 1015–1026.

Sawamoto, N., Piccini, P., Hotton, G., Pavese, N., Thielemans, K., & Brooks, D. J. (2008). Cognitive deficits and striato-frontal dopamine release in Parkinson's disease. *Brain, 131*, 1294–1302.

Segura, B., Ibarretxe-Bilbao, N., Sala-Llonch, R., Baggio, H. C., Martí, M. J., Valldeoriola, . . . Junque, C. (2013). Progressive changes in a recognition memory network in Parkinson's disease. *Journal of Neurology, Neurosurgery and Psychiatry, 84*, 370–378.

Shmuel, A., Augath, M., Oeltermann, A., & Logothetis, N. K. (2006). Negative functional MRI response correlates with decreases in neuronal activity in monkey visual area V1. *Nature Neuroscience, 9*(4), 569–577.

Sperling, R. A., Dickerson, B. C., Pihlajamaki, M., Vannini, P., LaViolette, P. S., Vitolo, O. V.,...Johnson, K. A. (2010). Functional alterations in memory networks in early Alzheimer's disease. *Neuromolecular Medicine, 12*(1), 27–43.

Summerfield, C., Junque, C., Tolosa, E., Salgado-Pineda, P., Gomez-Anson, B., Marti, M. J.,...Mercader, J. (2005). Structural brain changes in Parkinson disease with dementia: A voxel-based morphometry study. *Archives of Neurology, 62*(2), 281–285.

Tessitore, A., Hariri, A. R., Fera, F., Smith, W. G., Chase, T. N., Hyde, T. M.,.... (2002). Dopamine modulates the response of the human amygdala: A study in Parkinson's disease. *Journal of Neuroscience, 22*(20), 9099–9103.

Tinaz, S., Courtney, M. G., & Stern, C. E. (2011). Focal cortical and subcortical atrophy in early Parkinson's disease. *Movement Disorders, 26*(3), 436–441.

Tinaz, S., Schendan, H. E., Schon, K., & Stern, C. E. (2006). Evidence for the importance of basal ganglia output nuclei in semantic event sequencing: An fMRI study. *Brain Research, 1067*(1), 239–249.

Vaillancourt, D. E., Spraker, M. B., Prodoehl, J., Abraham, I., Corcos, D. M., Zhou, X. J.,... (2009). High-resolution diffusion tensor imaging in the substantia nigra of de novo Parkinson disease. *Neurology, 72*(16), 1378–1384.

van Beilen, M., Portman, A. T., Kiers, H. A., Maguire, R. P., Kaasinen, V., Koning, M.,... (2008). Striatal FDOPA uptake and cognition in advanced non-demented Parkinson's disease: A clinical and FDOPA-PET study. *Parkinsonism & Related Disorders, 14*(3), 224–228.

van den Heuvel, M. P., & Hulshoff Pol, H. E. (2010). Exploring the brain network: A review on resting-state fMRI functional connectivity. *European Neuropsychopharmacology, 20*(8), 519–534.

van Eimeren, T., Monchi, O., Ballanger, B., & Strafella, A. P. (2009). Dysfunction of the default mode network in Parkinson disease: A functional magnetic resonance imaging study. *Archives of Neurology, 66*(7), 877–883.

Wallin, A., Ekberg, S., Lind, K., Milos, V., Granerus, A. K., & Granerus, G. (2007). Posterior cortical brain dysfunction in cognitively impaired patients with Parkinson's disease--a rCBF scintigraphy study. *Acta Neurologica Scandinavica, 116*(6), 347–354.

Wattendorf, E., Welge-Lussen, A., Fiedler, K., Bilecen, D., Wolfensberger, M., Fuhr, P.,...Westermann B (2009). Olfactory impairment predicts brain atrophy in Parkinson's disease. *Journal of Neuroscience, 29*(49), 15410–15413

Wermke, M., Sorg, C., Wohlschlager, A. M., & Drzezga, A. (2008). A new integrative model of cerebral activation, deactivation and default mode function in Alzheimer's disease. *European Journal of Nuclear Medicine and Molecular Imaging, 35*(Suppl 1), S12–24.

Wu, T., & Hallett, M. (2008). Neural correlates of dual task performance in patients with Parkinson's disease. *Journal of Neurology, Neurosurgery and Psychiatry, 79*(7), 760–766.

Wu, T., Wang, L., Chen, Y., Zhao, C., Li, K., & Chan, P. (2009). Changes of functional connectivity of the motor network in the resting state in Parkinson's disease. *Neuroscience Letters, 460*(1), 6–10.

Zhang, K., Yu, C., Zhang, Y., Wu, X., Zhu, C., Chan, P.,...Li, K. (2011). Voxel-based analysis of diffusion tensor indices in the brain in patients with Parkinson's disease. *European Journal of Radiology, 77*(2), 269–273.

7 Genetics and Cognition in Parkinson's Disease

Madeleine E. Sharp and Roy N. Alcalay

INTRODUCTION

Cognitive performance among people affected by Parkinson's disease (PD) is highly variable. Although some have little or almost no cognitive impairment, others develop dementia within a few years of disease onset. The factors best correlated with cognitive impairment in PD are older age and longer PD duration. However, even these factors may affect people differently. Nearly 20% of patients do not develop dementia even after 20 years of disease (Hely et al., 2008). It is hypothesized that patients' genetic profiles may explain this variability. The goal of this chapter is to review the literature examining the association between cognition in PD and genetic profiles.

We will briefly review the clinical, epidemiological, and anatomical aspects of cognition in PD that are necessary for a better understanding of the contribution of genetics to the cognitive profile of PD patients. We will then provide an introduction to the basic concepts of genetics relevant to PD. The rest of the chapter is dedicated to a review of the literature on each of the genes linked to cognitive performance in PD, including genes associated with rare genetic forms of PD and genetic risk factors that are more common in idiopathic (nongenetic) PD (iPD).

FACTORS TO CONSIDER IN UNDERSTANDING THE GENETIC CONTRIBUTION TO COGNITION IN PD

Heterogeneity of Cognition in PD

At the time of PD motor-symptom onset, patients may present with no, subtle, or mild cognitive impairment (MCI) (Aarsland et al., 2009). By definition, if dementia is present within a year of onset of motor symptoms a diagnosis of Dementia with Lewy bodies (DLB) is made. The cognitive domains that are involved early in the disease are variable, but difficulties often include a dysexecutive syndrome that causes problems with complex attention, decision making, learning, and set-shifting.

MCI is common and may be present at the onset of PD in some individuals (Aarsland et al., 2009). In one pooled analysis, the overall prevalence of MCI was 25.8% among PD patients (Aarsland et al., 2010). Loss of executive function is the most common domain affected in PD patients, as opposed to memory domain among the pre-Alzheimer's patient population (Caviness et al., 2007; Goldman, Weis, Stebbins, Bernard, & Goetz, 2012; Janvin, Larsen, Aarsland, & Hugdahl, 2006), but some patients also exhibit visuospatial, language or memory difficulties (Poletti, Emre, & Bonuccelli, 2011).

Finally, dementia can complicate PD, especially later in the disease. Prevalence of dementia in PD patients 10 years after diagnosis is estimated around 75% (Aarsland & Kurz, 2010), and in an Australian cohort 86% of participants who were alive 20 years after disease onset were demented (Hely, Reid, Adena, Halliday, & Morris, 2008). Even at the time of diagnosis, rates of dementia range from 8–17% (Aarsland & Kurz, 2010), but these studies probably included patients with DLB. Overall, the average, estimated time for PD patients to develop dementia is 10 years. Both older age and longer disease duration are associated with cognitive impairment and are closely correlated to one another; however, the general effect age seems to predominate (Aarsland et al., 2007). This is a key detail to keep in mind as we will show later that most studies of dementia in genetic PD probably do not include patients with either sufficiently long duration of disease or sufficiently advanced age.

In summary, the cognitive profile of PD patients is variable. The cognitive domains that are affected early in the disease differ among patients, and the rate of progression to dementia also varies.

Risk Factors for Cognitive Decline

It is worth taking a closer look at risk factors for cognitive decline. First, identification of risk factors could help establish a link between genetics and dementia in PD if certain features of the genetic forms of PD could also be found to predict incipient dementia in sporadic PD. Second, published data comparing mutation carriers and noncarriers should ideally take into account these risk factors as they represent potential confounders for the rates of dementia in both groups. As we will show in the next section, the number of patients with genetic PD is quite small, making it difficult to adjust analyses for these factors while retaining statistical power.

The strongest risk factors for developing dementia are age (Aarsland et al., 2007; Levy et al., 2002), disease duration (Aarsland et al., 2010), motor severity, and motor phenotype of parkinsonism (postural instability and gait difficulty is associated with higher risk of dementia than the tremor-predominant form of PD) (Burn et al., 2006; Marder, Tang, Cote, Stern, & Mayeux, 1995; Zetusky, Jankovic, & Pirozzolo, 1985), presence of hallucinations (Aarsland, Andersen, Larsen, Lolk, & Kragh-Sørensen, 2003; Aarsland et al., 2004; Ramirez-Ruiz, Junque, Marti,

Valldeoriola, & Tolosa, 2007) and the presence of mild cognitive impairment (Janvin et al., 2006; Williams-Gray, Foltynie, Brayne, Robbins, & Barker, 2007). The issue of age and disease duration has been particularly difficult to control for since patients with genetic forms of PD usually have early PD onset and are quite young at the time of enrollment despite having a long disease duration; this makes it difficult to adequately compare them to a group of sporadic PD patients.

Pathophysiology

Different aspects of dementia in PD can be assigned to separate neuroanatomical substrates.

Early dopaminergic loss in the dorsal striatum, the starting point of the frontostriatal projections (Damier, Hirsch, Agid, & Graybiel, 1999), likely explains why executive function is affected earliest in nondemented PD patients. Deficits in other neurotransmitter systems also contribute to cognitive dysfunction in PD. For instance, PET imaging studies have shown that loss of cholinergic rather than dopaminergic input best parallels cognitive decline (Bohnen et al., 2006; Hilker et al., 2005; Klein et al., 2010). If and how genetic mutations specifically affect signaling in the different brain networks subserving cognition is not known.

In addition to synaptic dysfunction, certain key pathological changes in PD likely also contribute to the pathogenesis of dementia (Braak et al., 2006). Lewy bodies are abnormal intraneuronal aggregates of protein primarily made up of α-synuclein typically found in the substantia nigra of patients with PD. In addition to substantia nigra Lewy bodies, PD patients with dementia also have Lewy bodies in the cortex, an infrequent finding in patients without dementia (Aarsland, Perry, Brown, Larsen, & Ballard, 2005; Apaydin, Ahlskog, Parisi, Boeve, & Dickson, 2002; Hurtig et al., 2000). There are no clear pathological differences between autopsies of patients with PD-dementia and DLB. Neuropathological changes of Alzheimer's disease are also common in PD patients with dementia suggesting a possible overlap between PD and AD (Mattila, Rinne, Helenius, Dickson, & Röyttä, 2000). When autopsies of 92 patients with PD and dementia were examined, all patients with dementia had either limbic (16%) or neocortical (84%) Lewy bodies and 38% also had neuropathologic features consistent with a diagnosis of Alzheimer's disease. This is in contrast to a group of 48 PD patients without dementia, of similar age, where 6% had Lewy bodies that had not spread beyond the brainstem, only 45% had reached the neocortical stage, and only 9.1% had neuropathological changes consistent with Alzheimer's disease (Irwin et al., 2012). Common genetic risk factors for other dementias including Alzheimer's have, therefore, also been investigated as possible contributions to dementia in PD, as will be discussed in a later section.

GENETICS OF PARKINSON'S DISEASE

Although most cases of PD present sporadically, 10–15% of patients have a family history of PD suggesting a strong genetic contribution to disease in these patients.

Recent discoveries in the genetics of PD have led to major advances in our understanding of the pathogenesis of the disease. Genetic risk factors for PD can be defined as alterations in the genetic code that are associated with higher risk for PD. These genetic risk factors can be divided crudely into two categories: (1) genetic alterations that are associated with a high risk for PD, which we, for didactic purposes, will refer to as "monogenic PD" (although the term is slightly misleading because carrying a mutation would not necessarily lead to PD), and (2) genetic alterations that increase the risk for PD only modestly (up to twofold), which we will refer to as "genetic risk factors." Monogenic PD genes are often identified through family-based genetic studies (linkage studies) and are quite rare. Risk factors are more common and often identified through case-control studies. Eighteen genetic loci that are linked to PD have been identified and named PARK1-18.

Monogenic PD

Mutations in at least seven genes (*SNCA, LRRK2, PARKIN, PINK1, DJ-1, GBA,* and *VPS35*) are confirmed to be strongly associated with PD. These genes cause either autosomal dominant (*SNCA, LRRK2, VPS35*) or autosomal recessive (*PARKIN, PINK1, DJ-1*) inheritance of PD. Though these genes are considered to cause monogenic PD, the inheritance is quite complex, because not all mutation carriers will develop the disease. This is defined as incomplete penetrance. For example, only 30–80% of carriers of the most common *LRRK2* mutation in Caucasians, the G2019S, develop PD (Goldwurm et al., 2011). Incomplete penetrance probably results from interaction between the affected gene, other genes, and unknown environmental factors. This inherent heterogeneity among mutation carriers can make it difficult to make generalizations about the clinical characteristics of carriers of certain mutations.

Other factors can also influence the clinical presentation. Most of the genes already listed have been found to have various mutations, not all of which have the same effect. The *PARKIN* and *SNCA* genes, for instance, can either harbor a *mutation* (such as the replacement or deletion of a DNA base pair) or a variation in *copy number* (a deletion, an insertion or a multiplication—either duplication or triplication—of the entire gene or parts of the gene). In the case of *PARKIN,* as will be discussed later, copy number variations are thought to carry a higher risk of disease than simple mutations.

Other Genetic Risk Factors

In addition to the well-defined genes already listed, other genetic variants, or polymorphisms, have been found to confer susceptibility to PD; carriers of these risk factors are at a mildly increased risk of PD. Polymorphisms differ from mutations because they are common, present in at least 1% of the general population, but often in 10–30% of the general population. Though individuals harboring one or more of these polymorphisms have an increased risk of PD, additional factors are necessarily required, and the vast majority of carriers will never develop PD. Polymorphisms in *MAPT, COMT, BDNF, ApoE,* and PARK16 have been identified as risk factors for PD. In some cases, these polymorphisms are located in the genome very close to the location of a gene that causes monogenic-PD. This phenomenon has been reported in the cases of *LRRK2,* and *SNCA.*

In the following sections, we will summarize the studies that focused on the cognitive characteristics of patients with different forms of monogenic PD and those with genetic risk factors for PD. Our review excludes genes that cause atypical PD like *PLA2G6* (PARK 14) which causes dystonia-parkinsonism, *ATP13A2* (PARK9) which causes Kufor-Rakeb syndrome, and *FBX07* (PARK15) which causes early-onset parkinsonian-pyramidal syndrome. *VPS35* is not discussed in further detail either; mutations in this gene have only very recently been discovered (Zimprich et al., 2011), and there are no reports detailing cognitive function.

GENES WITH A STRONG ASSOCIATION TO PD

LRRK2

Background

Mutations in the leucine-rich repeat kinase 2 (*LRRK2*) are a common cause of genetic PD. They account for 4% of hereditary cases and 1% of sporadic PD in one worldwide analysis (Healy et al., 2008).

There are at least six mutations with definite pathogenicity, of which G2019S is the most common, accounting for up to 39% of cases in North African Arabs and up to 18% in Ashkenazi Jews (Clark et al., 2006; Healy et al., 2008; Ozelius et al., 2006). In addition, there are variants in the gene that also convey a risk (albeit lower) for PD. The most prevalent variant is the G2385R, which was reported in 3.6% of a healthy Chinese population from Singapore, *and* in 7.3% of Chinese patients with sporadic PD (Tan et al., 2006). The lifetime penetrance of *LRRK2* mutations is controversial and ranges from 31% to 74% by age 80 (Healy et al., 2008). The protein product of *LRRK2* is Lrrk2, and though its role in the pathogenesis of PD is incompletely understood, some studies suggest that the mutated form shows increased phosphorylation (the addition of phosphorous molecules to the protein) of α -synuclein, one of the major components of Lewy bodies, and that this may interfere with normal degradation (Qing, Zhang, Deng, McGeer, & McGeer, 2009). Other roles for *LRRK2* are also emerging. Neuropathologic features of *LRRK2*-associated PD are highly variable, but Lewy body deposition is common and cortical involvement has been identified in some (Poulopoulos et al., 2012). Clinically, patients are often indistinguishable from idiopathic PD (Healy et al., 2008).

Cognitive Function in LRRK2 Carriers

There are no longitudinal cognitive studies comparing *LRRK2* carriers and noncarriers. Most studies that compared carriers to noncarriers included only the

Mini-Mental State Examination (MMSE) and showed inconsistent results. Although Alcalay and Aasly reported similar MMSE performance, Healy and Lesage reported worse performance among *LRRK2* carriers (Aasly et al., 2005; Alcalay et al., 2010; Healy et al., 2008; Lesage et al., 2006). However, only Alcalay and colleagues corrected for common confounders of cognitive function, including age, disease duration and level of education. Only one study (from Belgium) investigated the prevalence of *LRRK2* mutations in a group of PD patients with dementia, either PD-dementia (PDD, *n* = 75) or DLB (*n* = 99) and found a mutation in only one patient with PDD (Meeus, Verstraeten, et al., 2012).

LRRK2 mutations have also been very rarely reported in patients with primarily dementing conditions typically classified as "cortical" dementias: 3.5% of Alzheimer's patients in one sample had a genetic variant, but this variant was also present in 1.6% of controls (Zhao et al., 2011); one patient with corticobasal syndrome and one with primary progressive aphasia had the G2019S mutation (Chen-Plotkin et al., 2008).

Studies that included more in-depth neuropsychological evaluations of PD patients who are *LRRK2* carriers and noncarriers are summarized in Table 7-1. All studies were cross-sectional (rather than longitudinal) and included participants with variable disease durations. In summary, studies have not shown a consistent difference between mutation carriers and noncarriers, but given their small sample sizes, they were underpowered to detect small differences between groups. Larger studies comparing neuropsychological performance between carriers and noncarriers are currently under way in the Michael J. Fox Foundation LRRK2 consortium.

SNCA

Background

SNCA mutations were the first to be linked to genetic PD. Both mutations and copy number variations have been identified, but, overall, *SNCA* mutations remain an extremely rare cause of hereditary PD, accounting for approximately 2% of autosomal dominant cases. Polymorphisms in *SNCA* have also shown a strong association with idiopathic PD. Linking *SNCA* to PD led to the discovery that α-synuclein, the protein product of *SNCA,* is a major component of Lewy Bodies in PD. Though its function remains incompletely understood, α-synuclein localizes to the presynaptic membrane and is thought to have a role in neurotransmitter release into the synapse.

Three mutations (PARK1) as well as copy-number variations (a duplication and a triplication; PARK4), cause autosomal dominant PD with variable penetrance and a variable phenotype. The A53T and A30P mutations cause typical PD with dopamine-responsive parkinsonism but an earlier age of onset, whereas the E46K mutation can cause a phenotype more typical of DLB. The clinical features of *SNCA* duplications are also similar to sporadic PD except for the earlier age of onset. In addition to variable penetrance, there appears to be a gene dosage

Table 7-1 Neuropsychological evaluations of patients with *LRRK2* PD

Report	*Sample*	*Cognitive measures*	*Findings*	*Comments*
Ben Sassi et al., 2012	55 *LRRK2* PD (all G2019S) 55 non-carrier PD Tunisian cohort.	MMSE MoCA (*n* = 20 *LRRK2*) FAB 6-picture test (*n* = 35 *LRRK2*)	No significant difference: • MoCA <=26 in 65% *LRRK2* and 69% NC • FAB < 13 in 54% *LRRK2* and 66% NC	Visuospatial and executive subscores were particularly low in both groups; however, this could be due to high illiteracy rates in both groups.
Shanker et al., 2011	21 *LRRK2* PD (all G2019S) 21 non-carrier PD Ashkenazi Jewish cohort. Patients were matched for age, sex, disease duration and AAO.	MMSE Hopkins Verbal Learning Test Judgment Line Orientation Test FAB	No significant difference in cognition between carriers and non-carriers.	Psychiatric evaluation revealed that lifetime risk for pre-morbid mood disorder was increased in *LRRK2*
Belarbi et al., 2010	23 *LRRK2* PD (all G2019S) 48 non-carrier PD Algerian cohort. Groups were stratified according to median and high levels of education vs. low level of education.	MMSE MDRS FAB Nine picture test* Associative memory test* Verbal fluency (phonemic and semantic) Trail making (A/B) Isaac's test Stroop Color-Word test Clock drawing test	No significant difference between groups. (In the low educational level subgroup (*n* = 16), a low MMSE was more common in *LRRK2* but this was no longer significant after adjusting for disease duration)	Extensive executive function testing. Neuropsychiatric evaluations revealed a higher prevalence of depression, hallucinations and sleep disturbances in the *LRRK2* group

(*continued*)

Table 7-1 Continued

Report	*Sample*	*Cognitive measures*	*Findings*	*Comments*
Lohman et al., 2009	8 *LRRK2* PD (all G2019S) 10 unaffected carriers from one French Caucasian family.	Medical chart of deceased patients (*n* = 3) MMSE (*n* = 4) MDRS (*n* = 1) FAB (*n* = 1) Trail Making Test A/B (*n* = 1)	Cognitive impairment in 6/8 patients but specific details not available. Avg MMSE 20.7+/−6.1 in carriers compared to 26.7 in nonaffected carriers.	
Goldwurm et al., 2006	17 *LRRK2* PD (all G2019S) Italian cohort	MMSE; FAB Clock Drawing Task Rey Auditory Verbal Learning Test Verbal fluencies Raven's Colored Progressive Matrices Attentive matrices	5/17 (29%) had abnormal MMSE (<24) 6/17 (35%) had abnormal FAB (<13.5)	Significant behavioral abnormalities present in 14/16 carriers

PD, Parkinson's disease; NC, noncarriers; MMSE, Mini-Mental State Examination; MoCA, Montreal Cognitive Assessment; FAB, Frontal Assessment Battery; AAO, age at onset; MDRS, Mattis Dementia Rating Scale.

*novel tests with verbalized visual material used in cases of illiteracy.

effect within the *PARK4* spectrum; in other words, more copies of the gene cause a more severe phenotype: compared to duplications, *SNCA* triplications cause an earlier onset of symptoms, a more aggressive course, more prominent autonomic symptoms and earlier dementia (Fuchs et al., 2007; Meeus, Theuns, & van Broeckhoven, 2012; Sekine et al., 2010).

Cognitive Function in *SNCA* Carriers

Due to the very small number of patients with *SNCA*-associated PD, only limited conclusions can be drawn about their clinical presentation. Though most patients reported have some degree of cognitive decline, neuropsychiatric evaluations have been limited in scope. In some reports of both *PARK1* and

PARK4, patients are simply described as demented without mention of the diagnostic tests used (Ahn et al., 2008; Duda et al., 2002; Farrer et al., 2004; Golbe, DiIorio, Bonavita, Miller, & Duvoisin, 1990; Gwinn-Hardy et al., 2000; Ikeuchi et al., 2008; Markopoulou et al., 2008; Seidel et al., 2010; Spira, Sharpe, Halliday, Cavanagh, & Nicholson, 2001; Wakabayashi et al., 1998; Waters & Miller, 1994; Zarranz et al., 2004), whereas others used the MMSE (Nishioka et al., 2006; Nishioka et al., 2009). The exact profile of cognitive changes in *SNCA*-associated PD cannot be drawn from these reports since none used more detailed neuropsychological testing, except for one family with the E56K mutation that showed early visuospatial deficits and later executive function deficits based on poor performance on the Wisconsin card-sorting test (Muenter et al., 1998). Two patients with dementia underwent advanced neuroimaging: in the first, SPECT imaging showed hypoperfusion of the frontotemporal lobes (Nishioka et al., 2006) and in the second, FDG-PET showed hypometabolism in the occipital lobes reminiscent of dementia with Lewy bodies (Nishioka et al., 2009).

Autopsy studies show that overall, the pathological characteristics of PARK1 and PARK4 are similar—both show typical LB pathology. Neuronal loss is also frequently seen in cortical areas, particularly the hippocampus. In addition to the typical changes of PD, tau-positive neurofibrillary tangles are present but not in sufficient concentrations to fulfill the criteria for a diagnosis of Alzheimer's disease (Poulopoulos, Levy, & Alcalay, 2012).

In summary, both mutations and multiplications of the *SNCA* gene can cause dementia, probably at a higher rate than among mutation-noncarriers. Less clear is whether they have a particular cognitive profile and whether the type of mutation plays a role in their exact cognitive phenotype.

PARKIN

Background

More than 100 different mutations in the *PARKIN* gene (PARK2) have been identified to date. *PARKIN*-associated PD remains the most common cause of autosomal recessive, EOPD. In one systematic review of autosomal recessive PD that looked at more than 5,800 patients with EOPD, 8.6% were found to have a *PARKIN* mutation (Kilarski et al., 2012). Both mutations and copy-number variations have been described but copy-number variations are associated with a higher risk and severity of disease (Pankratz et al., 2009). In addition to the clear risk conveyed by inheriting two mutations in *PARKIN* (a homozygous state), there is some debate that one mutation (a heterozygous state) could also confer increased susceptibility to PD (Pankratz et al., 2009). The gene codes for the parkin protein, a ubiquitin E3 ligase that plays a role in the proteasome degradation pathway. Mutant parkin shows loss of this function with the resulting protein accumulation causing selective neuronal loss without Lewy body formation (Shimura et al., 2000). Affected individuals may develop juvenile (defined as younger than 21) or EOPD. In addition, some patients are described to have foot dystonia, an excellent response to levodopa, and dose-sensitive motor and psychiatric complications of levodopa therapy (Khan et al., 2003; Lohmann et al., 2003). Certain pathological characteristics differentiate them from sporadic PD: Lewy Bodies are uncommon and most reports show more involvement of the substantia nigra than the locus coeruleus (Poulopoulos et al., 2012).

Cognitive Functioning in *PARKIN* Carriers

Several studies have focused on the neuropsychological features of *PARKIN* PD. Of great interest is the fact that, in contrast to sporadic PD, few carriers with dementia have been reported (Benbunan, Korczyn, & Giladi, 2004; Hedrich et al., 2002; Macedo et al., 2009). Given the general clinical impression that *PARKIN* carriers are less likely to develop cognitive impairment (Khan et al., 2003; Lücking et al., 2000), three studies investigated this question using two cohorts.

Lohman and colleagues compared 21 EOPD *PARKIN* carriers to 23 EOPD noncarriers and 9 asymptomatic *PARKIN* carriers in France using the Mattis Dementia Rating Scale (MDRS) (Lohmann, Thobois, et al., 2009). Performance did not differ between the groups, and the authors mention that four of the *PARKIN* EOPD patients had impaired performance on the MDRS.

Alcalay and colleagues investigated an American EOPD cohort, CORE-PD. First, Alcalay and colleagues compared self-reported cognitive impairment between carriers of different genetic mutations (Alcalay et al., 2010). They used the Unified Parkinson's Disease Rating Scale (UPDRS), which asked patients about any signs of intellectual impairment such as forgetfulness, disorientation or difficulty handling complex problems. *PARKIN* carriers reported similar cognitive impairment as noncarriers; however, this cohort was truncated as only nondemented participants were included. In a follow-up examination, participants were evaluated with a comprehensive battery of neuropsychological tests administered to 43 EOPD *PARKIN* carriers (23 heterozygotes and 20 homozygotes or compound heterozygotes) who were compared to 52 noncarrier EOPD and 217 healthy controls (Caccappolo et al., 2011). The battery included tests designed to evaluate each of 5 domains deemed to be predictors of later cognitive decline in PD: psychomotor speed, attention, memory, visuospatial function and executive function. No significant differences were found in neuropsychological performance across the groups and, even when examining individual scores for the *PARKIN* EOPD patients, all were within normal limits. It is worth noting patients had a mean disease duration of at least 10 years; those with two copies of the mutation, who generally have a more benign (albeit early) presentation, had PD on average for 22 years. It is possible that an even longer follow-up is required to identify a cognitive difference between *PARKIN* carriers and noncarriers because carriers develop the disease at a young age when dementia is not prevalent regardless of genetic status (Klein & Lohmann, 2009).

In summary, the data for evaluating cognition in *PARKIN* carriers are more robust than other autosomal recessive PD cases. Although the overall clinical impression is that carriers are less likely to have dementia than noncarriers, this was not confirmed in two independent studies comparing carriers and noncarriers with neuropsychological tools. It is possible the effect is apparent only after a longer disease duration (Alcalay et al., 2013). This observation is particularly interesting given PD patients with two *PARKIN* mutations typically do not show accumulation of Lewy Bodies, suggesting Lewy Bodies are somehow specifically implicated in cognitive decline in sporadic PD and other non-*PARKIN* genetic PD.

PINK1

Background

Mutations of *PINK1* (in the PARK6 locus) were initially identified in 2004 in a large consanguineous Sicilian family (Valente et al., 2004) and though rare, they are an important cause of *PARKIN*-negative autosomal recessive EOPD, especially in European populations (Valente et al., 2002). Like *PARKIN*, heterozygous and homozygous mutations have been associated with PD, but asymptomatic heterozygotes have also been described (Ferraris et al., 2009). *PINK1* localizes to the mitochondria and is thought to play a role in protecting neurons against stress-induced mitochondrial damage (Valente et al., 2004). There have been only a few reports describing the clinical characteristics of patients with *PINK1*-associated PD. The typical phenotype is one of early-onset parkinsonism (as early as the teenage years), levodopa responsiveness, and a protracted course.

Cognitive Functioning in *PINK1* Carriers

Few reports detail the cognitive and neuropsychiatric features of the illness. Though patients seem prone to psychiatric comorbidities such as anxiety and psychotic symptoms (Ephraty et al., 2007; Steinlechner et al., 2007), only a few patients are reported to have dementia. In these studies carriers were assessed at various points in their illness and at various ages. Of 17 patients with homozygous mutations described in the literature and for whom cognition was described, only two developed dementia, and in one case, only 20 years after disease onset (Ephraty et al., 2007; Healy, Abou-Sleiman, Gibson, et al., 2004). Of 13 patients with heterozygous mutations and PD (Bonifati et al., 2005; Ferraris et al., 2009; Healy, Abou-Sleiman, Gibson, et al., 2004; Klein et al., 2005), one developed dementia 11 years after onset of first PD symptoms (Healy, Abou-Sleiman, Gibson, et al., 2004). Only two studies (three patients) used a full neuropsychological battery as part of the clinical assessment (Albanese et al., 2005; Ephraty et al., 2007), which led to the diagnosis of a frontal-type dementia in one patient.

In summary, though there are very few reports of patients with *PINK1* PD, and fewer still for whom cognition was evaluated, it is possible dementia is less frequent among carriers than in sporadic PD. Longitudinal studies with long follow-up periods will be necessary to accurately characterize cognition in this subgroup of patients.

DJ-I

Background

DJ-1 was first identified as a cause of autosomal recessive EOPD in two consanguineous families, one Dutch and one Italian (Bonifati et al., 2003). Mutations of *DJ-1* are very rare and account for less than 1% of EOPD. Heterozygous carriers are probably not affected suggesting *DJ-1* loss of function is pathogenic (Lockhart et al., 2004). The mechanism underlying *DJ-1*-associated PD is not clear, but the protein product appears to play a role in the antioxidative stress reaction. (Taira et al., 2004). In a recent rat model, it was shown to protect dopaminergic neurons by increasing antioxidant capacity and inhibiting α -synuclein formation (Sun, An, & Pu, 2012). The clinical phenotype is that of early-onset, slowly progressive parkinsonism with resting tremor and good response to levodopa (Bonifati et al., 2003; Guo et al., 2010).

Cognitive Functioning in *DJ-1* Carriers

Most patients described were evaluated early in the course of their illness. Given the slow progression of motor symptoms, it is possible that, if present, cognitive changes would follow the same temporal pattern. Macedo and colleagues reported three patients with a *DJ-1* mutation among a Dutch cohort; one had cognitive problems 4.7 years after disease onset as identified by the Cognitive Scale for Outcomes in Parkinson's disease (SCOPA-COG; http://www.scopa-propark.eu) (Macedo et al., 2009). Three brothers have also been reported with *DJ-1* mutations who had a clinical phenotype resembling the PD-Dementia-Amyotrophic Lateral Sclerosis complex; all three had dementia within 10 years of disease onset (Annesi et al., 2005). Overall, PD patients with *DJ-1* mutations have been rarely described and cognitive impairment was occasionally described as part of the phenotype.

GBA

Background

Recessive mutations in the *GBA* gene, which codes for the enzyme glucocerebrosidase, cause Gaucher's disease, an autosomal recessive lysosomal storage disorder. The milder form of Gaucher, Type-1, can present with liver failure, splenomegaly, anemia, and bony involvement. The connection between *GBA* mutations and PD was first discovered when clinicians reported higher frequency of parkinsonism in Gaucher patients. *GBA* mutations are now known to be the most common genetic risks for PD, especially in Ashkenazi Jewish populations (Sidransky et al., 2009). Both carriers of a single mutation (heterozygotes) and carriers of two mutations (by definition, Gaucher patients) are at an increased risk for PD (Chetrit et al., 2012). However, the majority of *GBA* carriers will not develop PD (Rana, Balwani, Bier, & Alcalay, 2013). A pooled analysis found *GBA* mutations in 15% of Ashkenazi Jewish patients with PD and in 7% of non-Ashkenazi PD patients compared to 3% of healthy controls (Sidransky et al., 2009). The mechanism for *GBA*-associated PD remains elusive, but some hypothesize it could be linked to excessive accumulation of α-synuclein. Mutations in *GBA* have also been linked to DLB, and autopsy studies have shown that mutations are associated with a higher load of cortical Lewy bodies (Clark et al., 2009).

Cognitive Function in Gaucher Patients with PD

Patients with Gaucher's disease and PD may have an earlier age of onset, more frequent hallucinations, and exhibit a higher rate of cognitive decline (Goker-Alpan et al., 2008; Neumann et al., 2009). Even in the absence of motor parkinsonism, Gaucher patients and *GBA*-carriers were found to have more cognitive deficits as measured by a two-point difference on the MoCA (McNeill et al., 2012) or by the clinical dementia rating scale (CDR; Biegstraaten et al., 2012).

Cognitive Function in GBA Carriers

When looking at *GBA*-carriers with PD, one report found that the odds of dementia (defined as a score of ≥ 1 on the CDR) was 5.8 in carriers compared to noncarrier PD patients after adjusting for age at onset of motor symptoms, disease duration, and sex (Setó-Salvia, Pagonbarraga, et al., 2011). When using only the MMSE to evaluate cognition, no difference was seen between *GBA* mutation carriers and noncarriers (Alcalay et al., 2010; Clark et al., 2007; Nichols et al., 2009), except for one report that showed worse performance on the MMSE in those with a *GBA* mutation after a mean disease duration of 15.4 years (Alcalay et al., 2012). Studies that used either self-reported cognitive decline (Alcalay et al., 2010) or more sensitive tests of cognitive function such as the Montreal Cognitive Assessment (MoCA) (Brockmann et al., 2011; McNeill et al., 2012), the CDR (Alcalay et al., 2012; Setó-Salvia, Pagonbarraga, et al., 2011), and a battery of neuropsychological tests exploring various cognitive domains (Alcalay et al., 2012) showed significant differences between *GBA* carriers and noncarriers. The most detailed neuropsychological evaluation of patients with *GBA* mutations performed in the CORE PD study included 33 EOPD *GBA* mutation carriers and 60 EOPD noncarrier patients matched for disease duration (15 years in both groups), age (59 and 58 years old, respectively), and gender. Five domains were examined: psychomotor speed and attention using the Trail-Making and Stroop tests; memory and visuospatial function using the California verbal learning test, the Wechsler Memory Scale (WMS), and the Benton Visual Retention Test (BVRT); and executive function using the Controlled Oral Word Association test, the Category Fluency test and delayed recognition. *GBA* carriers did significantly worse on tests of visuospatial function (BVRT) and nonverbal memory (WMS and BVRT). *GBA* mutation carriers were also significantly more likely to receive a clinical diagnosis of MCI or dementia by a consensus meeting based on clinical data, neuropsychological performance, and CDR.

Autopsy studies further support the association between *GBA* mutations and dementia in PD. Among patients who were clinically diagnosed with PD, mutation carriers were more likely to have Lewy body cortical involvement, a pathological finding that may correspond with dementia (Neumann et al., 2009) even after adjusting for age and clinical diagnosis of dementia (Clark et al., 2009). *GBA* mutations were not associated with the presence of Alzheimer's changes. In one report, 7.6% of pathologically proven dementia with diffuse Lewy body disease cases were found to harbor a *GBA* mutation whereas the proportion of Alzheimer's disease cases with a *GBA* mutation was no different than the control group (Tsuang et al., 2012).

Overall, patients with *GBA* mutations appear to exhibit higher rates of Lewy body dementia suggesting *GBA* mutation status could be an independent risk factor for developing cognitive impairment in PD patients, and could be used to distinguish between synucleinopathy and Alzheimer's changes. Further larger scale studies are required to better define the exact neuropsychological profile in these patients and to examine the progression over time of cognitive decline in these patients.

COMMON VARIANTS

Common variants as described earlier are genetic alterations that can be quite common (1–49% of the population) and may be associated with disease risk. There are hundreds of thousands of common variants in the genome; testing each one for an association with cognition in PD would be impractical. Therefore, those that have been investigated for an association with cognition in PD can be divided into three categories: the variants that are already linked to an increased risk for PD (e.g., *SNCA*), those that are already identified as risk factors for other dementing illnesses (e.g., *APOE* and *MAPT*) (Farrer et al., 1997; Galpern & Lang, 2006) and those that are located in genes biologically linked to dopamine function (e.g., *COMT* and *BDNF*) (Bath & Lee, 2006; Foltynie et al., 2005).

APOE

The *APOE* gene has 3 different alleles: ε2, ε3, and ε4. Most people carry two copies of the ε3 allele; individuals with an ε4 allele are at higher risk of developing Alzheimer's disease (relative risk 2.2 in Whites; Tang et al., 1998). Results in PD patients, however, have been mixed. Several cross-sectional studies have shown that the ε4 allele also increases the risk of dementia in PD patients (Pankratz et al., 2006; Parsian, Racette, Goldsmith, & Perlmutter, 2002), as supported by two meta-analyses: one which showed an odds ratio=1.6 for developing dementia in patients carrying the ε4 allele (Huang, Chen, Kaufer, Tröster, & Poole, 2006) and another that showed an overrepresentation of ε4 allele carriers among PD patients with dementia compared to nondementia cases (OR 1.74; Williams-Gray, Goris, et al., 2009). However, others have failed to show this association (Ezquerra et al., 2008; Marder et al., 1994; Ryu & Kwon, 2010) probably because *APOE* is associated with Alzheimer's dementia, which accounts for some but not all cases of PD dementia. Three prospective cohort studies also attempted to answer this question: two found no association between *APOE* genotype and the development of dementia (Kurz et al., 2009) or rate of change on the MMSE (Williams-Gray, Goris, et al., 2009) whereas the third, which used rate of change on the MDRS, found that the ε4 allele was associated with a more rapid decline in MDRS scores (Hazard ratio 2.8; Morley et al., 2012).

COMT

Results from studies investigating the effect of *COMT*, *MAPT*, or *BDNF* polymorphisms on cognition also offer conflicting results. The *COMT* met/met polymorphism leads to a lower level of *COMT* activity and thus higher levels of dopamine. This polymorphism was shown to cause impairment on a task of attention in a small group of patients (Williams-Gray, Hampshire, Barker, & Owen, 2008) and was associated with lower scores on the MDRS attention subscale in a prospective cohort of 212 patients (Morley et al., 2012). However, two other studies: a prospective cohort that screened for dementia using the MMSE (Williams-Gray, Evans, et al., 2009) and a cross-sectional study that used an extensive battery of attention and executive function tests (Hoogland et al., 2010) did not show an association between the *COMT* genotype and cognitive function.

MAPT

Polymorphisms in the *MAPT* gene (specifically, a combination of polymorphisms labeled the H1/H1 haplotype) are linked to tau formation, an important neuropathological finding in other neurodegenerative disorders such as Alzheimer's disease and Progressive Supranuclear Palsy. The H1/H1 haplotype was shown to be associated with cognitive decline in two studies (Goris et al., 2007; Setó-Salvia, Clarimón, et al., 2011), but this was not replicated in a larger cross-sectional cohort (Ezquerra et al., 2008). Longitudinal studies have offered equally conflicting results. Williams-Gray and colleagues followed a group of patients early in the course of their illness over five years and found that the H1/H1 haplotype was a very strong predictor of dementia (OR 12.1; Williams-Gray, Evans, et al., 2009). Another study that followed MDRS scores over an average of three years in a group of slightly older subjects with a longer disease duration showed that, although *MAPT* status was not associated with overall rate of cognitive decline, it was associated with decline in memory (Morley et al., 2012). Morley and colleagues suggested that these conflicting results could be attributed to the longer disease duration in their group and the fact that ultimately, different genetic mechanisms might differentially drive early- versus late-onset dementia.

BDNF

Polymorphisms in the *BDNF* gene, which are thought to influence the function of dopaminergic neurons, were shown in a cohort of 294 PD patients and 233 controls

Table 7-2 Summary of genetic risk factors and reported cognitive features

Genetic risk factors	*Frequency in general population*	*Frequency in PD*	*Association with cognition in PD*
APOE ε4 allele	25% of healthy controls	30% Williams-Gray, Goris, et al., 2009).	OR for dementia 1.6 (Huang et al., 2006).
COMT met/met[#]	28% of healthy controls (Voutilainen et al., 2007).	24% (Hoogland et al., 2010).	Conflicting results, possible effect on attention.
MAPT H1/H1	most common genotype, present in >50% of healthy controls.	65% (Healy, Abou-Sleiman, Lees, et al., 2004).	Conflicting results but probably confers an increased risk for dementia (OR 3.7 to 12.1).
BDNF A/A genotype	4% of healthy controls.	5%	Not clear.

[#] Not all studies specified whether subjects had 1 or 2 copies of the SNP.

to be associated with an increased risk of PD and an increased risk of cognitive dysfunction based on MMSE scores (Guerini et al., 2009). However, later studies in similarly large cohorts did not find this association (Foltynie et al., 2005; Gao et al., 2010; Karakasis, Kalinderi, Katsarou, Fidani, & Bostantjopoulou, 2011).

In summary, the role of known genetic variants in cognition in PD remains unclear (Table 7-2).

SUMMARY, CONCLUSIONS, AND FUTURE DIRECTIONS

In this chapter we summarized the literature on the contribution of genetic profiles to cognitive function in PD (Table 7-3). When compared to iPD, monogenic PD cases may have lower rates of dementia (probably in the case of *PARKIN*), similar rates of dementia (probably in the case of *LRRK2*), or higher rates of dementia (probably in the case of *GBA*). The association between genetic risk factors and dementia is controversial.

There are limitations to the published studies evaluating cognition in mutation carriers. First, very few were longitudinal studies and most evaluated patients relatively early in the course of their illness, when dementia is less likely. Second, patients in the genetic PD groups were often quite young, again limiting the generalizability of results. Third, few studies carried out in-depth neuropsychological evaluations, which is the only way to detect subtle changes in executive function. Instead, the most widely used tool was the MMSE, which lacks sensitivity and is not tailored to detect the subcortical deficits most often present in PD. Finally, many of these monogenic forms of PD are very rare and the number of patients studied is still very small.

Table 7-3 Summary of all monogenic PD and reported cognitive features

Gene	*Mode of inheritance*	*Epidemiology*	*Clinical Features*	*Studies examining cognitive function*
LRRK2 PARK8	AD	Common cause of genetic PD, accounts for 4% of familial cases. Most common in North-African Arabs and Ashkenazi Jews.	Similar to idiopathic PD.	Similar to idiopathic PD.
SNCA PARK1/4	AD	Extremely rare, selected families from Europe. Variable penetrance.	EOPD, rapid progression, dysautonomia. Triplications have more severe course than duplications.	Studies include only small case series but suggest a higher frequency of dementia in mutation carriers.
PARKIN PARK2	AR[#]	Most common cause of AR PD, up to 8.6% of EOPD. More common in Hispanics.	EOPD, dystonia, good levodopa response, higher rate of dyskinesias. Probably slower motor progression than EOPD	Overall impression that dementia is less common in carriers than in noncarriers but detailed cognitive testing performed in two large cohorts showed no difference.
PINK1 PARK6	AR[#]	Very rare, mostly in European populations.	EOPD, similar to *PARKIN.*	Very few reports of cognitive testing in *PINK1* but cognitive decline seems less frequent than in sporadic PD.
DJ-1 PARK7	AR	Extremely rare.	Often EOPD with levodopa-responsiveness but psychiatric and motor neuron disease also reported.	Very few patients described and cognitive decline was identified in some at various points in the illness.
GBA	AD	Most common genetic risk factor for PD, especially in Ashkenazi Jews.	Indistinguishable from idiopathic PD, but can present with more rapid motor progression.	Cognitive decline seems to be more prevalent and perhaps more profound than in sporadic PD.

[#] Heterozygote mutations in this gene may also increase the risk for PD.

Based on autopsy and clinical studies, it is very possible the causes of cognitive impairment in PD are heterogeneous; some cases are a result of Lewy Body pathology progressing to the cortex (e.g., *SNCA* mutations) and others result from concomitant Alzheimer's changes (e.g., *APOE*).

Future research will be required to:

1. Find additional genetic risk factors for PD.
2. Longitudinally study larger groups of patients to more accurately describe, using in depth neuropsychological assessments, their cognitive profile over the course of their illness.
3. Study sufficiently large samples to allow adjustment for important confounders such as age, disease duration, sex, and education.
4. Determine if there is a genetic basis for the difference between patients with mild or severe and early or late cognitive impairment.
5. Evaluate individuals who are asymptomatic mutation carriers to determine if, independent of PD-related changes, there may be an effect of these mutations on cognition.
6. Follow these asymptomatic carriers to determine whether poor performance on cognitive testing precedes (and perhaps predicts) the onset of motor symptoms.

REFERENCES

Aarsland, D., Andersen, K., Larsen, J. P., Lolk, A., & Kragh-Sørensen, P. (2003). Prevalence and characteristics of dementia in Parkinson disease: An 8-year prospective study. *Archives of Neurology, 60*(3), 387–392.

Aarsland, D., Andersen, K., Larsen, J. P., Perry, R., Wntzel-Larsen, T., Lolk, A., & Kragh-Sorensen, P. (2004). The rate of cognitive decline in Parkinson disease. *Archives of Neurology, 61*(12), 1906–1911.

Aarsland, D., Bronnick, K., Larsen, J. P., Tysnes, O. B., Alves, G., & Group, F. t. N. P. S. (2009). Cognitive impairment in incident, untreated Parkinson disease: The Norwegian ParkWest Study. *Neurology, 72*(13), 1121–1126.

Aarsland, D., Bronnick, K., Williams-Gray, C., Weintraub, D., Marder, K., Kulisevsky, J., . . . Emre, M. (2010). Mild cognitive impairment in Parkinson disease: A multicenter pooled analysis. *Neurology, 75*(12), 1062–1069.

Aarsland, D., & Kurz, M. W. (2010). The epidemiology of dementia associated with Parkinson disease. *Journal of the Neurological Sciences, 289*(1–2), 18–22.

Aarsland, D., Kvaløy, J. T., Andersen, K., Larsen, J. P., Tang, M. X., Lolk, A., . . . Marder, K. (2007). The effect of age of onset of PD on risk of dementia. *Journal of Neurology, 254*(1), 38–45.

Aarsland, D., Perry, R., Brown, A., Larsen, J. P., & Ballard, C. (2005). Neuropathology of dementia in Parkinson's disease: A prospective, community-based study. *Annals of Neurology, 58*(5), 773–776.

Aasly, J. O., Toft, M., Fernandez-Mata, I., Kachergus, J., Hulihan, M., White, L. R., & Farrer, M. (2005). Clinical features of LRRK2-associated Parkinson's disease in central Norway. *Annals of Neurology, 57*(5), 762–765.

Ahn, T. B., Kim, S. Y., Kim, J. Y., Park, S. S., Lee, D. S., Min, H. J., . . . Jeon, B. S. (2008). Synuclein gene duplication is present in sporadic Parkinson disease. *Neurology, 70*(1), 43–49.

Albanese, A., Valente, E. M., Romito, L. M., Bellacchio, E., Elia, A. E., & Dallapiccola, B. (2005). The PINK1 phenotype can be indistinguishable from idiopathic Parkinson disease. *Neurology, 64*(11), 1958–1960.

Alcalay, R. N., Caccappolo, E., Mejia-Santana, H., Tang, M. X., Rosado, L., Orbe Reilly, M., . . . Marder, K. (2012). Cognitive performance of GBA mutation carriers with early-onset PD: The CORE-PD study. *Neurology, 78*(18), 1434–1440.

Alcalay, R. N., Caccappolo, E., Mejia-Santana, H., Tang, M. X., Rosado, L., Orbe Reilly, M., . . . Marder, K. (2013). Cognitive and motor function in long duration *PARKIN*-associated Parkinson Disease. *JAMA Neurology, 71*(1), 62–67.

Alcalay, R. N., Mejia-Santana, H., Tang, M.-X., Ratkin, B., Rosado, L., Ross, B., . . . Caccappolo, E. (2010). Self-report of cognitive impairment and mini-mental state examination performance in PRKN, LRRK2, and GBA carriers with early onset Parkinson's disease. *Journal of Clinical and Experimental Neuropsychology, 32*(7), 775–779.

Annesi, G., Savettieri, G., Pugliese, P., D'Amelio, M., Tarantine, P., Ragonese, P., . . . Quattrone, A. (2005). DJ-1 mutations and parkinsonism-dementia-amyotrophic lateral sclerosis complex. *Annals of Neurology, 58*(5), 803–807.

Apaydin, H., Ahlskog, J. E., Parisi, J. E., Boeve, B. F., & Dickson, D. W. (2002). Parkinson disease neuropathology: Later-developing dementia and loss of the levodopa response. *Archives of Neurology, 59*(1), 102–112.

Bath, K. G., & Lee, F. S. (2006). Variant BDNF (Val66Met) impact on brain structure and function. *Cognitive, Affective, & Behavioral Neuroscience, 6*(1), 79–85.

Belarbi, S., Hecham, N., Lesage, S., Kediha, M. I., Smail, N., Benhassine, T., . . . Tazir, M. (2010). LRRK2 G2019S mutation in Parkinson's disease: A neuropsychological and neuropsychiatric study in a large Algerian cohort. *Parkinsonism & Related Disorders, 16*(10), 676–679.

Ben Sassi, S., Nabli, F., Hentati, E., Nahdi, H., Trabelsi, M., Ben Ayed, H., . . . Hentati, F. (2012). Cognitive dysfunction in Tunisian LRRK2 associated Parkinson's disease. *Parkinsonism & Related Disorders, 18*(3), 243–246.

Benbunan, B. R., Korczyn, A. D., & Giladi, N. (2004). Parkin mutation associated parkinsonism and cognitive decline, comparison to early onset Parkinson's disease. *Journal of Neural Transmission (Vienna, Austria: 1996), 111*(1), 47–57.

Biegstraaten, M., Wesnes, K. A., Luzy, C., Petakov, M., Mrsic, M., Niederau, C., . . . Schaik, I. N. (2012). The cognitive profile of type 1 Gaucher disease patients. *Journal of Inherited Metabolic Disease, 35*(6), 1093–1099.

Bohnen, N. I., Kaufer, D. I., Hendrickson, R., Ivanco, L. S., Lopresti, B. J., Constantine, G. M., . . . Dekosky, S. T. (2006). Cognitive correlates of cortical cholinergic denervation in Parkinson's disease and parkinsonian dementia. *Journal of Neurology, 253*(2), 242–247.

Bonifati, V., Rizzu, P., van Baren, M. J., Schaap, O., Breedveld, G. J., Krieger, E., . . . Heutink, P. (2003). Mutations in the DJ-1 gene associated with autosomal recessive early-onset parkinsonism. *Science, 299*(5604), 256–259.

Bonifati, V., Rohé, C. F., Breedveld, G. J., Fabrizio, E., De Mari, M., Tassorelli, C., . . . Network, I. P. G. (2005). Early-onset parkinsonism associated with PINK1 mutations: Frequency, genotypes, and phenotypes. *Neurology, 65*(1), 87–95.

Braak, H., Bohl, J. R., Müller, C. M., Rüb, U., de Vos, R. A. I., & Del Tredici, K. (2006). Stanley Fahn Lecture 2005: The staging procedure for the inclusion body pathology associated with sporadic Parkinson's disease reconsidered. *Movement Disorders, 21*(12), 2042–2051.

Brockmann, K., Srulijes, K., Hauser, A. K., Schulte, C., Csoti, I., Gasser, T., & Berg, D. (2011). GBA-associated PD presents with nonmotor characteristics. *Neurology, 77*(3), 276–280.

Burn, D. J., Rowan, E. N., Allan, L. M., Molloy, S., O'Brien, J. T., & McKeith, I. G. (2006). Motor subtype and cognitive decline in Parkinson's disease, Parkinson's disease with dementia, and dementia with Lewy bodies. *Journal of Neurology, Neurosurgery and Psychiatry, 77*(5), 585–589.

Caccappolo, E., Alcalay, R. N., Mejia-Santana, H., Tang, M.-X., Rakitin, B., Rosado, L.,... Marder, K. S. (2011). Neuropsychological Profile of Parkin Mutation Carriers with and without Parkinson Disease: The CORE-PD Study. *Journal of the International Neuropsychological Society: JINS, 17*(01), 91–100.

Caviness, J. N., Driver-Dunckley, E., Connor, D. J., Sabbagh, M. N., Hentz, J. G., Noble, B.,... Adler, C. H. (2007). Defining mild cognitive impairment in Parkinson's disease. *Movement Disorders, 22*(9), 1272–1277.

Chen-Plotkin, A. S., Yuan, W., Anderson, C., Wood, E. M., Hurtig, H. I., Clark, C. M.,... Deerlin, V. M. V. (2008). Corticobasal syndrome and primary progressive aphasia as manifestations of LRRK2 gene mutations. *Neurology, 70*(7), 521–527.

Chetrit, E. B., Alcalay, R. N., Steiner-Birmanns, B., Altarescu, G., Phillips, M., Elstein, D., & Zimran, A. (2012). Phenotype in patients with Gaucher disease and Parkinson disease. *Blood Cells, Molecules, and Diseases, 50*(3), 218–221.

Clark, L. N., Kartsaklis, L. A., Wolf Gilbert, R., Dorado, B., Ross, B. M., Kisselev, S.,... Marder, K. (2009). Association of glucocerebrosidase mutations with dementia with lewy bodies. *Archives of Neurology, 66*(5), 578–583.

Clark, L. N., Ross, B. M., Wang, Y., Mejia-Santana, H., Harris, J., Louis, E. D.,... Marder, K. (2007). Mutations in the glucocerebrosidase gene are associated with early-onset Parkinson disease. *Neurology, 69*(12), 1270–1277.

Clark, L. N., Wang, Y., Karlins, E., Saito, L., Mejia-Santana, H., Harris, J.,... Marder, K. (2006). Frequency of LRRK2 mutations in early- and late-onset Parkinson disease. *Neurology, 67*(10), 1786–1791.

Damier, P., Hirsch, E. C., Agid, Y., & Graybiel, A. M. (1999). The substantia nigra of the human brain. II. Patterns of loss of dopamine-containing neurons in Parkinson's disease. *Brain, 122*(Pt 8), 1437–1448.

Duda, J. E. J., Giasson, B. I. B., Mabon, M. E. M., Miller, D. C. D., Golbe, L. I. L., Lee, V. M.-Y. V., & Trojanowski, J. Q. J. (2002). Concurrence of alpha-synuclein and tau brain pathology in the Contursi kindred. *Acta Neuropathologica, 104*(1), 7–11.

Ephraty, L., Porat, O., Israeli, D., Cohen, O. S., Tunkel, O., Yael, S.,... Hassin-Baer, S. (2007). Neuropsychiatric and cognitive features in autosomal-recessive early parkinsonism due to PINK1 mutations. *Movement Disorders, 22*(4), 566–569.

Ezquerra, M., Campdelacreu, J., Gaig, C., Compta, Y., Muñoz, E., Martí, M. J.,... Tolosa, E. (2008). Lack of association of APOE and tau polymorphisms with dementia in Parkinson's disease. *Neuroscience Letters, 448*(1), 20–23.

Farrer, L. A., Cupples, L. A., Haines, J. L., Hyman, B., Kukull, W. A., Mayeux, R.,... van Duijn, C. M. (1997). Effects of age, sex, and ethnicity on the association between apolipoprotein E genotype and Alzheimer disease. A meta-analysis. APOE and Alzheimer Disease Meta Analysis Consortium. *JAMA, 278*(16), 1349–1356.

Farrer, M., Kachergus, J., Forno, L., Lincoln, S., Wang, D.-S., Hulihan, M.,...Langston, J. W. (2004). Comparison of kindreds with parkinsonism and alpha-synuclein genomic multiplications. *Annals of Neurology, 55*(2), 174–179.

Ferraris, A., Ialongo, T., Passali, G. C., Pellecchia, M. T., Brusa, L., Laruffa, M.,...Bentivoglio, A. R. (2009). Olfactory dysfunction in Parkinsonism caused by PINK1 mutations. *Movement Disorders, 24*(16), 2350–2357.

Foltynie, T., Lewis, S. G. J., Goldberg, T. E., Blackwell, A. D., Kolachana, B. S., Weinberger, D. R.,...Barker, R. A. (2005). The BDNF Val66Met polymorphism has a gender specific influence on planning ability in Parkinson's disease. *Journal of Neurology, 252*(7), 833–838.

Fuchs, J., Nilsson, C., Kachergus, J., Munz, M., Larsson, E. M., Schule, B.,...Farrer, M. J. (2007). Phenotypic variation in a large Swedish pedigree due to SNCA duplication and triplication. *Neurology, 68*(12), 916–922.

Galpern, W. R., & Lang, A. E. (2006). Interface between tauopathies and synucleinopathies: A tale of two proteins. *Annals of Neurology, 59*(3), 449–458.

Gao, L., Díaz-Corrales, F. J., Carrillo, F., Díaz-Martín, J., Caceres-Redondo, M. T., Carballo, M.,...Mir, P. (2010). Brain-derived neurotrophic factor G196A polymorphism and clinical features in Parkinson's disease. *Acta Neurologica Scandinavica, 122*(1), 41–45.

Goker-Alpan, O., Lopez, G., Vithayathil, J., Davis, J., Hallett, M., & Sidransky, E. (2008). The spectrum of parkinsonian manifestations associated with glucocerebrosidase mutations. *Archives of Neurology, 65*(10), 1353–1357.

Golbe, L. I., Di Iorio, G., Bonavita, V., Miller, D. C., & Duvoisin, R. C. (1990). A large kindred with autosomal dominant Parkinson's disease. *Annals of Neurology, 27*(3), 276–282.

Goldman, J. G., Weis, H., Stebbins, G., Bernard, B., & Goetz, C. G. (2012). Clinical differences among mild cognitive impairment subtypes in Parkinson's disease. *Movement Disorders, 27*(9), 1129–1136.

Goldwurm, S., Tunesi, S., Tesei, S., Zini, M., Sironi, F., Primignani, P.,...Pezzoli, G. (2011). Kin-cohort analysis of LRRK2-G2019S penetrance in Parkinson's disease. *Movement Disorders, 26*(11), 2144–2145.

Goldwurm, S., Zini, M., Di Fonzo, A., De Gaspari, D., Siri, C., Simons, E. J.,...Pezzoli, G. (2006). LRRK2 G2019S mutation and Parkinson's disease: a clinical, neuropsychological and neuropsychiatric study in a large Italian sample. *Parkinsonism & Related Disorders, 12*(7), 410–419.

Goris, A., Williams-Gray, C. H., Clark, G. R., Foltynie, T., Lewis, S. J. G., Brown, J.,...Sawcer, S. J. (2007). Tau and α-synuclein in susceptibility to, and dementia in, Parkinson's disease. *Annals of Neurology, 62*(2), 145–153.

Guerini, F. R., Beghi, E., Riboldazzi, G., Zangaglia, R., Pianezzola, C., Bono, G.,...Martignoni, E. (2009). BDNF Val66Met polymorphism is associated with cognitive impairment in Italian patients with Parkinson's disease. *European Journal of Neurology, 16*(11), 1240–1245.

Guo, J.-f., Zhang, X.-w., Nie, L.-l., Zhang, H.-n., Liao, B., Li, J.,...Tang, B.-s. (2010). Mutation analysis of Parkin, PINK1 and DJ-1 genes in Chinese patients with sporadic early onset parkinsonism. *Journal of Neurology, 257*(7), 1170–1175.

Gwinn-Hardy, K., Mehta, N. D., Farrer, M., Maraganore, D., Muenter, M., Yen, S. H.,...Dickson, D. W. (2000). Distinctive neuropathology revealed by alpha-synuclein antibodies in hereditary parkinsonism and dementia linked to chromosome 4p. *Acta Neuropathologica, 99*(6), 663–672.

Healy, D. G., Abou-Sleiman, P. M., Gibson, J. M., Ross, O. A., Jain, S., Gandhi, S., . . . Lynch, T. (2004). PINK1 (PARK6) associated Parkinson disease in Ireland. *Neurology, 63*(8), 1486–1488.

Healy, D. G., Abou-Sleiman, P. M., Lees, A. J., Casas, J. P., Quinn, N., Bhatia, K., . . . Wood, N. W. (2004). Tau gene and Parkinson's disease: a case-control study and meta-analysis. *Journal of Neurology, Neurosurgery and Psychiatry, 75*(7), 962–965.

Healy, D. G., Falchi, M., O'Sullivan, S. S., Bonifati, V., Dürr, A., Bressman, S., . . . Wood, N. W. (2008). Phenotype, genotype, and worldwide genetic penetrance of LRRK2-associated Parkinson's disease: a case-control study. *Lancet Neurology, 7*(7), 583–590.

Hedrich, K., Marder, K., Harris, J., Kann, M., Lynch, T., Meija Santana, H., . . . Fahn, S. (2002). Evaluation of 50 probands with early-onset Parkinson's disease for Parkin mutations. *Neurology, 58*(8), 1239–1246.

Hely, M. A., Reid, W. G. J., Adena, M. A., Halliday, G. M., & Morris, J. G. L. (2008). The Sydney multicenter study of Parkinson's disease: The inevitability of dementia at 20 years. *Movement Disorders, 23*(6), 837–844.

Hilker, R., Thomas, A. V., Klein, J. C., Weisenbach, S., Kalbe, E., Burghaus, L., . . . Heiss, W. D. (2005). Dementia in Parkinson disease: Functional imaging of cholinergic and dopaminergic pathways. *Neurology, 65*(11), 1716–1722.

Hoogland, J., de Bie, R. M. A., Williams-Gray, C. H., Muslimović, D., Schmand, B., & Post, B. (2010). Catechol-O-methyltransferase val158met and cognitive function in Parkinson's disease. *Movement Disorders, 25*(15), 2550–2554.

Huang, X., Chen, P., Kaufer, D. I., Tröster, A. I., & Poole, C. (2006). Apolipoprotein E and dementia in Parkinson disease: A meta-analysis. *Archives of Neurology, 63*(2), 189–193.

Hurtig, H. I., Trojanowski, J. Q., Galvin, J., Ewbank, D., Schmidt, M. L., Lee, V. M., . . . Arnold, S. E. (2000). Alpha-synuclein cortical Lewy bodies correlate with dementia in Parkinson's disease. *Neurology, 54*(10), 1916–1921.

Ikeuchi, T., Kakita, A., Shiga, A., Kasuga, K., Kaneko, H., Tan, C.-F., . . . Ishikawa, A. (2008). Patients homozygous and heterozygous for SNCA duplication in a family with parkinsonism and dementia. *Archives of Neurology, 65*(4), 514–519.

Irwin, D. J., White, M. T., Toledo, J. B., Xie, S. X., Robinson, J. L., Van Deerlin, V., . . . Trojanowski, J. Q. (2012). Neuropathologic substrates of Parkinson disease dementia. *Annals of Neurology, 72*(4), 587–598.

Janvin, C. C., Larsen, J. P., Aarsland, D., & Hugdahl, K. (2006). Subtypes of mild cognitive impairment in parkinson's disease: Progression to dementia. *Movement Disorders, 21*(9), 1343–1349.

Karakasis, C., Kalinderi, K., Katsarou, Z., Fidani, L., & Bostantjopoulou, S. (2011). Association of brain-derived neurotrophic factor (BDNF) Val66Met polymorphism with Parkinson's disease in a Greek population. *Journal of Clinical Neuroscience, 18*(12), 1744–1745.

Khan, N. L., Graham, E., Critchley, P., Schrag, A. E., Wood, N. W., Lees, A. J., . . . Quinn, N. (2003). Parkin disease: a phenotypic study of a large case series. *Brain, 126*(6), 1279–1292.

Kilarski, L. L., Pearson, J. P., Newsway, V., Majounie, E., Knipe, M. D. W., Misbahuddin, A., . . . Morris, H. R. (2012). Systematic Review and UK-Based Study of PARK2 (parkin), PINK1, PARK7 (DJ-1) and LRRK2 in early-onset Parkinson's disease. *Movement Disorders, 27*(12), 1522–1529.

Klein, C., Djarmati, A., Hedrich, K., Schäfer, N., Scaglione, C., Marchese, R., ... Pramstaller, P. P. (2005). PINK1, Parkin, and DJ-1 mutations in Italian patients with early-onset parkinsonism. *European Journal of Human Genetics: EJHG, 13*(9), 1086–1093.

Klein, C., & Lohmann, K. (2009). Parkinson disease(s): Is "Parkin disease" a distinct clinical entity? *Neurology, 72*(2), 106–107.

Klein, J. C., Eggers, C., Kalbe, E., Weisenbach, S., Hohmann, C., Vollmar, S., ... Hilker, R. (2010). Neurotransmitter changes in dementia with Lewy bodies and Parkinson disease dementia in vivo. *Neurology, 74*(11), 885–892.

Kurz, M. W., Dekomien, G., Nilsen, O. B., Larsen, J. P., Aarsland, D., & Alves, G. (2009). APOE alleles in Parkinson disease and their relationship to cognitive decline: A population-based, longitudinal study. *Journal of Geriatric Psychiatry and Neurology, 22*(3), 166–170.

Lesage, S., Dürr, A., Tazir, M., Lohmann, E., Leutenegger, A.-L., Janin, S., ... Group, F. P. a. s. D. G. S. (2006). LRRK2 G2019S as a cause of Parkinson's disease in North African Arabs. *The New England Journal of Medicine, 354*(4), 422–423.

Levy, G., Schupf, N., Tang, M.-X., Cote, L. J., Louis, E. D., Mejia, H., ... Marder, K. (2002). Combined effect of age and severity on the risk of dementia in Parkinson's disease. *Annals of Neurology, 51*(6), 722–729.

Lockhart, P. J., Lincoln, S., Hulihan, M., Kachergus, J., Wilkes, K., Bisceglio, G., ... Farrer, M. J. (2004). DJ-1 mutations are a rare cause of recessively inherited early onset parkinsonism mediated by loss of protein function. *Journal of Medical Genetics, 41*(3), e22.

Lohmann, E., Leclere, L., De Anna, F., Lesage, S., Dubois, B., Agid, Y., ... Group, F. P. a. s. D. G. S. (2009). A clinical, neuropsychological and olfactory evaluation of a large family with LRRK2 mutations. *Parkinsonism & Related Disorders, 15*(4), 273–276.

Lohmann, E., Periquet, M., Bonifati, V., Wood, N. W., De Michele, G., Bonnet, A.-M., ... Disease, E. C. o. G. S. i. P. a. s. (2003). How much phenotypic variation can be attributed to parkin genotype? *Annals of Neurology, 54*(2), 176–185.

Lohmann, E., Thobois, S., Lesage, S., Broussolle, E., du Montcel, S. T., Ribeiro, M.-J., ... Group, F. P. a. s. D. G. S. (2009). A multidisciplinary study of patients with early-onset PD with and without parkin mutations. *Neurology, 72*(2), 110–116.

Lücking, C. B., Dürr, A., Bonifati, V., Vaughan, J., De Michele, G., Gasser, T., ... Disease, E. C. o. G. S. i. P. s. (2000). Association between early-onset Parkinson's disease and mutations in the parkin gene. *The New England Journal of Medicine, 342*(21), 1560–1567.

Macedo, M. G., Verbaan, D., Fang, Y., van Rooden, S. M., Visser, M., Anar, B., ... Heutink, P. (2009). Genotypic and phenotypic characteristics of Dutch patients with early onset Parkinson's disease. *Movement Disorders, 24*(2), 196–203.

Marder, K., Maestre, G., Cote, L., Mejia, H., Alfaro, B., Halim, A., ... Mayeux, R. (1994). The apolipoprotein epsilon 4 allele in Parkinson's disease with and without dementia. *Neurology, 44*(7), 1330–1331.

Marder, K., Tang, M. X., Cote, L., Stern, Y., & Mayeux, R. (1995). The frequency and associated risk factors for dementia in patients with Parkinson's disease. *Archives of Neurology, 52*(7), 695–701.

Markopoulou, K., Dickson, D. W., McComb, R. D., Wszolek, Z. K., Katechalidou, L., Avery, L., ... Chase, B. A. (2008). Clinical, neuropathological and genotypic variability in SNCA A53T familial Parkinson's disease. Variability in familial Parkinson's disease. *Acta Neuropathologica, 116*(1), 25–35.

Mattila, P. M., Rinne, J. O., Helenius, H., Dickson, D. W., & Röyttä, M. (2000). Alpha-synuclein-immunoreactive cortical Lewy bodies are associated with cognitive impairment in Parkinson's disease. *Acta Neuropathologica, 100*(3), 285–290.

McNeill, A., Duran, R., Proukakis, C., Bras, J., Hughes, D., Mehta, A., . . . Schapira, A. H. V. (2012). Hyposmia and cognitive impairment in Gaucher disease patients and carriers. *Movement Disorders, 27*(4), 526–532.

Meeus, B., Theuns, J., & Van Broeckhoven, C. (2012). The genetics of dementia with Lewy bodies: what are we missing? *Archives of Neurology, 69*(9), 1113–1118.

Meeus, B., Verstraeten, A., Crosiers, D., Engelborghs, S., Van den Broeck, M., Mattheijssens, M., . . . Theuns, J. (2012). DLB and PDD: a role for mutations in dementia and Parkinson disease genes? *Neurobiology of Aging, 33*(3), 629.e625–629.e618.

Morley, J. F., Xie, S. X., Hurtig, H. I., Stern, M. B., Colcher, A., Horn, S., . . . Siderowf, A. (2012). Genetic influences on cognitive decline in Parkinson's disease. *Movement Disorders, 27*(4), 512–518.

Muenter, M. D., Forno, L. S., Hornykiewicz, O., Kish, S. J., Maraganore, D. M., Caselli, R. J., . . . Calne, D. B. (1998). Hereditary form of parkinsonism--dementia. *Annals of Neurology, 43*(6), 768–781.

Neumann, J., Bras, J., Deas, E., O'Sullivan, S. S., Parkkinen, L., Lachmann, R. H., . . . Wood, N. W. (2009). Glucocerebrosidase mutations in clinical and pathologically proven Parkinson's disease. *Brain, 132*(7), 1783–1794.

Nichols, W. C., Pankratz, N., Marek, D. K., Pauciulo, M. W., Elsaesser, V. E., Halter, C. A., . . . Investigators, F. t. P. S. G.-P. (2009). Mutations in GBA are associated with familial Parkinson disease susceptibility and age at onset. *Neurology, 72*(4), 310–316.

Nishioka, K., Hayashi, S., Farrer, M. J., Singleton, A. B., Yoshino, H., Imai, H., . . . Hattori, N. (2006). Clinical heterogeneity of α-synuclein gene duplication in Parkinson's disease. *Annals of Neurology, 59*(2), 298–309.

Nishioka, K., Ross, O. A., Ishii, K., Kachergus, J. M., Ishiwata, K., Kitagawa, M., . . . Hattori, N. (2009). Expanding the clinical phenotype of SNCA duplication carriers. *Movement Disorders, 24*(12), 1811–1819.

Ozelius, L. J., Senthil, G., Saunders-Pullman, R., Ohmann, E., Deligtisch, A., Tagliati, M., . . . Bressman, S. B. (2006). LRRK2 G2019S as a cause of Parkinson's disease in Ashkenazi Jews. *The New England Journal of Medicine, 354*(4), 424–425.

Pankratz, N., Byder, L., Halter, C., Rudolph, A., Shults, C. W., Conneally, P. M., . . . Nichols, W. C. (2006). Presence of an APOE4 allele results in significantly earlier onset of Parkinson's disease and a higher risk with dementia. *Movement Disorders, 21*(1), 45–49.

Pankratz, N., Kissell, D. K., Pauciulo, M. W., Halter, C. A., Rudolph, A., Pfeiffer, R. F., . . . Nichols, W. C. (2009). Parkin dosage mutations have greater pathogenicity in familial PD than simple sequence mutations. *Neurology, 73*(4), 279–286.

Parsian, A., Racette, B., Goldsmith, L. J., & Perlmutter, J. S. (2002). Parkinson's Disease and Apolipoprotein E: Possible Association with Dementia but not Age at Onset. *Genomics, 79*(3), 458–461.

Poletti, M., Emre, M., & Bonuccelli, U. (2011). Mild cognitive impairment and cognitive reserve in Parkinson's disease. *Parkinsonism & Related Disorders, 17*(8), 579–586.

Poulopoulos, M., Cortes, E., Vonsattel, J.-P. G., Fahn, S., Waters, C., Cote, L. J., . . . Alcalay, R. N. (2012). Clinical and pathological characteristics of LRRK2 G2019S patients with PD. *Journal of Molecular Neuroscience : MN, 47*(1), 139–143.

Poulopoulos, M., Levy, O. A., & Alcalay, R. N. (2012). The neuropathology of genetic Parkinson's disease. *Movement Disorders, 27*(7), 831–842.

Qing, H., Zhang, Y., Deng, Y., McGeer, E. G., & McGeer, P. L. (2009). Lrrk2 interaction with α-synuclein in diffuse Lewy body disease. *Biochemical and Biophysical Research Communications, 390*(4), 1229–1234.

Ramirez-Ruiz, B., Junque, C., Martí, M. J., Valldeoriola, F., & Tolosa, E. (2007). Cognitive changes in Parkinson's disease patients with visual hallucinations. *Dementia and Geriatric Cognitive Disorders, 23*(5), 281–288.

Rana, H. Q., Balwani, M., Bier, L., & Alcalay, R. N. (2013). Age-specific Parkinson disease risk in GBA mutation carriers: information for genetic counseling. *Genetics in Medicine 15*(2), 146–149.

Ryu, H. G., & Kwon, O. D. (2010). Apolipoprotein E epsilon 4 allele is not associated with age at onset or MMSE of Parkinson's disease in a Korean study. *Parkinsonism & Related Disorders, 16*(9), 615–617.

Seidel, K., Schöls, L., Nuber, S., Petrasch-Parwez, E., Gierga, K., Wszolek, Z., . . . Krüger, R. (2010). First appraisal of brain pathology owing to A30P mutant alpha-synuclein. *Annals of Neurology, 67*(5), 684–689.

Sekine, T., Kagaya, H., Funayama, M., Li, Y., Yoshino, H., Tomiyama, H., & Hattori, N. (2010). Clinical course of the first Asian family with Parkinsonism related to SNCA triplication. *Movement Disorders, 25*(16), 2871–2875.

Setó-Salvia, N., Clarimón, J., Pagonabarraga, J., Pascual-Sedano, B., Campolongo, A., Combarros, O., . . . Kulisevsky, J. (2011). Dementia risk in Parkinson disease: Disentangling the role of MAPT haplotypes. *Archives of Neurology, 68*(3), 359–364.

Setó-Salvia, N., Pagonabarraga, J., Houlden, H., Pascual-Sedano, B., Dols-Icardo, O., Tucci, A., . . . Clarimón, J. (2011). Glucocerebrosidase mutations confer a greater risk of dementia during Parkinson's disease course. *Movement Disorders, 27*(3), 393–399.

Shanker, V., Groves, M., Heiman, G., Palmese, C., Saunders-Pullman, R., Ozelius, L., . . . Bressman, S. (2011). Mood and cognition in leucine-rich repeat kinase 2 G2019S Parkinson's disease. *Movement Disorders, 26*(10), 1875–1880.

Shimura, H., Hattori, N., Kubo, S. i., Mizuno, Y., Asakawa, S., Minoshima, S., . . . Suzuki, T. (2000). Familial Parkinson disease gene product, parkin, is a ubiquitin-protein ligase. *Nature Genetics, 25*(3), 302–305.

Sidransky, E., Nalls, M. A., Aasly, J. O., Aharon-Peretz, J., Annesi, G., Barbosa, E. R., . . . Ziegler, S. G. (2009). Multicenter analysis of glucocerebrosidase mutations in Parkinson's disease. *The New England Journal of Medicine, 361*(17), 1651–1661.

Spira, P. J., Sharpe, D. M., Halliday, G., Cavanagh, J., & Nicholson, G. A. (2001). Clinical and pathological features of a Parkinsonian syndrome in a family with an Ala53Thr alpha-synuclein mutation. *Annals of Neurology, 49*(3), 313–319.

Steinlechner, S., Stahlberg, J., Völkel, B., Djarmati, A., Hagenah, J., Hiller, A., . . . Lencer, R. (2007). Co-occurrence of affective and schizophrenia spectrum disorders with PINK1 mutations. *Journal of Neurology, Neurosurgery and Psychiatry, 78*(5), 532–535.

Sun, S.-Y., An, C.-N., & Pu, X.-P. (2012). DJ-1 protein protects dopaminergic neurons against 6-OHDA/MG-132-induced neurotoxicity in rats. *Brain Research Bulletin, 88*(6), 609–616.

Taira, T., Saito, Y., Niki, T., Iguchi-Ariga, S. M. M., Takahashi, K., & Ariga, H. (2004). DJ-1 has a role in antioxidative stress to prevent cell death. *EMBO Reports, 5*(2), 213–218.

Tan, E. K., Zhao, Y., Skipper, L., Tan, M. G., Di Fonzo, A., Sun, L.,... Liu, J. J. (2006). The LRRK2 Gly2385Arg variant is associated with Parkinson's disease: genetic and functional evidence. *Human Genetics, 120*(6), 857–863.

Tang, M. X., Stern, Y., Marder, K., Bell, K., Gurland, B., Lantigua, R.,... Mayeux, R. (1998). The APOE-epsilon4 allele and the risk of Alzheimer disease among African Americans, whites, and Hispanics. *JAMA, 279*(10), 751–755.

Tsuang, D., Leverenz, J. B., Lopez, O. L., Hamilton, R. L., Bennett, D. A., Schneider, J. A.,... Zabetian, C. P. (2012). GBA mutations increase risk for Lewy body disease with and without Alzheimer disease pathology. *Neurology, 79*(19), 1944–1950.

Valente, E. M., Brancati, F., Ferraris, A., Graham, E. A., Davis, M. B., Breteler, M. M. B.,... Disease, E. C. o. G. S. i. P. a. s. (2002). PARK6-linked parkinsonism occurs in several European families. *Annals of Neurology, 51*(1), 14–18.

Valente, E. M. E., Abou-Sleiman, P. M. P., Caputo, V. V., Muqit, M. M. K. M., Harvey, K. K., Gispert, S. S.,... Wood, N. W. N. (2004). Hereditary early-onset Parkinson's disease caused by mutations in PINK1. *Science, 304*(5674), 1158–1160.

Voutilainen, S., Tuomainen, T.-P., Korhonen, M., Mursu, J., Virtanen, J. K., Happonen, P.,... Salonen, J. T. (2007). Functional COMT Val158Met polymorphism, risk of acute coronary events and serum homocysteine: The Kuopio ischaemic heart disease risk factor study. *PLoS ONE, 2*(1), e181.

Wakabayashi, K., Hayashi, S., Ishikawa, A., Hayashi, T., Okuizumi, K., Tanaka, H.,... Takahashi, H. (1998). Autosomal dominant diffuse Lewy body disease. *Acta Neuropathologica, 96*(2), 207–210.

Waters, C. H., & Miller, C. A. (1994). Autosomal dominant Lewy body parkinsonism in a four-generation family. *Annals of Neurology, 35*(1), 59–64.

Williams-Gray, C. H., Evans, J. R., Goris, A., Foltynie, T., Ban, M., Robbins, T. W.,... Barker, R. A. (2009). The distinct cognitive syndromes of Parkinson's disease: 5 year follow-up of the CamPaIGN cohort. *Brain, 132*(Pt 11), 2958–2969.

Williams-Gray, C. H., Foltynie, T., Brayne, C. E. G., Robbins, T. W., & Barker, R. A. (2007). Evolution of cognitive dysfunction in an incident Parkinson's disease cohort. *Brain, 130*(Pt 7), 1787–1798.

Williams-Gray, C. H., Goris, A., Saiki, M., Foltynie, T., Compston, D. A. S., Sawcer, S. J., & Barker, R. A. (2009). Apolipoprotein E genotype as a risk factor for susceptibility to and dementia in Parkinson's disease. *Journal of Neurology, 256*(3), 493–498.

Williams-Gray, C. H., Hampshire, A., Barker, R. A., & Owen, A. M. (2008). Attentional control in Parkinson's disease is dependent on COMT val158met genotype. *Brain, 131*(2), 397–408.

Zarranz, J. J., Alegre, J., Gómez-Esteban, J. C., Lezcano, E., Ros, R., Ampuero, I.,... de Yebenes, J. G. (2004). The new mutation, E46K, of alpha-synuclein causes Parkinson and Lewy body dementia. *Annals of Neurology, 55*(2), 164–173.

Zetusky, W. J., Jankovic, J., & Pirozzolo, F. J. (1985). The heterogeneity of Parkinson's disease: clinical and prognostic implications. *Neurology, 35*(4), 522–526.

Zhao, Y., Ho, P., Yih, Y., Chen, C., Lee, W. L., & Tan, E. K. (2011). LRRK2 variant associated with Alzheimer's disease. *Neurobiology of Aging, 32*(11), 1990–1993.

Zimprich, A., Benet-Pagès, A., Struhal, W., Graf, E., Eck, S. H., Offman, M. N.,... Strom, T. M. (2011). A mutation in VPS35, encoding a subunit of the retromer complex, causes late-onset Parkinson disease. *American Journal of Human Genetics, 89*(1), 168–175.

8 Earliest Cognitive Changes and Mild Cognitive Impairment in Parkinson's Disease

Ben Schmand and Alexander I. Tröster

It took more than half a century after James Parkinson published his Essay on the Shaking Palsy (Parkinson, 1817, 2002) before neurologists began to realize that the disease is more than a movement disorder. It took another full century before neuropsychologists started to study the cognitive and behavioral symptoms of Parkinson's disease (PD). Hans-Lukas Teuber and his coworkers at the Massachusetts Institute of Technology were pioneers during the 1960s, soon followed by Florry Bowen with Margaret Hoehn and Melvin Yahr at the Parkinson Research Center of Columbia University. The neuropsychological work that has been carried out since then has been summarized in a number of influential review papers by Taylor et al., Brown and Marsden, Dubois and Pillon, Owen, Zgaljardic et al., and many more (Brown & Marsden, 1990; Dubois & Pillon, 1997; Owen, 2004; Taylor, Saint-Cyr, & Lang, 1988; Zgaljardic, Borod, Foldi, & Mattis, 2003). Levin and Katzen thoroughly reviewed cognitive and behavioral changes during the first five years of the disease (Levin & Katzen, 2005).

Although some authors expressed nuances, this literature was dominated by the fronto-striatal dopamine depletion hypothesis (Albert, 1978; Bowen, Kamienny, Burns, & Yahr, 1975), that is, the view that cognitive symptoms in PD are mainly due to failure of dopaminergic innervation in fronto-striatal networks. The ensuing cognitive impairments supposedly are of a frontal-dysexecutive nature, whereas impairments in other cognitive domains, such as memory and visuospatial functioning, if present, were thought to be secondary to the executive deficits. One cannot deny that there is much evidence in favor of this hypothesis. However, with time, it has come under attack. Other neurotransmitter systems than the dopamine system, such as cholinergic and serotonergic systems, and other networks than fronto-striatal circuitry, such as temporal cortical areas, appeared to be involved in PD also (e.g., Hawkes, Del Tredici, & Braak, 2010). Moreover, the accumulation of Lewy bodies in various parts of the brain gradually gained recognition as another cause of cognitive impairment (Jellinger, 2008; Lippa et al., 2007). Consequently, recent overviews tend to give a more refined picture of cognitive impairments in early PD (Aarsland, Bronnick, & Fladby, 2011; Kehagia, Barker, & Robbins, 2010; Litvan et al., 2011; Marder, 2010; Tröster, 2011).

The first part of this chapter focuses on cognitive changes in newly diagnosed patients. We will first review three recent population-based studies of incident PD and one of neurological disorders in general, including PD. We will also briefly consider a population-based study aimed at detecting future PD, that is, subjects who are in the premotor stage of the disease. Next, we will discuss several clinic-based studies that were conducted in newly diagnosed PD patients and that used a sufficiently large battery of neuropsychological tests to draw a cognitive profile. The aim in this part of the chapter is to describe the very first cognitive alterations of the disease. The second part of the chapter reviews studies on mild cognitive impairment (MCI) in PD, also considering patients who are in later disease stages. Finally, we will attempt to determine the consequences of early cognitive changes for the course of the disease.

POPULATION-BASED STUDIES IN NEWLY DIAGNOSED PATIENTS

The best way to study the characteristics and natural history of a disease is to start with new cases, preferably all new cases in a circumscribed area or population, and to follow them during the course of the disease (Altman, 2001). Such research is expensive. Not surprisingly, this strategy has not been used very often in research on cognitive changes in PD. Most longitudinal studies of cognition in PD have been conducted in clinical samples of patients who have had the disease for a number of years (Muslimovic, Schmand, Speelman, & de Haan, 2007).

There are three large population-based studies that follow cognitive changes in new PD patients. One is the CamPaIGN study in Cambridgeshire, England (Foltynie, Brayne, Robbins, & Barker, 2004), the second is the ParkWest study in southwestern Norway (Alves et al., 2009), and the third is a study in Umeå in central Sweden, the NYPUM-project [NY (new) Parkinsonism in UMeå] (Elgh et al., 2009; Linder, Stenlund, & Forsgren, 2010) (Table 8-1). These three studies aimed to establish the incidence of PD, and to examine the cognitive and behavioral evolution over several years. These studies tried to trace all new PD patients in the area by recruitment via general practitioners, neurologic and geriatric outpatient services, and nursing homes. Participation rates for the longitudinal parts of the studies were 77% in England, 80% in Norway, and 79% in Sweden. Age-standardized to the European population of 1991, the incidence was 10.8 per 100,000 inhabitants per year in England (Foltynie et al., 2004), and

Table 8-1 Demographic and clinical characteristics of patients in population based studies. Mean (standard deviation or range) unless otherwise stated

	CamPaIGN, England	*ParkWest, Norway*	*NEDICES, Spain*	*NYPUM Umeå, Sweden*
Number of patients	159	196	46	88
Age	70.6 (37–90)	67.6 (9.2)	78.1 (5.7)	68.1 (9.3)
Education years	–	11.0 (3.3)	–	9.9 (4.1)
Premorbid IQ	109 (86–126)	–	–	–
Symptom duration years	2.8 (1–23)	2.3 (1.8)	1.9 (1.0)	1.9
UPDRS motor score	25.9 (4–61)	22.8 (11.1)	–	23.8 (9.7)
Hoehn & Yahr stage	2.0 (1–5)	–	2.4 (0.8)	–
MMSE score	27.3 (11–30)	27.9 (2.3)	–	28.7 (1.4)
% on medication	47	0	65	2

12.6 in Norway (Alves et al., 2009). These figures are representative for incidence studies worldwide, although the strategy of case finding via health-care providers probably resulted in some underestimation of the actual incidence (de Lau & Breteler, 2006). The Swedish study reported a relatively high-incidence figure of 21.5 per 100,000, age-adjusted to the Swedish population (Linder, Stenlund, & Forsgren, 2010). A fourth population-based study has been conducted since 1994 in central Spain. This study, NEDICES, is aimed at various neurological diseases in the elderly of 65 years and older. The age-adjusted annual incidence rate of PD in this study is 187 per 100,000 inhabitants (Benito-Leon et al., 2004). This figure is much higher than in the other studies due to the selected age range of 65 years and older.

The CamPaIGN study included 201 newly diagnosed patients satisfying the UKPDS brain-bank criteria between 2000 and 2003 (Foltynie et al., 2004). Mean age was 70 years, and although the patients had been diagnosed a few months before the evaluation, symptom onset had been around three years earlier. Fifty-three percent were drug naïve. At baseline, cognitive functions of 79% of the patients were evaluated. They were tested with the MMSE, the National Adult Reading Test (an estimator of premorbid verbal intelligence), letter and category fluency, and three subtests of the CANTAB battery, namely pattern recognition memory, spatial recognition memory, and the Tower of London. Also the Beck depression inventory was administered.

Eight percent of the patients scored below 24 points on the MMSE, 19% scored at least one standard deviation below the normative mean on the pattern-recognition test, and 9% scored below this cut-off on the Tower of London test. The authors, therefore, concluded that 36% of the patients showed some form of cognitive impairment. About one-third of this subgroup of impaired patients was considered to have fronto-striatal deficits defined by an abnormal performance on the Tower of London Test, about a quarter was considered to have a temporal-lobe-type deficit indicated by a low pattern-recognition score, and the remainder showed both types of deficits, since they scored low on both tests. The impaired patients were older than the cognitively intact patients, had more severe motor symptoms, had lower premorbid intelligence, and scored less on the spatial recognition and fluency tests. Fourteen percent of the patients scored above cut-off on the depression scale, but depression was unrelated to cognitive impairment. At group level, there was no clearly discernible profile of cognitive impairments. The percentages of impaired scores on each test varied between ±20% for the pentagon copy item of the MMSE and ±30% for animal fluency (Williams-Gray, Foltynie, Brayne, Robbins, & Barker, 2007a). Although half the patients were on medication, no mention was made of correlations with test performance.

At follow-up after a mean of 3.5 years, 9% of the patients had deceased and 10% had become demented (Williams-Gray et al., 2007). The remaining patients showed a degree of impairment on the neuropsychological tests similar to baseline. Higher age, nontremor dominant motor symptoms (postural imbalance and gait dysfunctions, PIGD), lower semantic fluency, and inability to copy the MMSE intersecting pentagons at baseline were predictive of subsequent cognitive decline (Williams-Gray et al., 2007). Levodopa dose at baseline did not predict decline. The authors concluded that dementia is not heralded by the dopaminergic fronto-striatal dysfunction typical for PD, but by PIGD and cognitive deficits with a posterior cortical basis.

At a second follow-up five years from baseline, 50% of the patients were still available for assessment (Williams-Gray et al., 2009). These findings were corroborated. Together, the same three characteristics, that is, PIGD, inability to copy pentagons, low semantic fluency, predicted dementia within five years with an odds ratio of 88 (95% CI 8-962). When a genetic factor was entered in the analysis, namely the gene for microtubule-associated tau protein (MAPT), it replaced PIGD as predictor of dementia. Almost all demented patients were carriers of the MAPT H1/H1 genotype. Tau proteins play a role in the stabilization of axonal microtubules in the normal nervous system. However, they may undergo chemical changes and get misfolded, which results in the formation of cerebral tangles. Carriers of the H1 allele are particularly subject to this misfolding process, and consequently, they are at increased risk of neurodegenerative disease. Another gene, COMT, was not related to dementia but to fronto-striatal function as measured by the Tower of London test (Williams-Gray et al., 2009). These findings were largely corroborated at follow-ups after 6.6 and 10 years. Age at onset, MAPT H1/H1 haplotype and impaired semantic fluency predicted dementia (Evans et al., 2011; Williams-Gray et al., 2013).

From an epidemiological point of view, CamPaIGN is a well-conducted study with thorough case ascertainment, a respectable sample size, a longitudinal design, and a broad range of clinical assessments. However, the cognitive evaluation is limited. As a result, the conclusion that dementia is predicted by cognitive deficits with a posterior cortical basis, although plausible by itself, seems to be based on fragile evidence. This conclusion was derived from only two test results, namely impaired animal fluency and impaired pentagon copy.

The ParkWest study identified 295 incident PD cases between 2004 and 2006, most of who participated in the longitudinal part of the study (Alves et al., 2009). Most patients were drug naïve. Mean age was 67 years; onset of motor symptoms was typically two to three years earlier. All drug naïve patients (after exclusion of a few subjects with dementia or depression) were compared to a demographically matched control group of friends and spouses of the patients (Aarsland, Bronnick, Larsen, Tysnes, Alves, et al., 2009). The cognitive tests used were MMSE, Stroop Color-Word Test, California Verbal Learning Test, category fluency, and the Silhouettes and Cube Subtests of the Visual Object and Space Perception battery. These tests were considered to cover three cognitive domains: memory (CVLT), attention and executive functions (Stroop test, fluency, and serial sevens of the MMSE), and visuospatial functioning (VOSP). Depression was measured with Montgomery and Åsberg's depression rating scale.

All cognitive tests showed statistically significant differences between patients and controls, but similar to the CamPaIGN study, the effect sizes were moderate. As in the British study, there was not a clearly discernible profile of impairments at group level. Mean performance of the patients was between 0.3 and 0.5 standard deviations below the control group (Glass's delta; 0.3 for the silhouettes subtest and 0.5 word reading speed on the Stroop test). Correction for depressive symptoms changed this pattern slightly. The differences on speeded tests were moderated, and memory impairment came more to the front.

Brønnick et al. studied memory performance of these patients in more depth (Bronnick, Alves, Aarsland, Tysnes, & Larsen, 2011). They analyzed the encoding, storage and retrieval parameters of the California verbal learning test in a subgroup of 133 drug naïve patients and individually matched controls. The patients learned fewer words than the controls; the slope of their learning curves was less steep. However, after controlling for learning performance, there were no group differences in free and cued recall, or in recognition. In a multivariate regression analysis learning performance was explained by disease status and executive functioning, namely verbal fluency, Stroop interference, and a learning strategy of semantic clustering. Brønnick et al. concluded that the memory impairment in PD is an encoding deficit due to executive dysfunction. However, a subsequent analysis showed that delayed recall and recognition were related to hippocampal atrophy (Beyer et al., 2013).

Nineteen percent of the patients and about half as many controls in the ParkWest study satisfied criteria of mild cognitive impairment (MCI). This was defined as a mean domain score of more than 1.5 standard deviations below the demographically corrected mean; subjective or informant report of cognitive decline was not required. About one-third of the affected patients had amnestic MCI, and two thirds had nonamnestic forms of MCI. There were no correlations of cognitive impairment with severity or duration of motor symptoms, neither with depression or use of antidepressants or sedative medication. After three years, 27% of the MCI patients had developed dementia (Pedersen et al., 2013).

The smaller NEDICES study identified 46 PD patients, of whom 23 were incident cases (Benito-Leon et al., 2011; Sanchez-Ferro et al., 2011). Mean age of the patients was 78 years, and their mean level of education was very low. Only 40% had received some formal education. At follow-up after three years, the performance of the PD group on a brief series of cognitive tests was compared to a control group matched on demographic characteristics, comorbidity, and premorbid intelligence. The patients scored less than controls on an adapted version of the MMSE (0.4 standard deviation below controls; Glass's delta), semantic fluency (0.3 to 0.5 SD below controls), and delayed recall of a memory task (0.3 SD below controls), but not on naming of common objects nor on the Trail-Making test part A (Benito-Leon et al., 2011). The latter finding is remarkable, given that mean disease onset was almost two years at baseline, and consequently, disease duration was almost five years at the moment of evaluation in this Spanish study.

The NYPUM study in Umeå, Sweden, included 111 new PD patients between 2004 and 2008 (Elgh et al., 2009). Eighty-eight patients (79%) participated in the neuropsychological evaluation. They were drug naïve, except two patients. Thirty healthy volunteers were recruited as control subjects. They were sex and age matched to the patients, but had a higher level of education. An extensive battery of 12 neuropsychological tests was administered covering psychomotor speed, working memory, attention, language, executive functions, visuospatial function, and memory (Figure 8-1). Most conspicuous were slow performances on tests of psychomotor speed. The patients needed almost twice as much time as controls to complete the Trail-Making test, and their finger-tapping speed was 25% below the control group. Significant group differences were found in all cognitive domains except working memory. After correction for finger-tapping speed, the differences in the executive and visuospatial domains were no longer significant. After this correction, what remained were differences in episodic memory (free recall tasks), attention (Trail-Making test A and B), and category fluency. If Trail-Making and Finger Tapping Tests were not considered, 30% of the patients were impaired in at least one domain and 16% in two or more domains. Impairment was defined as scores less than 1.5 SD below the normative mean on more than half the tests in a domain. Impaired patients had longer disease duration and more severe motor symptoms, in particular rigidity, bradykinesia, impaired speech, and reduced facial expression. At follow-up after a year, increase in bradykinesia was related to a decline in working memory and mental flexibility, whereas worsening of PIGD was associated with decline in visuospatial memory (Domellöf, Forsgren, & Elgh, 2013).

Comparison of Population-Based Studies

Except for the Spanish study, these studies are comparable with respect to methods of case finding and ascertainment, and demographic and clinical characteristics of the patients. The English and Norwegian studies reported similar incidence figures, whereas the Spanish incidence was much higher due to the older age range of the participants. The mean profiles of cognitive functions in all three projects were rather flat and the impairments were mild.

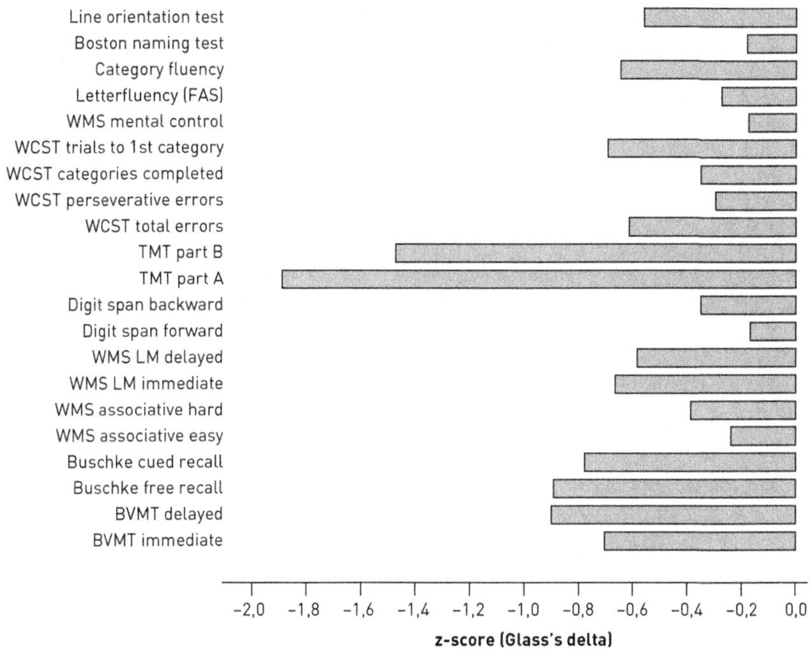

FIGURE 8-1

Mean performance of 88 newly diagnosed PD patients on neuropsychological tests (Umeå, Sweden) (Elgh et al., 2009). Bars represent Glass's delta, that is, mean difference between patient and control groups divided by the standard deviation of the control group. Glass's delta is equivalent to *z*-scores, that is, number of standard deviations below the control mean. Controls were healthy subjects ($n = 30$) who were sex and age matched to the patients. WMS = Wechsler Memory Scale; WCST = Wisconsin Card Sorting Test; TMT = Trail Making test; BVMT = Brief Visuospatial Memory test. Source: Derived from Table 3 of Elgh et al. (2009). Finger tapping test not shown (z-score = −2.5).

In the Swedish study, a more complete cognitive profile was obtained, with conspicuous impairments in psychomotor functioning, memory, card sorting, and category fluency.

The percentages of cognitively impaired patients varied considerably across the studies. It was twice as high in the English (36%) than in the Norwegian study (19%), with the Swedish study in between (30%). The Spanish study made no mention of the number of impaired patients.

The most plausible explanation of this divergence is the way impairment was defined. The English figure was obtained by summation of patients with low MMSE scores, and patients with scores less than one standard deviation below normative means on one or two other cognitive tests. This latter criterion is rather liberal, since it implies that 16% of the normal population is incorrectly classified as impaired if only one test is used. If two tests are used, as in this case, the percentage may increase to 29% (if the tests are uncorrelated[1]).

When considering the percentages of impaired patients, one also has to keep in mind that 20–33% of the subjects did not participate in the cognitive assessment (except in the Spanish study, where all patients participated). In general, this kind of selection is not random. The participating patients mostly are relatively well functioning and less ill than the subjects who refuse. Consequently, the figures mentioned earlier may be underestimated.

Other explanations for the diverging percentages of impairment are the presence of a control group, the use of medication, and the choice of cognitive tests. In the Norwegian study, impairment was based on comparison to data of a large control group. This is probably more precise and more sensitive than using fixed cut-off scores (without correction for demographic characteristics of the subjects), as was done in the CamPaIGN study. The Swedish study used demographically corrected normative data to decide which patients were impaired. Given the limited size of the control group (*n*=30) this was the best way to handle the data, although probably less precise than the method used in the Norwegian study.

About half of the English group and two-thirds of the Spanish group were on dopaminergic medication, which, in theory, may have affected their cognitive performance. However, no relation was found between levodopa dose and cognitive decline (Williams-Gray et al., 2007a). Also, the Swedish patients were without dopaminergic treatment, and yet a similar percentage was impaired.

Finally, the CANTAB tests might be more sensitive to cognitive impairment than the conventional neuropsychological tests used in the ParkWest and Umeå projects. Judging from the mean MMSE scores, however, severity of cognitive impairment was about equal in all samples (Table 8-1). Consequently, the CamPaIGN estimate of cognitive impairment may have been too high. The ParkWest study, on the other hand, may have underestimated the impairments. It used a limited battery containing several tests that are not very sensitive due to ceiling effects. Thus, it may have missed impaired patients. The Umeå study used 13 tests, most of which are quite sensitive to cognitive impairment. Its impairment estimate seems to be the most trustworthy of the three.

Notwithstanding these disparities, the English and Norwegian studies concurred in the finding that the majority of the cognitively impaired patients had fronto-striatal or nonamnestic symptoms, whereas a minority had temporal lobe or amnestic symptoms. The Swedish investigators were in the best position to analyze the profile of cognitive impairments, given their extensive battery, but their early report did not convey this information. It only stated that memory, executive, and language domains were equally affected in impaired patients (Elgh et al., 2009, pg. 1281). In a later study they also reported two pathways of decline, one cluster of increasing bradykinesia and executive decline, and another cluster of worsening PIGD and memory decline (Domellöf et al., 2013). These authors corrected all group differences for motor speed, but for the untimed tests this may have been an overcorrection. If we disregard this correction for untimed tests, the largest and most robust differences are found in the memory domain, followed by visuospatial and executive functioning (line orientation and many of the Wisconsin test parameters; Figure 8-1). In this respect the Umeå study seems to deviate from the other two projects, although the ParkWest study also found its largest group difference in the memory test. In the Spanish study, fluency was most affected, and delayed verbal memory to a lesser extent. Motor slowness is an unlikely explanation for the decrease in fluency, because patients and controls performed equally on the Trail-Making test.

Provisional Conclusions

Overlooking these population-based studies, it is evident that mild cognitive deficits are quite common in incident PD, that is, in the first few years after appearance of motor symptoms, and very soon after the formal PD diagnosis. The exact percentage of patients showing these mild deficits is not yet clear, but it may be as high as 30%. Apart from psychomotor speed, the most severely affected domain seems to be memory, immediately followed by executive and visuospatial functioning. These studies found no indications that mild depression or dopaminergic medication greatly influences cognitive functioning in early patients. Higher age of onset, however, as well as negative motor symptoms such as bradykinesia, postural imbalance and gait disorders, are related to faster cognitive decline.

PREMOTOR COGNITIVE IMPAIRMENT?

Given the considerable proportion of patients who show subtle cognitive impairments around the moment of diagnosis, the question rises whether these impairments might have been present already before motor symptoms emerged. In hindsight, many patients report a long history of prodromal signs, but cognitive symptoms do not rank particularly high in the list (Gaenslen, Swid, Liepelt-Scarfone, Godau, & Berg, 2011).

The same question was prospectively investigated in the population-based Parkinson At-Risk Syndrome (PARS) study, and its preliminary results seem to suggest otherwise. PARS aims at finding ways to screen large cohorts of subjects for prodromal signs of PD (Stern & Siderowf, 2010). One of the risk factors for PD is impaired olfaction or hyposmia. People with hyposmia relatively frequently report other PD risk factors, such as REM sleep behavior disorders, constipation, and subtle changes in motor function (Siderowf et al., 2012). Moreover, hyposmic persons perform slightly lower than nonhyposmic controls on cognitive tasks, namely verbal fluency and psychomotor speed, especially when they also show loss of dopamine transporters on b-CIT SPECT scanning (Hawkins et al., 2010). This suggests the existence of prodromal cognitive impairments in PD, although follow-up is necessary to corroborate this. The Spanish NEDICES investigators were unable to support this hypothesis, however. They retrospectively compared the incident PD cases to demographically matched control subjects who remained healthy. The baseline global cognition scores of both groups, three years before the PD diagnosis, were not different (Sanchez-Ferro et al., 2011). The patients did not show accelerated cognitive decline per MMSE during the years before PD diagnosis (Sánchez Ferro et al., 2013).

CLINIC-BASED STUDIES IN NEWLY DIAGNOSED PATIENTS

From an epidemiological point of view, studies that recruit patients in clinical settings are less informative than population-based studies, because it is unclear to what extent a clinic-based sample is representative for the patient population. The assessments, on the other hand, are often more thorough and reliable in clinic-based than in population-based studies.

In this section we review neuropsychological studies that were conducted in early PD patients, and that used a sufficiently large battery of neuropsychological tests to draw a cognitive profile. We will not consider studies that used a small set of tests to examine a specific hypothesis.

Lees and Smith conducted one of the first neuropsychological studies in newly diagnosed PD patients (Lees & Smith, 1983). They compared idiopathic PD patients (Table 8-2) to patient controls, who were waiting for elective surgery. All patients were under age 65, had normal CT scans, and were not depressed. The PD patients were not on antiparkinsonian medication. Both groups were comparable with respect to premorbid and current intelligence (NART and WAIS, respectively). Apart from these intelligence tests, the Warrington recognition memory tests for words and faces, Nelson's modified Wisconsin Card Sorting Test, and Benton's Letter Fluency Test were given to the patient groups. Their scores on the recognition memory tests were equal. However, the PD patients scored less than

Table 8-2 Demographic and clinical characteristics of newly diagnosed PD patients in clinic based studies. Mean (standard deviation or range) unless otherwise stated

	Lees & Smith 1983, London	*Levin et al. 1989, Miami*	*Owen et al. 1992, London*	*Cooper et al. 1991, Sheffield*	*Muslimovic et al. 2005, Amsterdam*
Number of patients	30	41	15	60	115
Age	59 (7)	63.4 (11.4)	55.7 (2.9)	59.8 (37–77)	66.2 (10.1)
Education yrs	–	13.4 (3.0)	–	9.9 (9–17)	11.7 (2.4)
Premorbid IQ	110 (9)	–	112 (3)	107 (88–124)	104 (21)
Symptom duration yrs	2.4	1.9 (0.8)	1.5 (4.2)	1.3 (0.2–4.0)	1.5 (0.9)
UPDRS motor score	–	–	–	–	16.8 (7.8)
Hoehn & Yahr score	1.8 (0.7)	1.9 (0.8)	1.9 (0.6)	–	1.8 (0.7)
MMSE score	–	–	–	–	27.9 (1.6)
% on medication	0	89	0	0	68

the controls on the Card Sorting Test and on Letter Fluency. Some PD patients (20–30%) showed a remarkable perseverative tendency.

Lees and Smith (1983) interpreted these results as an indication of problems with set shifting and mental flexibility, and related these to destruction of dopaminergic mesocorticolimbic pathways that causes PD, and that deprives the frontal lobe from its dopaminergic input. They pointed at "the striking resemblance [of these findings] to those reported with frontal lobe damage" (p. 265). They saw this as support for the "fronto-subcortical" hypothesis of PD, which had been proposed in the preceding years (Albert, 1978; Bowen et al., 1975).

The group differences in this study were generally small, however. The largest difference was found for the number of categories completed in the card-sorting task (mean = 4.3, SD = 1.7 for PD patients, and mean = 5.2, SD = 1.1 for controls; Glass's delta = 0.8). Moreover, the control subjects were, on average, five years younger than the PD patients, and the statistical analyses were not corrected for demographic characteristics. Consequently, the differences between both groups in this study may have been somewhat exaggerated. The absence of differences on the memory tests may have been due to the recognition format, which is less sensitive to impairment than free recall.

Owen and coworkers examined three groups of nondemented PD patients and a group of research volunteers matched to the patients on age and premorbid IQ (Owen et al., 1992). One of the groups consisted of early PD patients who were not yet on medication. The other patient groups had long-standing mild or severe PD, and were medicated; we will not consider them here. Five subtests of the CANTAB battery were given: a spatial short-term memory test, a spatial working-memory test, the Tower of London, a pattern recognition task, and an attentional set-shifting test. The latter test became later known as the "intra-extra dimensional set-shift test." Devised as an analogue to the Wisconsin Card Sorting Test, it consists of discrimination and reversal learning tasks of increasing difficulty. The early PD patients performed at the same level as controls on all tests, except on this set-shifting test. Some patients failed already at relatively easy stages of the test. This replicated findings with this test in another small study of early PD (Downes et al., 1989).

According to Owen et al., their results showed a resemblance to those of neurosurgical patients with frontal lobe excisions. They saw this resemblance evolving across the three PD groups, with the early PD patients showing the first signs of similarity to frontal patients. Similar to Lees and Smith (1983), they ascribed it to progressive fronto-striatal damage and/or frontostriatal dopamine depletion.

Cooper et al. arrived at a somewhat different conclusion (Cooper et al., 1992; Cooper, Sagar, Jordan, Harvey, & Sullivan, 1991). They thoroughly evaluated a group of consecutive, early and untreated PD patients, without clinical dementia or major depression. The patients were compared to an age- and sex-matched control group that was not different with respect to premorbid or current intelligence. The authors used a much larger test battery than Lees and Smith and Owen and colleagues.

Impairments were found in the patient group on the Brown-Petersen short-term memory test and on the Wechsler memory scale subtests of mental control, digit-span backwards, logical memory, visual reproduction, and paired associate learning. Cooper et al. thought these memory impairments were most likely due to a reduced efficiency of working memory, not to a faster rate of forgetting, because there was no disproportionately worse delayed recall in the PD patients.

Executive impairments were found with a digit-ordering task, the WAIS picture arrangement subtest (both standard and untimed administration), and the Wisconsin Card Sorting Test. On the latter test, patients showed a trend toward inferior performance on all test parameters, but only the number of cards sorted to complete the first category was significant. Self-generated aspects of expressive language were slightly impaired, especially category and alternating fluency, whereas naming and language comprehension were intact. No visuospatial impairments were found with tests of matchsticks construction and perception of incomplete (degraded) pictures. Patients did worse than controls on copying, but not on delayed recall of Rey's and Taylor's complex figures. The problems with copying were ascribed to poor motor control, given the absence of abnormalities on the other visuospatial tests.

One-third of the patients had an abnormal score on the Blessed dementia scale. When these patients were removed from the analyses, group differences remained significant for logical memory, digit ordering, and the Brown-Petersen test. Depressive and motor symptoms correlated modestly with each other ($r = 0.46$), but did not substantially correlate with the cognitive test results.

Unlike Lees and Smith (1983) and Owen et al. (1992), Cooper and colleagues reasoned that the cognitive and motor symptoms of early PD are dissociated, and, therefore, concluded that the cognitive impairments of PD cannot completely be explained by fronto-striatal dopamine deficiency, but probably involve other brain areas and neurotransmitter systems as well. This conclusion seemed to be corroborated by a subsequent study, conducted after the patients were put on medication (Cooper et al., 1992). Motor symptoms were alleviated in both groups, but patients who were taking anticholinergics deteriorated on short-term memory tests, whereas working-memory performance improved in patients who were on levodopa treatment. Cooper et al. took this as an indication that both dopaminergic and cholinergic systems are involved in the cognitive deterioration of PD. They also suspected that the formation of cortical Lewy bodies would play a role, which by now is generally recognized (Hawkes et al., 2010; Jellinger, 2008; Lippa et al., 2007).

Levin et al. conducted an equally thorough, but smaller study in early PD patients (Levin, Llabre, & Weiner, 1989). They compared the patients to a demographically matched control group of healthy volunteers. Most patients were on medication (Table 8-2), with a high percentage (68%) using anticholinergics. An extensive battery of tests was administered, covering language, visuospatial, attention, memory, and executive functions. The largest group differences (up to one standard deviation; Glass's delta) were found in the memory domain, especially with the Wechsler memory scale, logical memory subtest. Visual perception tests of embedded figures and overlapping line drawings of objects also showed clear impairments. The mean scores of the patients were 0.5–0.8 standard deviations below the mean of controls (i.e., Glass's delta). Visuospatial tests of line orientation and visual organization were not different, however. In the language domain category fluency and proverb recognition showed differences, but letter fluency and naming did not. Attention tests (digit and spatial span, and an auditory vigilance task) also showed no impairments. The authors compared the patients who were on anticholinergics to the remaining patients and found no differences. However, the statistical power was small to detect effects of medication in these subgroups. Thus, it remains conceivable that the memory impairment may have been partly due to medication effects. Nevertheless, the authors concluded that the early cognitive changes in PD cannot totally be explained by fronto-striatal dysfunction, but probably reflect more widespread pathology.

Muslimovic et al. conducted another study with an extensive cognitive evaluation (Muslimovic, Post, Speelman, De Haan, & Schmand, 2009a; Muslimovic, Post, Speelman, & Schmand, 2005). They recruited newly diagnosed cases in outpatient clinics in Amsterdam and surrounding regions in the Netherlands. Demented patients and subjects older than 85 years were excluded. Spouses and relatives volunteered as controls. Patients were evaluated a few months after diagnosis. The majority were already on medication (Table 8-2). The assessment covered psychomotor speed, attention, executive functions, memory, language, and visuo-spatial functions. Patients scored worse than controls on all tests except digit span forward (Figure 8-2). Large differences were found on speeded tests of psychomotor function and attention (digit symbol test and trail making test part B), but also on immediate and delayed memory tests, and several executive tests (Tower of London and modified Wisconsin Card Sorting). After correction for psychomotor speed, differences on timed tests were reduced but most remained significant (Muslimovic et al., 2005). The numbers of abnormal test scores (defined as more than 2 SD below demographically corrected mean) were tallied for each participant. Four percent of the controls had three or more abnormal test results. This was taken as the cut-off for cognitive impairment in the patient group. Twenty-four percent of the patients were impaired by this criterion. All impaired patients had at least one abnormal test in the attention or executive domain, and 45–60% of these patients had at least one other abnormal test in the psychomotor, memory, or visuo-spatial domain. The impaired patients were older and had a later disease onset, had more severe motor symptoms (axial symptoms in particular, i.e., PIGD), were more often male, and showed more symptoms of depression. When tested in a multivariate way, only age at onset remained significant. Levodopa dose did not correlate with cognitive impairment.

After three years, nine percent of the patients had become demented, and cognition had declined significantly faster in 48% of the patients than in controls (Muslimovic et al., 2009a). Psychomotor and attention domains showed the greatest decline, with a more modest worsening in memory, and visuo-spatial and executive functions declined least. Again, patients who declined had more severe

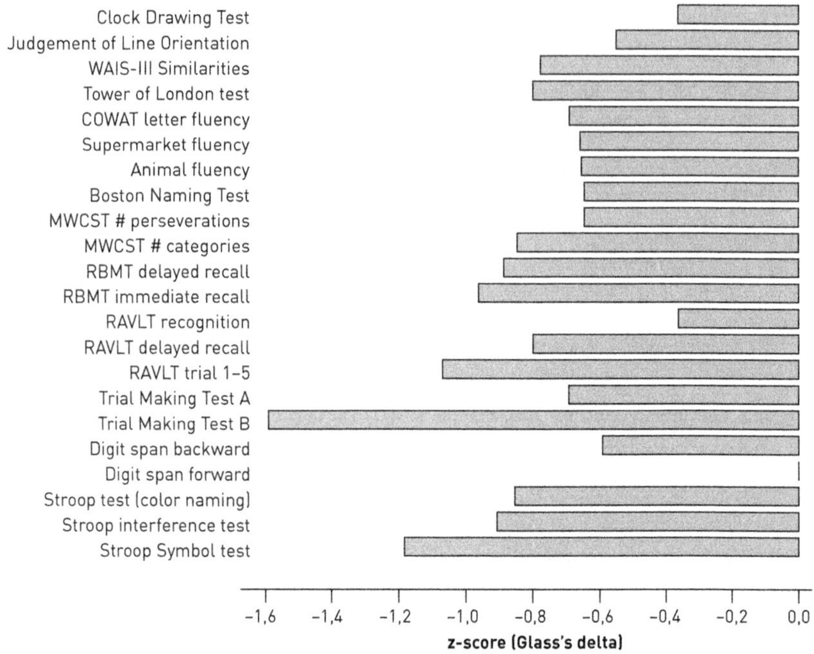

FIGURE 8-2
Mean performance of 115 newly diagnosed PD patients on neuropsychological tests. Controls are demographically matched healthy subjects ($n = 70$). WAIS = Wechsler Adult Intelligence Scale; MWCST = modified WCST; RBMT = Rivermead Behavioral Memory Test; RAVLT = Rey's Auditory Verbal Memory Test. Source: Based on Table E1 of Muslimovic et al. (2005). Bars represent Glass's delta (for explanation: see legend Figure 8-1).

motor symptoms at baseline, especially PIGD. After five years, 17% had dementia and about half of the remaining patients showed faster decline than controls (Broeders, de Bie, et al., 2013; Broeders, Velseboer, et al., 2013). Not only their cognitive functioning had deteriorated, but also their functional status, that is, instrumental and basic activities of daily living (Velseboer et al., 2013).

Comparison and Interpretation of Clinic-Based Studies

A conspicuous similarity of the clinic-based studies is that they all reported at least some cognitive impairment, and that the executive domain was always involved. Impairments in memory and visuospatial functions were less consistently reported, and in the language domain only subtle abnormalities were found, apart from decreased verbal fluency, which is a speeded measure. However, if a study did find memory impairment, it was often the domain with the largest effect sizes (Cooper et al., 1991; Levin et al., 1989; Muslimovic et al., 2005).

In two of these three studies, the mean age of the patients was relatively high, whereas it was lower in the other studies that primarily reported executive deficits.

Another conclusion that emerges from these studies is that the mild depressive symptoms in newly diagnosed PD patients do not seem to worsen their cognitive functioning. Medication also seems to be well tolerated in the early phase of the disease. The diverging cognitive effects of anticholinergics and levodopa reported by Cooper et al. (1992) were small and were not replicated in the other studies discussed here. Apparently, the deleterious and ameliorating effects of antiparkinson medication reported in the literature for a review see (Kehagia et al., 2010) surface only at later disease stages or at higher dosages than in the current studies.

Integrating Population-Based and Clinic-Based Findings

The proportion of patients who are already cognitively impaired when the PD diagnosis is established is around 25–30%. Both types of studies seem to concur on this figure. One has to keep in mind, however, that the proportion is age-dependent. It is based on samples of patients with a mean age of 65–70 years. In older samples, the prevalence of cognitive impairment is probably higher, in younger samples lower.

With the detailed cognitive profiles depicted in Figures 8-1 and 8-2 at our disposal, we may attempt to draw conclusions about the fronto-striatal dopamine depletion hypothesis. If the hypothesis were valid, one would expect effect sizes for executive tests to be larger than for tests that do not (or less heavily) tax executive functions. For example, among tests that are not speeded, the Wisconsin Card Sorting Test should show larger group differences than memory or visuospatial tests. Within the visuospatial domain, construction tasks with a strong executive character, such as clock drawing, should show more severe impairments than visuospatial perception tasks. Similarly, one would expect letter fluency to be more impaired than category fluency, because the former is of a more frontal-executive character (Henry & Crawford, 2004). None of these predictions seems to be confirmed by the data, at least not consistently so across studies. Even in the ParkWest study, in which Brønnick et al. concluded that memory impairment in PD is secondary to executive dysfunction, the differences between patients and controls were larger in memory than in executive performance (about 0.4 versus about 0.3 standard deviation) (Bronnick et al., 2011).

Instead, the picture that emerges from this research seems to point at the existence of a continuum of cognitive symptoms with two clusters marking the extremes (Figure 8-3). The first cluster is of a frontal-executive nature, and is primarily found in patients with a relatively young age of onset. It conforms to the fronto-striatal dopamine depletion hypothesis. The motor symptoms of these patients respond well to dopaminergic medication. Behavioral and cognitive symptoms are mostly of the frontal-executive type, and do not lead to dementia. With increasing age of onset, and with increasing age in patients with long-standing disease, the second cluster of memory and visuospatial symptoms encroaches on the first, probably due to the gradual involvement of posterior brain areas. The motor symptoms of these older patients are of a more axial nature and are less responsive to medication (Kempster et al., 2007). This adds to and interacts with the first cluster, complicates the clinical presentation of cognitive impairments, and ultimately deteriorates into dementia. This clinical

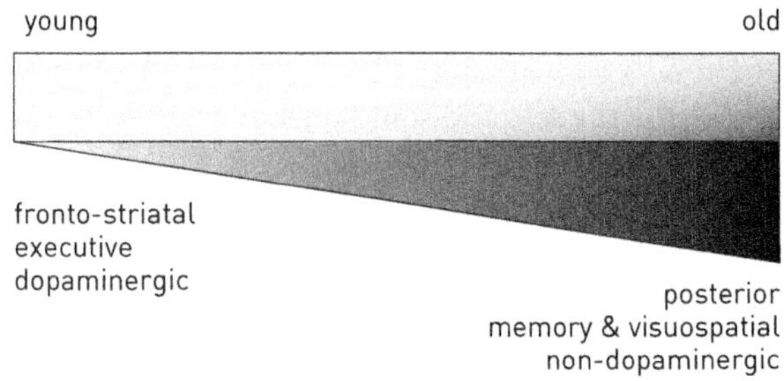

FIGURE 8-3
Relations between age of onset, affected brain regions, type of cognitive impairments, and neurotransmitters involved.

course parallels the neuropathological progression of the disease (Halliday & McCann, 2010; Jellinger, 2013; Kempster, O'Sullivan, Holton, Revesz, & Lees, 2010).

MILD COGNITIVE IMPAIRMENT

The studies reviewed thus far concerning cognitive changes in early and newly diagnosed PD are instructive with regard to types of cognitive functions affected and their potential neural and chemical bases. The study of the earliest cognitive changes, given their subtlety, may require large samples to identify group differences between patients and unaffected control subjects. As has been pointed out (Tröster, 2011), such studies are liable to have combined persons with PD, those with intact cognition, and those with mild impairments into a single group, thus perhaps obscuring changes. In addition, although group comparisons can be helpful in identifying impairments and treatment effects, such comparisons do not inform one about either the clinical significance of changes (i.e., whether the changes constitute a clinical syndrome or treatment effects are functionally meaningful) or about impairments in individual patients. In the last 5 years, in particular, greater attention has been devoted to cognitive syndromes in individuals with PD without dementia. In earlier parts of this chapter, for example, attention has been paid not only to the nature of cognitive change in early PD, but also to the frequency with which such impairments occur. Another issue is that studies of cognition in PD have sometimes interchangeably used the terms of early and mild cognitive impairment, yet these terms are not synonymous. This chapter clarifies this distinction by discussing first impairments in newly diagnosed/early PD and then MCI. The severity of cognitive impairment in early PD is variable and, indeed, some patients may develop dementia within a few years of disease diagnosis, whereas a minority shows only mild cognitive changes even after 15–20 years of disease progression (Hely, Reid, Adena, Halliday, & Morris, 2008; Williams-Gray, Foltynie, Brayne, Robbins, & Barker, 2007b). One issue that has faced clinicians and researchers is the definition of what mild impairment means. The recent attempt to define a syndrome of MCI in PD makes clear that the syndrome should not be considered synonymous with "mild" cognitive impairment in which the adjective may describe a wide range of impairments and impairment severities in the samples studied, ranging from cognitive *changes* or *declines* of minimal clinical significance to *impairments* of clinical significance. Indeed, studies speaking of "mild" cognitive impairment often compare groups of PD and healthy control subjects, and the statistically (albeit not necessarily clinically) significant differences between group mean test scores do not always imply that MCI is present in the PD group.

Mild cognitive impairment (MCI) is considered to be an intermediate stage between normal cognitive aging and dementia. The concept, which derives from studies of cognitive aging and dementia, in its most recent reiteration, has four subtypes defined on the basis of whether memory is impaired and whether one or more domains of cognition are impacted. Early studies defining MCI in PD have paralleled studies of MCI in the general population, often defining only amnestic MCI, or amnestic and nonamnestic MCI on the basis of performance on a limited number of tests and a rigid criterion (e.g., 1.5 SD below normative means). The tests used, the cut-off score defining impairment, and ancillary MCI criteria (for example, a requirement that a patient or caregiver offers a complaint of cognitive impairment) varied across studies. These studies were reviewed in detail (Litvan et al., 2011; Tröster, 2011) and because new criteria were recently proposed, we will only briefly discuss them here.

Early Studies of MCI in Parkinson's Disease

Recent reviews reported that the prevalence of MCI in PD ranged from 19% to 38% when studies with larger samples but loosely defined MCI criteria (and studies of "mild cognitive impairment") were included (Litvan et al., 2011). Prevalence range in another review was 15–62% when smaller studies were included but more precise quantitative definitions of MCI were required for inclusion (Tröster, 2011). The lowest rates tend to be reported in studies of incident cases of yet untreated PD (Aarsland, Bronnick, Larsen, Tysnes, & Alves, 2009). In an analysis of pooled data from multiple centers, the average MCI prevalence was about 26% (Aarsland et al., 2010). Early studies generally agree that the nonamnestic and single-domain subtypes are the most common forms of MCI (Monastero et al., 2012; Sollinger, Goldstein, Lah, Levey, & Factor, 2010), although memory may the most commonly impaired single domain of cognition when all single and multiple domain forms of MCI are considered together (Aarsland et al., 2010). Single- and multiple-domain amnestic MCI subtypes are sufficiently frequent to deserve close attention; they were reported to be present in 5% and 9% of persons, respectively, in one study (Aarsland et al., 2010) and in 24% and 19% in a second study (Goldman, Weis, Stebbins, Bernard, & Goetz, 2012).

The pathology underlying MCI in PD is likely to be heterogeneous (Jellinger, 2013), although this topic has received scant attention. One study of eight patients found that all had either neocortical and/or limbic or brainstem Lewy bodies;

however the two cases with amnestic MCI met neuropathologic criteria for Alzheimer's disease and cerebrovascular pathology was observed in three cases (Adler et al., 2010). Whether this heterogeneity in neuropathology reflects heterogeneity of the MCI phenotype and potentially different risk for or progression rates to dementia remains to be studied. Metabolic imaging studies have shown posterior cortical hypometabolism to be associated with amnestic (Nobili et al., 2009) and multiple domain MCI (Huang et al., 2008). Similarly, a gradient of greater reduction of posterior relative to frontal acetylcholinesterase activity has been observed in PD with dementia than PD (Klein et al., 2010; Shimada et al., 2009), although the role of cholinergic dysfunction in PD-MCI has not been explicitly explored. Parkinson Disease is associated with reduced dopamine uptake in the striatum. A recent study showed that in PD-MCI presynaptic dopamine uptake in the right caudate as assessed with SPECT is further reduced in comparison to PD, and that this finding correlates with the reduced striatal functional MRI BOLD (blood oxygen level dependent) signal in PD-MCI. Furthermore, the same study observed under-recruitment of right caudate and bilateral anterior cingulate in response to a working-memory task (2-back) on functional MRI in PD-MCI compared to PD (Ekman et al., 2012).

It is generally found that Lewy body pathology is a stronger determinant of cognitive impairment in PD than is amyloid pathology, especially plaques that are a hallmark of Alzheimer's disease (Compta et al., 2011). Nonetheless there has been interest in amyloid abnormalities as possible biomarkers of cognitive impairment in PD. Although some studies have found the cerebrospinal fluid (CSF) reductions in $A\beta_{42}$ that are present in about one-third of PD-MCI subjects (Montine et al., 2010) to be associated with some neuropsychological test performances (Leverenz et al., 2011) and more rapid cognitive decline (Siderowf et al., 2010), amyloid imaging studies have been less successful in showing a relationship between brain amyloid deposition and cognition in PD patients without dementia (Gomperts et al., 2012).

Only one early study of explicitly defined MCI examined its role in the evolution of dementia in PD (Janvin, Larsen, Aarsland, & Hugdahl, 2006). That study found that single domain *non*amnestic and multiple domain MCI were associated with progression to dementia four years later. The study, like many early MCI studies in PD, was limited in sample size and the number of tests used to define MCI. Thus, it is unclear how these findings can be reconciled with other recent studies, the CamPaIGN study in particular, showing amnestic MCI and posterior cerebral cognitive deficits to be predictive of dementia (Williams-Gray et al., 2007). More recent work, using new diagnostic criteria may be instructive in this regard, clarifying some apparent inconsistencies in the early PD-MCI literature.

Diagnostic Criteria for MCI

Because early studies used a variety of definitions and assessment methods to establish the presence of MCI, Tröster (2011) proposed preliminary research criteria for MCI that considered two classification categories based on whether the cognitive impairment was probabilistically linked to PD. The Movement Disorder Society (MDS) recently established clinical diagnostic criteria for MCI that are instead based on the breadth and depth of cognitive assessment in persons in whom the etiology of cognitive impairment is probably PD. Thus, the level of evaluation or ascertainment defines the certainty with which specific domains of cognition can be inferred to be compromised or not (Litvan et al., 2012). These criteria are detailed later and then recent research using and evaluating the criteria is discussed. As in more recent conceptualizations of MCI (Petersen, 2011), MCI in PD can be subtyped along two dimensions, namely the presence/absence of memory impairment (amnestic versus nonamnestic), and the number of cognitive domains affected (single domain versus multiple domains). This classification yields four subtypes, although some recommend a clear specification of the nonamnestic domains affected (Tröster, 2011).

Tröster (2011) proposed preliminary research criteria for PD-MCI (Parkinson's disease with mild cognitive impairment) that allow cognitive impairment in PD to be due to a variety of etiologies (e.g., depression, PD, chronic cerebral microvascular disease). By contrast, the criteria for PCI (Parkinson cognitive impairment) required that the etiology of the deficits probably be PD (largely by exclusion of comorbid conditions). This second set of criteria is essentially the starting point for the MDS criteria (Litvan et al., 2012) which require that the observed MCI be due to PD. The MDS criteria envision assessments being conducted at two levels, namely Levels I and II. The Level I assessment facilitates especially the needs of busy clinicians and clinical trialists, for whom subtyping of MCI is less important, but rapid, reliable assessment is of paramount concern in diagnosis or in defining study entry criteria and outcomes. Level II assessment, which is more time consuming and onerous, seeks to meet the researcher's need for subtyping of MCI because the subtype (phenotype) of MCI might be of importance in predicting progression to dementia, treatment outcomes, and identification of biomarkers of early cognitive compromise in PD. Table 8-3 outlines the criteria for MCI in PD. Level II assessment requires assessment of 5 domains: (1) attention/working memory, (2) executive functions, (3) language, (4) visuospatial, and (5) memory. Theoretically, 2 tests should be administered for each domain, although per criteria it is possible to subtype PD MCI with fewer tests if one domain has already been shown to be impaired by two tests, or one test in each of at least 2 domains has revealed impairment. Although such an approach might be clinically expedient, research studies would do well to administer the same, full set of tests to all participants.

Studies of MCI Prevalence and Dementia Progression Using the Tröster or MDS Criteria

Due to the youthfulness of the MDS criteria, only a handful of studies has examined a limited number of issues (e.g., MCI prevalence and progression) using these or the Tröster criteria. All these studies are retrospective analyses involving

Table 8-3 PD-MCI criteria and assessment strategies based on movement disorder society task force guidelines

Inclusion criteria	*Exclusion criteria*
• Diagnosis of PD per UK PD Brain Bank Criteria	• Diagnosis of dementia
• Gradual cognitive decline reported by patient, informant, or observed by clinician	• Other potential explanation for impairment (e.g., medication, medical condition)
• Cognitive decline evident on neuropsychological testing and/or Parkinson's disease-appropriate cognitive screening instrumentor global cognitive measure	• Conditions co-morbid with PD that impact neuropsychological test performance (e.g., motor impairment, fatigue, psychosis)
• Cognitive decline may make activities of daily living more effortful or challenging but does not compromise functional independence	
Level I-Abbreviated assessment	**Level II-Comprehensive assessment**
• Impairment on PD-appropriate global cognitive ability scale (e.g., Dementia Rating Scale) or	• Neuropsychological testing includes 2 tests per domain (attention and working memory, executive functions, language, memory, and visuospatial skills)
• Impairment on at least 2 neuropsychological tests when a limited set of tests is used (less than 2 tests per domain or less than 5 cognitive domains assessed)	• Impairment on 2 tests in one domain or impairment on 1 test in 2 different domains
	• Impairment shown by: score 1-2 SD below norms, or significant decline on serial testing, or significant decline from estimated premorbid functioning
PD-MCI Subtype classification (comprehensive, Level II assessment required) • Single-domain: Impairment on 2 tests in one domain • Multiple-domain: Impairment on at least 1 test in each of 2 or more domains	

existing databases rather than prospective studies, and the specific tests used to confirm the MCI criteria have varied considerably, as has the allocation of specific tests to given domains of cognition.

Despite some variability in tests used and the source of samples (community, hospital), prevalence figures of MCI have been generally comparable. A study using a modification of Tröster's criteria and assessing 5 domains of cognition (language, executive, function, praxis, and visuospatial), albeit with only one test for some domains, found that 14.8% of newly diagnosed, drug-naïve PD patients had MCI (Poletti et al., 2012). The authors of that study also reported that PD-MCI was associated with greater bradykinesia, whereas patients with tremor-predominant motor symptoms generally performed better on cognitive tests.

The first study using the MDS criteria was the Norwegian ParkWest population study, which was discussed earlier. The sample consists of newly diagnosed patients, almost all drug-naïve. Of the 182 subjects followed for 3 years, 20.3% had MCI at baseline (Pedersen, Larsen, Tysnes, & Alves, 2013). Mild cognitive impairment was presumably defined using Level I criteria because not enough neuropsychological tests were given and only four of the five prescribed cognitive domains were evaluated (language tests were not given and the semantic verbal fluency task was counted as an executive function test). Patients with MCI at baseline were at much greater risk (relative risk 39.2) of developing dementia during the follow-up than were those without MCI. Whereas 27% of those with MCI progressed to dementia, less than 1% of those without MCI developed dementia in 3 years. Patients with MCI who demented performed more poorly than those who did not, especially on tests of memory and attention, with a trend seen on executive tests. Of note, the performance of MCI patients developing dementia did not differ on "posterior" visuospatial tests.

In a cross-sectional study of 139 patients from 6 North American movement-disorder centers, on average more than 5 years after PD diagnosis, a prevalence of MCI of 33% using MDS Level II criteria was observed (Marras et al., 2013). Of those with MCI, 93% had multidomain MCI. Among those with multidomain MCI, the most common impairments involved executive function (84%), visuospatial tasks (79%), and memory (47%). Less common were impairments in attention (26%) and language (19%).

The third published study using MCI criteria was a re-analysis of the Dutch study we described earlier (Muslimovic, Post, Speelman, De Haan, & Schmand, 2009b; Muslimovic et al., 2005). This study also used a hospital sample and Level II criteria, but followed newly diagnosed patients for 5 years (Broeders, de Bie, et al., 2013). At baseline, 35% of patients had MCI, and of those 65% had multidomain MCI. The proportion of multidomain MCI as a function of all MCI remained quite stable over the first years of follow-up (64% at Year 3) but declined at year 5 (43%), presumably because more of those with multidomain than single domain MCI had progressed to dementia. One difficulty faced in interpreting progression to MCI and dementia in this study is that the attrition rate from the neuropsychological study was quite high: 24% at year 3 versus 8% in the ParkWest study at year 3. Similarly, a further 25% attrition occurred between years 3 and 5. Thus, it is likely that progression estimates are conservatively biased. Indeed, attrition analyses indicated that those not continuing in the study were older and had greater cognitive problems per MMSE score than those who remained without MCI. Bearing these rates in mind, of the survivors, 53% had MCI at year

3. Of 43 patients with MCI at baseline, 6 (14%) developed dementia at year 3. Of the 47 patients with MCI at year 3, 8 (17%) developed dementia by year 5, and overall, of patients with formal neuropsychological testing, 14 patients with MCI had developed dementia between baseline and final follow-up. The study authors noted that, when clinical data were considered as well, however, 20 patients with prior MCI (including those developing MCI between baseline and year 3) had developed dementia by year 5.

Other Issues Addressed by Recent Studies on MCI

One issue concerning the new criteria is their reliability, particularly since reliability is a precondition for validity. There are multiple types of reliability, but those most often considered are test-retest reliability (the extent to which repeat assessment yields similar results), and intra- and inter-rater reliability (the extent to which one rater obtains a result when given the same data repeatedly, and the extent to which two or more raters agree on a diagnosis when given the same data).

The Dutch MCI study is the only one to have examined intra- and inter-rater reliability of the new MCI criteria (Broeders, de Bie, et al., 2013). That study found adequate intrarater reliability for each of two raters using the MDS criteria and Level II assessments (ranging from r = 0.85 to 0.96). Inter-rater reliability was also excellent (kappa = 0.91).

Concern has been expressed regarding the stability of the MCI diagnosis, not only generally, but also in PD (Yarnall, Rochester, & Burn, 2013). Neuropsychological test results might a priori be expected to have lesser test-retest reliability in a neurodegenerative condition that progresses in heterogeneous and nonlinear fashion. However, some might argue that although progression from MCI to dementia is an acceptable and logical reason for lack of stability of MCI diagnosis, reversion from MCI to normal is less expected and aberrant. Such an argument has merit, so long as one accepts that MCI attribution to a neurodegenerative condition requires clinical judgment, and MCI, even in PD, might reflect co-morbid conditions such as depression, medical illness, or indeed, a multitude of factors rather than just one. It is for this very reason that some have argued that MCI criteria should be available that consider the certainty of the etiologic attribution (Tröster, 2011). Theoretically, if a treatment is available for a condition impacting cognition, then MCI might normalize if that condition is treated, much as might blood pressure in a hypertensive prescribed antihypertensive agents. Another possibility is that MCI diagnosis varies because the course of disease progression is characterized by an undulating rather than a straight line. The idea that MCI reversion to normality is aberrant has merit if the condition is assumed to be progressive and no significant treatment changes or changes in comorbid conditions have been evidenced during the period of MCI normalization. Furthermore, it should be borne in mind that reversion from MCI to normalcy may occur more often in community or population epidemiological studies in which MCI may be less rigorously ascertained than in clinical settings.

Two of the more recent studies have considered the stability of MCI diagnosis. In the Dutch study (Broeders, de Bie, et al., 2013), 4/47 (8.5%) between baseline and year 3, and 3/47 (6%) between year 3 and year 5 reverted from MCI to normal. In the ParkWest Study (Pedersen et al., 2013) 8/37 (21.6%) of patients with MCI at baseline had reverted to normal cognition by 3-year follow-up. Of note, 6 of those 8 patients had less than 2 neuropsychological test impairments, highlighting perhaps the shortcomings inherent in making a diagnosis of MCI based on Level I criteria or on the basis of one among several tests, a procedure that would naturally be expected to be associated with a high false positive rate. It is unclear how patients with only one impaired test qualified for MDS MCI criteria and it is possible that criteria were not properly applied in that study. Indeed, the MDS criteria indicate that scores highly correlated on a single test should not be used to infer MCI. It is also worth noting that, if consistency in MCI diagnosis at baseline and year 1 was considered, only 9% reverted to normal by year 3.

Another issue is how one determines whether a test score reflects a decline or impairment. The traditional method has been to compare a patient's tests score to a normative sample, and to infer a decline/impairment if the score is 1–2 SD (most frequently 1.5 SD in the case of PD; Yarnall et al., 2013) below the normative mean. A problem with this approach is that the distributions of cognitive test scores in the normal population are often assumed to approach normal curves. In the normal distribution, 16% of scores fall 1 or more SD below the mean. If test scores are not corrected for factors such as education, it is likely then that a considerable number of scores reflecting no change from premorbid level (i.e., among the lowest 16% to begin with) might be inferred to reflect MCI. If one uses a cut-off of 1.5 SD, then only 9% of scores are below this level in a normally distributed collection of scores. Because the detection of MCI is primarily concerned with the early detection and treatment of cognitive decline, the more egregious errors might be a false negative rather than a false positive (assuming no or minimal psychological or treatment ill effects of a false positive). Yet, if test scores are normally distributed in a normative sample, 30% of scores are 0.5 SD or more above the mean. Such scores would have to decline *at least* 1.5 SD to even reach the 1 SD below the mean cut-off, and 2 SD to reach the 1.5 SD below the mean cut-off (and most of those scores would have to decline even more since this number considers only those scores at the 0.5 SD mark above the mean). Consequently, persons with high premorbid functioning might show signs of MCI (cognitive decline) long before meeting strict psychometric criteria for MCI and fail to be detected. Given this scenario, the MDS criteria allow for declines from estimated premorbid levels. The impact on diagnostic rates of using declines from premorbid levels rather than normative cut-offs has not been widely investigated. The North American study (Marras et al., 2013) did find that, when using test scores uncorrected for education, normative standards for MCI yielded a prevalence rate of 33%. When each test score was compared to an index of premorbid function (oral word reading test score), the rate increased to 79%. One possibility is that this higher rate reflects false positive errors, a possibility that must be considered since premorbid estimates usually are associated with a sizeable error, and this study compared the score to the premorbid point estimate rather than the lower bound of the confidence interval. Issues such as test score scatter and correlations between test scores, as well as base rates of differences between pairs of scores in the population also need to be considered. Another possibility is that this higher rate is actually more (though not completely) accurate than the normative based MCI rate, something that seems reasonable seeing how well educated the sample was (on average, almost 16 years of education, or the equivalent of a first university degree).

In clinical settings, there is a need for efficient cognitive screening instruments. The reasons for the desirability of such instruments, and their shortcomings in use with PD, have been well described in the past (Kulisevsky & Pagonabarraga, 2009; Tröster & Fields, 2008). The evaluation of screening instruments is particularly desirable in PD-MCI given that Movement Disorder Society (MDS) Level I criteria can be met using such scales. Using neuropsychologically defined MCI (Level II) as the gold standard, one study evaluated the sensitivity and specificity of several screening instruments vis-à-vis that gold standard (Marras et al., 2013). When screening for a condition of interest, high sensitivity rather than specificity is desirable. Setting a goal of 80% sensitivity (the MMSE failed to attain this sensitivity), the Montreal Cognitive Assessment (MoCA) had a specificity of 44% when the cut-off score of 26 or less was used; the SCOPA-Cog (cut-off 30 or less) had specificity of 33%. Diagnostic accuracy, that is, the overall percentage correctly classified, using these scores was 57% for the MoCA and 50% for the SCOPA-Cog.

When seeking a diagnostic instrument, specificity is valued over sensitivity. The highest cut-off scores providing at least 80% specificity were 23 for the MoCA, 26 for the MMSE, and 24 for the SCOPA-Cog. These scores provided sensitivities of only 35–44%, and diagnostic accuracy ranging from 68% to 73%. These somewhat discouraging figures are worth bearing in mind when using Level I criteria and a cognitive screening instrument or global cognitive function scale to define MCI.

An issue in evaluating the new MDS criteria is that they often might be considered to represent the gold standard against which to evaluate other criteria and diagnostic instruments. One avenue of evaluating the criteria might be to obtain quantitative, empirical evidence that clusters of test scores correspond to domains of MCI impairment. Although a recent study did not provide a direct test of the criteria, used too few tests to address Level II evaluation, and did not evaluate language, the statistical clustering of scores defined groups with intact cognition, nonamnestic single and multidomain and amnestic multidomain MCI, and dementia (Dujardin et al., 2013). Thus, there is tentative independent quantitative support for the subgrouping of MCI proposed in the MDS criteria.

Another issue that has been debated is whether patient report (subjective complaint) of cognitive dysfunction should be required to diagnose MCI. The MDS criteria have provided some leeway from the original Petersen criteria in that they allow for patient report, caregiver report, or clinician observation. All three studies of the MDS criteria have required such confirmation, although they have used different rating scales to derive this report. One study has determined how using or not using this requirement impacts MCI prevalence. Specifically, the North American study found that prevalence of MCI increased from 33% to 41% when cognitive complaint was not required. Indeed, literature findings support the use of report of disability or cognitive problems (though not in isolation) in cognitive diagnosis except when the reporting patient has considerable cognitive impairment (Brown, MacCarthy, Jahanshahi, & Marsden, 1989; Dujardin et al., 2010; Naismith, Pereira, Shine, & Lewis, 2011; Sitek, Soltan, Wieczorek, Robowski, & Slawek, 2011).

A final issue is whether everyday functioning is truly intact in MCI. The original MCI criteria of Petersen required instrumental activities of daily living to be uncompromised, whereas recent iterations of the criteria, and those of the MDS, acknowledge that functioning might not be fully preserved. Although the MDS MCI criteria require that functional impairments cannot be of the extent to compromise independence, the criteria do allow that day-to-day functions and activities of daily living be more effortful or challenging. Indeed, recent studies have shown that global measures of cognition are related to scores on ADL scales (Rosenthal et al., 2010) and that the presence of MCI per MDS criteria is associated with a decrement in ADLs (Leroi, McDonald, Pantula, & Harbishettar, 2012). Recent studies have also begun to examine more specific instrumental ADLs in PD-MCI. For example, financial abilities such as basic money skills, investment decision making and knowledge of financial concepts may be poorer in PD-MCI than in elderly controls and 50% of PD-MCI patients may show impairments in overall financial capacity (Martin et al., 2013). It is of note that this study was based on a small sample, the majority of which had multidomain, and especially amnestic multidomain MCI. Whether the findings generalize to persons with less severe MCI is unknown. Perhaps of greater concern is that a recent study of PD found the group with borderline impaired cognition to frequently lack capacity to consent to research: at least one third of the borderline cognitively impaired group (defined by the Mattis Dementia Rating Scale) were deemed to have trouble providing informed consent for drug and surgery trials (Karlawish et al., 2013). These findings, if replicated, suggest that capacity to consent should be scrutinized rather than assumed in potential research participants with PD-MCI.

TREATMENT OF MILD COGNITIVE IMPAIRMENT

Surprisingly little attention has been paid to the treatment of nondementia cognitive impairment. Two broad strategies have received attention: pharmacologic and cognitive rehabilitation. The role of cholinergic mechanisms in Parkinson's disease dementia is well established. The recent studies we reviewed that suggest cholinergic deficits to be apparent in milder cognitive impairments in PD provide a rational basis for targeting the cholinergic system. Several trials evaluated the use of cholinesterase inhibitors (e.g., donepezil, rivastigmine, galantamine) or glutamatergic agents such as memantine. A recent Cochrane review (Rolinski, Fox, Maidment, & McShane, 2012) supports the use of cholinesterase inhibitors in PD dementia given positive effects on ADL, cognition and behavior, but their use in nondementia cognitive impairment was not supported at time of review. Two small, preliminary studies have shown that atomoxetine (a selective norepinephrine reuptake inhibitor used to treat attention deficit disorder) might have a beneficial effect on cognition, specifically executive function (Marsh, Biglan, Gerstenhaber, & Williams, 2009; Weintraub et al., 2010).

Very little data are available regarding nonpharmacologic treatment of cognition in PD, and in particular cognitive rehabilitation (Hindle, Petrelli, Clare, & Kalbe, 2013). Two studies that have relatively poorly described their interventions suggest that executive functions might improve with cognitive rehabilitation (Sammer, Reuter, Hullmann, Kaps, & Vaitl, 2006; Sinforiani, Banchieri, Zucchella, Pacchetti, & Sandrini, 2004). Although three other small studies reported cognitive improvements with training (McKinlay, Grace, Dalrymple-Alford, & Roger, 2010; Mohlman, Chazin, & Georgescu, 2011; Nombela et al., 2011), another study found that computerized cognition-specific and non-specific sports game programs yielded similar cognitive benefits in four cognitive domains, and the non-specific program yielded superior gains in attention (Zimmerman et al., 2014). Overall, there are few data supporting such cognitive training interventions (Calleo et al., 2012). Indeed, a recent evidence-based review concluded that although there were some positive results of cognitive rehabilitation on executive functions and memory, there was insufficient evidence to recommend this type of intervention in PD (Langenbahn, Ashman, Cantor, & Trott, 2013).

CONCLUSIONS AND FUTURE DIRECTIONS

Cognition is impaired earlier in the course of PD than once assumed, and one-quarter to one- third of persons with newly diagnosed PD may have subtle cognitive changes or definable MCI. Persons with MCI are at greater risk of developing dementia within one to two years, in one estimate having a 39-fold risk. Dementia risk may be especially heightened in those demonstrating consistent MCI over at least two annual assessments. Probably fewer than 10% of persons with confirmed MCI revert to normal status. It remains unclear, however, whether a particular subtype of MCI confers greater dementia risk than others. It is thought that, early on, attention and executive dysfunction is prominent (and largely mediated by dopaminergic abnormalities), whereas disease progression is associated with emergence of multidomain MCI and amnestic and visuospatial abnormalities (mediated by additional cholinergic and noradrenergic) abnormalities. The neuropathology of MCI is poorly studied and likely heterogeneous, involving brain alpha synuclein deposition (Lewy bodies), amyloid deposition (plaques), multiple neurotransmitter abnormalities, and cerebrovascular pathology.

Recent MCI criteria appear reliable, consonant with quantitatively established groupings of cognitive impairment, and predictive of dementia. However, future research is needed to identify the prognostic value of MCI subtypes more clearly, their neuropathological basis, and their functional impact and treatment. MCI, once thought to be benign from a functional standpoint, may not be completely benign given its impact on quality of life and several activities of daily living, including financial management. These functional changes in MCI do not compromise a patient's independence, but they do make life more difficult and demand adaptation and/or accommodations. Future research that more clearly separates cognitive and physical determinants of ADL impairments is needed if we are to better understand the causes of initial functional changes in PD. Given that MCI produces functional changes that are not benign, and may be a harbinger of dementia, much more research into MCI treatment should be demanded.

NOTE

1. This is called family-wise error. When based on one variable, the error of incorrect classification using this criterion is 16%, because this percentage of the Gaussian normal distribution is below –1 standard deviation. With two uncorrelated variables and the same 16% criterion, the error increases to $1 - (1 - 0.16)^2 = 0.29$.

REFERENCES

Aarsland, D., Bronnick, K., & Fladby, T. (2011). Mild cognitive impairment in Parkinson's disease. *Current Neurology and Neuroscience Reports, 11*(4), 371–378. doi: 10.1007/s11910-011-0203-1

Aarsland, D., Bronnick, K., Larsen, J. P., Tysnes, O. B., & Alves, G. (2009). Cognitive impairment in incident, untreated Parkinson disease: the Norwegian ParkWest study. *Neurology, 72*(13), 1121–1126. doi: 01.wnl.0000338632.00552.cb [pii] 10.1212/01.wnl.0000338632.00552.cb

Aarsland, D., Bronnick, K., Larsen, J. P., Tysnes, O. B., Alves, G., & Norwegian Park-West Study, G. (2009). Cognitive impairment in incident, untreated Parkinson disease: the Norwegian ParkWest study. *Neurology,* 72(13), 1121–1126. doi: 10.1212/01.wnl.0000338632.00552.cb

Aarsland, D., Bronnick, K., Williams-Gray, C., Weintraub, D., Marder, K., Kulisevsky, J.,... Emre, M. (2010). Mild cognitive impairment in Parkinson disease: a multicenter pooled analysis. *Neurology,* 75(12), 1062–1069. doi: 75/12/1062 [pii] 10.1212/WNL.0b013e3181f39d0e

Adler, C. H., Caviness, J. N., Sabbagh, M. N., Shill, H. A., Connor, D. J., Sue, L.,... Beach, T. G. (2010). Heterogeneous neuropathological findings in Parkinson's disease with mild cognitive impairment. *Acta Neuropathologica, 120*(6), 827–828. doi: 10.1007/s00401-010-0744-4

Albert, M. L. (1978). Subcortical dementia. In R. Katzman, R. D. Terry, & K. L. Bick (Eds.), *Alzheimer's Disease, Senile dementia and related disorders* (pp. 173–180). New York, NY: Raven Press.

Altman DG. Systematic reviews of evaluations of prognostic variables. *BMJ.* 2001;323(7306):224–228.

Alves, G., Muller, B., Herlofson, K., HogenEsch, I., Telstad, W., Aarsland, D.,... Norwegian ParkWest Study Group. (2009). Incidence of Parkinson's disease in Norway: the Norwegian ParkWest study. *Journal of Neurology, Neurosurgery, and Psychiatry, 80*(8), 851–857. doi: 10.1136/jnnp.2008.168211

Benito-Leon, J., Bermejo-Pareja, F., Morales-Gonzalez, J. M., Porta-Etessam, J., Trincado, R., Vega, S.,... Neurological Disorders in Central Spain Study Group. (2004). Incidence of Parkinson disease and parkinsonism in three elderly populations of central Spain. *Neurology, 62*(5), 734–741.

Benito-Leon, J., Louis, E. D., Posada, I. J., Sanchez-Ferro, A., Trincado, R., Villarejo, A.,... Bermejo-Pareja, F. (2011). Population-based case-control study of cognitive function in early Parkinson's disease (NEDICES). *Journal of the Neurological Sciences, 310*(1–2), 176–182. doi: 10.1016/j.jns.2011.06.054

Beyer, M. K., Bronnick, K. S., Hwang, K. S., Bergsland, N., Tysnes, O. B., Larsen, J. P., ... Apostolova, L. G. (2013). Verbal memory is associated with structural hippocampal changes in newly diagnosed Parkinson's disease. *Journal of Neurology, Neurosurgery & Psychiatry, 84*(1), 23–28. doi: 10.1136/jnnp-2012-303054

Bowen, F. P., Kamienny, R. S., Burns, M. M., & Yahr, M. (1975). Parkinsonism: effects of levodopa treatment on concept formation. *Neurology, 25*(8), 701–704.

Broeders, M., de Bie, R. M., Velseboer, D. C., Speelman, J. D., Muslimovic, D., & Schmand, B. (2013). Evolution of mild cognitive impairment in Parkinson disease. *Neurology, 81*(4), 346–352. doi: 10.1212/WNL.0b013e31829c5c86

Broeders, M., Velseboer, D. C., de Bie, R., Speelman, J. D., Muslimovic, D., Post, B.,... Schmand, B. (2013). Cognitive change in newly-diagnosed patients with Parkinson's disease: a 5-year follow-up study. *Journal of the International Neuropsychological Society, 19*(6), 695–708. doi: 10.1017/S1355617713000295

Bronnick, K., Alves, G., Aarsland, D., Tysnes, O. B., & Larsen, J. P. (2011). Verbal memory in drug-naive, newly diagnosed Parkinson's disease. The retrieval deficit hypothesis revisited. *Neuropsychology, 25*(1), 114–124. doi: 10.1037/a0020857

Brown, R. G., MacCarthy, B., Jahanshahi, M., & Marsden, C. D. (1989). Accuracy of self-reported disability in patients with parkinsonism. *Archives of Neurology, 46*(9), 955–959.

Brown, R. G., & Marsden, C. D. (1990). Cognitive function in Parkinson's disease: from description to theory. *Trends in Neurosciences, 13*(1), 21–29.

Calleo, J., Burrows, C., Levin, H., Marsh, L., Lai, E., & York, M. K. (2012). Cognitive rehabilitation for executive dysfunction in Parkinson's disease: application and current directions. *Parkinsons Disorders, 2012*, 512892. doi: 10.1155/2012/512892

Compta, Y., Parkkinen, L., O'Sullivan, S. S., Vandrovcova, J., Holton, J. L., Collins, C.,... Revesz, T. (2011). Lewy- and Alzheimer-type pathologies in Parkinson's disease dementia: which is more important? *Brain, 134*(Pt 5), 1493–1505. doi: 10.1093/brain/awr031

Cooper, J. A., Sagar, H. J., Doherty, S. M., Jordan, N., Tidswell, P., & Sullivan, E. V. (1992). Different effects of dopaminergic and anticholinergic therapies on cognitive and motor function in Parkinson's disease. A follow-up study of untreated patients. *Brain, 115 (Pt 6)*(Pt 6), 1701–1725.

Cooper, J. A., Sagar, H. J., Jordan, N., Harvey, N. S., & Sullivan, E. V. (1991). Cognitive impairment in early, untreated Parkinson's disease and its relationship to motor disability. *Brain, 114 (Pt 5)*(Pt 5), 2095–2122.

de Lau, L. M., & Breteler, M. M. (2006). Epidemiology of Parkinson's disease. *Lancet Neurology, 5*(6), 525–535. doi: 10.1016/s1474-4422(06)70471-9

Domellöf, M. E., Forsgren, L., & Elgh, E. (2013). Persistence of associations between cognitive impairment and motor dysfunction in the early phase of Parkinson's disease. *Journal of Neurology, 260*(9), 2228–2236. doi: 10.1007/s00415-013-6971-6

Downes, J. J., Roberts, A. C., Sahakian, B. J., Evenden, J. L., Morris, R. G., & Robbins, T. W. (1989). Impaired extra-dimensional shift performance in medicated and unmedicated Parkinson's disease: evidence for a specific attentional dysfunction. *Neuropsychologia, 27*(11–12), 1329–1343.

Dubois, B., & Pillon, B. (1997). Cognitive deficits in Parkinson's disease. *Journal of Neurology, 244*(1), 2–8.

Dujardin, K., Duhamel, A., Delliaux, M., Thomas-Anterion, C., Destee, A., & Defebvre, L. (2010). Cognitive complaints in Parkinson's disease: its relationship with objective cognitive decline. *Journal of Neurology, 257*(1), 79–84. doi: 10.1007/s00415-009-5268-2

Dujardin, K., Leentjens, A. F., Langlois, C., Moonen, A. J., Duits, A. A., Carette, A. S., & Duhamel, A. (2013). The spectrum of cognitive disorders in Parkinson's disease: A data-driven approach. *Movement Disorders, 28*(2), 183–189. doi: 10.1002/mds.25311

Ekman, U., Eriksson, J., Forsgren, L., Mo, S. J., Riklund, K., & Nyberg, L. (2012). Functional brain activity and presynaptic dopamine uptake in patients with Parkinson's disease and mild cognitive impairment: a cross-sectional study. *Lancet Neurology, 11*(8), 679–687. doi: 10.1016/S1474-4422(12)70138-2

Elgh, E., Domellof, M., Linder, J., Edstrom, M., Stenlund, H., & Forsgren, L. (2009). Cognitive function in early Parkinson's disease: a population-based study. *European Journal of Neurology, 16*(12), 1278–1284. doi: 10.1111/j.1468-1331.2009.02707.x

Evans, J. R., Mason, S. L., Williams-Gray, C. H., Foltynie, T., Brayne, C., Robbins, T. W., & Barker, R. A. (2011). The natural history of treated Parkinson's disease in an incident, community based cohort. *Journal of Neurology, Neurosurgery & Psychiatry, 82*(10), 1112–1118. doi: 10.1136/jnnp.2011.240366

Foltynie, T., Brayne, C. E., Robbins, T. W., & Barker, R. A. (2004). The cognitive ability of an incident cohort of Parkinson's patients in the UK. The CamPaIGN study. *Brain, 127*(Pt 3), 550–560. doi: 10.1093/brain/awh067

Gaenslen, A., Swid, I., Liepelt-Scarfone, I., Godau, J., & Berg, D. (2011). The patients' perception of prodromal symptoms before the initial diagnosis of Parkinson's disease. *Movement Disorders, 26*(4), 653–658. doi: 10.1002/mds.23499; 10.1002/mds.23499

Goldman, J. G., Weis, H., Stebbins, G., Bernard, B., & Goetz, C. G. (2012). Clinical differences among mild cognitive impairment subtypes in Parkinson's disease. *Movement Disorders, 27*(9), 1129–1136. doi: 10.1002/mds.25062

Gomperts, S. N., Locascio, J. J., Marquie, M., Santarlasci, A. L., Rentz, D. M., Maye, J., . . . Growdon, J. H. (2012). Brain amyloid and cognition in Lewy body diseases. *Movement Disorders, 27*(8), 965–973. doi: 10.1002/mds.25048

Halliday, G. M., & McCann, H. (2010). The progression of pathology in Parkinson's disease. *Annals of the New York Academy of Sciences, 1184*, 188–195. doi: 10.1111/j.1749-6632.2009.05118.x

Hawkes, C. H., Del Tredici, K., & Braak, H. (2010). A timeline for Parkinson's disease. *Parkinsonism & Related Disorders, 16*(2), 79–84. doi: 10.1016/j.parkreldis.2009.08.007

Hawkins, K., Jennings, D., Marek, K., Siderowf, A., Stern, M., & Investigators, P. S. (2010). Cognitive deficits associated with dopamine transporter loss in the pre-motor subjects in the PARS cohort [Abstract]. *Movement Disorders, 25*(Suppl 3), S690-S691.

Hely, M. A., Reid, W. G., Adena, M. A., Halliday, G. M., & Morris, J. G. (2008). The Sydney multicenter study of Parkinson's disease: The inevitability of dementia at 20 years. *Movement Disorders, 23*(6), 837–844. doi: 10.1002/mds.21956

Henry, J. D., & Crawford, J. R. (2004). A meta-analytic review of verbal fluency performance following focal cortical lesions. *Neuropsychology, 18*(2), 284–295.

Hindle, J. V., Petrelli, A., Clare, L., & Kalbe, E. (2013). Nonpharmacological enhancement of cognitive function in Parkinson's disease: A systematic review. *Movement Disorders, 28*(8), 1034–1049. doi: 10.1002/mds.25377

Huang, C., Mattis, P., Perrine, K., Brown, N., Dhawan, V., & Eidelberg, D. (2008). Metabolic abnormalities associated with mild cognitive impairment in Parkinson disease. *Neurology, 70*(16 Pt 2), 1470–1477. doi:10.1212/01.wnl.0000304050.05332.9c

Janvin, C. C., Larsen, J. P., Aarsland, D., & Hugdahl, K. (2006). Subtypes of mild cognitive impairment in Parkinson's disease: progression to dementia. *Movement Disorders, 21*(9), 1343–1349.

Jellinger, K. A. (2008). A critical reappraisal of current staging of Lewy-related pathology in human brain. *Acta Neuropathologica, 116*(1), 1–16. doi: 10.1007/s00401-008-0406-y

Jellinger, K. A. (2013). Mild cognitive impairment in Parkinson disease: Heterogenous mechanisms. *Journal of Neural Transmission, 120*(1), 157–167. doi:10.1007/s00702-012-0771-5

Karlawish, J., Cary, M., Moelter, S. T., Siderowf, A., Sullo, E., Xie, S., & Weintraub, D. (2013). Cognitive impairment and PD patients' capacity to consent to research. *Neurology*. doi: 10.1212/WNL.0b013e3182a05ba5

Kehagia, A. A., Barker, R. A., & Robbins, T. W. (2010). Neuropsychological and clinical heterogeneity of cognitive impairment and dementia in patients with Parkinson's disease. *Lancet Neurology, 9*(12), 1200–1213. doi: 10.1016/S1474-4422(10)70212-X

Kempster, P. A., O'Sullivan, S. S., Holton, J. L., Revesz, T., & Lees, A. J. (2010). Relationships between age and late progression of Parkinson's disease: A clinico-pathological study. *Brain, 133*(Pt 6), 1755–1762. doi: 10.1093/brain/awq059

Kempster, P. A., Williams, D. R., Selikhova, M., Holton, J., Revesz, T., & Lees, A. J. (2007). Patterns of levodopa response in Parkinson's disease: a clinico-pathological study. *Brain, 130*(Pt 8), 2123–2128. doi: 10.1093/brain/awm142

Klein, J. C., Eggers, C., Kalbe, E., Weisenbach, S., Hohmann, C., Vollmar, S., . . . Hilker, R. (2010). Neurotransmitter changes in dementia with Lewy bodies and Parkinson disease dementia in vivo. *Neurology, 74*(11), 885–892. doi: WNL.0b013e3181d55f61 [pii] 10.1212/WNL.0b013e3181d55f61

Kulisevsky, J., & Pagonabarraga, J. (2009). Cognitive impairment in Parkinson's disease: tools for diagnosis and assessment. *Movement Disorders, 24*(8), 1103–1110. doi: 10.1002/mds.22506

Langenbahn, D. M., Ashman, T., Cantor, J., & Trott, C. (2013). An evidence-based review of cognitive rehabilitation in medical conditions affecting cognitive function. *Archives of Physical Medicine and Rehabilitation, 94*(2), 271–286. doi: 10.1016/j.apmr.2012.09.011

Lees, A. J., & Smith, E. (1983). Cognitive deficits in the early stages of Parkinson's disease. *Brain, 106 (Pt 2)*(Pt 2), 257–270.

Leroi, I., McDonald, K., Pantula, H., & Harbishettar, V. (2012). Cognitive impairment in Parkinson disease: impact on quality of life, disability, and caregiver burden. *Journal of Geriatric Psychiatry and Neurology, 25*(4), 208–214. doi: 10.1177/0891988712464823

Leverenz, J. B., Watson, G. S., Shofer, J., Zabetian, C. P., Zhang, J., & Montine, T. J. (2011). Cerebrospinal fluid biomarkers and cognitive performance in non-demented patients with Parkinson's disease. *Parkinsonism & Related Disorders, 17*(1), 61–64. doi: 10.1016/j.parkreldis.2010.10.003

Levin, B. E., & Katzen, H. L. (2005). Early cognitive changes and nondementing behavioral abnormalities in Parkinson's disease. *Advances in Neurology, 96*, 84–94.

Levin, B. E., Llabre, M. M., & Weiner, W. J. (1989). Cognitive impairments associated with early Parkinson's disease. *Neurology, 39*(4), 557–561.

Linder, J., Stenlund, H., & Forsgren, L. (2010). Incidence of Parkinson's disease and parkinsonism in northern Sweden: a population-based study. *Movement Disorders, 25*(3), 341–348. doi: 10.1002/mds.22987

Lippa, C. F., Duda, J. E., Grossman, M., Hurtig, H. I., Aarsland, D., Boeve, B. F., ... Group, D. P. W. (2007). DLB and PDD boundary issues: diagnosis, treatment, molecular pathology, and biomarkers. *Neurology, 68*(11), 812–819. doi: 10.1212/01.wnl.0000256715.13907.d3

Litvan, I., Aarsland, D., Adler, C. H., Goldman, J. G., Kulisevsky, J., Mollenhauer, B., ... Weintraub, D. (2011). MDS task force on mild cognitive impairment in Parkinson's disease: Critical review of PD-MCI. *Movement Disorders,* 26(10), 1814–1824. doi: 10.1002/mds.23823

Litvan, I., Goldman, J. G., Troster, A. I., Schmand, B. A., Weintraub, D., Petersen, R. C., ... Emre, M. (2012). Diagnostic criteria for mild cognitive impairment in Parkinson's disease: Movement Disorder Society Task Force guidelines. *Movement Disorders, 27*(3), 349–356. doi: 10.1002/mds.24893

Marder, K. (2010). Cognitive impairment and dementia in Parkinson's disease. *Movement disorders, 25*(Suppl 1), S110–116. doi: 10.1002/mds.22787

Marras, C., Armstrong, M. J., Meaney, C. A., Fox, S., Rothberg, B., Reginold, W., ... Duff-Canning, S. (2013). Measuring mild cognitive impairment in patients with Parkinson's disease. *Movement Disorders, 28*(5), 626–633. doi: 10.1002/mds.25426

Marsh, L., Biglan, K., Gerstenhaber, M., & Williams, J. R. (2009). Atomoxetine for the treatment of executive dysfunction in Parkinson's disease: a pilot open-label study. *Movement Disorders, 24*(2), 277–282. doi: 10.1002/mds.22307

Martin, R. C., Triebel, K. L., Kennedy, R. E., Nicholas, A. P., Watts, R. L., Stover, N. P., ... Marson, D. C. (2013). Impaired financial abilities in Parkinson's disease patients with mild cognitive impairment and dementia. *Parkinsonism & Related Disorders*. doi: 10.1016/j.parkreldis.2013.06.017

McKinlay, A., Grace, R. C., Dalrymple-Alford, J. C., & Roger, D. (2010). Characteristics of executive function impairment in Parkinson's disease patients without dementia. *Journal of the International Neuropsychological Society: JINS, 16*(2), 268–277. doi: 10.1017/S1355617709991299

Mohlman, J., Chazin, D., & Georgescu, B. (2011). Feasibility and acceptance of a nonpharmacological cognitive remediation intervention for patients with Parkinson disease. *Journal of Geriatric Psychiatry and Neurology, 24*(2), 91–97. doi: 10.1177/0891988711402350

Monastero, R., Di Fiore, P., Ventimiglia, G. D., Ventimiglia, C. C., Battaglini, I., Camarda, R., & Camarda, C. (2012). Prevalence and profile of mild cognitive impairment in Parkinson's disease. *Neurodegenerative Disorders, 10*(1–4), 187–190. doi: 10.1159/000335909

Montine, T. J., Shi, M., Quinn, J. F., Peskind, E. R., Craft, S., Ginghina, C., ... Zhang, J. (2010). CSF Abeta(42) and tau in Parkinson's disease with cognitive impairment. *Movement Disorders, 25*(15), 2682–2685. doi: 10.1002/mds.23287

Muslimovic, D., Post, B., Speelman, J. D., De Haan, R. J., & Schmand, B. (2009a). Cognitive decline in Parkinson's disease: a prospective longitudinal study. *Journal of the International Neuropsychological Society: JINS, 15*(3), 426–437. doi: 10.1017/s1355617709090614

Muslimovic, D., Post, B., Speelman, J. D., De Haan, R. J., & Schmand, B. (2009b). Cognitive decline in Parkinson's disease: a prospective longitudinal study. *Journal of the International Neuropsychological Society: JINS, 15*(3), 426–437. doi: S1355617709090614 [pii] 10.1017/S1355617709090614

Muslimovic, D., Post, B., Speelman, J. D., & Schmand, B. (2005). Cognitive profile of patients with newly diagnosed Parkinson disease. *Neurology, 65*(8), 1239–1245.

Muslimovic, D., Schmand, B., Speelman, J. D., & de Haan, R. J. (2007). Course of cognitive decline in Parkinson's disease: A meta-analysis. *Journal of the International Neuropsychological Society: JINS, 13*(6), 920–932. doi: 10.1017/s1355617707071160

Naismith, S. L., Pereira, M., Shine, J. M., & Lewis, S. J. (2011). How well do caregivers detect mild cognitive change in Parkinson's disease? *Movement Disorders, 26*(1), 161–164. doi: 10.1002/mds.23331

Nobili, F., Abbruzzese, G., Morbelli, S., Marchese, R., Girtler, N., Dessi, B.,... Rodriguez, G. (2009). Amnestic mild cognitive impairment in Parkinson's disease: a brain perfusion SPECT study. *Movement Disorders, 24*(3), 414–421. doi: 10.1002/mds.22381

Nombela, C., Bustillo, P. J., Castell, P. F., Sanchez, L., Medina, V., & Herrero, M. T. (2011). Cognitive rehabilitation in Parkinson's disease: evidence from neuroimaging. *Frontiers in Neurology, 2*, 82. doi: 10.3389/fneur.2011.00082

Owen, A. M. (2004). Cognitive dysfunction in Parkinson's disease: the role of frontostriatal circuitry. *Neuroscientist, 10*(6), 525–537. doi: 10.1177/1073858404266776

Owen, A. M., James, M., Leigh, P. N., Summers, B. A., Marsden, C. D., Quinn, N. P.,... Robbins, T. W. (1992). Fronto-striatal cognitive deficits at different stages of Parkinson's disease. *Brain, 115 (Pt 6)*(Pt 6), 1727–1751.

Parkinson, J. (1817). *An essay on the shaking palsy.* London, England: Sherwood, Neely & Jones.

Parkinson, J. (2002). An essay on the shaking palsy. [originaly published in 1817]. *Journal of Neuropsychiatry & Clinical Neuroscience, 14*(2), 223–236; discussion 222.

Pedersen, K. F., Larsen, J. P., Tysnes, O. B., & Alves, G. (2013). Prognosis of mild cognitive impairment in early Parkinson disease: The Norwegian ParkWest study. *JAMA Neurology, 70*(5), 580–586. doi: 10.1001/jamaneurol.2013.2110

Petersen, R. C. (2011). Clinical practice. Mild cognitive impairment. *New England Journal of Medicine, 364*(23), 2227–2234. doi: 10.1056/NEJMcp0910237

Poletti, M., Frosini, D., Pagni, C., Baldacci, F., Nicoletti, V., Tognoni, G.,... Bonuccelli, U. (2012). Mild cognitive impairment and cognitive-motor relationships in newly diagnosed drug-naive patients with Parkinson's disease. *Journal of Neurology, Neurosurgery and Psychiatry, 83*(6), 601–606. doi: 10.1136/jnnp-2011-301874

Rolinski, M., Fox, C., Maidment, I., & McShane, R. (2012). Cholinesterase inhibitors for dementia with Lewy bodies, Parkinson's disease dementia and cognitive impairment in Parkinson's disease. *Cochrane Database Systematic Review, 3*, CD006504. doi: 10.1002/14651858.CD006504.pub2

Rosenthal, E., Brennan, L., Xie, S., Hurtig, H., Milber, J., Weintraub, D.,... Siderowf, A. (2010). Association between cognition and function in patients with Parkinson disease with and without dementia. *Movement Disorders, 25*(9), 1170–1176. doi: 10.1002/mds.23073

Sammer, G., Reuter, I., Hullmann, K., Kaps, M., & Vaitl, D. (2006). Training of executive functions in Parkinson's disease. *Journal of Neurological Science, 248*(1–2), 115–119. doi: S0022-510X(06)00224-3 [pii] 10.1016/j.jns.2006.05.028

Sánchez-Ferro, Á., Benito-León, J., Louis, E. D., Mitchell, A. J., Molina-Arjona, J. A., Trincado, R., . . . Bermejo-Pareja, F. (2013). Rate of cognitive decline in premotor

Parkinson's disease: a prospective study (NEDICES). *Movement Disorders, 28*(2), 161–168. doi: 10.1002/mds.25148

Sanchez-Ferro, A., Benito-Leon, J., Mitchell, A. J., Louis, E. D., Posada, I. J., Trincado, R.,... Bermejo-Pareja, F. (2011). Premotor cognitive status in a cohort of incident Parkinson disease patients (NEDICES). *Journal of the Neurological Sciences, 310*(1–2), 211–215. doi: 10.1016/j.jns.2011.05.007

Shimada, H., Hirano, S., Shinotoh, H., Aotsuka, A., Sato, K., Tanaka, N.,... Irie, T. (2009). Mapping of brain acetylcholinesterase alterations in Lewy body disease by PET. *Neurology, 73*(4), 273–278. doi: WNL.0b013e3181ab2b58 [pii] 10.1212/WNL.0b013e3181ab2b58

Siderowf, A., Jennings, D., Eberly, S., Oakes, D., Hawkins, K. A., Ascherio, A.,... the, P. I. (2012). Impaired olfaction and other prodromal features in the Parkinson At-Risk Syndrome study. *Movement Disorders, 27*(3), 406–412. doi: 10.1002/mds.24892; 10.1002/mds.24892

Siderowf, A., Xie, S. X., Hurtig, H., Weintraub, D., Duda, J., Chen-Plotkin, A.,... Clark, C. (2010). CSF amyloid {beta} 1–42 predicts cognitive decline in Parkinson disease. *Neurology, 75*(12), 1055–1061. doi: WNL.0b013e3181f39a78 [pii] 10.1212/WNL.0b013e3181f39a78

Sinforiani, E., Banchieri, L., Zucchella, C., Pacchetti, C., & Sandrini, G. (2004). Cognitive rehabilitation in Parkinson's disease. *Archives of Gerontology & Geriatrics* (Suppl 9), 387–391.

Sitek, E. J., Soltan, W., Wieczorek, D., Robowski, P., & Slawek, J. (2011). Self-awareness of memory function in Parkinson's disease in relation to mood and symptom severity. *Aging & Mental Health,15*(2), 150–156. doi: 10.1080/13607863.2010.508773

Sollinger, A. B., Goldstein, F. C., Lah, J. J., Levey, A. I., & Factor, S. A. (2010). Mild cognitive impairment in Parkinson's disease: subtypes and motor characteristics. *Parkinsonism & Related Disorders, 16*(3), 177–180. doi: S1353-8020(09)00274-0 [pii] 10.1016/j.parkreldis.2009.11.002

Stern, M. B., & Siderowf, A. (2010). Parkinson's at risk syndrome: can Parkinson's disease be predicted? *Movement Disorders, 25* (Suppl 1), S89–93. doi: 10.1002/mds.22719

Taylor, A. E., Saint-Cyr, J. A., & Lang, A. E. (1988). Idiopathic Parkinson's disease: revised concepts of cognitive and affective status. *The Canadian Journal of Neurological Sciences. [Le journal canadien des sciences neurologiques], 15*(2), 106–113.

Tröster, A. I. (2011). A precis of recent advances in the neuropsychology of mild cognitive impairment(s) in Parkinson's disease and a proposal of preliminary research criteria. *Journal of the International Neuropsychological Society, 17*(3), 393–406. doi: 10.1017/S1355617711000257

Tröster, A. I., & Fields, J. A. (2008). Parkinson's disease, progressive supranuclear palsy, corticobasal degeneration, and related disorders of the frontostriatal system. In J. E. Morgan & J. H. Ricker (Eds.), *Textbook of clinical neuropsychology* (pp. 536–577). New York, NY: Psychology Press.

Velseboer, D. C., Broeders, M., Post, B., van Geloven, N., Speelman, J. D., Schmand, B.,... de Bie, R. M. (2013). Prognostic factors of motor impairment, disability, and quality of life in newly diagnosed PD. *Neurology, 80*(7), 627–633. doi: 10.1212/WNL.0b013e318281cc99

Weintraub, D., Mavandadi, S., Mamikonyan, E., Siderowf, A. D., Duda, J. E., Hurtig, H. I.,... Stern, M. B. (2010). Atomoxetine for depression and other neuropsychiatric symptoms in Parkinson disease. *Neurology, 75*(5), 448–455. doi: 75/5/448 [pii] 10.1212/WNL.0b013e3181ebdd79

Williams-Gray, C. H., Evans, J. R., Goris, A., Foltynie, T., Ban, M., Robbins, T. W., . . . Barker, R. A. (2009). The distinct cognitive syndromes of Parkinson's disease: 5 year follow-up of the CamPaIGN cohort. *Brain, 132*(Pt 11), 2958–2969. doi: 10.1093/brain/awp245

Williams-Gray, C. H., Foltynie, T., Brayne, C. E., Robbins, T. W., & Barker, R. A. (2007). Evolution of cognitive dysfunction in an incident Parkinson's disease cohort. *Brain, 130*(Pt 7), 1787–1798. doi: 10.1093/brain/awm111

Williams-Gray, C. H., Mason, S. L., Evans, J. R., Foltynie, T., Brayne, C., Robbins, T. W., & Barker, R. A. (2013). The CamPaIGN study of Parkinson's disease: 10-year outlook in an incident population-based cohort. *Journal of Neurology, Neurosurgery and Psychiatry, 84*(11), 1258–1264. doi: 10.1136/jnnp-2013-305277

Yarnall, A. J., Rochester, L., & Burn, D. J. (2013). Mild cognitive impairment in Parkinson's disease. *Age and Ageing, 42*(5), 567–576. doi: 10.1093/ageing/aft085

Zgaljardic, D. J., Borod, J. C., Foldi, N. S., & Mattis, P. (2003). A review of the cognitive and behavioral sequelae of Parkinson's disease: relationship to frontostriatal circuitry. *Cognitive and Behavioral Neurology, 16*(4), 193–210.

Zimmerman, R., Gschwandtner, U., Benz, N., Hatz, F., Schindler, C. Taub, E., & Fuhr, P. (2014). Cognitive training in Parkinson disease: Cognition-specific vs nonspecific computer training. *Neurology, 82*, 1219–1226.

9 Dementia in Parkinson's Disease

Arvid Rongve, Eirik Auning, Astrid Haram, and Dag Aarsland

INTRODUCTION

Parkinson's disease dementia (PDD) belongs to the α-synucleinopathies (Table 9-1), pathologically characterized by aggregation of α-synuclein in Lewy bodies and Lewy neurites, spreading from the brainstem to the cortex. Clinically, PD is defined by the gradual occurrence of motor symptoms such as rigidity (stiffness), bradykinesia (slowness of movements), resting tremor, and postural and gait disturbances, usually with unilateral onset. Significant cognitive decline and dementia typically develops several years after the start of motor symptoms. Per definition, a diagnosis of PDD cannot be made if dementia occurs before, simultaneously with, or within one year after onset of motor symptoms. Such patients will be more likely to receive a diagnosis of dementia with Lewy bodies (DLB). However, in a subgroup of Parkinson's disease (PD) patients, mild cognitive impairment (MCI) has been found from the start of motor symptoms and the risk for dementia is increased in these patients. By convention, these early impaired cases are currently labeled PD-MCI. The cognitive profile of PDD is characterized by attentional, executive, and visuospatial impairment, but memory impairment is also common (Emre et al., 2007). In addition, as is the case in DLB, patients with PDD typically have sleep disturbances, neuropsychiatric symptoms, autonomic dysfunction, tendency to fall, which all result in admission to a nursing home, impaired quality of life, high costs, and caregiver burden, underlining the clinical importance of the condition. Some of these patients have particularly good response to treatment with cholinesterase inhibitors, and there is an increased risk for neuroleptic hypersensitivity reactions, and thus an accurate diagnosis of PDD is essential in clinical practice.

Table 9-1 The α-synucleinopathies

Name	*Clinical features*
Parkinson's disease	Tremor, rigidity, akinesia, and gait disturbance
Parkinson's disease dementia	Dementia developed after more than 1 year of parkinsonian motor symptoms
Dementia with Lewy bodies	Dementia prior to parkinsonism, visual hallucinations, fluctuating cognition, and REM sleep behavior disorder (RBD)
Multiple system atrophy	Autonomic dysfunction, parkinsonism and ataxia
Idiopathic REM sleep behavior disorder	Acting out dream content during REM sleep
Pure autonomic failure	Orthostatic hypotension, constipation, sweating and impotence

Table 9-2 Staging and Grouping of Lewy body pathology in the human brain

Reference	*Year*	*Comment*
(Kosaka, Yoshimura, Ikeda, & Budka, 1984)	1984	*Group A*: Diffuse type of LBD; cerebral cortex, basal ganglia, diencephalon and brainstem affected by Lewy body pathology *Group B*: Transitional type between A and C *Group C*: Brainstem and diencephalon affected like in PD
(Braak et al., 2003)	2003	*Stages 1-2*: Presymptomatic; pathology confined to medulla oblongata and olfactory bulb *Stages 3-4*: Symptomatic phase; affection of the substantia nigra, midbrain and basal forebrain *Stages 5-6*: Cognitive failure and dementia, cortex affected
(G. Halliday et al., 2008)	2008	*Group 1*: Younger patients with distribution of pathology according to the Braak staging *Group 2*: Early malignant dementia dominant syndrome *Group 3*: Older onset, shorter survival and more pronounced Lewy related pathology
(Beach et al., 2009)	2009	*Stage I* Olfactory Bulb *Stage IIa* Brainstem Predominant *Stage IIb* Limbic Predominant *Stage III* Brainstem and Limbic *Stage IV* Neocortical

MOLECULAR PATHOLOGY

The Lewy body diseases share aggregation of α-synuclein and formation of Lewy bodies and Lewy neurites as their common hallmarks of pathology. The normal structure and function of α-synuclein is at present unknown, but it is believed to be involved in synaptic plasticity. Increased expression of α-synuclein will inhibit synaptic reclustering after neurotransmitter release and thus inhibit neurotransmitter release in the synaptic cleft (Nemani et al., 2010). Pathological phosphorylation and aggregation into toxic oligomers consisting of several monomers of α-synuclein and pathological spread of oligomers from one neuron to adjacent neurons have been suggested as possible mechanisms for spreading of the α-synuclein pathology within the CNS (Danzer, Krebs, Wolff, Birk, & Hengerer, 2009).

NEUROPATHOLOGY

Most studies report that Lewy bodies and Lewy neurites are the main pathological correlate of dementia in PD (Aarsland, Perry, Brown, Larsen, & Ballard, 2005; Irwin et al., 2012). However, Alzheimer-type pathologies also contribute, and a synergistic effect of amyloid, tau, and Lewy-type pathology on both the severity and quality of cognitive impairment and dementia in PD has been reported (Compta et al., 2011). The role of other pathologies such as synaptic loss, inflammation, and cerebrovascular disease is not yet known. Staging and phenomenological groupings of the Lewy body pathology for PD and DLB have been proposed (see Table 9-2) (Leverenz et al., 2008; Muller et al., 2005). Three distinctive groups have been described: One group with younger onset PD and longer duration of disease with neuropathology distribution beginning in the brain stem and olfactory nucleus and progressing rostrally; a second group, characterized by an early malignant dementia-dominant syndrome and severe neocortical disease as described in DLB. The third group consists of persons with older onset of PD, shorter survival, and a more complex disease with additional pathologies, including vascular and Alzheimer-type changes, and higher Lewy body loads in the brain (G. Halliday, Hely, Reid, & Morris, 2008).

THE PREVALENCE AND INCIDENCE OF PARKINSON'S DISEASE DEMENTIA

PDD is recognized as a common subtype of dementia. Cross-sectional epidemiological studies have reported that the proportion of PD patients with dementia is approximately 30%, suggesting that PDD represents 3–5 % of all dementia cases (Aarsland, Zaccai, & Brayne, 2005). Longitudinal studies have reported a sixfold risk of developing dementia in PD compared to people without PD of the same age, with an incidence of dementia of 100 per 100.000 patient-years leading to a cumulative proportion of up to 80% dementia in PD (Aarsland, Andersen, Larsen, Lolk, & Kragh-Sorensen, 2003; Buter et al., 2008; Hely, Reid, Adena, Halliday,

& Morris, 2008). These studies have, however, been based on prevalent samples, and a lower incidence has been reported during the first 5-10 years after diagnosis in incident samples. In a longitudinal study based on an incidence PD-cohort, a dementia incidence of 30 per 100 000 person-years was reported and slightly less than 50% of the cohort had developed dementia 8 years after diagnosis, with a mean time period to dementia of 6.2 years (Evans et al., 2011).

CLINICAL DIAGNOSTIC CRITERIA FOR PDD

The clinical profile of PDD differs from that of Alzheimer's disease and other dementias. A Movement Disorders Society Task Force defined clinical criteria for probable and possible PDD (Emre et al., 2007) and an operationalization of these criteria for practical administration in the clinic with cognitive tests has been published (Dubois et al., 2007). The criteria define core and associated clinical features: The two core features are (1) a diagnosis of PD according to Queen Square Brain Bank Criteria (Hughes, Daniel, Blankson, & Lees, 1993), and (2) a dementia syndrome with insidious onset and slow progression with cognitive impairment in more than one domain representing a decline from previous level and impairment in activities of daily living (ADL) independent of motor or autonomic symptoms. Associated clinical features are (1) cognitive features: impaired attention, executive functions, visuospatial functions, memory, or language functions, and (2) behavioral features: apathy, changes in personality or mood like depression or anxiety, hallucinations, delusions, and excessive daytime sleepiness. Practical procedures for cognitive testing at different levels of diagnostic accuracy, that is, Level I for a clinician without particular expertise in neuropsychological procedures, and a more advanced Level II are defined. Level I includes simple bedside tests like Mini-Mental State Examination (MMSE) (score below 26) as a global cognitive measure, reversed-months test for attention, lexical fluency, and clock drawing for executive function, MMSE pentagons for visuospatial functions, and three-word recall from the MMSE as a test for memory. The authors suggest the Neuropsychiatric Inventory (NPI) to detect behavioral features and a clinical interview with a caregiver to diagnose excessive daytime sleepiness and explore ADL abilities. Unfortunately, the suggested MMSE is probably suboptimal for DLB and PDD assessment due to minimal focus on executive functions, and scales such as the Montreal Cognitive Assessment (MOCA) and PD-Cognitive Rating Scale have been validated and recommended (Kulisevsky & Pagonabarraga, 2009).

CLINICAL DIFFERENTIAL DIAGNOSIS

The clinical diagnosis of dementia is based on an interview with both the person with dementia and the caregiver, and an active approach to the clinical features (Table 9-3) by applying appropriate cognitive and neuropsychiatric tests and ADL interview is important to detect dementia in PD. In addition to a clinical examination including physical and neurological examination and cognitive testing, supplemental blood tests, magnetic resonance imaging (MRI) and cerebrospinal fluid (CSF) analysis to exclude other intracranial pathology might be indicated. Important differential diagnoses include drugs, systemic disease, depression, and apathy, and motor symptoms such as bradykinesia and masked facies. Although MRI and CSF can support a dementia diagnosis, these techniques cannot reliably distinguish between dementia subtypes including AD, PDD, and DLB. Of note, both β-CIT dopamine transporter SPECT (DaTSCAN) and cardiac scintigraphy (MIBG) have shown a high sensitivity and specificity in differentiating between

Table 9-3 Clinical symptoms in PDD

Cognitive impairment	Attentional
	Visuospatial
	Executive
	Memory
	Language
Cognition/consciousness	Fluctuating
Neuropsychiatric and behavioural symptoms	Depression
	Apathy
	Anxiety
	Hallucinations
	Delusions
	Agitation
	Somatoform disorder
	Obsessive compulsive disorder
Sleep disturbances	REM sleep behavior disorder
	Excessive daytime sleepiness
	Insomnia
	Restless legs syndrome
	Nocturnal leg cramps
	Obstructive sleep apnea
	Sleep walking
	Periodic leg movements during sleep
	Sleep attacks
	Unintended sleep episodes
Motor	Symmetrical or asymmetrical parkinsonian symptoms
	Postural instability
	Gait disorder
Autonomic	Orthostatic hypotension
	Syncope
	Incontinence
	Obstipation
	Impotence

Lewy body dementias and Alzheimer's disease, but only DaTSCAN is at present approved for routine diagnostics.

DLB is differentiated from PDD based on the 1-year rule: in DLB parkinsonian motor symptoms can start after, simultaneously with, or within one year before the dementia syndrome. If motor parkinsonian symptoms start more than 1 year before dementia, the condition is diagnosed as PDD. Whether this is a biologically valid distinction, or whether PDD and DLB are merely syndromes on a continuum of Lewy body disease is not known. Currently, unlike the distinction between DLB and AD, there are no major prognostic or therapeutic consequences related to the distinction between PDD and DLB, although the severity of AD-type pathology is more pronounced in DLB compared to PDD.

Parkinsonism can occur in AD, vascular dementia, and frontotemporal dementia, but these syndromes can, in most cases, be differentiated from PDD and DLB based on the history, clinical examination, and supplemental tests like MRI, perfusion SPECT, and DaTSCAN. MRI can assist in identifying vascular parkinsonism. Progressive supranuclear palsy is a tauopathy and characterized by axial parkinsonism, early tendency to fall backward and impaired vertical eye movements, and can be complicated by subcortical dementia. Corticobasal degeneration also has tau pathology and is characterized by more severe motor impairment with apraxia, agnosia, parkinsonism, aphasia, and alien-hand syndrome with poor response to L-dopa. New diagnostic criteria for probable and possible CBD were recently proposed (Armstrong et al., 2013). Multiple system atrophy, an α-synucleinopathy, is characterized clinically by the early development of ataxia, autonomic failure, and symmetrical parkinsonism with rigidity and bradykinesia without tremor. Patients have poor response to L-dopa treatment and poor prognosis. DaTSCAN is abnormal in these three atypical parkinsonian disorders, but MRI can, in many cases, inform the clinical diagnosis. Parkinsonism and impaired cognition can be caused by neuroleptic medication and thus a drug history must be taken during the diagnostic process. DaTSCAN can be used to differentiate brain-stem parkinsonism from other motor impairments like essential tremor and vascular parkinsonism (Contrafatto et al., 2011; Vlaar et al., 2008).

NEUROPSYCHIATRIC SYMPTOMS

Neuropsychiatric and behavioral symptoms are common in PD, and were found in 89% of patients in one study, with depression (58%), apathy (54%), anxiety (49%), and visual hallucinations (44%) emerging as the most common symptoms (Aarsland et al., 2007). Neuropsychiatric symptoms are particularly common in PDD. Apathy, and, in particular, hallucinations and delusions are more common and severe in PDD compared to PD without dementia. In nondemented patients, impulse-control disorders like pathological gambling, hypersexuality and compulsive buying have been described in PD and found to be associated with dopamine-agonist treatment (Weintraub, Koester, et al., 2010), but their frequency in PDD is less explored.

SLEEP DISTURBANCES

Up to 80% of patients with mild DLB or PDD have a sleep disturbance, as compared to 56% of age matched cognitively normal controls and 64% of patients diagnosed with mild AD. The most common sleep symptoms are insomnia (47%), sleep-related leg cramps (42%), excessive daytime sleepiness (41%), REM-sleep behavioral disorder (RBD) (39%), restless legs syndrome (31%), obstructive sleep apnea (26%) and periodic leg movements during sleep (21%) (Rongve, Boeve, & Aarsland, 2010).

In PD without dementia, a wide range of different sleep disturbances have been described including insomnia, excessive daytime sleepiness, sleep attacks or unintended sleep episodes, RBD, restless legs syndrome, sleep related leg cramps, periodic leg movements during sleep, obstructive sleep apnoea and sleep walking/somnambulism (Jauregui-Barrutia, Tijero-Merino, Gomez-Esteban, & Zarranz, 2010; Mondragon-Rezola, Arratibel-Echarren, Ruiz-Martinez, & Marti-Masso, 2010).

Sleep disturbances in dementia have been found to relate to pathology in specific brain areas such as the suprachiasmatic nucleus, hypothalamus, the brainstem and pons area. Neurochemical changes including in melatonin and acetylcholine tend to differ in relation to the specific brain pathology and type of dementia involved (Claassen et al., 2010). Of note, the occurrence of RBD is a significant predictor for early dementia in PD.

AUTONOMIC FAILURE

Autonomic failure can be an early and prominent feature of PDD as a consequence of involvement of the ganglia and peripheral nervous system. Symptoms of autonomic failure are more common in PDD and DLB than in AD and include orthostatic hypotension, cardiac arrhythmias, syncope, constipation, impotence, urinary retention and excessive sweating (Allan et al., 2007; Sonnesyn et al., 2009). Orthostatic hypotension is associated with compensatory vascular mechanisms and can lead to white matter lesions, and thus can also contribute to cognitive impairment (Kim et al., 2012).

RISK FACTORS FOR EARLY COGNITIVE DECLINE

There is a wide variation in the time from onset of PD to dementia. Whereas some patients develop dementia within a few years of the diagnosis, others remain without dementia for more than 20 years (Aarsland et al., 2007). The mean rate of cognitive decline in PD is approximately 1 point each year on the MMSE scale (Aarsland et al., 2004), but there are large inter- and intra-individual variations in the rate of decline. Typically, in an individual PD patient, a period of no or very little decline is followed by an inflexion point after which a much more rapid decline occurs, with large interindividual variation in the time period to this inflexion point (Aarsland, Muniz, & Matthews, 2011; Johnson & Galvin, 2011). After onset of dementia in PD, the progression to the terminal stage of the illness is less variable, and there is an average of 3 years with increasing disability leading to death, whatever the age of onset (Kempster, O'Sullivan, Holton, Revesz, & Lees, 2010).

Identifying predictors of time to dementia and of the rate of cognitive decline is thus a key clinical and research priority. A shorter time to cognitive impairment in PD is associated with older age and older age at diagnosis, nontremor dominant motor subtypes with significant postural instability and gait disturbances (Alves, Larsen, Emre, Wentzel-Larsen, & Aarsland, 2006; Evans et al., 2011; G. M. Halliday & McCann, 2010), visual hallucinations, RBD (Boot et al., 2012; Postuma et al., 2009), and olfactory dysfunction (Baba et al., 2012).

GENETIC CONTRIBUTIONS TO COGNITIVE IMPAIRMENT

Mutations in the genes coding for α-synuclein (*SNCA*), tau (*MAPT*), leucine-rich repeat kinase2 (*LRRK2*), glucocerebrosidase (*GBA*), and human leukocyte antigen (*HLA*) have been found to increase the risk for PD, and, together with new genetic findings from genome wide- association studies (GWAS), explain about half the genetic risk to develop this disease (Hardy, 2010; Nalls et al., 2011). The genetics of PDD have been much less studied, but increased dementia risk in family members of people with PD has been reported (Kurz, Schlitter, Larsen, Ballard, & Aarsland, 2006), and associations between dementia and mutations in *MAPT* (Seto-Salvia et al., 2011) and *PSEN2* (Meeus et al., 2011) have been reported. Previously known mutations in AD and PD have been found in both PDD and DLB and suggests genetic overlap in these conditions (Meeus et al., 2011). Most PDD cases occur sporadically, although families have been described having many affected members with gene alterations in different locations of which some overlap with DLB (Nervi et al., 2011). Traditional genetic studies have identified multiplications (Chartier-Harlin et al., 2004; Singleton et al., 2003) and mutations (Polymeropoulos et al., 1997; Yamaguchi et al., 2005; Zarranz et al., 2004) in SNCA and β-synuclein genes (*SNCB*; Ohtake et al., 2004). PD patients with glucocerebrosidase (GBA) mutations have more frequent and severe cognitive impairments when compared to sporadic cases of PD (Neumann et al., 2009), and GBA mutation status may be an independent risk factor for cognitive impairment in patients with PD (Lyoo, Ryu, & Lee, 2010). Other typical PD mutations such as *LRRK2* and Parkin-mutations do not seem to be associated with cognitive impairment (Alcalay et al., 2010). Mutations of the *COMT* gene were associated with dopamine-related cognitive deficits in one study, such as attention, but do not seem be associated with increased risk of dementia. These findings have not been replicated in other studies (Williams-Gray, Evans, et al., 2009). Butyrylcholinesterase K (BCHE-K) is associated with increased risk of developing Alzheimer's disease (AD) in apolipoprotein ε (APOE4) carriers, whereas, among APOE4 noncarriers, BCHE-K appears to be protective. In PD, however, inconsistent results have been found regarding the associations between APOE and (BCHE-K) genotypes and risk of dementia (Kurz et al., 2009; Lane & He, 2009; Williams-Gray, Goris, et al., 2009). Genome wide association studies have been presented in PD and at least 10 different genes have been confirmed to be associated with PD including *HLA*, but such studies have not yet been presented in PDD (Nalls et al., 2011).

MILD COGNITIVE IMPAIRMENT

During the last 5 years, researchers have focused on MCI in PD (PD-MCI), that is, cognitive impairment without significant functional consequences (also, see Schmand & Tröster, Chapter 8 in this volume). The exact time when dementia should be diagnosed can be difficult to determine due to the fact that ADL difficulties can be caused by motor, sleep, and autonomic problems in addition to the cognitive failure. Although there is variation between studies, about 20–25% of PD patients without dementia have PD-MCI (Aarsland et al., 2010). At the time of PD diagnosis, MCI is observed in 15–20% of these people, even in nontreated patients (Aarsland, Bronnick, Larsen, Tysnes, & Alves, 2009). One reason for the variation is the use of different criteria for MCI. Tröster proposed two sets of criteria (Troster, 2011). MCI-PD outlines criteria when cognitive impairment occurring in PD may be due to a variety of factors, whereas PCI (Parkinson cognitive impairment) requires the etiology of the cognitive deficits to be PD. More elaborate criteria for this second group of PD patients with cognitive impairment have been developed. Specifically, The Movement Disorders Society seated a task force (MDS-TF) that published the first clinical consensus criteria for MCI in PD (Litvan et al., 2012). The criteria require a diagnosis of PD, gradual decline in cognitive ability reported by either the patient or informant, or observed by the clinician, which can be measured by either a cognitive screening scale, which is validated for PD (see earlier), (Level 1) or formal neuropsychological testing (Level 2). For Level 2 classification, at least 2 tests for each of five cognitive domains are required. In contrast to dementia, cognitive deficits in MCI are not sufficient to interfere significantly with functional independence.

Typically, attentional, visuospatial, and executive deficits occur early, but there is interindividual heterogeneity in the cognitive profile (Barone et al., 2011; Litvan et al., 2011). Memory impairment is also common, even independent of executive and attentional deficits (Bronnick, Alves, Aarsland, Tysnes, & Larsen, 2011), and it correlates with hippocampal atrophy (Beyer et al., 2012) and microstructural alterations in both hippocampi as measured by diffusor-tensor imaging (Carlesimo et al., 2012). The clinical significance of PD-MCI is highlighted by findings that PD-MCI is associated with shorter time to PDD (C. C. Janvin, Aarsland, & Larsen, 2005). There is some evidence that patients with different cognitive profiles differ in dementia risk, that is, that those with attention and executive deficits, usually due to fronto-subcortical dopaminergic lesions, may have a lower dementia risk than those with visuoconstructive and semantic memory impairment, which is more associated with posterior and possibly nondopaminergic lesions (Williams-Gray, Evans, et al., 2009; Williams-Gray, Foltynie, Brayne, Robbins, & Barker, 2007). One interpretation of these findings is that frontal-type deficits are more related to dopaminergic lesions causing mild cognitive deficits, whereas the more posteriorly based cognitive deficits may be associated with structural pathologies such as temporoparietal Lewy bodies and plaque pathology leading to more rapid decline and dementia and early cognitive changes in PD.

The cognitive deficits broaden with advancing PD, and in PDD there is typically a mixture of a frontal-subcortical profile (attentional and executive dysfunction), and cortical cognitive impairment (memory, visuoconstruction, and language deficits) (C. Janvin et al., 2004; Pagonabarraga et al., 2008). Thus, in PDD, most cognitive domains are impaired. Important from a diagnostic perspective, patients may complain of "memory problems" initially, although detailed testing show the typical attention and executive deficits.

BIOMARKERS PREDICTING COGNITIVE DECLINE

Biomarkers to detect and quantitatively predict cognitive impairment and dementia in PD have not yet been made available in clinical settings. However, markers of brain atrophy on MRI and of amyloid abnormalities in CSF have been associated with cognitive impairment in PD, and, recently, several longitudinal studies have suggested that biomarkers like quantitative EEG, CSF amyloid β 1-42, and plasma epidermal growth factor can indeed predict future cognitive decline (Chen-Plotkin et al., 2011; Klassen et al., 2011; Siderowf et al., 2010). A complicating factor, however, is the heterogeneous brain pathology in PD and the considerable overlap between neuropathological changes and clinical presentation in PD and other dementias, especially AD.

Structural Imaging

Atrophy of the parietotemporal lobe, entorinal cortex, hippocampus, prefrontal cortex, and posterior cingulate cortex demonstrated on MRI are associated with dementia in Parkinson's disease (Burton, McKeith, Burn, Williams, & JT, 2004; Kenny, Burton, & O'Brien, 2008; Lyoo et al., 2010; Song et al., 2011; Weintraub et al., 2011). In PD-MCI, similar changes of a lesser degree have been identified (Beyer, Janvin, Larsen, & Aarsland, 2007). Atrophy of the hippocampus and parietal-temporal cortex was found to be related to cognitive performance in PD and these changes prospectively predicted a global cognitive decline in nondemented patients over a 2-year follow-up period (Weintraub et al., 2012). Recently, studies using diffusion tensor imaging (DTI) suggest that white matter integrity can more sensitively detect brain changes underlying early cognitive decline than volumetric MRI (Hattori et al., 2012).

Functional Imaging

Fluorodeoxyglucose-positron emission tomography (FDG-PET) PET has shown reduced glucose metabolism in both frontal and parietal cortex, which is associated with cognitive decline in PD-MCI (Huang et al., 2008). Hypometabolism in temporal cortices has been associated with verbal memory, whereas hypometabolism in frontal cortex is associated with executive changes and parietal hypometabolism is associated with visuospatial deficits (Jokinen et al., 2010). A recent longitudinal study suggested that early metabolic changes in visual association and posterior cingulate cortices could predict incident dementia in PD (Bohnen et al., 2011). Cross-sectional studies using SPECT have reported hypoperfusion in lateral parietal and frontal cortex in PD patients without dementia, which correlated with cognitive impairment (Firbank, Colloby, Burn, McKeith, & O'Brien, 2003). Bilateral hypoperfusion in posterior parietal lobes and in the right occipital lobe were seen in PD-MCI, which differed from the pattern seen in non-PD-MCI (Nobili et al., 2009). Few studies have used functional MRI (fMRI) to study brain responses underlying cognitive functioning. This was recently done during a verbal working-memory task. Compared with controls, denovo PD patients had under-recruitment in an extensive brain network including bilateral striatal and frontal regions. Within the PD-group, patients with MCI had additional under-recruitment in the right dorsal caudate nucleus and the bilateral anterior cingulate cortex compared with those without MCI (Ekman et al., 2012). Another fMRI study identified progressive changes in networks involved in recognition memory in early PD (Segura et al., 2012). In addition, PET can be used to identify neurotransmitter correlates of cognitive impairment in PD. Several studies have demonstrated reduced cholinergic activity. Such changes are heterogeneous, but cortical cholinergic deficits correlate with cognition, whereas thalamic cholinergic deficits seem to be associated with more frequent falls (Bohnen et al., 2012). For amyloid imaging, please see the following section.

Cerebrospinal Fluid

Low CSF concentrations of aβ42 have been found to be indicative of incident Alzheimer's disease, and have also been found to be reduced in early PD and to correlate with memory impairment (Alves et al., 2010). Recently this finding was confirmed in a longitudinal study showing that low CSF levels of aβ42 predicted significant cognitive decline during the next two years (Siderowf et al., 2010). A recent study showed an association between low aβ42 an postural instability and gait instability (PIGD) symptoms (Alves et al., 2013), consistent with the association of postural and gait disturbance and more rapid cognitive decline (Alves et al., 2006). Amyloid imaging using Pittsburg compound B (PIB) usually finds low amyloid load in PDD compared to AD and DLB (Jokinen et al., 2010) and increased PIB binding was found in only 15% of PD patients at risk for dementia (Petrou et al., 2012). Despite this, amyloid binding was significantly associated with cognitive impairment. These observations suggest that amyloid pathology contributes to cognitive impairment in PD.

Much interest has recently focused on measuring alpha-synuclein species in CSF. Patients with PD have shown reduced CSF α-synuclein levels compared to patients with AD and controls (Mollenhauer et al., 2011). Correlations between cognitive status and lower CSF α-synuclein have been reported in DLB, but, up to now, not in PD (Ballard et al., 2010). Alpha-synuclein oligomers or phospho-alpha-synuclein (129p) in CSF have also been reported to be higher in patients with PD compared to patients with AD or controls (Tokuda et al., 2010). An important future research area is to further explore the association between potentially neurotoxic alpha-synuclein species and cognitive decline in PD.

TREATMENT

Cholinesterase Inhibitors

There is good evidence linking cognitive changes in PD to disease-related disturbances of dopaminergic, cholinergic, and possibly noradrenergic and glutamatergic activity (Klein et al., 2010) and thus transmitter-based treatments might be expected to improve cognition in PD. In 2011 the Movement Disorders Society commissioned an evidence-based review of treatment of cognitive and other nonmotor symptoms (Seppi et al., 2011). In this review, it was concluded that there was good evidence that rivastigmine is of clinical use for PDD, but that other antidementia drugs, that is, donepezil, galantamine and the NMDA-receptor antagonist memantine were of investigational use. In 2012, a Cochrane analysis concluded that there is good evidence for the use of cholinesterase inhibitors in patients with PDD, with a positive impact on global clinical functioning, cognition, neuropsychiatric symptoms and activities of daily living rating scales (Rolinski, Fox, Maidment, & McShane, 2012). The pivotal study was a large, 24-week randomized, placebo controlled trial, the EXPRESS trial (Emre et al., 2004), demonstrating significant improvement by rivastigmine of both primary outcomes (global cognition and clinical impression) and all secondary outcomes (including attention, executive functions, neuropsychiatric symptoms), and activities of daily living. An open-label extension phase suggested that rivastigmine may provide sustained benefits for up to 48 weeks (Poewe et al., 2006). A detailed analysis of the motor effects in the EXPRESS study indicates that although first exposure of rivastigmine can cause transient increase in tremor, there is no worsening of PD over 48 weeks (Oertel et al., 2008). There are major individual differences in the response, that is, some patients experienced marked (4.3%) or moderate (15.5%) improvements on rivastigmine (compared to 2.4% and 12.1% in the placebo group), whereas others worsened. Cholinergic side effects are relatively common, in particular gastro-intestinal effects such as nausea, which occurred in 29% of the rivastigmine group compared to 11% in the placebo group. These symptoms were usually mild and transient, and the proportion with serious side effects did not differ between the group: 13% in the rivastigmine and 14.5% in the placebo group. Still, side effects lead to 45% not reaching the target dose level of 9 or 12 mg per day. Worsening of parkinsonism was reported more commonly in the rivastigmine (27%) compared to the placebo (16%) group, but only 1.7% of the rivastigmine group withdrew from the study due to worsening of parkinsonism, and there was no worsening of motor symptoms as measured by a standardized motor scale. In AD, the use of a rivastigmine patch, which leads to a more stable serum-concentration of the drug, is associated with fewer side effects and thus a higher dose can be achieved (Cummings et al., 2012). A placebo-controlled study with rivastigmine capsules in DLB also reported improvement of neuropsychiatric symptoms and cognitive tests (McKeith et al., 2000), supporting the concept that rivastigmine is useful in Lewy-body dementias. As a result, the use of rivastigmine is approved for PDD in the United States and the EU.

Currently there are no established clinical or biological markers that can predict which patients will improve with cholinesterase inhibitors, but there is some evidence that those with visual hallucinations (Burn et al., 2006) and hyperhomocysteinemia (Barone et al., 2008) respond particularly well. The response of attention (Wesnes, McKeith, Edgar, Emre, & Lane, 2005) and executive functioning (Schmitt et al., 2010) indicate a beneficial effect on frontal subcortical circuits, which has been supported in two small studies showing increased brain perfusion using SPECT (Ceravolo et al., 2006) and increased alpha-activity on quantitative EEG (Fogelson et al., 2003) in frontal regions during successful treatment with rivastigmine.

The evidence is less robust for the other cholinesterase inhibitors, although several small placebo-controlled studies have reported significant benefits of donepezil. However, in the only large trial, the EDON study, 550 patients were randomized to placebo or to a daily dose of 5 or 10 mg of donepezil, once daily (Dubois et al., 2012). Only one of the two primary efficacy measures, the clinical global impression, differed significantly between active and placebo groups, although the difference was small (3.9 versus 3.7), compared to 4.3 and 3.8 in the rivastigmine trial. The Alzheimer's Disease Assessment Scale–cognitive subscale (ADAS-COG) measures cognitive changes in AD and was specifically designed for drug trials. ADAS-COG scores did not differ significantly according to the preplanned analyses, but became significant when the treatment-by-country interaction was removed. The effect size on ADAS-COG for 10mg donepezil versus placebo was 0.49, by convention a moderate effect and similar to the difference reported in the EXPRESS study. The proportion reporting adverse events did not differ between the three groups, but the incidence of nausea was higher in the 10 mg (21%) and 5 mg (17%) compared to placebo (7%) group. In summary, the findings in the EDON study, although somewhat less convincing than those in the EXPRESS study, support the usefulness of cholinesterase inhibitors for PDD.

Memantine

Three placebo-controlled trials of the effects of the partial NMDA-receptor antagonist memantine on cognition in PDD (Aarsland, Ballard, et al., 2009; Emre et al., 2010; Leroi, Overshott, Byrne, Daniel, & Burns, 2009) and one in PD (Ondo et al., 2011) have been reported (Table 9-4). The results are somewhat inconsistent, although some significant benefits were reported in all studies, and memantine was well tolerated. Only one study showed significant effect on the predefined primary outcome, clinical global impression of change (Aarsland, Ballard, et al., 2009), as well as on global cognition, quality of life (Larsson et al., 2011), and sleep disturbances (Larsson, Aarsland, Ballard, Minthon, & Londos,

Table 9-4 Placebo-controlled treatment studies* of PD cognitive impairment

Study	*Inclusion criteria*	*Drug*	*N*	*Primary outcome*	*Result*	*Comment*
EXPRESS (Emre, 2004)	PDD, MMSE 10-24	Rivastigmine	541	CGIC, ADAS-COG	Effect on both	Effect on all secondary outcomes as well
EDON (Dubois, 2012)	PDD, MMSE 10-26	Donepezil	550	CGIC, ADAS-COG	Effect on ADAS-Cog	Effect on ADAS-COG became significant when the treatment-by-country interaction was removed
Aarsland et al., 2009	PDD and DLB; ChEI allowed, MMSE > 12	Memantine	72	CGIC	Significant	In subgroup analysis significant effect was found in PDD only
Emre, 2010	PDD and DLB; ChEIs not allowed, MMSE 10-24	memantine	199	No predefined primary outcome	No significant effect	Significant effect reported on selected outcomes in DLB, but not in PDD
Ondo, 2011	PD, MMSE > 23	memantine	40[1]	No predefined primary outcome	No significant results found	Scales of fatigue, attention, sedation, depression, and quality of life
Weintraub et al., 2010	Depressed PD, MMSE > 14	Atomoxetine	55[1]	Depression scale	Positive effect on MMSE	Cognition was a secondary outcome measure
Hanagasi, 2011	PD without dementia	Rasagiline	55[2]	Neuropsychological tests	Effect on executive tests	Selected effects on some of many tests performed

*With $n > 50$.

PD = Parkinson's disease; PDD = dementia associated with Parkinson's disease; DLB = Dementia with Lewy-bodies; MME = Mini-Mental State Examination; CGIC = Clinical Global Impression of Change; ADAS-COG = Alzheimer's Disease Assessment Scale, cognitive scale.

Duration was 24 weeks in most; [1] 8 weeks; [2] 12 weeks.

2010). Two studies included both DLB and PDD, although they were not powered to assess efficacy in PDD and DLB separately. In one study, a significant improvement was found only in PDD (Aarsland, Ballard, et al., 2009), whereas significant effect was found only in DLB in the other trial (Emre et al., 2010). Another difference is that cholinesterase inhibitors were allowed in one (Aarsland, Ballard, et al., 2009) but not the other (Emre et al., 2010) study.

Table 9-4 summarizes the four largest antidementia agent trials in PD. In one study, including 40 nondemented PD patients, without a predefined primary outcome, no significant differences were found on scales of fatigue, attention, sedation, depression, and overall quality of life between memantine and placebo (Ondo et al., 2011).

Other Agents

In addition to acetylcholine and glutamate, several other neurotransmitters are probably involved in various aspects of the pathophysiology underlying MCI and dementia. Noradrenaline is likely involved in attention modulation (Kehagia, Barker, & Robbins, 2010). Indeed, in a study of atomoxetine, a noradrenergic reuptake inhibitor, there were indications of improved cognitive functioning as a secondary outcome measure in nondemented PD patients with depression (Weintraub, Mavandadi, et al., 2010).

Anti-Parkinson Treatments and Cognition

Dopaminergic depletion is associated with fronto-executive deficits, and treatment with dopaminergic treatments used to treat the motor symptoms of the disease may thus improve some aspects of cognitive functioning. Cognitive functions such as flexibility and working memory may improve, whereas other functions, such as attentional set shifting, associative learning, and verbal, pattern, and spatial-recognition memories, remain unaffected (Cooper et al., 1992; Kehagia et al., 2010). The effect depends on the dopamine level in the structure involved in the task (Kehagia et al., 2010), and on the metabolic activity in a specific network associated with cognitive dysfunction in PD (Mattis, Tang, Ma, Dhawan, & Eidelberg, 2011). A clinically significant effect of L-dopa on cognition is usually not seen. However, the monoamine oxidase type-B inhibitor, rasagiline, was found to have some beneficial effects on aspects of attention and executive functions in patients with PD without dementia (Hanagasi et al., 2011). At higher concentrations, L-dopa as well as D2 receptor agonists may cause cognitive deterioration with deficits in reversal learning, decision making, and impulse control (Kehagia et al., 2010). Among the D2 receptor agonists, there is some evidence that pramipexole, a D2/D3 agonist, has more harmful effects than pergolide, a D1/D2 agonist (Kehagia et al., 2010).

With regards to nondopaminergic antiparkinsonian treatments, it has been found that amantadine may delay the onset of dementia in PD, but can also induce severe confusion and hallucinations (Inzelberg et al., 2006). It is well-known that the use of antimuscarinic compounds in PD is limited by their liability to cause cognitive impairments, including executive dysfunctions and memory encoding (Bedard et al., 1999; Cooper et al., 1992; Kehagia et al., 2010).

Subthalamic deep brain stimulation (DBS) is frequently used for medication-resistant motor complications in PD. A meta-analysis of 28 cohort studies on cognitive performance after subthalamic DBS revealed moderate declines in semantic and verbal fluency and smaller, but significant, decreases in executive functions and verbal learning and memory (Parsons, Rogers, Braaten, Woods, & Troster, 2006). The authors concluded that subthalamic DBS in PD patients appears relatively safe from a cognitive standpoint. However, subsequent studies have shown that PD patients with a borderline global cognitive impairment have less benefit on quality of life scores after subthalamic DBS than PD patients with high cognitive performance. It has also been reported that subthalamic DBS is associated with a more rapid decline of executive functions (Daniels et al., 2010).

Cognitive Training

Cognitive intervention programs have been shown to be useful in AD and MCI (Jean et al., 2010), and might be particularly relevant in PD due to the enhanced dopamine release demonstrated after cognitive training (Backman et al., 2011). After some positive preliminary reports, the first randomized controlled study recently suggested that intensive cognitive training leads to improvement in a range of cognitive tasks immediately after the training procedure compared to the control group (Paris et al., 2011). Whether such positive effects can be maintained over time remains to be demonstrated.

CONCLUSIONS

Cognitive impairment is a common and important aspect of PD. The majority of patients who survive more than 10 years will eventually develop dementia, with key functional consequences. In addition, mild cognitive changes can be found already at time of diagnosis, and frequently progress to dementia. Consensus clinical diagnostic criteria exist for dementia and MCI in PD. Emerging biomarkers such as imaging and CSF analyses may help in predicting which patients are at highest risk for early and rapid cognitive decline. Dementia can be treated with rivastigmine, but there are yet no treatment options for MCI in PD, and there are yet no disease-modifying agents that can prevent or reduce the progression from normal cognition to MCI and dementia.

REFERENCES

Aarsland, D., Andersen, K., Larsen, J. P., Lolk, A., & Kragh-Sorensen, P. (2003). Prevalence and characteristics of dementia in Parkinson disease: an 8-year prospective study. *Archives of Neurology, 60*(3), 387–392.

Aarsland, D., Andersen, K., Larsen, J. P., Perry, R., Wentzel-Larsen, T., Lolk, A., & Kragh-Sorensen, P. (2004). The rate of cognitive decline in Parkinson disease. *Archives of Neurology, 61*(12), 1906–1911.

Aarsland, D., Ballard, C., Walker, Z., Bostrom, F., Alves, G., Kossakowski, K.,... Londos, E. (2009). Memantine in patients with Parkinson's disease dementia or dementia with Lewy bodies: a double-blind, placebo-controlled, multicentre trial. *Lancet Neurology, 8*(7), 613–618.

Aarsland, D., Bronnick, K., Ehrt, U., De Deyn, P. P., Tekin, S., Emre, M., & Cummings, J. L. (2007). Neuropsychiatric symptoms in patients with Parkinson's disease and dementia: frequency, profile and associated care giver stress. *Journal of Neurology, Neurosurgery and Psychiatry, 78*(1), 36–42.

Aarsland, D., Bronnick, K., Larsen, J. P., Tysnes, O. B., & Alves, G. (2009). Cognitive impairment in incident, untreated Parkinson disease: The Norwegian ParkWest study. *Neurology, 72*(13), 1121–1126.

Aarsland, D., Bronnick, K., Williams-Gray, C., Weintraub, D., Marder, K., Kulisevsky, J.,... Emre, M. (2010). Mild cognitive impairment in Parkinson disease: a multicenter pooled analysis. *Neurology, 75*(12), 1062–1069. doi: 10.1212/WNL.0b013e3181f39d0e

Aarsland, D., Muniz, G., & Matthews, F. (2011). Nonlinear decline of mini-mental state examination in Parkinson's disease. *Movement Disorders, 26*(2), 334–337. doi: 10.1002/mds.23416

Aarsland, D., Perry, R., Brown, A., Larsen, J. P., & Ballard, C. (2005). Neuropathology of dementia in Parkinson's disease: a prospective, community-based study. *Annals of Neurology, 58*(5), 773–776. doi: 10.1002/ana.20635

Aarsland, D., Zaccai, J., & Brayne, C. (2005). A systematic review of prevalence studies of dementia in Parkinson's disease. *Movement Disorders, 20*(10), 1255–1263.

Alcalay, R. N., Mejia-Santana, H., Tang, M. X., Rakitin, B., Rosado, L., Ross, B.,... Caccappolo, E. (2010). Self-report of cognitive impairment and mini-mental state examination performance in PRKN, LRRK2, and GBA carriers with early onset Parkinson's disease. *Journal of Clinical & Experimental Neuropsychology, 32*(7), 775–779. doi: 10.1080/13803390903521018

Allan, L. M., Ballard, C. G., Allen, J., Murray, A., Davidson, A. W., McKeith, I. G., & Kenny, R. A. (2007). Autonomic dysfunction in dementia. *Journal of Neurology, Neurosurgery and Psychiatry, 78*(7), 671–677. doi: 10.1136/jnnp.2006.102343

Alves, G., Bronnick, K., Aarsland, D., Blennow, K., Zetterberg, H., Ballard, C.,... Mulugeta, E. (2010). CSF amyloid-beta and tau proteins, and cognitive performance, in early and untreated Parkinson's disease: the Norwegian ParkWest study. *Journal of Neurology, Neurosurgery and Psychiatry, 81*(10), 1080–1086. doi: 10.1136/jnnp.2009.199950

Alves, G., Larsen, J. P., Emre, M., Wentzel-Larsen, T., & Aarsland, D. (2006). Changes in motor subtype and risk for incident dementia in Parkinson's disease. *Movement Disorders 21*(8), 1123–1130.

Alves, G., Pedersen, K. F., Bloem, B. R., Blennow, K., Zetterberg, H., Borm, G. F.,... Andreasson, U. (2013). Cerebrospinal fluid amyloid-β and phenotypic heterogeneity in de novo Parkinson's disease. *Journal of Neurology, Neurosurgery & Psychiatry, 84*(5), 537–543.

Armstrong, M. J., Litvan, I., Lang, A. E., Bak, T. H., Bhatia, K. P., Borroni, B.,... Weiner, W. J. (2013). Criteria for the diagnosis of corticobasal degeneration. *Neurology, 80*(5), 496–503. doi: 10.1212/WNL.0b013e31827f0fd1

Baba, T., Kikuchi, A., Hirayama, K., Nishio, Y., Hosokai, Y., Kanno, S.,... Takeda, A. (2012). Severe olfactory dysfunction is a prodromal symptom of dementia associated with Parkinson's disease: a 3 year longitudinal study. *Brain, 135*(Pt 1), 161–169. doi: 10.1093/brain/awr321

Backman, L., Karlsson, S., Fischer, H., Karlsson, P., Brehmer, Y., Rieckmann, A.,... Nyberg, L. (2011). Dopamine D(1) receptors and age differences in brain activation during working memory. *Neurobiology & Aging, 32*(10), 1849–1856. doi: 10.1016/j.neurobiolaging.2009.10.018

Ballard, C., Jones, E. L., Londos, E., Minthon, L., Francis, P., & Aarsland, D. (2010). alpha-Synuclein antibodies recognize a protein present at lower levels in the CSF of patients with dementia with Lewy bodies. *International Psychogeriatrics, 22*(2), 321–327. doi: 10.1017/S1041610209991049

Barone, P., Aarsland, D., Burn, D., Emre, M., Kulisevsky, J., & Weintraub, D. (2011). Cognitive impairment in nondemented Parkinson's disease. *Movement Disorders, 26*(14), 2483–2495. doi: 10.1002/mds.23919

Barone, P., Burn, D. J., van Laar, T., Hsu, C., Poewe, W., & Lane, R. M. (2008). Rivastigmine versus placebo in hyperhomocysteinemic Parkinson's disease dementia patients. *Movement Disorders, 23*(11), 1532–1540. doi: 10.1002/mds.21997

Beach, T. G., Adler, C. H., Lue, L., Sue, L. I., Bachalakuri, J., Henry-Watson, J.,... Walker, D. G. (2009). Unified staging system for Lewy body disorders: correlation with nigrostriatal degeneration, cognitive impairment and motor dysfunction. *Acta Neuropathologica, 117*(6), 613–634. doi: 10.1007/s00401-009-0538-8

Bedard, M. A., Pillon, B., Dubois, B., Duchesne, N., Masson, H., & Agid, Y. (1999). Acute and long-term administration of anticholinergics in Parkinson's disease: specific effects on the subcortico-frontal syndrome. *Brain & Cognition, 40*(2), 289–313.

Beyer, M. K., Bronnick, K. S., Hwang, K. S., Bergsland, N., Tysnes, O. B., Larsen, J. P.,... Apostolova, L. G. (2012). Verbal memory is associated with structural hippocampal changes in newly diagnosed Parkinson's disease. *Journal of Neurology, Neurosurgery and Psychiatry, 84*(1), 23–28. doi: 10.1136/jnnp-2012-303054

Beyer, M. K., Janvin, C. C., Larsen, J. P., & Aarsland, D. (2007). A magnetic resonance imaging study of patients with Parkinson's disease with mild cognitive impairment and dementia using voxel-based morphometry. *Journal of Neurology, Neurosurgery and Psychiatry, 78*(3), 254–259.

Bohnen, N. I., Koeppe, R. A., Minoshima, S., Giordani, B., Albin, R. L., Frey, K. A., & Kuhl, D. E. (2011). Cerebral glucose metabolic features of Parkinson disease and incident dementia: longitudinal study. *Journal of Nuclear Medicine, 52*(6), 848–855. doi: 10.2967/jnumed.111.089946

Bohnen, N. I., Muller, M. L., Kotagal, V., Koeppe, R. A., Kilbourn, M. R., Gilman, S.,... Frey, K. A. (2012). Heterogeneity of cholinergic denervation in Parkinson's disease without dementia. *J Cereb Blood Flow Metab, 32*(8), 1609–1617. doi: 10.1038/jcbfm.2012.60

Boot, B. P., Boeve, B. F., Roberts, R. O., Ferman, T. J., Geda, Y. E., Pankratz, V. S.,... Petersen, R. C. (2012). Probable rapid eye movement sleep behavior disorder increases risk for mild cognitive impairment and Parkinson disease: a population-based study. *Annals of Neurology, 71*(1), 49–56. doi: 10.1002/ana.22655

Braak, H., Del Tredici, K., Rub, U., de Vos, R. A., Jansen Steur, E. N., & Braak, E. (2003). Staging of brain pathology related to sporadic Parkinson's disease. *Neurobiology & Aging, 24*(2), 197–211.

Bronnick, K., Alves, G., Aarsland, D., Tysnes, O. B., & Larsen, J. P. (2011). Verbal memory in drug-naive, newly diagnosed Parkinson's disease. The retrieval deficit hypothesis revisited. *Neuropsychology, 25*(1), 114–124. doi: 10.1037/a0020857

Burn, D., Emre, M., McKeith, I., De Deyn, P. P., Aarsland, D., Hsu, C., & Lane, R. (2006). Effects of rivastigmine in patients with and without visual hallucinations in dementia associated with Parkinson's disease. *Movement Disorders, 21*(11), 1899–1907.

Burton, E. J., McKeith, I. G., Burn, D. J., Williams, E. D., & JT, O. Brien. (2004). Cerebral atrophy in Parkinson's disease with and without dementia: a comparison with Alzheimer's disease, dementia with Lewy bodies and controls. *Brain, 127*(Pt 4), 791–800.

Buter, T. C., van den Hout, A., Matthews, F. E., Larsen, J. P., Brayne, C., & Aarsland, D. (2008). Dementia and survival in Parkinson disease: A 12-year population study. *Neurology, 70*(13), 1017–1022. doi: 70/13/1017 [pii] 10.1212/01.wnl.0000306632.43729.24

Carlesimo, G. A., Piras, F., Assogna, F., Pontieri, F. E., Caltagirone, C., & Spalletta, G. (2012). Hippocampal abnormalities and memory deficits in Parkinson disease: a multimodal imaging study. *Neurology, 78*(24), 1939–1945. doi: 10.1212/WNL.0b013e318259e1c5

Ceravolo, R., Volterrani, D., Frosini, D., Bernardini, S., Rossi, C., Logi, C., ... Bonuccelli, U. (2006). Brain perfusion effects of cholinesterase inhibitors in Parkinson's disease with dementia. *Journal of Neural Transmission, 113*(11), 1787–1790. doi: 10.1007/s00702-006-0478-6

Chartier-Harlin, M. C., Kachergus, J., Roumier, C., Mouroux, V., Douay, X., Lincoln, S., ... Destee, A. (2004). Alpha-synuclein locus duplication as a cause of familial Parkinson's disease. *Lancet, 364*(9440), 1167–1169.

Chen-Plotkin, A. S., Hu, W. T., Siderowf, A., Weintraub, D., Goldmann Gross, R., Hurtig, H. I., ... Trojanowski, J. Q. (2011). Plasma epidermal growth factor levels predict cognitive decline in Parkinson disease. *Annals of Neurology, 69*(4), 655–663. doi: 10.1002/ana.22271

Claassen, D. O., Josephs, K. A., Ahlskog, J. E., Silber, M. H., Tippmann-Peikert, M., & Boeve, B. F. (2010). REM sleep behavior disorder preceding other aspects of synucleinopathies by up to half a century. *Neurology, 75*(6), 494–499. doi: 10.1212/WNL.0b013e3181ec7fac

Compta, Y., Parkkinen, L., O'Sullivan, S. S., Vandrovcova, J., Holton, J. L., Collins, C., ... Revesz, T. (2011). Lewy- and Alzheimer-type pathologies in Parkinson's disease dementia: which is more important? *Brain, 134*(Pt 5), 1493–1505. doi: 10.1093/brain/awr031

Contrafatto, D., Mostile, G., Nicoletti, A., Dibilio, V., Raciti, L., Lanzafame, S., ... Zappia, M. (2011). [(123) I]FP-CIT-SPECT asymmetry index to differentiate Parkinson's disease from vascular parkinsonism. *Acta Neurologica Scandinavica, 126*(1), 12–16. doi: 10.1111/j.1600-0404.2011.01583.x

Cooper, J. A., Sagar, H. J., Doherty, S. M., Jordan, N., Tidswell, P., & Sullivan, E. V. (1992). Different effects of dopaminergic and anticholinergic therapies on cognitive and motor function in Parkinson's disease. A follow-up study of untreated patients. *Brain, 115* (Pt 6), 1701–1725.

Cummings, J., Froelich, L., Black, S. E., Bakchine, S., Bellelli, G., Molinuevo, J. L., ... Strohmaier, C. (2012). Randomized, double-blind, parallel-group, 48-week study for efficacy and safety of a higher-dose rivastigmine patch (15 vs. 10 cm(2))

in Alzheimer's disease. *Dementia and Geriatric Cognitive Disorders, 33*(5), 341–353. doi: 10.1159/000340056

Daniels, C., Krack, P., Volkmann, J., Pinsker, M. O., Krause, M., Tronnier, V.,... Witt, K. (2010). Risk factors for executive dysfunction after subthalamic nucleus stimulation in Parkinson's disease. *Movement Disorders, 25*(11), 1583–1589. doi: 10.1002/mds.23078

Danzer, K. M., Krebs, S. K., Wolff, M., Birk, G., & Hengerer, B. (2009). Seeding induced by alpha-synuclein oligomers provides evidence for spreading of alpha-synuclein pathology. *Journal of Neurochemistry, 111*(1), 192–203.

Dubois, B., Burn, D., Goetz, C., Aarsland, D., Brown, R. G., Broe, G. A.,... Emre, M. (2007). Diagnostic procedures for Parkinson's disease dementia: recommendations from the movement disorder society task force. *Movement Disorders, 22*(16), 2314–2324.

Dubois, B., Tolosa, E., Katzenschlager, R., Emre, M., Lees, A. J., Schumann, G.,... Moline, M. L. (2012). Donepezil in Parkinson's disease dementia: a randomized, double-blind efficacy and safety study. *Movement Disorders, 27*(10), 1230–1238. doi: 10.1002/mds.25098

Ekman, U., Eriksson, J., Forsgren, L., Mo, S. J., Riklund, K., & Nyberg, L. (2012). Functional brain activity and presynaptic dopamine uptake in patients with Parkinson's disease and mild cognitive impairment: A cross-sectional study. *Lancet Neurology, 11*(8), 679–687. doi: 10.1016/S1474-4422(12)70138-2

Emre, M., Aarsland, D., Albanese, A., Byrne, E. J., Deuschl, G., De Deyn, P. P.,... Lane, R. (2004). Rivastigmine for dementia associated with Parkinson's disease. *New England Journal of Medicine, 351*(24), 2509–2518.

Emre, M., Aarsland, D., Brown, R., Burn, D. J., Duyckaerts, C., Mizuno, Y.,... Dubois, B. (2007a). Clinical diagnostic criteria for dementia associated with Parkinson's disease. *Movement Disorders, 22*(12), 1689–1707; quiz 1837. doi: 10.1002/mds.21507

Emre, M., Tsolaki, M., Bonuccelli, U., Destee, A., Tolosa, E., Kutzelnigg, A.,... Jones, R. (2010). Memantine for patients with Parkinson's disease dementia or dementia with Lewy bodies: a randomised, double-blind, placebo-controlled trial. *Lancet Neurology, 9*(10), 969–977. doi: 10.1016/S1474-4422(10)70194-0

Evans, J. R., Mason, S. L., Williams-Gray, C. H., Foltynie, T., Brayne, C., Robbins, T. W., & Barker, R. A. (2011). The natural history of treated Parkinson's disease in an incident, community based cohort. *Journal of Neurology, Neurosurgery and Psychiatry, 82*(10), 1112–1118. doi: 10.1136/jnnp.2011.240366

Firbank, M. J., Colloby, S. J., Burn, D. J., McKeith, I. G., & O'Brien, J. T. (2003). Regional cerebral blood flow in Parkinson's disease with and without dementia. *Neuroimage, 20*(2), 1309–1319.

Fogelson, N., Kogan, E., Korczyn, A. D., Giladi, N., Shabtai, H., & Neufeld, M. Y. (2003). Effects of rivastigmine on the quantitative EEG in demented Parkinsonian patients. *Acta Neurologica Scandinavica, 107*(4), 252–255.

Halliday, G., Hely, M., Reid, W., & Morris, J. (2008). The progression of pathology in longitudinally followed patients with Parkinson's disease. *Acta Neuropathologica, 115*(4), 409–415. doi: 10.1007/s00401-008-0344-8

Halliday, G. M., & McCann, H. (2010). The progression of pathology in Parkinson's disease. *Annals of the New York Academy of Science, 1184*, 188–195. doi: NYAS5118 [pii] 10.1111/j.1749-6632.2009.05118.x

Hanagasi, H. A., Gurvit, H., Unsalan, P., Horozoglu, H., Tuncer, N., Feyzioglu, A.,... Emre, M. (2011). The effects of rasagiline on cognitive deficits in Parkinson's disease patients without dementia: a randomized, double-blind, placebo-controlled, multicenter study. *Movement Disorders, 26*(10), 1851–1858. doi: 10.1002/mds.23738

Hardy, J. (2010). Genetic analysis of pathways to Parkinson disease. *Neuron, 68*(2), 201–206. doi: 10.1016/j.neuron.2010.10.014

Hattori, T., Orimo, S., Aoki, S., Ito, K., Abe, O., Amano, A.,... Mizusawa, H. (2012). Cognitive status correlates with white matter alteration in Parkinson's disease. *Human Brain Mapping, 33*(3), 727–739. doi: 10.1002/hbm.21245

Hely, M. A., Reid, W. G., Adena, M. A., Halliday, G. M., & Morris, J. G. (2008). The Sydney multicenter study of Parkinson's disease: the inevitability of dementia at 20 years. *Movement Disorders, 23*(6), 837–844. doi: 10.1002/mds.21956

Huang, C., Mattis, P., Perrine, K., Brown, N., Dhawan, V., & Eidelberg, D. (2008). Metabolic abnormalities associated with mild cognitive impairment in Parkinson disease. *Neurology, 70*(16 Pt 2), 1470–1477. doi: 10.1212/01.wnl.0000304050.05332.9c

Hughes, A. J., Daniel, S. E., Blankson, S., & Lees, A. J. (1993). A clinicopathologic study of 100 cases of Parkinson's disease. *Archives of Neurology, 50*(2), 140–148.

Inzelberg, R., Bonuccelli, U., Schechtman, E., Miniowich, A., Strugatsky, R., Ceravolo, R.,... Rabey, J. M. (2006). Association between amantadine and the onset of dementia in Parkinson's disease. *Movement Disorders, 21*(9), 1375–1379. doi: 10.1002/mds.20968

Irwin, D. J., White, M. T., Toledo, J. B., Xie, S. X., Robinson, J. L., Van Deerlin, V.,... Trojanowski, J. Q. (2012). Neuropathologic substrates of Parkinson disease dementia. *Annals of Neurology, 72*(4), 587–598. doi: 10.1002/ana.23659

Janvin, C. C., Aarsland, D., & Larsen, J. P. (2005). Cognitive predictors of dementia in Parkinson's disease: a community-based, 4-year longitudinal study. *Journal of Geriatric Psychiatry and Neurology, 18*(3), 149–154.

Janvin, C., Larsen, J.P., Salmon, D., Galasko, D., Hugdahl, K., & Aarsland, D. (2004, Oct 24-27). *Cognitive profiles of individual patients with Parkinson's disease and dementia: comparison with dementia with Lewy bodies and Alzheimer's disease.* Paper presented at the Mental dysfunctions in Parkinson's disease, Salzburg, Austria.

Jauregui-Barrutia, A., Tijero-Merino, B., Gomez-Esteban, J. C., & Zarranz, J. J. (2010). [Sleep disorders in Parkinson's disease: REM sleep behaviour disorder and restless legs syndrome]. *Review of Neurology, 50*(Suppl 2), S15–19. doi: rn2010054 [pii]

Jean, L., Simard, M., Wiederkehr, S., Bergeron, M. E., Turgeon, Y., Hudon, C.,... van Reekum, R. (2010). Efficacy of a cognitive training programme for mild cognitive impairment: Results of a randomised controlled study. *Neuropsychology Rehabilitation, 20*(3), 377–405. doi: 10.1080/09602010903343012

Johnson, D. K., & Galvin, J. E. (2011). Longitudinal changes in cognition in Parkinson's disease with and without dementia. *Dementia & Geriatric Cognitive Disorders, 31*(2), 98–108. doi: 10.1159/000323570

Jokinen, P., Scheinin, N., Aalto, S., Nagren, K., Savisto, N., Parkkola, R.,... Rinne, J. O. (2010). [(11)C]PIB-, [(18)F]FDG-PET and MRI imaging in patients with Parkinson's disease with and without dementia. *Parkinsonism Related Disorders, 16*(10), 666–670. doi: 10.1016/j.parkreldis.2010.08.021

Kehagia, A. A., Barker, R. A., & Robbins, T. W. (2010). Neuropsychological and clinical heterogeneity of cognitive impairment and dementia in patients with Parkinson's disease. *Lancet Neurology, 9*(12), 1200–1213. doi: 10.1016/S1474-4422(10)70212-X

Kempster, P. A., O'Sullivan, S. S., Holton, J. L., Revesz, T., & Lees, A. J. (2010). Relationships between age and late progression of Parkinson's disease: a clinico-pathological study. *Brain, 133*(Pt 6), 1755–1762. doi: 10.1093/brain/awq059

Kenny, E. R., Burton, E. J., & O'Brien, J. T. (2008). A volumetric magnetic resonance imaging study of entorhinal cortex volume in dementia with lewy bodies. A comparison with Alzheimer's disease and Parkinson's disease with and without dementia. *Dementia & Geriatric Cognitive Disorders, 26*(3), 218–225. doi: 10.1159/000153432

Kim, J. S., Oh, Y. S., Lee, K. S., Kim, Y. I., Yang, D. W., & Goldstein, D. S. (2012). Association of cognitive dysfunction with neurocirculatory abnormalities in early Parkinson disease. *Neurology, 79*(13), 1323–1331. doi: 10.1212/WNL.0b013e31826c1acd

Klassen, B. T., Hentz, J. G., Shill, H. A., Driver-Dunckley, E., Evidente, V. G., Sabbagh, M. N.,... Caviness, J. N. (2011). Quantitative EEG as a predictive biomarker for Parkinson disease dementia. *Neurology, 77*(2), 118–124. doi: 10.1212/WNL.0b013e318224af8d

Klein, J. C., Eggers, C., Kalbe, E., Weisenbach, S., Hohmann, C., Vollmar, S.,... Hilker, R. (2010). Neurotransmitter changes in dementia with Lewy bodies and Parkinson disease dementia in vivo. *Neurology, 74*(11), 885–892. doi: 10.1212/WNL.0b013e3181d55f61

Kosaka, K., Yoshimura, M., Ikeda, K., & Budka, H. (1984). Diffuse type of Lewy body disease: progressive dementia with abundant cortical Lewy bodies and senile changes of varying degree—a new disease? *Clinical Neuropathology, 3*(5), 185–192.

Kulisevsky, J., & Pagonabarraga, J. (2009). Cognitive impairment in Parkinson's disease: tools for diagnosis and assessment. *Movement Disorders, 24*(8), 1103–1110. doi: 10.1002/mds.22506

Kurz, M. W., Dekomien, G., Nilsen, O. B., Larsen, J. P., Aarsland, D., & Alves, G. (2009). APOE alleles in Parkinson disease and their relationship to cognitive decline: A population-based, longitudinal study. *Journal of Geriatric Psychiatry & Neurology, 22*(3), 166–170.

Kurz, M. W., Schlitter, A. M., Larsen, J. P., Ballard, C., & Aarsland, D. (2006). Familial occurrence of dementia and parkinsonism: a systematic review. *Dementia & Geriatric Cognitive Disorders, 22*(4), 288–295. doi: DEM2006022004288 [pii] 10.1159/000095159

Lane, R. M., & He, Y. (2009). Emerging hypotheses regarding the influences of butyrylcholinesterase-K variant, APOE epsilon 4, and hyperhomocysteinemia in neurodegenerative dementias. *Medical Hypotheses, 73*(2), 230–250. doi: 10.1016/j.mehy.2009.01.050

Larsson, V., Aarsland, D., Ballard, C., Minthon, L., & Londos, E. (2010). The effect of memantine on sleep behaviour in dementia with Lewy bodies and Parkinson's disease dementia. *International Journal of Geriatric Psychiatry, 25*(10), 1030–1038. doi: 10.1002/gps.2506

Larsson, V., Engedal, K., Aarsland, D., Wattmo, C., Minthon, L., & Londos, E. (2011). Quality of life and the effect of memantine in dementia with Lewy bodies and Parkinson's disease dementia. *Dementia & Geriatric Cognitive Disorders, 32*(4), 227–234. doi: 10.1159/000334523

Leroi, I., Overshott, R., Byrne, E. J., Daniel, E., & Burns, A. (2009). Randomized controlled trial of memantine in dementia associated with Parkinson's disease. *Movement Disorders, 24*(8), 1217–1221. doi: 10.1002/mds.22495

Leverenz, J. B., Hamilton, R., Tsuang, D. W., Schantz, A., Vavrek, D., Larson, E. B.,... Montine, T. J. (2008). Empiric refinement of the pathologic assessment of Lewy-related pathology in the dementia patient. *Brain Pathology, 18*(2), 220–224. doi: BPA117 [pii] 10.1111/j.1750-3639.2007.00117.x

Litvan, I., Aarsland, D., Adler, C. H., Goldman, J. G., Kulisevsky, J., Mollenhauer, B.,... Weintraub, D. (2011). MDS task force on mild cognitive impairment in Parkinson's disease: Critical review of PD-MCI. *Movement Disorders, 26*(10), 1814–1824. doi: 10.1002/mds.23823

Litvan, I., Goldman, J. G., Tröster, A. I., Schmand, B.A., Weintraub, D., Petersen, R.,... Emre, M. (2012). Diagnostic criteria for mild cognitive impairment in Parkinson's disease: Movement Disorder Society Task Force Guidelines. *Movement Disorders, 27*(3), 349–356.

Lyoo, C. H., Ryu, Y. H., & Lee, M. S. (2010). Topographical distribution of cerebral cortical thinning in patients with mild Parkinson's disease without dementia. *Movement Disorders, 25*(4), 496–499. doi: 10.1002/mds.22975

Mattis, P. J., Tang, C. C., Ma, Y., Dhawan, V., & Eidelberg, D. (2011). Network correlates of the cognitive response to levodopa in Parkinson disease. *Neurology, 77*(9), 858–865. doi: 10.1212/WNL.0b013e31822c6224

McKeith, I., Del Ser, T., Spano, P., Emre, M., Wesnes, K., Anand, R.,... Spiegel, R. (2000). Efficacy of rivastigmine in dementia with Lewy bodies: a randomised, double-blind, placebo-controlled international study. *Lancet, 356*(9247), 2031–2036.

Meeus, B., Verstraeten, A., Crosiers, D., Engelborghs, S., Van den Broeck, M., Mattheijssens, M.,... Theuns, J. (2011). DLB and PDD: a role for mutations in dementia and Parkinson disease genes? *Neurobiology & Aging, 33*(3), e625–e629. doi: 10.1016/j.neurobiolaging.2011.10.014

Mollenhauer, B., Locascio, J. J., Schulz-Schaeffer, W., Sixel-Doring, F., Trenkwalder, C., & Schlossmacher, M. G. (2011). alpha-Synuclein and tau concentrations in cerebrospinal fluid of patients presenting with parkinsonism: A cohort study. *Lancet Neurology, 10*(3), 230–240. doi: 10.1016/S1474-4422(11)70014-X

Mondragon-Rezola, E., Arratibel-Echarren, I., Ruiz-Martinez, J., & Marti-Masso, J. F. (2010). [Sleep disorders in Parkinson's disease: Insomnia and sleep fragmentation, daytime hypersomnia, alterations to the circadian rhythm and sleep apnea syndrome]. *Review of Neurology, 50*(Suppl 2), S21–26. doi: rn2009735 [pii]

Muller, C. M., de Vos, R. A., Maurage, C. A., Thal, D. R., Tolnay, M., & Braak, H. (2005). Staging of sporadic Parkinson disease-related alpha-synuclein pathology: Inter- and intra-rater reliability. *Journal of Neuropathology and Experimental Neurology, 64*(7), 623–628.

Nalls, M. A., Plagnol, V., Hernandez, D. G., Sharma, M., Sheerin, U. M., Saad, M.,... Wood, N. W. (2011). Imputation of sequence variants for identification of genetic risks for Parkinson's disease: a meta-analysis of genome-wide association studies. *Lancet, 377*(9766), 641–649. doi: 10.1016/S0140-6736(10)62345-8

Nemani, V. M., Lu, W., Berge, V., Nakamura, K., Onoa, B., Lee, M. K.,... Edwards, R. H. (2010). Increased expression of alpha-synuclein reduces neurotransmitter release by inhibiting synaptic vesicle reclustering after endocytosis. *Neuron, 65*(1), 66–79. doi: 10.1016/j.neuron.2009.12.023

Nervi, A., Reitz, C., Tang, M. X., Santana, V., Piriz, A., Reyes, D.,... Mayeux, R. (2011). Familial aggregation of dementia with Lewy bodies. *Archives of Neurology, 68*(1), 90–93. doi: 10.1001/archneurol.2010.319

Neumann, J., Bras, J., Deas, E., O'Sullivan, S. S., Parkkinen, L., Lachmann, R. H.,... Wood, N. W. (2009). Glucocerebrosidase mutations in clinical and pathologically proven Parkinson's disease. *Brain, 132*(Pt 7), 1783–1794. doi: 10.1093/brain/awp044

Nobili, F., Abbruzzese, G., Morbelli, S., Marchese, R., Girtler, N., Dessi, B.,... Rodriguez, G. (2009). Amnestic mild cognitive impairment in Parkinson's disease: a brain perfusion SPECT study. *Movement Disorders, 24*(3), 414–421. doi: 10.1002/mds.22381

Oertel, W., Poewe, W., Wolters, E., De Deyn, P. P., Emre, M., Kirsch, C.,...Lane, R. (2008). Effects of rivastigmine on tremor and other motor symptoms in patients with Parkinson's disease dementia: A retrospective analysis of a double-blind trial and an open-label extension. *Drug Saf, 31*(1), 79–94.

Ohtake, H., Limprasert, P., Fan, Y., Onodera, O., Kakita, A., Takahashi, H.,...La Spada, A. R. (2004). Beta-synuclein gene alterations in dementia with Lewy bodies. *Neurology, 63*(5), 805–811.

Ondo, W. G., Shinawi, L., Davidson, A., & Lai, D. (2011). Memantine for non-motor features of Parkinson's disease: a double-blind placebo controlled exploratory pilot trial. *Parkinsonism Related Disorders, 17*(3), 156–159. doi: 10.1016/j.parkreldis.2010.12.003

Pagonabarraga, J., Kulisevsky, J., Llebaria, G., Garcia-Sanchez, C., Pascual-Sedano, B., & Gironell, A. (2008). Parkinson's disease-cognitive rating scale: A new cognitive scale specific for Parkinson's disease. *Movement Disorders, 23*(7), 998–1005. doi: 10.1002/mds.22007

Paris, A. P., Saleta, H. G., de la Cruz Crespo Maraver, M., Silvestre, E., Freixa, M. G., Torrellas, C. P.,...Bayes, A. R. (2011). Blind randomized controlled study of the efficacy of cognitive training in Parkinson's disease. *Movement Disorders, 26*(7), 1251–1258. doi: 10.1002/mds.23688

Parsons, T. D., Rogers, S. A., Braaten, A. J., Woods, S. P., & Tröster, A. I. (2006). Cognitive sequelae of subthalamic nucleus deep brain stimulation in Parkinson's disease: a meta-analysis. *Lancet Neurology, 5*(7), 578–588. doi: 10.1016/S1474-4422(06)70475-6

Petrou, M., Bohnen, N. I., Muller, M. L., Koeppe, R. A., Albin, R. L., & Frey, K. A. (2012). Abeta-amyloid deposition in patients with Parkinson disease at risk for development of dementia. *Neurology, 79*(11), 1161–1167. doi: 10.1212/WNL.0b013e3182698d4a

Poewe, W., Wolters, E., Emre, M., Onofrj, M., Hsu, C., Tekin, S.,...Investigators, Express. (2006). Long-term benefits of rivastigmine in dementia associated with Parkinson's disease: an active treatment extension study. *Movement Disorders, 21*(4), 456–461. doi: 10.1002/mds.20700

Polymeropoulos, M. H., Lavedan, C., Leroy, E., Ide, S. E., Dehejia, A., Dutra, A.,...Nussbaum, R. L. (1997). Mutation in the alpha-synuclein gene identified in families with Parkinson's disease. *Science, 276*(5321), 2045–2047.

Postuma, R. B., Gagnon, J. F., Vendette, M., Fantini, M. L., Massicotte-Marquez, J., & Montplaisir, J. (2009). Quantifying the risk of neurodegenerative disease in idiopathic REM sleep behavior disorder. *Neurology, 72*(15), 1296–1300. doi: 10.1212/01.wnl.0000340980.19702.6e

Rolinski, M., Fox, C., Maidment, I., & McShane, R. (2012). Cholinesterase inhibitors for dementia with Lewy bodies, Parkinson's disease dementia and cognitive impairment in Parkinson's disease. *Cochrane Database Systematic Review*, 3, CD006504. doi: 10.1002/14651858.CD006504.pub2

Rongve, A., Boeve, B. F., & Aarsland, D. (2010). Frequency and correlates of caregiver-reported sleep disturbances in a sample of persons with early dementia. *Journal of the American Geriatric Society, 58*(3), 480–486. doi: JGS2733 [pii] 10.1111/j.1532-5415.2010.02733.x

Schmitt, F. A., Aarsland, D., Bronnick, K. S., Meng, X., Tekin, S., & Olin, J. T. (2010). Evaluating rivastigmine in mild-to-moderate Parkinson's disease dementia using

ADAS-cog items. *American Journal of Alzheimers Disease & Other Dementias, 25*(5), 407–413. doi: 10.1177/1533317510367486

Segura, B., Ibarretxe-Bilbao, N., Sala-Llonch, R., Baggio, H. C., Marti, M. J., Valldeoriola, F.,...Junque, C. (2012). Progressive changes in a recognition memory network in Parkinson's disease. *Journal of Neurology, Neurosurgery and Psychiatry, 84*(4), 370–378. doi: 10.1136/jnnp-2012-302822

Seppi, K., Weintraub, D., Coelho, M., Perez-Lloret, S., Fox, S. H., Katzenschlager, R.,...Sampaio, C. (2011). The Movement Disorder Society Evidence-Based Medicine Review Update: Treatments for the non-motor symptoms of Parkinson's disease. *Movement Disorders, 26* (Suppl 3), S42–80. doi: 10.1002/mds.23884

Seto-Salvia, N., Clarimon, J., Pagonabarraga, J., Pascual-Sedano, B., Campolongo, A., Combarros, O.,...Kulisevsky, J. (2011). Dementia risk in Parkinson disease: disentangling the role of MAPT haplotypes. *Archives of Neurology, 68*(3), 359–364. doi: 10.1001/archneurol.2011.17

Siderowf, A., Xie, S. X., Hurtig, H., Weintraub, D., Duda, J., Chen-Plotkin, A.,...Clark, C. (2010). CSF amyloid {beta} 1-42 predicts cognitive decline in Parkinson disease. *Neurology, 75*(12), 1055–1061. doi: 10.1212/WNL.0b013e3181f39a78

Singleton, A. B., Farrer, M., Johnson, J., Singleton, A., Hague, S., Kachergus, J.,...Gwinn-Hardy, K. (2003). alpha-Synuclein locus triplication causes Parkinson's disease. *Science, 302*(5646), 841.

Song, S. K., Lee, J. E., Park, H. J., Sohn, Y. H., Lee, J. D., & Lee, P. H. (2011). The pattern of cortical atrophy in patients with Parkinson's disease according to cognitive status. *Movement Disorders, 26*(2), 289–296. doi: 10.1002/mds.23477

Sonnesyn, H., Nilsen, D. W., Rongve, A., Nore, S., Ballard, C., Tysnes, O. B., & Aarsland, D. (2009). High prevalence of orthostatic hypotension in mild dementia. *Dementia & Geriatric Cognitive Disorders, 28*(4), 307–313. doi: 000247586 [pii] 10.1159/000247586

Tokuda, T., Qureshi, M. M., Ardah, M. T., Varghese, S., Shehab, S. A., Kasai, T.,...El-Agnaf, O. M. (2010). Detection of elevated levels of alpha-synuclein oligomers in CSF from patients with Parkinson disease. *Neurology, 75*(20), 1766–1772. doi: 10.1212/WNL.0b013e3181fd613b

Tröster, A. I. (2011). A precis of recent advances in the neuropsychology of mild cognitive impairment(s) in Parkinson's disease and a proposal of preliminary research criteria. *Journal of the International Neuropsychological Society, 17*, 1–14. doi: 10.1017/S1355617711000257

Vlaar, A. M., de Nijs, T., Kessels, A. G., Vreeling, F. W., Winogrodzka, A., Mess, W. H.,...Weber, W. E. (2008). Diagnostic value of 123I-ioflupane and 123I-iodobenzamide SPECT scans in 248 patients with parkinsonian syndromes. *European Neurology, 59*(5), 258–266. doi: 10.1159/000115640

Weintraub, D., Dietz, N., Duda, J. E., Wolk, D. A., Doshi, J., Xie, S. X.,...Siderowf, A. (2011). Alzheimer's disease pattern of brain atrophy predicts cognitive decline in Parkinson's disease. *Brain, 135*(Pt 1), 170–180. doi: 10.1093/brain/awr277

Weintraub, D., Dietz, N., Duda, J. E., Wolk, D. A., Doshi, J., Xie, S. X.,...Siderowf, A. (2012). Alzheimer's disease pattern of brain atrophy predicts cognitive decline in Parkinson's disease. *Brain, 135*(Pt 1), 170–180. doi: 10.1093/brain/awr277

Weintraub, D., Koester, J., Potenza, M. N., Siderowf, A. D., Stacy, M., Voon, V.,...Lang, A. E. (2010). Impulse control disorders in Parkinson disease: A cross-sectional study of 3090 patients. *Archives of Neurology, 67*(5), 589–595. doi: 10.1001/archneurol.2010.65

Weintraub, D., Mavandadi, S., Mamikonyan, E., Siderowf, A. D., Duda, J. E., Hurtig, H. I., ... Stern, M. B. (2010). Atomoxetine for depression and other neuropsychiatric symptoms in Parkinson disease. *Neurology, 75*(5), 448–455. doi:10.1212/WNL.0b013e3181ebdd79

Wesnes, K. A., McKeith, I., Edgar, C., Emre, M., & Lane, R. (2005). Benefits of rivastigmine on attention in dementia associated with Parkinson disease. *Neurology, 65*(10), 1654–1656.

Williams-Gray, C. H., Evans, J. R., Goris, A., Foltynie, T., Ban, M., Robbins, T. W., ... Barker, R. A. (2009). The distinct cognitive syndromes of Parkinson's disease: 5 year follow-up of the CamPaIGN cohort. *Brain, 132*(Pt 11), 2958–2969. doi: awp245 [pii] 10.1093/brain/awp245

Williams-Gray, C. H., Foltynie, T., Brayne, C. E., Robbins, T. W., & Barker, R. A. (2007). Evolution of cognitive dysfunction in an incident Parkinson's disease cohort. *Brain, 130*(Pt 7), 1787–1798. doi: 10.1093/brain/awm111

Williams-Gray, C. H., Goris, A., Saiki, M., Foltynie, T., Compston, D. A., Sawcer, S. J., & Barker, R. A. (2009). Apolipoprotein E genotype as a risk factor for susceptibility to and dementia in Parkinson's disease. *Journal of Neurology, 256*(3), 493–498. doi: 10.1007/s00415-009-0119-8

Yamaguchi, K., Cochran, E. J., Murrell, J. R., Polymeropoulos, M. H., Shannon, K. M., Crowther, R. A., ... Ghetti, B. (2005). Abundant neuritic inclusions and microvacuolar changes in a case of diffuse Lewy body disease with the A53T mutation in the alpha-synuclein gene. *Acta Neuropathologica, 110*(3), 298–305. doi: 10.1007/s00401-005-1042-4

Zarranz, J. J., Alegre, J., Gomez-Esteban, J. C., Lezcano, E., Ros, R., Ampuero, I., ... de Yebenes, J. G. (2004). The new mutation, E46K, of alpha-synuclein causes Parkinson and Lewy body dementia. *Annals of Neurology, 55*(2), 164–173.

10 Depression and Anxiety in Parkinson's Disease

Laura Marsh and Roseanne D. Dobkin

INTRODUCTION

Defined by its motor triad of tremor, rigidity, and bradykinesia, Parkinson's disease (PD) is conceptualized as a movement disorder. However, nonmotor complications, such as depression, anxiety, sleep disturbance, psychosis, and cognitive changes, affect most individuals with PD (Aarsland, Marsh, & Schrag, 2009; Kulisevsky, Pagonabarraga, Pascual-Sedano, Garcia-Sanchez, & Gironell, 2008). These neuropsychiatric disturbances contribute significantly to disability and distress for both individuals with PD and their families, and by some accounts, are more impairing than motor features (Carter, Stewart, Lyons, & Archbold, 2008; Forsaa, Larsen, Wentzel-Larsen, Herlofson, & Alves, 2008)

Depression and anxiety are two of the most common and functionally relevant psychiatric complications observed in PD. This chapter reviews the prevalence, phenomenology, clinical characteristics, and impact of these two nonmotor disturbances. We also highlight pathophysiology, and pharmacological and nonpharmacological interventions for depression and anxiety in PD. The complex relationships between depression, anxiety, and cognitive function in PD receive particular emphasis throughout the chapter.

DEPRESSION

Prevalence

Depression is one of the most frequently cited neuropsychiatric symptoms in PD, though it is under-recognized in clinical settings (Shulman, Taback, Rabinstein, & Weiner, 2002). Variations in reported prevalence are related to methodological differences, for example, subject selection procedures, diagnostic criteria, the types of depressive disorders included, and statistical methods. Nonetheless, it is generally accepted that up to 50% of people with PD experience clinically significant depressive disturbances (Reijnders, Ehrt, Weber, Aarsland, & Leentjens, 2008). Incidence of depression in PD is more than double that observed in the general population and significantly higher than the rates reported in other medical conditions (Dooneief et al., 1992; Tandberg, Larsen, Aarsland, & Cummings, 1996).

Phenomenology

Depressive diagnoses in PD include major depressive disorder (MDD) and non-major depressive disturbances: dysthymia, minor depression, and subsyndromal depression. Fundamentally, depressive disorders involve a persistent and pervasive abnormal disturbance in mood or affective regulation that is accompanied by a predictable symptom complex, course, and response to treatment. Adjustment disorders, reactive emotional states, and bereavement also involve depressed moods, but these are not generally regarded as affective disorders. Major and non-major forms of depression involve similar phenomena, but the latter have milder and fewer symptoms. Even subsyndromal depressive disturbances cause significant suffering, distress, and functional impairment. Therefore, the diagnosis of a depressive disorder should be considered when self-reported disability and distress exceed what is expected from the clinical examination.

Typical emotional symptoms of a depressive disorder include a persistent or pervasive low or sad mood, diminished ability to enjoy otherwise enjoyable activities (anhedonia), and a decline in interests from baseline levels. Motor symptoms of PD can limit select activities, for example, needlepoint, but depressed individuals fail to seek alternate activities to enjoy. Other nonsomatic features of depression, such as negative ruminations, tearfulness, helplessness, hopelessness, worthlessness, decreased self-attitude, suicidal ideation, and excessive pessimism or guilt, help distinguish depressed from nondepressed PD patients.

Many symptoms of depressive disturbances overlap with physical features of PD (Table 10-1), that is, fatigue, psychomotor retardation, and sleep disturbances. To avoid under-diagnosing depressive disorders in PD, a National Institutes of Health (NIH) workgroup on depression in PD recommended an inclusive diagnostic approach; this attributes overlapping somatic and neurovegetative symptoms as features of the depressive disorder rather than of PD (Marsh, McDonald, Cummings, & Ravina, 2006).

A separate validation study of depressive syndromes in PD supports the applicability of *DSM-IV* diagnostic criteria for major depression, minor depression, and dysthymia in PD patients, as well as the NIH workgroup's assessment recommendations (Starkstein et al., 2008). In that study sample, anhedonia, loss of interest or pleasure, appetite and weight changes, insomnia, fatigue, worthlessness and inappropriate guilt, concentration problems, psychomotor retardation and agitation, and suicidal ideation were all significantly associated with the *DSM-IV* depressed mood criterion for major depression (Starkstein et al., 2008). Similar patterns were observed for dysthymia, underscoring the validity of *DSM-IV* diagnostic criteria in PD, irrespective of presence of a chronic medical condition, that is, PD. Of note, clinician and self-report rating scales facilitate

Table 10-1 Overlapping clinical features of major depression and Parkinson's disease

<table>
<tr><th></th><th>Major depression</th><th>Parkinson's disease</th></tr>
<tr><td>Motor Phenomena</td><td>Psychomotor retardation
Stooped posture
Restricted/depressed affect
Agitation</td><td>Bradykinesia
Stooped posture
Masked face/hypomimia
Tremor</td></tr>
<tr><td>Other Somatic Complaints</td><td colspan="2">Physical Complaints
Muscle tension
Gastrointestinal symptoms
Sexual dysfunction</td></tr>
<tr><td>Vegetative Changes</td><td colspan="2">Decreased energy
Fatigue
Sleep and appetite changes</td></tr>
<tr><td>Cognitive disturbances</td><td colspan="2">Poor concentration
Decreased memory
Impaired problem-solving</td></tr>
</table>

screening and identification of a depressive disorder in PD, but are not substitutes for a diagnostic clinical exam (Williams, 2012).

Clinical Course and Correlates

Depressive disturbances frequently predate the onset of motor symptoms and diagnosis of PD (Ishihara & Brayne, 2006; Leentjens, Van den Akker, Metsemakers, Lousberg, & Verhey, 2003). After the onset of PD, new onset depressive disorders can develop at any phase in the continuum of the disease. In many cases, depressive episodes are chronic or recurrent (Brown, MacCarthy, Gotham, Der, & Marsden, 1988; Ravina et al., 2007; Starkstein, Mayberg, Leiguarda, Preziosi, & Robinson, 1992). In a study of patients early in the course of PD, depressive symptoms resolved by 6 months in nearly half the subjects who had clinically significant depressive symptoms at baseline (Ravina et al., 2009). However, compared to subjects with no depression at baseline, those with mild depression also had a six-fold higher rate of developing moderate to severe depressive symptoms during the follow-up period. Depression in PD is characterized by greater cognitive dysfunction along with high rates of executive dysfunction and additional psychiatric comorbidities (Menza, Robertson-Hoffman, & Bonapace, 1993) and somatic complaints (Dobkin, Menza, Bienfait, et al., 2011). As in the general population, this complex neuropsychiatric presentation may predict nonresponse to treatment and lead to high rates of disability, relapse, and recurrence (Alexopoulos et al., 2005; Andreescu et al., 2007; Dobkin et al., 2010; Mohlman & Gorman, 2005).

Studies investigating other clinical correlates of depression in PD have produced inconsistent findings. Identified risk factors for PD-depression include motor disability (Riedel, Heuser, Klotsche, Dodel, & Wittchen, 2010; Rojo et al., 2003), female gender (Rojo et al., 2003), past psychiatric history (Starkstein, Bolduc, Mayberg, Preziosi, & Robinson, 1990), (Leentjens, Lousberg, & Verhey, 2002), early-onset PD (i.e., prior to age 55; Cole et al., 1996), neuropsychiatric comorbidities (i.e., psychosis, anxiety, fatigue, insomnia, cognitive decline; Aarsland, Larsen, Cummings, & Laake, 1999; Caap-Ahlgren & Dehlin, 2001; Lou, Kearns, Oken, Sexton, & Nutt, 2001; Marsh et al., 2004), right-side predominant motor symptoms (Starkstein et al., 1990), and atypical parkinsonism (i.e., prominent rigidity or balance problems versus tremor) (Starkstein et al., 1998). However, other studies have not confirmed such results (Frisina, Borod, Foldi, & Tenenbaum, 2008; Weintraub & Burn, 2011). Furthermore, there is no evidence of consistent relationships between PD age of onset, duration, severity, stage, or subtype, or the timing of when depressive episodes commence or depression severity (Marsh et al., 2006).

Impact

Depression in PD is linked with significant negative effects for individuals with PD as well as their family members. Specifically, depression in PD is associated with faster physical and cognitive deterioration (Starkstein et al., 1992), poorer quality of life (Forsaa et al., 2008), greater impairment in activities of daily living (Ravina et al., 2007), earlier initiation of dopaminergic replacement therapy (Ravina et al., 2007), and increased caregiver distress (Carter et al., 2008). The detrimental impact of depression is compounded by the fact that this common nonmotor disturbance is often undetected (Shulman et al., 2002) and insufficiently managed in clinical settings (Ravina et al., 2007; Weintraub, Moberg, Duda, Katz, & Stern, 2003).

The negative impact of depression on cognition in PD has received substantial attention. In a seminal paper involving subjects from a movement disorders treatment program (Starkstein et al., 1990), PD patients who were depressed at the time of their initial evaluation showed significantly greater cognitive deficits in global cognition and memory over the next three to four years, compared to PD patients without depression. Depression has since been identified as a risk factor for dementia in PD in both longitudinal and cross-sectional investigations (Marder, Tang, Cote, Stern, & Mayeux, 1995; Riedel, Klotsche, et al., 2010). It is also well-documented that depression may exacerbate the wide range of cognitive deficits frequently observed in most PD patients, including impaired global cognition, executive functions, memory, attention, language, and visuoconstructional skills (Fernandez et al., 2009; Kummer et al., 2009; Kuzis et al., 2001; Norman, Tröster, Fields, & Brooks, 2002; Tröster, Stalp, Paolo, Fields, & Koller, 1995; Uekermann et al., 2003). Dozens of studies have addressed this important topic over the past few decades, and a handful of more recent findings will be highlighted below.

Prevailing evidence suggests that both the extent and pattern of cognitive dysfunction is influenced by depression severity (Stefanova et al., 2006). In a cross-sectional study, all PD patients showed greater deficits on executive tasks such as category fluency and visuospatial organization compared to matched controls (Stefanova et al., 2006); the impairments were more profound in those with depression (major depression or dysthymia). In addition to these executive difficulties, PD patients with major depression were more impaired in the areas of episodic visuospatial memory, spatial working memory, and language. These findings remained significant after accounting for potential confounds such as general intellectual abilities and motor slowness. Importantly, in this sample of early PD patients, depression predicted cognitive impairment more robustly than PD disease severity, age of PD onset, and PD treatment regimen.

PD-depression is also associated with both global cognitive impairment, as measured by Mini-mental State Exam (MMSE) and Dementia Rating Scale, and specific cognitive impairments (i.e., naming, verbal memory, language) (Fernandez et al., 2009). For example, Santangelo and colleagues (Santangelo et al., 2009) demonstrated that depressed patients performed worse on the Frontal Assessment Battery, as well as semantic fluency, copying, and Stroop tasks, compared to nondepressed PD patients. Of note, impairments in visuoconstructional and frontal functions were most severe in depressed PD patients who displayed apathy and anhedonia (with or without depressed mood) versus depressed mood alone (Santangelo et al., 2009). Others have confirmed the role of apathy in exacerbating cognitive dysfunction in PD (Butterfield, Cimino, Oelke, Hauser, & Sanchez-Ramos, 2010; Oguru, Tachibana, Toda, Okuda, & Oka, 2010). It is also suggested that cognitive deficits may be most profound in depressed patients with lower levels of education (Klepac & Trkulja, 2009; Kummer et al., 2009).

Finally, additional research suggests that a history of pre-PD depression (i.e., before onset of motor symptoms) may render nondemented individuals particularly vulnerable to cognitive decline throughout the course of the illness. It was also observed that depression that predated the diagnosis of PD had a negative, direct, and independent effect on executive function tasks, even when controlling for current level of depressive symptoms (Klepac, Hajnsek, & Trkulja, 2010). Furthermore, pre-PD depression was also strongly related to current level of depression severity and indirectly influenced several other cognitive domains, including verbal fluency, verbal memory, and color naming via this mechanism (Klepac et al., 2010).

Pathophysiology

Discrete mechanisms for depression in PD have not been identified. The clinical phenotype of depressive syndromes in PD is attributed to a combination of psychosocial issues, genetic factors, and neuropathological changes associated with PD, along with other somatic factors (Mayberg & Solomon, 1995). Depressive phenomena can develop as a reaction to the diagnosis of PD, its psychosocial consequences, and perceived or actual disability (Brown et al., 1988). In addition to the impact of the disease itself, major life events are also associated with development of depression in PD patients and are further modulated by coping abilities and social supports (Rod, Bordelon, Thompson, Marcotte, & Ritz, 2013).

Whereas this evidence supports use of interventions that address important psychosocial issues, biological factors in PD provide an important context for predisposition to mood disorders. For example, depressive syndromes and mood dysregulation often precede the diagnosis of PD (Ishihara & Brayne, 2006), the natural history of depression in PD does not parallel disease progression (Huber, Freidenberg, Paulson, Shuttleworth, & Christy, 1990), and depressive symptoms in PD patients are more severe compared to conditions with comparable disability (Ehmann, Beninger, Gawel, & Riopelle, 1990). Research on genetic factors associated with PD-depression is limited. None of the genetic forms of PD appears to be associated with depression (Kasten et al., 2010). However, higher rates of depression in first-degree relatives of patients with PD suggest shared familial susceptibility with PD (Arabia et al., 2007).

Neuropathologically, PD is characterized by discrete loss of dopaminergic neurons as well as noradrenergic and serotonergic neurons, all of which are associated with regulation of mood and reward systems as well as mood disturbances in PD and in the general population (Aarsland, Pahlhagen, Ballard, Ehrt, & Svenningsson, 2012). A prevailing model for development of depression in PD proposes that degeneration of mesocortical and mesolimbic dopaminergic neurons causes orbitofrontal dysfunction, which leads to disruption of serotonergic neurons in the dorsal raphe and to dysfunction of the depression-related orbitofrontal-basal ganglia-thalamic circuits (Mayberg & Solomon, 1995). Neuroimaging, cerebrospinal fluid, and postmortem brain tissue studies provide support for this conceptualization in PD patients with depression, who demonstrate reduced striatal dopamine transporter activity, frontal blood flow, and caudate-frontal glucose metabolism and relative to nondepressed PD patients (Matsui, Nishinaka, et al., 2006; Mayberg et al., 1990; Weintraub et al., 2005). Consistent with this are structural neuroimaging studies associating PD-depression with white matter loss in cortical-limbic circuits (Kostic et al., 2010; Matsui et al., 2007). Functional imaging studies provide consistent associations between PD-depression and dopamine and noradrenergic neuronal dysfunction, whereas there is less substantiation of the role of serotonin (Aarsland et al., 2012).

Analyses of outcomes after deep brain stimulation (DBS) for treatment of motor symptoms in PD provide additional perspectives on the many potential explanations for mood changes in PD. Affective and behavioral changes, including aggression, suicide, depression, and mania, are also described as complications after DBS, especially subthalamic (STN) relative to pallidal or thalamic stimulation (Bronstein et al., 2009). It is thought that STN stimulation leads to serotonin inhibition via interconnected regions (e.g., substantia nigra pars reticulate, medial prefrontal cortex, and ventral pallidum) (Tan, Hartung, Sharp, & Temel, 2011). Stimulation-related mood changes could be related to spread of the stimulation field to adjacent nonmotor circuits, deviant electrode placement, or activation of inappropriate electrode contacts. The role of the nigrostriatal pathway in the pathophysiology of depression is highlighted by case reports describing PD patients with acute depressive states following stimulation to the substantia nigra (Bejjani et al., 1999; Blomstedt et al., 2008). For some patients, modification of contact selection can resolve mood changes. Depressive phenomena can also emerge as part of dopamine withdrawal syndrome when antiparkinsonian medications are reduced postoperatively (Rabinak & Nirenberg, 2010). In many instances, post-DBS mood disorders were unrecognized as pre-existing conditions, though disappointment over the results or impact of the surgery can also contribute to reactive mood changes, which can evolve into a persistent depressive disorder.

Treatment

To date, antidepressants have received the most preliminary support in randomized controlled trials (RCTs) of treatments for PD-depression (dPD) (Table 10-2;

Table 10-2 Randomized, Placebo-controlled Treatment Trials for PD-Depression

Study	*Treatment*	*Diagnosis*	*Sample size*	*Trial duration*	*Significant findings re reduced depressive symptoms*
Devos et al. 2008	~Desipramine 75 mg Citalopram 20 mg Placebo	Major Depression	*N*=48	30 days	14 days posttreatment: Desipramine> Citalopram, Placebo 30 days posttreatment Desipramine= Citalopram> Placebo
Menza et al. 2009a	~Nortriptyline 64 mg Paroxetine 32 mg Placebo	*DSM-IV* Depressive disorders*	*N*=52	8 weeks	Nortriptyline> Paroxetine, Placebo
Richard et al. 2012	~Paroxetine 24 mg Venlafaxine XR 121 mg Placebo	DSM-IV Depressive disorders**	*N*=115 (17 sites)	12 weeks	Paroxetine, Venlafaxine > Placebo
Psychotherapeutic interventions					
Veazey et al. 2009	CBT versus Support group	Depressive or Anxiety symptom ratings	*N*=14	9 weeks	CBT>Support Group for anxiety symptoms
Dobkin et al. 2011	CBT versus Treatment as Usual (TAU)	DSM-IV Depressive disorders*	*N*=80	10–14 weeks	CBT>TAU

~Average doses.

*DSM-IV Depressive disorders: Major Depression, Dysthymia, Depression NOS.

**also includes subsyndromal depression.

Devos et al., 2008; Menza et al., 2009a; Richard et al., 2012). In general, all the antidepressants evaluated were safe and well tolerated, with efficacy, relative to placebo, demonstrated for nortriptyline, venlafaxine XR, desipramine, citalopram, and paroxetine, though the time course of the antidepressant response varied. For example, nortriptyline was superior to placebo for the acute treatment (i.e., 8 weeks) of PD-depression, whereas both nortiptyline and paroxetine were associated with the long-term maintenance (i.e., 6 months) of treatment gains (Menza et al., 2009b). Whereas initial findings suggested a preferential response with serotonin-norepinephrine reuptake inhibitors, a current meta-analysis offers support for the efficacy and acceptability of selective serotonin reuptake inhibitors, as a class, for the treatment of PD-depression (Skapinakis et al., 2010). Finally, in an open-label, randomized, prospective, parallel group study, the augmentation of levodopa with selegiline, an MAO-B inhibitor, appeared to prevent the aggravation of minor depression in PD, over a one-year period (Imamura, Okayasu, & Nagatsu, 2011).

In addition to traditional antidepressant medications, other somatic treatments are being investigated. Dopamine agonists have also been explored as a primary treatment for PD-depression with mixed results in select double-blind RCTs (Leentjens, 2011). Although effect sizes were small, the dopamine agonist pramipexole was associated with reduced depressive symptoms in PD versus placebo over 12-weeks (Barone et al., 2010). Randomized, open-label trials of pramipexole also noted antidepressant effects in PD (Barone et al., 2006; Rektorova et al., 2003). Other blinded trials reported inconclusive (Pahwa et al., 2007) or negative findings regarding depression, though the studies were not designed with mood measures as the primary outcome (Navan, Findley, Jeffs, Pearce, & Bain, 2003). Alternative treatment approaches such as omega-3 fatty acids (da Silva et al., 2008) and left prefrontal repetitive transcranial magnetic stimulation (Pal, Nagy, Aschermann, Balazs, & Kovacs, 2010; Boggio et al., 2005; Fregni et al., 2004) have also been explored in small RCTs with encouraging results.

In contrast, psychosocial interventions, such as cognitive-behavioral therapy (CBT), have received less scientific attention in this patient group (Dobkin, Menza, Allen, Gara, et al., 2011; Sproesser, Viana, Quagliato, & de Souza, 2010) despite their demonstrated success in other geriatric (Serfaty et al., 2009) and neurological populations (Mohr et al., 2000). In the only randomized-controlled trial of CBT for PD-depression reported to date (Dobkin, Menza, Allen, Gara, et al., 2011), a 10-session CBT protocol that incorporated behavioral activation, cognitive restructuring, anxiety-management techniques, sleep-hygiene approaches, and caregiver support was associated with notable improvements in PD-depression over a 14-week period, compared to usual clinical management. Furthermore, there were significantly more treatment responders in the CBT group (i.e., number needed to treat 2.1; absolute risk reduction 48%), and large effect sizes were observed on all depression outcome measures. Several uncontrolled pilot trials and case series designs specific to CBT for PD-depression produced similar results (Armento et al., 2012), as did a 10-session phone-based CBT approach (Dobkin, Menza, Allen, Tiu, et al., 2011). A small (N=16) randomized study of a

12-session group psychotherapy, incorporating a psychodrama intervention (i.e., role-playing daily situations and discussing their meaning and psychosocial implications), was also associated with significant improvements in PD-depression over 6-months (Sproesser et al., 2010). Finally, one case study documented beneficial effects of problem-solving therapy for depression in PD patient with mild cognitive impairment (Mackin, Arean, & Elite-Marcandonatou, 2006).

Effect of Depression Treatment on Cognition

Cognitive outcomes have not been examined systematically in the pharmacological or nonpharmacological treatment trials for PD-depression referenced earlier. Studies on the impact of improved depression on neuropsychological functioning have yielded mixed results, and evidence for improved cognitive functioning following successful depression treatment is inconclusive (Price et al., 2011). Although some authors report posttreatment improvements in global cognitive functioning (Weintraub et al., 2010), as well as memory and executive functioning (Dobkin et al., 2014), others emphasize that the treatment under study was associated with no negative effects on cognition or any other cognitive changes (Devos et al., 2008). In some instances, baseline neuropsychological status was found to predict treatment response, though cognitive improvement did not coincide with amelioration of depression (Dobkin et al., 2010; Weintraub et al., 2006). Thus, the extent to which cognitive symptoms in PD may improve following successful depression treatment is unclear.

Several methodological issues are implicated in the inconsistent neuropsychological data from treatment outcomes studies for PD-depression. One important influence on results is that the MMSE, a dementia-screening tool with insensitivity to the neuropsychological complexity of PD, was the cognitive outcome measure in many depression trials. Furthermore, interpretation of neuropsychological effects of depression treatment is confounded by the short follow-up period in most reported trials. For example, the finding of "no change" in cognition in the acute treatment of depression may be interpreted as a disappointing result (apart from ruling out adverse events of a study drug), but maintenance of cognitive skills over a period of a few years may prove meaningful in a population such as PD that is vulnerable to cognitive decline (Tröster, Woods, & Morgan, 2007). However, few treatment trials are of sufficient duration to assess the clinical significance of any observed cognitive effects. In addition, many trials did not include no-treatment comparison conditions to control for the contribution of practice effects of repeat neuropsychological testing over time (Boggio et al., 2005; Fregni et al., 2004). Last, not all trials required a discrete depressive diagnosis, based on a structured clinical interview, for study entry (Sproesser et al., 2010). This last approach may bias sample selection to reflect a less severely depressed group; in such a cohort, cognitive effects, at least partially attributable to depression, may be less profound, and, therefore, contribute to under-reporting of cognitive outcomes. Specific findings from PD-depression treatment trials that incorporated cognitive outcomes are reviewed next.

Antidepressants. Studies regarding the impact of antidepressant treatment on cognition in dPD have been equivocal. Weintraub and colleagues reported that the selective norepinephrine reuptake inhibitor (SNRI) atomoxetine was associated with significant improvements in global cognition (MMSE) versus placebo, despite a very modest antidepressant effect for atomoxetine (Weintraub et al., 2010). In two RCTs comparing fluoxetine to repetitive transcranial magnetic stimulation, both active treatments were associated with improvements in depression and either global cognition (Fregni et al., 2004) or tests of executive function and visual-spatial ability (Boggio et al., 2005). In contrast, two separate RCTs observed no effect on cognition (i.e., global cognition, executive functions, memory, attention, or language) following the successful acute treatment of depression (Devos et al., 2008; M. Menza et al., 2009a). Related to this, acute open label trials of both citalopram (Menza, Marin, Kaufman, Mark, & Lauritano, 2004) and escitalopram (Weintraub et al., 2006) yielded no notable gains in cognition despite a clear antidepressant effect for both drugs.

Some cognitive benefits to treatment have been observed in the few antidepressant studies that employed longer follow-up periods. For example, improvements in verbal memory and language were observed for PD patients whose depression was at least "minimally improved" after 8-weeks of antidepressant treatment and remained on the study drug for an additional 6 months (Dobkin et al., 2010).[1] Imamura and colleagues (Imamura et al., 2011) also reported that PD patients (with *DSM-IV* minor depression) taking levodopa and selegiline (an MAO-B inhibitor) experienced less cognitive decline over a 1-year period, as assessed by the MMSE, compared to those taking levodopa only. Related to this, depressed patients taking levodopa only showed significant reductions in regional cerebral blood flow in several brain regions, including the frontal lobe, cingulate, hippocampus, parahippocampus, superior parietal lobe, middle temporal lobe, premotor area, and supplementary motor area, compared to those taking the levodopa-selegiline combination after one year.

Two of the previously referenced antidepressant trials also observed that baseline neuropsychological status predicted depression treatment response in PD. Weintraub and coworkers (Weintraub et al., 2006) noted that higher baseline scores on verbal memory were associated with increased rates of treatment response to escitalopram. Similarly, Dobkin and colleagues (Dobkin et al., 2010) found that treatment responders had higher baseline scores on measures of memory, speed of processing, and executive functioning compared to nonresponders. In this study, executive functioning, but not memory, was also a significant predictor of treatment response in logistic regression models, controlling for baseline depression severity, age, PD duration, and drug (paroxetine, nortriptyline, or placebo). Specifically, individuals who scored in the lowest quartile on the Stroop test were over 10 times less likely to be a treatment responder than patients who performed better on this measure (Dobkin et al., 2010).

Dopamine agonists. The effect of dopamine agonists on cognitive functioning in PD-depression remains unclear and probably depends on multiple factors, including cognitive task demands, the characteristics of the PD sample under study (i.e., de novo patients, motor fluctuations, presence of cognitive decline or dementia) and genetic factors, among others (Rektorova, 2010). However, limited data suggest that the cognitive performance of people with PD does not improve following the successful treatment of mild-to-moderate depression with dopamine agonists as an adjunctive treatment to levodopa therapy. In a randomized-prospective multicenter study (Rektorova et al., 2005) neither pramipexole nor pergolide were associated with improvements on a neuropsychological battery that predominantly assessed executive functions and working memory (i.e., Trails, Stroop, and arithmetic, picture completion, digit symbols, and similarities subtests of the Wechsler Adult Intelligence Scale), despite meaningful improvements in depression. As discussed (Rektorova, 2010), these results are also consistent with those observed in the EWO study (Epidemiology of Wearing Off Phenomenon in PD) in which the total daily dose of dopaminergic treatment had no effect on global cognition (as assessed by the Montreal Cognitive Assessment Battery), controlling for level of depression.

Nonpharmacological Trials

Repetitive Transcranial Magnetic Stimulation (rTMS). Pal and colleagues (Pal et al., 2010) observed that the accuracy of patient performance on an executive function task (i.e., Stroop test) was improved at both 1 and 30 days post rTMS over the left dorsolateral prefrontal cortex for PD-depression. However, the treatment group did not demonstrate meaningful changes on measures of global cognition (MMSE) or alternative measures of executive skills (Trails). No cognitive effects were observed in the control group, which received sham rTMS. As described earlier, two additional studies explored the efficacy of rTMS (compared to antidepressant medication) for dPD and noted improvements in global cognition, executive function, and spatial ability (Boggio et al., 2005; Fregni et al., 2004).

Cognitive Behavioral Therapy (Table 10-3) In a follow-up study to the first RCT of CBT for PD-depression described earlier (Dobkin, Menza, Allen, Gara, et al., 2011), executive functioning (as assessed by Trails B-A) was a significant predictor of treatment response in the CBT group at one-month posttreatment (Dobkin et al., 2012). Executive functioning also predicted depression symptom change, as assessed by the Beck Depression Inventory, for all participants over time (Dobkin et al., 2012). Moreover, depression improvement over the course of the CBT trial was associated with improvements in memory and executive function (Dobkin et al., 2014). These results remained significant when controlling for baseline scores on each respective cognitive measure, PD severity as assessed by the Unified Parkinson's Disease Rating Scale, age, and education (Dobkin et al.,

Table 10-3 Components of cognitive behavior therapy (CBT) trials for depression and anxiety in PD

Basic CBT components:
Address automatic thoughts and triggers that contribute to mood symptoms
PD-specific adaptations to account for bradyphrenia, memory and executive dysfunction
Problem-solving
Breathing strategies
Exposure to anxiety triggers
Activity scheduling
Stress management
Behavior modification
Sleep hygiene
Relaxation
Cognitive restructuring
Caregiver strategies to reinforce therapy for patient
Self-monitoring
Health promotion
Symptom (depression/anxiety) management
Social and communication skills training
Written strategies

2014). Similarly, improvements in memory were also observed following 10 sessions of phone-based CBT for PD-depression (Dobkin, 2014).

ANXIETY DISTURBANCES IN PARKINSON'S DISEASE

Prevalence

Like depression, anxiety disorders are commonly observed in PD and may predate the onset of the motor symptoms (Jacob, Gatto, Thompson, Bordelon, & Ritz, 2010). One recent estimate suggests that approximately half of people with PD will experience significant anxiety at some point during the course of their lives (Pontone et al., 2009). For example, in a community sample of patients with idiopathic PD (Pontone et al., 2009), current and lifetime prevalence of at least one anxiety disorder diagnosis were 43% and 49%, respectively, based on expert panel diagnostic consensus. Of the individuals surveyed, 20% also reported a lifetime prevalence of two or more anxiety disorders. Other recent reports documented prevalence of 34% and 25%, respectively, for the presence one *DSM-IV* anxiety disorder diagnosis (Dissanayaka et al., 2010; Leentjens, Dujardin, Marsh, Martinez-Martin, et al., 2011). Though these rates differ somewhat between studies based on the diagnostic procedures (Leentjens, Dujardin, Marsh, Martinez-Martin, et al., 2011), prevalence of anxiety disorders in PD is nonetheless high and of a greater magnitude compared to that observed in age- and illness-matched controls (Menza et al., 1993).

Phenomenology

Anxiety disorders in PD are heterogeneous in nature. Common symptoms include excessive worry, fatigue, concentration problems, sleep disturbance, restlessness, panic, fear of specific objects or situations, and phobic avoidance. In a community-based investigation (Pontone et al., 2009), the most prevalent anxiety disorder disturbance did not meet criteria for a specific *DSM-IV* categorical diagnosis, that is, current and lifetime prevalence of Anxiety Disorder Not Otherwise Specified (NOS) was 25% and 30%, respectively (Table 10-4). For example, it is common for anxiety symptoms in PD to fluctuate rapidly throughout the day and parallel changes in motor function for people (Maricle, Nutt, & Carter, 1995); such clinically significant disturbances are classified as Anxiety Disorder, NOS. After the nonspecific anxiety disturbances, the most common diagnoses, in order,

Table 10-4 Prevalence of specific anxiety disorders in studies on Parkinson's disease

Diagnostic category	*Reported prevalence*				
	Previous PD studies	*Pontone 2011*	*Dissanayaka 2010*	*Leentjens 2011*	*General population Kessler 2005*
Panic disorder	13–30%	7.1% Current (C) 10% Lifetime (L)	8%	4%	1%
Specific Phobia	–	13% C 19% L	–	–	5.5%
Generalized Anxiety Disorder	0–40%	3.2% C 3.2% L	3%	21%	1.6%
Social phobia	15%	7.9% C 8.7% L	13%	10%	4.5%
Agoraphobia	–	1.6% C 4% L	–	16%	2.3%
Post-traumatic stress disorder	–	0% C 1.6% L	–	–	–
Anxiety Disorder NOS	–	25% C* 30% L*	–	11%**	–

Anxiety Disorder NOS criteria based on *DSM-IV-TR.

** Neuropsychiatric Inventory Anxiety subscale cut-off> 3.

were specific phobia, social phobia, and panic disorder. Panic disorder, generalized anxiety disorder, and social phobia were the most frequent anxiety disorders observed in an Australian cohort of PD patients (Dissanayaka et al., 2010); others reported similar results (Leentjens, Dujardin, Marsh, Richard, et al., 2011; Menza et al., 1993).

Clinical Characteristics

Female sex, motor fluctuations, family psychiatric history, antidepressant use, and previous history of an anxiety or depressive disorder have been identified as markers or correlates of anxiety disorders in PD (Leentjens, Dujardin, Marsh, Martinez-Martin, et al., 2011; Pontone et al., 2009). PD severity, postural instability, gait dysfunction, the experience of dyskinesias or on-off fluctuations, and young onset PD are also significantly associated with anxiety (Dissanayaka et al., 2010). Of note, females, as well as individuals with longer disease duration, younger age of onset, higher daily levodopa equivalent dose, and greater motor complications of antiparkinsonian therapy are more likely to experience anxiety specifically associated with motor fluctuations (Pontone, Williams, et al., 2011). Anxiety disorders frequently co-occur with depressive disorders in PD and a number of publications have documented high comorbidity rates (Leentjens, Dujardin, Marsh, Martinez-Martin, et al., 2011; Leentjens, Dujardin, Marsh, Richard, et al., 2011; Menza et al., 1993; Pontone et al., 2009). As discussed earlier with regards to depression, this psychiatric comorbidity can complicate the course and management of both the motor and nonmotor aspects of the disease.

Impact

Anxiety has a widespread negative impact on quality of life in PD. Anxiety is associated with increased problems with mobility, activities of daily living, stigma, and isolation, as well as a diminished sense of emotional well-being in individuals with PD (Marinus, Leentjens, Visser, Stiggelbout, & van Hilten, 2002). Anxiety was also found to be stronger predictor of health-related quality of life specific to the quality of interpersonal interactions, health satisfaction, and overall well-being (bodily pain, mental health) than either physical symptoms of PD or depression (Chrischilles, Rubenstein, Voelker, Wallace, & Rodnitzky, 2002).

Additionally, state-dependent anxiety associated with motor fluctuations has also been shown to independently predict perceived health status among PD patients, even when controlling for comorbid depression and other relevant motor, nonmotor, and psychiatric variables, including age, symptom severity, medication side effects, and disability in activities of daily living (Pontone, Williams, et al., 2011).

Very few studies have examined the independent effect of anxiety on cognition in PD. In a cross-sectional investigation, (Ryder et al., 2002) demonstrated that anxiety accounted for a greater proportion of variance on a standardized cognitive performance battery than either depression or neurological variables.

Anxiety has also been found to have an independent influence on executive functions, visual-verbal substitution speed, visual-motor memory, attention, sequencing, information processing, and motor speed in nondemented PD patients (Klepac et al., 2010). Finally, anxiety has explained unique variance in delayed recall (verbal memory), even when controlling for depression, motor disability, age, and education, in people with PD (Dobkin et al., 2014). Additional research is needed to expand upon this limited data regarding the relationship between anxiety and cognition in PD, though it likely exerts a deleterious effect.

Pathophysiology

As with depression in PD, mechanisms underlying anxiety disturbances in PD are likely to involve multiple medical, neurochemical, genetic, and psychosocial factors, but a definitive explanation is not known. When considering anxiety in PD, it is important to distinguish anxiety, the everyday emotion, from anxiety disturbances. Anxiety is a common and understandable emotional reaction in the setting of uncertainty for all individuals, including situations such as receiving the diagnosis of PD or anticipating how one will overcome impending challenges in the context of motor and cognitive deficits. However, relative to non-PD patients with chronic illnesses and similar disability, anxiety in patients with PD is significantly more severe (Schiffer, Kurlan, Rubin, & Boer, 1988). Accordingly, in PD, several lines of evidence suggest that the pathophysiology of clinically significant anxiety disturbances is related to the underlying pathophysiology of PD itself.

Multiple epidemiologic studies indicate that individuals in the general population with anxiety disorders have a higher relative risk of developing PD later in life (Shiba et al., 2000; Weisskopf, Chen, Schwarzschild, Kawachi, & Ascherio, 2003). These findings suggest that anxiety may be an early nonmotor phenotype of PD and that disability, though it may contribute to anxiety, is not the sole etiologic determinant.

Among the anxiety disturbances, panic disorder and panic-like disturbances may be a marker for a discrete phenotype in PD that is associated with underlying PD pathology. Episodic anxiety is associated with motor fluctuations (Racette et al., 2002; Witjas et al., 2002), though not exclusively (Richard et al., 2004). Occurrence of panic disorder as well as panic-like phenomena also appears to be associated with earlier age of onset and motor fluctuations related to antiparkinson therapy (Pontone et al., 2009). During "off" phases, patients may experience feelings of despair, hopelessness, and panic that dissipate during the "on" phases (Vazquez, Jimenez-Jimenez, Garcia-Ruiz, & Garcia-Urra, 1993). Frequency of freezing is also highly correlated with presence of panic disorders and secondary panic attacks (Lauterbach, Freeman, & Vogel, 2003).

Further study of PD patients suggests that panic and "panic-like" disorders are familial disorders in PD and associated with significantly greater lifetime prevalence of similar phenomena in their first-degree relatives, as compared to PD patients without panic phenomena (Pontone, Palanci, et al., 2011). An association of panic onset further supports a role for common genetic factors before clinical motor symptoms develop in PD associated with *parkin* and *LRRK2* mutations (Khan et al., 2003; Khan et al., 2005; Matsui, Udaka, et al., 2006).

Emergence of anxiety disturbances later in life, but before onset of motor symptoms is consistent with Braak's theory that the earliest pathological processes in PD involve nondopaminergic systems in the lower brain stem (Braak, Ghebremedhin, Rub, Bratzke, & Del Tredici, 2004). In that model, damage to the locus coeruleus could account for a variety of nonmotor manifestations of PD, including sleep disturbances, autonomic symptoms, and anxiety (Fornai, di Poggio, Pellegrini, Ruggieri, & Paparelli, 2007).

Whether PD patients with anxiety represent a subgroup with disproportionate involvement of the locus coeruleus and noradrenergic system is unclear. Review of the experimental literature on anxiety in PD implicates degeneration of subcortical nuclei and ascending dopamine, norepinephrine, and serotonin pathways within the basal ganglia–frontal circuits (Prediger, Matheus, Schwarzbold, Lima, & Vital, 2012; Kano et al., 2011). Using (^{11}C)RTI-32, an *in vivo* marker of both dopamine and norepinephrine transporter binding and positron emission tomography (PET) in 8 depressed and 12 nondepressed PD patients matched for age, disease duration, and antiparkinsonian medication, Remy and coworkers (Remy, Doder, Lees, Turjanski, & Brooks, 2005) found that severity of anxiety in PD patients was inversely correlated with binding of (^{11}C)RTI-32 in the amygdala, locus coeruleus, and thalamus. These results support specific involvement of dopaminergic and noradrenergic innervation in the locus coeruleus and the limbic system that may be targets for discrete interventions.

Treatment

Few studies to date have examined the treatment of primary anxiety in PD. This paucity of available data stems from the exploration of anxiety as a secondary outcome in depression treatment trials. These secondary analyses suggest that anxiety that is comorbid with a primary depressive disturbance may respond well to either antidepressant medication (Devos et al., 2008; Menza et al., 2009a; Menza et al., 2004) or psychotherapy (Dobkin, Menza, Allen, Gara, et al., 2011; Sproesser et al., 2010).

To our knowledge, only three case studies to date have examined the impact of psychotherapeutic approaches on primary anxiety in PD. In a PD patient with generalized anxiety disorder (GAD), a 5-session CBT protocol, which included cognitive restructuring, relaxation training, and exposure based-techniques (augmented with a 5-session cognitive enhancement intervention), was associated with significant reductions in clinician-rated and self-reported measures of anxiety and maintained gains at 3-month follow-up (Mohlman et al., 2010). In a second case report regarding the psychosocial treatment of primary GAD in PD, a multi-component behavioral intervention consisting of relaxation training, imagery, and coping skills proved beneficial in the short-term reduction of generalized anxiety (Lundervold, Pahwa, & Lyons, 2009). Lastly, 12 weekly sessions of group CBT alleviated social anxiety in a 60-year-old male with PD, with gains maintained at 6-month follow-up (Heinrichs, Hoffman, & Hofmann, 2001).

Given the existing gaps in treatment of anxiety in Parkinson's disease, a pilot survey regarding treatment preferences for anxiety in PD was conducted among 33 expert neurologists affiliated with the National Parkinson Foundation (Palanci, Marsh, & Pontone, 2011). Although no consistent prescribing patterns were reported, first-line treatments included selective serotonin reuptake inhibitors (48%), benzodiazepines (24%), selective norepinephrine reuptake inhibitors (10%), and levodopa (5%). Psychosocial approaches, such as CBT, with a well-documented evidence base for the treatment of primary anxiety in older adults, were not referenced. At the current time, there is limited empirical data to support these treatment choices in PD. Additional research is needed to examine the efficacy of both pharmacological and nonpharmacological interventions for primary anxiety in PD, as well as the impact of those treatments on cognitive functioning, in this medical population.

EFFECT OF ANXIETY TREATMENT ON COGNITION

Cognitive Behavioral Therapy. No significant neuropsychological changes were observed following the CBT protocol described earlier (Mohlman et al., 2010) for primary GAD in PD. Measures of executive skills (i.e., Digits Forward and Backward, Trails B-A, Digit Symbol, Controlled Oral Word Association Test, Similarities) were administered pre- and posttreatment but did not improve over time. However, following treatment, the patient did report perceived improvements on a self-report measure of attention. To our knowledge, no additional treatment outcome studies for primary anxiety in PD assessed secondary cognitive outcomes.

SUMMARY, CONCLUSIONS, FUTURE DIRECTIONS

Depression and anxiety disturbances are common in PD and greatly affect overall morbidity. Substantial evidence indicates that these disturbances are related to the underlying neurodegenerative disease processes and related dysfunction of neural circuits. In addition, both depressive and anxiety disturbances appear to aggravate the inherent cognitive dysfunction evident in PD, adding another source of distress. Clinical treatments for depression have focused largely on pharmacological treatments, and there have been no controlled studies reported for anxiety disorders. A reactive element in patients with depression or anxiety exacerbates psychiatric distress and also provides a basis for psychosocial and behavioral interventions that ameliorate distress as well as enhance cognitive function overall. Although the need for research on treatment of mood disorders and cognitive dysfunction in PD continues, available and effective treatments, especially for depression, are often not utilized fully in clinical practice. Accordingly, in addition to development of specific pharmacological and nonpharmacological treatments, future directions must also address the implementation of mental health interventions for individuals with PD.

NOTE

1. Secondary analyses of neuropsychological data from the antidepressant trial conducted by Menza et al., 2009.

REFERENCES

Aarsland, D., Larsen, J. P., Cummings, J. L., & Laake, K. (1999). Prevalence and clinical correlates of psychotic symptoms in Parkinson disease: a community-based study. *Archives of Neurology, 56*(5), 595–601.

Aarsland, D., Marsh, L., & Schrag, A. (2009). Neuropsychiatric symptoms in Parkinson's disease.. *Movement Disorders, 24*(15), 2175–2186.

Aarsland, D., Pahlhagen, S., Ballard, C. G., Ehrt, U., & Svenningsson, P. (2012). Depression in Parkinson Disease—epidemiology, mechanisms, management. *Nature Reviews Neurology, 8*, 35–47.

Alexopoulos, G. S., Kiosses, D. N., Heo, M., Murphy, C. F., Shanmugham, B., & Gunning-Dixon, F. (2005). Executive dysfunction and the course of geriatric depression. *Biological Psychiatry, 58*(3), 204–210.

Andreescu, C., Lenze, E. J., Dew, M. A., Begley, A. E., Mulsant, B. H., Dombrovski, A. Y.,... Reynolds, C. F. (2007). Effect of comorbid anxiety on treatment response and relapse risk in late-life depression: controlled study. *British Journal of Psychiatry, 190*, 344–349.

Arabia, G., Grossardt, B. R., Geda, Y. E., Carlin, J. M., Bower, J. H., Ahlskog, J. E.,... Rocca, W. A. (2007). Increased risk of depressive and anxiety disorders in relatives of patients with Parkinson disease. *Archives of General Psychiatry, 64*(12), 1385–1392.

Armento, M., Stanley, M., Marsh, L., Kunik, M. E., York, M. K., Bush, A. L., & Calleo, J. (2012). Cognitive Behavioral Therapy (CBT) for Depression and Anxiety in Parkinson's Disease: A Clinical Review. *Journal of Parkinson's Disease, 2*(2), 135–151.

Barone, P., Poewe, W., Albrecht, S., Debieuvre, C., Massey, D., Rascol, O.,... Weintraub, D. (2010). Pramipexole for the treatment of depressive symptoms in patients with Parkinson's disease: a randomised, double-blind, placebo-controlled trial.. *Lancet Neurology, 9*(6), 573–580.

Barone, P., Scarzella, L., Marconi, R., Antonini, A., Morgante, L., Bracco, F.,... Musch, B. (2006). Pramipexole versus sertraline in the treatment of depression in Parkinson's disease: a national multicenter parallel-group randomized study.. *Journal of Neurology, 253*(5), 601–607.

Bejjani, B. P., Damier, P., Arnulf, I., Thivard, L., Bonnet, A. M., Dormont, D.,... Agid, Y. (1999). Transient acute depression induced by high-frequency deep-brain stimulation. *New England Journal of Medicine, 340*(19), 1476–1480.

Blomstedt, P., Hariz, M. I., Lees, A., Silberstein, P., Limousin, P., Yelnik, J., & Agid, Y. (2008). Acute severe depression induced by intraoperative stimulation of the substantia nigra: a case report.. *Parkinsonism & Related Disorders, 14*(3), 253–256.

Boggio, P. S., Fregni, F., Bermpohl, F., Mansur, C. G., Rosa, M., Rumi, D. O.,... Araujo Silva, M. T. (2005). Effect of repetitive TMS and fluoxetine on cognitive function in patients with Parkinson's disease and concurrent depression. *Movement Disorders, 20*(9), 1178–1184.

Braak, H., Ghebremedhin, E., Rüb, U., Bratzke, H., & Del Tredici. K. (2004). Stages in the development of Parkinson's disease-related pathology. *Cell and Tissue Research, 318*(1), 121–134.

Bronstein, J., Carvey, P., Chen, H., Cory-Slechta, D., DiMonte, D., Duda, J., ... Weisskopf, M. (2009). Meeting report: consensus statement-Parkinson's disease and the environment: collaborative on health and the environment and Parkinson's Action Network (CHE PAN) conference 26–28 June 2007.. *Environmental Health Perspectives, 117*(1), 117–121.

Brown, R. G., MacCarthy, B., Gotham, A. M., Der, G. J., & Marsden, C. D. (1988). Depression and disability in Parkinson's disease: a follow-up of 132 cases. *Psychological Medicine, 18*(1), 49–55.

Butterfield, L. C., Cimino, C. R., Oelke, L. E., Hauser, R. A., & Sanchez-Ramos, J. (2010). The independent influence of apathy and depression on cognitive functioning in Parkinson's disease. *Neuropsychology, 24*(6), 721–730.

Caap-Ahlgren, M., & Dehlin, O. (2001). Insomnia and depressive symptoms in patients with Parkinson's disease. Relationship to health-related quality of life. An interview study of patients living at home. *Archives in Gerontology & Geriatrics, 32*(1), 23–33.

Carter, J. H., Stewart, B. J., Lyons, K. S., & Archbold, P. G. (2008). Do motor and non-motor symptoms in PD patients predict caregiver strain and depression? *Movement Disorders, 23*(9), 1211–1216.

Chrischilles, E. A., Rubenstein, L. M., Voelker, M. D., Wallace, R. B., & Rodnitzky, R. L. (2002). Linking clinical variables to health-related quality of life in Parkinson's disease.. *Parkinsonism & Related Disorders, 8*(3), 199–209.

Cole, S. A., Woodard, J. L., Juncos, J. L., Kogos, J. L., Youngstrom, E. A., & Watts, R. L. (1996). Depression and disability in Parkinson's disease. *Journal of Neuropsychiatry & Clinical Neuroscience, 8*(1), 20–25.

da Silva, T. M., Munhoz, R. P., Alvarez, C., Naliwaiko, K., Kiss, A., Andreatini, R., & Ferraz, A. C. (2008). Depression in Parkinson's disease: a double-blind, randomized, placebo-controlled pilot study of omega-3 fatty-acid supplementation. *Journal of Affective Disorders, 111*(2-3), 351–359.

Devos, D., Dujardin, K., Poirot, I., Moreau, C., Cottencin, O., Thomas, P., ... Defebvre, L. (2008). Comparison of desipramine and citalopram treatments for depression in Parkinson's disease: A double-blind, randomized, placebo-controlled study.. *Movement Disorders, 23*(6), 850–857.

Dissanayaka, N. N., Sellbach, A., Matheson, S., O'Sullivan, J. D., Silburn, P. A., Byrne, G. J., ... Mellick, G. D. (2010). Anxiety disorders in Parkinson's disease: Prevalence and risk factors. *Movement Disorders, 25*(7), 838–845.

Dobkin, R. D. (2014). The relationship between telephone-administered cognitive-behavioral therapy for depression and neuropsychological functioning in Parkinson's disease. *Journal of Neuropsychiatry & Clinical Neuroscience, 26*, E10–E11. doi:10.1176/appi.neuropsych.13030065.

Dobkin, R. D., Menza, M., Allen, L. A., Gara, M. A., Mark, M. H., Tiu, J., ... Friedman, J. (2011). Cognitive-behavioral therapy for depression in Parkinson's disease: a randomized, controlled trial. *American Journal of Psychiatry, 168*(10), 1066–1074.

Dobkin, R. D., Menza, M., Allen, L. A., Tiu, J., Friedman, J., Bienfait, K. L., ... Mark, M. H. (2011). Telephone-based cognitive-behavioral therapy for depression in Parkinson disease.. *Journal of Geriatrics, Psychiatry & Neurology, 24*(4), 206–214.

Dobkin, R. D., Menza, M., Bienfait, K. L., Gara, M., Marin, H., Mark, M. H., ... Friedman, J. (2011). Depression in Parkinson's disease: Symptom improvement and residual symptoms after acute pharmacologic management.. *American Journal of Geriatric Psychiatry, 19*(3), 222–229.

Dobkin, R. D., Menza, M., Bienfait, K. L., Gara, M., Marin, H., Mark, M. H.,... Tröster, A. (2010). The impact of antidepressant treatment on cognitive functioning in depressed patients with Parkinson's disease.. *Journal of Neuropsychiatry & Clinical Neuroscience, 22*(2), 188–195.

Dobkin, R. D., Rubino, J. T., Allen, L. A., Friedman, J., Gara, M. A., Mark, M. H., & Menza, M. (2012). Predictors of treatment response to cognitive-behavioral therapy for depression in Parkinson's disease. *Journal of Consulting and Clinical Psychology, 80*(4), 694–699.

Dobkin, R. D., Tröster, A., Rubino, J. T., Allen, L. A., Gara, M., Mark, M. H., & Menza, M. (2014). Neuropsychological outcomes following psychosocial intervention for depression in Parkinson's disease. *Journal of Neuropsychiatry & Clinical Neuroscience, 26*, 57–63.

Dooneief, G., Mirabello, E., Bell, K., Marder, K., Stern, Y., & Mayeux, R. (1992). An estimate of the incidence of depression in idiopathic Parkinson's disease. *Archives of Neurology, 49*(3), 305–307.

Ehmann, T. S., Beninger, R. J., Gawel, M. J., & Riopelle, R. J. (1990). Depressive symptoms in Parkinson's disease: a comparison with disabled control subjects. *Journal of Geriatric Psychiatry and Neurology, 3*(1), 3–9.

Fernandez, H. H., See, R. H., Gary, M. F., Bowers, D., Rodriguez, R. L., Jacobson, C. t., & Okun, M. S. (2009). Depressive symptoms in Parkinson disease correlate with impaired global and specific cognitive performance. *Journal of Geriatric Psychiatry and Neurology, 22*(4), 223–227.

Forsaa, E. B., Larsen, J. P., Wentzel-Larsen, T., Herlofson, K., & Alves, G. (2008). Predictors and course of health-related quality of life in Parkinson's disease. *Movement Disorders, 23*(10), 1420–1427.

Fregni, F., Santos, C. M., Myczkowski, M. L., Rigolino, R., Gallucci-Neto, J., Barbosa, E. R.,... Marcolin, M. A. (2004). Repetitive transcranial magnetic stimulation is as effective as fluoxetine in the treatment of depression in patients with Parkinson's disease. *Journal of Neurology, Neurosurgery, and Psychiatry, 75*(8), 1171–1174.

Frisina, P. G., Borod, J. C., Foldi, N. S., & Tenenbaum, H. R. (2008). Depression in Parkinson's disease: health risks, etiology, and treatment options. *Neuropsychiatric Disease and Treatment, 4*(1), 81–91.

Fornai, F., di Poggio, A. B., Pellegrini, A., Ruggieri, S., & Paparelli, A. (2007). Norepinephrine in Parkinson's disease: from disease progression to current therapeutics. *Current Medical Chemistry, 14*, 2330–2334.

Heinrichs, N., Hoffman, E. C., & Hofmann, S. G. (2001). Cognitive-behavioral treatment for social phobia in Parkinson's disease: A single-case study. *Cognitive and Behavioral Practice, 8*(4), 328–335.

Huber, S. J., Freidenberg, D. L., Paulson, G. W., Shuttleworth, E. C., & Christy, J. A. (1990). The pattern of depressive symptoms varies with progression of Parkinson's disease. *Journal of Neurology, Neurosurgery & Psychiatry, 53*(4), 275–278.

Imamura, K., Okayasu, N., & Nagatsu, T. (2011). The relationship between depression and regional cerebral blood flow in Parkinson's disease and the effect of selegiline treatment. *Acta Neurologica Scandinavica, 124*(1), 28–39.

Ishihara, L., & Brayne, C. (2006). A systematic review of depression and mental illness preceding Parkinson's disease.. *Acta Neurologica Scandinavica, 113*(4), 211–220.

Jacob, E. L., Gatto, N. M., Thompson, A., Bordelon, Y., & Ritz, B. (2010). Occurrence of depression and anxiety prior to Parkinson's disease.. *Parkinsonism & Related Disorders, 16*(9), 576–581.

Kano, O., Ikeda, K., Cridebring, D., Takazawa, T., Yoshii, Y., & Iwasaki, Y. (2011). Neurobiology of depression and anxiety in Parkinson's disease. *Parkinsons Disease*, 143547.

Kasten, M., Kertelge, L., Bruggemann, N., van der Vegt, J., Schmidt, A., Tadic, V., ... Klein, C. (2010). Nonmotor symptoms in genetic Parkinson disease. *Archives of Neurology*, *67*(6), 670–676.

Kessler, R. C., Berglund, P., Demler, O., Jin, R., Merikangas, K. R., Walters, E. E. (2005). Lifetime prevalence and age-of-onset distributions of DSM-IV disorders in the National Comorbidity Survey Replication. *Archives of General Psychiatry*, *62*(6), 593–602.

Khan, N. L., Graham, E., Critchley, P., Schrag, A. E., Wood, N. W., Lees, A. J., ... Quinn, N. (2003). Parkin disease: a phenotypic study of a large case series. *Brain*, *126*(Pt 6), 1279–1292.

Khan, N. L., Jain, S., Lynch, J. M., Pavese, N., Abou-Sleiman, P., Holton, J. L., ... Wood, N. W. (2005). Mutations in the gene LRRK2 encoding dardarin (PARK8) cause familial Parkinson's disease: clinical, pathological, olfactory and functional imaging and genetic data. *Brain*, *128*(Pt 12), 2786–2796.

Klepac, N., Hajnsek, S., & Trkulja, V. (2010). Cognitive performance in nondemented nonpsychotic Parkinson disease patients with or without a history of depression prior to the onset of motor symptoms. *Journal of Geriatric Psychiatry and Neurology*, *23*(1), 15–26.

Klepac, N., & Trkulja, V. (2009). Education effect on depression and quality of life in nondemented Parkinson's disease patients. *Journal of Neuropsychiatry & Clinical Neuroscience*, *21*(3), 314–322.

Kostic, V. S., Agosta, F., Petrovic, I., Galantucci, S., Spica, V., Jecmenica-Lukic, M., & Filippi, M. (2010). Regional patterns of brain tissue loss associated with depression in Parkinson disease. *Neurology*, *75*(10), 857–863. doi:

Kulisevsky, J., Pagonabarraga, J., Pascual-Sedano, B., Garcia-Sanchez, C., & Gironell, A. (2008). Prevalence and correlates of neuropsychiatric symptoms in Parkinson's disease without dementia. *Movement Disorders*, *23*(13), 1889–1896.

Kummer, A., Harsanyi, E., Dias, F. M., Cardoso, F., Caramelli, P., & Teixeira, A. L. (2009). Depression impairs executive functioning in Parkinson disease patients with low educational level. *Cognitive Behavior & Neurology*, *22*(3), 167–172.

Kuzis, G., Sabe, L., Tiberti, C., Dorrego, F., Starkstein, S., & Merello, M. (2001). Neuropsychological effects of pallidotomy in patients with Parkinson's disease.. *Journal of Neurology, Neurosurgery and Psychiatry*, *71*(4), 563–564.

Lauterbach, E. C., Freeman, A., & Vogel, R. L. (2003). Correlates of generalized anxiety and panic attacks in dystonia and Parkinson disease. *Cognitive Behavior & Neurology*, *16*(4), 225–233.

Leentjens, A. F. (2011). The role of dopamine agonists in the treatment of depression in patients with Parkinson's disease: a systematic review. *Drugs*, *71*(3), 273–286.

Leentjens, A. F., Dujardin, K., Marsh, L., Martinez-Martin, P., Richard, I. H., & Starkstein, S. E. (2011). Symptomatology and markers of anxiety disorders in Parkinson's disease: A cross-sectional study. *Movement Disorders*, *26*(3), 484–492.

Leentjens, A. F., Dujardin, K., Marsh, L., Richard, I. H., Starkstein, S. E., & Martinez-Martin, P. (2011). Anxiety rating scales in Parkinson's disease: a validation study of the Hamilton anxiety rating scale, the Beck anxiety inventory, and the hospital anxiety and depression scale. *Movement Disorders*, *26*(3), 407–415.

Leentjens, A. F., Lousberg, R., & Verhey, F. R. (2002). Markers for depression in Parkinson's disease.. *Acta Psychiatrica Scandinavica, 106*(3), 196–201.

Leentjens, A. F., Van den Akker, M., Metsemakers, J. F., Lousberg, R., & Verhey, F. R. (2003). Higher incidence of depression preceding the onset of Parkinson's disease: a register study. *Movement Disorders, 18*(4), 414–418.

Lou, J. S., Kearns, G., Oken, B., Sexton, G., & Nutt, J. (2001). Exacerbated physical fatigue and mental fatigue in Parkinson's disease. *Movement Disorders, 16*(2), 190–196.

Lundervold, D. A., Pahwa, R., & Lyons, K. E. (2009). Effect of behavioral intervention on comorbid general anxiety disorder and Parkinson's disease. *Clinical Gerontologist, 32*, 104–117.

Mackin, R. S., Arean, P., & Elite-Marcandonatou, A. (2006). Problem solving therapy for the treatment of depression for a patient with Parkinson's disease and mild cognitive impairment: a case study. *Neuropsychiatric Disease and Treamentt, 2*(3), 375–379.

Marder, K., Tang, M. X., Cote, L., Stern, Y., & Mayeux, R. (1995). The frequency and associated risk factors for dementia in patients with Parkinson's disease. *Archives of Neurology, 52*(7), 695–701.

Maricle, R. A., Nutt, J. G., & Carter, J. H. (1995). Mood and anxiety fluctuation in Parkinson's disease associated with levodopa infusion: Preliminary findings. *Movement Disorders, 10*(3), 329–332.

Marinus, J., Leentjens, A. F., Visser, M., Stiggelbout, A. M., & van Hilten, J. J. (2002). Evaluation of the hospital anxiety and depression scale in patients with Parkinson's disease. *Clinical Neuropharmacology, 25*(6), 318–324.

Marsh, L., McDonald, W. M., Cummings, J., & Ravina, B. (2006). Provisional diagnostic criteria for depression in Parkinson's disease: Report of an NINDS/NIMH Work Group.. *Movement Disorders, 21*(2), 148–158.

Marsh, L., Williams, J. R., Rocco, M., Grill, S., Munro, C., & Dawson, T. M. (2004). Psychiatric comorbidities in patients with Parkinson disease and psychosis. *Neurology, 63*(2), 293–300.

Matsui, H., Nishinaka, K., Oda, M., Komatsu, K., Kubori, T., & Udaka, F. (2006). Minor depression and brain perfusion images in Parkinson's disease. *Movement Disorders, 21*(8), 1169–1174.

Matsui, H., Nishinaka, K., Oda, M., Niikawa, H., Komatsu, K., Kubori, T., & Udaka, F. (2007). Depression in Parkinson's disease. Diffusion tensor imaging study. *Journal of Neurology, 254*(9), 1170–1173.

Matsui, H., Udaka, F., Oda, M., Tamura, A., Kubori, T., Nishinaka, K., & Kameyama, M. (2006). Parkinson's disease following panic disorder. *Journal of Neuropsychiatry and Clinical Neuroscience, 18*(1), 130.

Mayberg, H. S., & Solomon, D. H. (1995). Depression in Parkinson's disease: a biochemical and organic viewpoint. *Advances in Neurology, 65*, 49–60.

Mayberg, H. S., Starkstein, S. E., Sadzot, B., Preziosi, T., Andrezejewski, P. L., Dannals, R. F., . . . Robinson, R. G. (1990). Selective hypometabolism in the inferior frontal lobe in depressed patients with Parkinson's disease.. *Annals of Neurology, 28*(1), 57–64.

Menza, M., Dobkin, R. D., Marin, H., Mark, M. H., Gara, M., Buyske, S., . . . Dicke, A. (2009a). A controlled trial of antidepressants in patients with Parkinson disease and depression. *Neurology, 72*(10), 886–892.

Menza, M., Dobkin, R. D., Marin, H., Mark, M. H., Gara, M., Buyske, S., . . . Dicke, A. (2009b). The impact of treatment of depression on quality of life, disability and relapse in patients with Parkinson's disease. *Movement Disorders, 24*(9), 1325–1332.

Menza, M., Marin, H., Kaufman, K., Mark, M., & Lauritano, M. (2004). Citalopram treatment of depression in Parkinson's disease: the impact on anxiety, disability, and cognition. *Journal of Neuropsychiatry and Clinical Neuroscience, 16*(3), 315–319.

Menza, M., Robertson-Hoffman, D. E., & Bonapace, A. S. (1993). Parkinson's disease and anxiety: comorbidity with depression. *Biological Psychiatry, 34*(7), 465–470.

Mohlman, J., & Gorman, J. M. (2005). The role of executive functioning in CBT: a pilot study with anxious older adults. *Behavioral Research and Therapy, 43*(4), 447–465.

Mohlman, J., Reel, D. H., Chazin, D., Ong, D., Georgescu, B., Tiu, J., & Dobkin, R. D. (2010). A novel approach to treating anxiety and enhancing executive skills in an older adult with Parkinson's disease. *Clinical Case Studies, 9*(1), 74–90.

Mohr, D. C., Likosky, W., Bertagnolli, A., Goodkin, D. E., Van Der Wende, J., Dwyer, P., & Dick, L. P. (2000). Telephone-administered cognitive-behavioral therapy for the treatment of depressive symptoms in multiple sclerosis. *Journal of Consulting and Clinical Psychology, 68*(2), 356–361.

Navan, P., Findley, L. J., Jeffs, J. A., Pearce, R. K., & Bain, P. G. (2003). Randomized, double-blind, 3-month parallel study of the effects of pramipexole, pergolide, and placebo on Parkinsonian tremor. *Movement Disorders, 18*(11), 1324–1331.

Norman, S., Tröster, A. I., Fields, J. A., & Brooks, R. (2002). Effects of depression and Parkinson's disease on cognitive functioning. *Journal of Neuropsychiatry and Clinical Neuroscience, 14*(1), 31–36.

Oguru, M., Tachibana, H., Toda, K., Okuda, B., & Oka, N. (2010). Apathy and depression in Parkinson disease. *Journal of Geriatric Psychiatry and Neurology, 23*(1), 35–41.

Pahwa, R., Stacy, M. A., Factor, S. A., Lyons, K. E., Stocchi, F., Hersh, B. P., . . . Earl, N. L. (2007). Ropinirole 24-hour prolonged release: Randomized, controlled study in advanced Parkinson disease.. *Neurology, 68*(14), 1108–1115.

Pal, E., Nagy, F., Aschermann, Z., Balazs, E., & Kovacs, N. (2010). The impact of left prefrontal repetitive transcranial magnetic stimulation on depression in Parkinson's disease: a randomized, double-blind, placebo-controlled study. *Movement Disorders, 25*(14), 2311–2317.

Palanci, J., Marsh, L., & Pontone, G. M. (2011). Gaps in treatment for anxiety in Parkinson disease. *American Journal of Geriatric Psychiatry, 19*(10), 907–908.

Pontone, G. M., Palanci, J., Bienvenu, O. J., Liang, K. Y., Nestadt, G., Rabins, P. V., . . . Marsh, L. (2011). Familial aggregation of panic disturbances in Parkinson's disease. *Journal of Neuropsychiatry and Clinical Neuroscience, 23*(4), 417–424.

Pontone, G. M., Williams, J. R., Anderson, K. E., Chase, G., Goldstein, S. A., Grill, S., . . . Marsh, L. (2009). Prevalence of anxiety disorders and anxiety subtypes in patients with Parkinson's disease. *Movement Disorders, 24*(9), 1333–1338.

Pontone, G. M., Williams, J. R., Anderson, K. E., Chase, G., Goldstein, S. R., Grill, S., . . . Marsh, L. (2011). Anxiety and self-perceived health status in Parkinson's disease.. *Parkinsonism & Related Disorders, 17*(4), 249–254.

Prediger, R. D., Matheus, F. C., Schwarzbold, M. L., Lima, M. M., & Vital, M. A. (2012). Anxiety in Parkinson's disease: a critical review of experimental and clinical studies. *Neuropharmacology, 62*(1), 115–124.

Price, A., Rayner, L., Okon-Rocha, E., Evans, A., Valsraj, K., Higginson, I. J., & Hotopf, M. (2011). Antidepressants for the treatment of depression in neurological disorders: a systematic review and meta-analysis of randomised controlled trials. *Journal of Neurology, Neurosurgery and Psychiatry, 82*(8), 914–923.

Rabinak, C. A., & Nirenberg, M. J. (2010). Dopamine agonist withdrawal syndrome in Parkinson disease. *Archives of Neurol, 67*(1), 58–63.

Racette, B. A., Hartlein, J. M., Hershey, T., Mink, J. W., Perlmutter, J. S., & Black, K. J. (2002). Clinical features and comorbidity of mood fluctuations in Parkinson's disease. *Journal of Neuropsychiatry & Clinical Neuroscience, 14*(4), 438–442.

Ravina, B., Camicioli, R., Como, P. G., Marsh, L., Jankovic, J., Weintraub, D., & Elm, J. (2007). The impact of depressive symptoms in early Parkinson disease. *Neurology, 69*(4), 342–347.

Ravina, B., Elm, J., Camicioli, R., Como, P. G., Marsh, L., Jankovic, J., & Weintraub, D. (2009). The course of depressive symptoms in early Parkinson's disease. *Movement Disorders, 24*(9), 1306–1311.

Reijnders, J. S., Ehrt, U., Weber, W. E., Aarsland, D., & Leentjens, A. F. (2008). A systematic review of prevalence studies of depression in Parkinson's disease. *Movement Disorders, 23*(2), 183–189;

Rektorova, I. (2010). Effects of dopamine agonists on neuropsychiatric symptoms of Parkinson's disease. *Neurodegenerative Diseases, 7*(1-3), 206–209.

Rektorova, I., Rektor, I., Bares, M., Dostal, V., Ehler, E., Fanfrdlova, Z.,... Veliskova, J. (2003). Pramipexole and pergolide in the treatment of depression in Parkinson's disease: A national multicentre prospective randomized study.. *European Journal of Neurology, 10*(4), 399–406.

Rektorova, I., Rektor, I., Bares, M., Dostal, V., Ehler, E., Fanfrdlova, Z.,... Veliskova, J. (2005). Cognitive performance in people with Parkinson's disease and mild or moderate depression: Effects of dopamine agonists in an add-on to L-dopa therapy. *European Journal of Neurology, 12*(1), 9–15.

Remy, P., Doder, M., Lees, A., Turjanski, N., & Brooks, D. (2005). Depression in Parkinson's disease: loss of dopamine and noradrenaline innervation in the limbic system. *Brain, 128*(Pt 6), 1314–1322.

Richard, I. H., Frank, S., McDermott, M. P., Wang, H., Justus, A. W., LaDonna, K. A., & Kurlan, R. (2004). The ups and downs of Parkinson disease: a prospective study of mood and anxiety fluctuations. *Cognitive Behavior and Neurology, 17*(4), 201–207.

Richard, I. H., McDermott, M. P., Kurlan, R., Lyness, J. M., Como, P. G., Pearson, N.,... McDonald, W. (2012). A randomized, double-blind, placebo-controlled trial of antidepressants in Parkinson disease. *Neurology, 78*(16), 1229–1236.

Riedel, O., Heuser, I., Klotsche, J., Dodel, R., & Wittchen, H. U. (2010). Occurrence risk and structure of depression in Parkinson disease with and without dementia: results from the GEPAD Study. *Journal of Geriatric Psychiatry Neurology, 23*(1), 27–34.

Riedel, O., Klotsche, J., Spottke, A., Deuschl, G., Forstl, H., Henn, F.,... Wittchen, H. U. (2010). Frequency of dementia, depression, and other neuropsychiatric symptoms in 1,449 outpatients with Parkinson's disease. *Journal of Neurology, 257*(7), 1073–1082.

Rod, N. H., Bordelon, Y., Thompson, A., Marcotte, E., & Ritz, B. (2013). Major life events and development of major depression in Parkinson's disease patients. *European Journal of Neurology, 20*(4), 663–670.

Rojo, A., Aguilar, M., Garolera, M. T., Cubo, E., Navas, I., & Quintana, S. (2003). Depression in Parkinson's disease: clinical correlates and outcome. *Parkinsonism & Related Disorders, 10*(1), 23–28.

Ryder, K. A., Gontkovsky, S. T., McSwan, K. L., Scott, J. G., Bharucha, K. J., & Beatty, W. W. (2002). Cognitive function in Parkinson's disease: association with anxiety but not depression. *Aging, Neuropsychology, and Cognition, 9*(2), 77–84.

Santangelo, G., Vitale, C., Trojano, L., Longo, K., Cozzolino, A., Grossi, D., & Barone, P. (2009). Relationship between depression and cognitive dysfunctions in Parkinson's disease without dementia. *Journal of Neurology, 256*(4), 632–638.

Schiffer, R. B., Kurlan, R., Rubin, A., & Boer, S. (1988). Evidence for atypical depression in Parkinson's disease. *American Journal of Psychiatry, 145*, 1020–1022.

Serfaty, M. A., Haworth, D., Blanchard, M., Buszewicz, M., Murad, S., & King, M. (2009). Clinical effectiveness of individual cognitive behavioral therapy for depressed older people in primary care: A randomized controlled trial. *Archives of General Psychiatry, 66*(12), 1332–1340.

Shiba, M., Bower, J. H., Maraganore, D. M., McDonnell, S. K., Peterson, B. J., Ahlskog, J. E.,... Rocca, W. A. (2000). Anxiety disorders and depressive disorders preceding Parkinson's disease: a case-control study. *Movement Disorders, 15*(4), 669–677.

Shulman, L. M., Taback, R. L., Rabinstein, A. A., & Weiner, W. J. (2002). Non-recognition of depression and other non-motor symptoms in Parkinson's disease. *Parkinsonism & Related Disorders, 8*(3), 193–197.

Skapinakis, P., Bakola, E., Salanti, G., Lewis, G., Kyritsis, A. P., & Mavreas, V. (2010). Efficacy and acceptability of selective serotonin reuptake inhibitors for the treatment of depression in Parkinson's disease: a systematic review and meta-analysis of randomized controlled trials. *BMC Neurology, 10*, 49.

Sproesser, E., Viana, M. A., Quagliato, E. M., & de Souza, E. A. (2010). The effect of psychotherapy in patients with PD: a controlled study. *Parkinsonism & Relate Disorderd, 16*(4), 298–300.

Starkstein, S. E., Bolduc, P. L., Mayberg, H. S., Preziosi, T. J., & Robinson, R. G. (1990). Cognitive impairments and depression in Parkinson's disease: a follow up study. *Journal of Neurology, Neurosurgery and Psychiatry, 53*(7), 597–602.

Starkstein, S. E., Mayberg, H. S., Leiguarda, R., Preziosi, T. J., & Robinson, R. G. (1992). A prospective longitudinal study of depression, cognitive decline, and physical impairments in patients with Parkinson's disease. *Journal of Neurology, Neurosurgery and Psychiatry, 55*(5), 377–382.

Starkstein, S. E., Merello, M., Jorge, R., Brockman, S., Bruce, D., Petracca, G., & Robinson, R. G. (2008). A validation study of depressive syndromes in Parkinson's disease. *Movement Disorders, 23*(4), 538–546.

Starkstein, S. E., Petracca, G., Chemerinski, E., Teson, A., Sabe, L., Merello, M., & Leiguarda, R. (1998). Depression in classic versus akinetic-rigid Parkinson's disease. *Movement Disorders, 13*(1), 29–33.

Stefanova, E., Potrebic, A., Ziropadja, L., Maric, J., Ribaric, I., & Kostic, V. S. (2006). Depression predicts the pattern of cognitive impairment in early Parkinson's disease. *Journal of Neurological Science, 248*(1-2), 131–137.

Tan, S. K., Hartung, H., Sharp, T., & Temel, Y. (2011). Serotonin-dependent depression in Parkinson's disease: A role for the subthalamic nucleus? *Neuropharmacology, 61*(3), 387–399.

Tandberg, E., Larsen, J. P., Aarsland, D., & Cummings, J. L. (1996). The occurrence of depression in Parkinson's disease. A community-based study. *Archives of Neurology, 53*(2), 175–179.

Tröster, A. I., Woods, S. P., & Morgan, E. E. (2007). Assessing cognitive change in Parkinson's disease: development of practice effect-corrected reliable change indices. *Archives of Clinical Neuropsychology, 22*(6), 711–718.

Uekermann, J., Daum, I., Peters, S., Wiebel, B., Przuntek, H., & Muller, T. (2003). Depressed mood and executive dysfunction in early Parkinson's disease. *Acta Neurologica Scandinavica, 107*(5), 341–348.

Vazquez, A., Jimenez-Jimenez, F. J., Garcia-Ruiz, P., & Garcia-Urra, D. (1993). "Panic attacks" in Parkinson's disease. A long-term complication of levodopa therapy. *Acta Neurologica Scandinavica, 87*(1), 14–18.

Veazey, C., Cook, K. F., Stanley, M., Lai, E.., Kunik, M. E. (2009). Telephone-administered cognitive behavioral therapy: a case study of anxiety and depression in Parkinson's disease (2009). *Journal of Clinical Psychology in Medical Settings,* 16(3), 243–53.

Weintraub, D., & Burn, D. J. (2011). Parkinson's disease: the quintessential neuropsychiatric disorder. *Movement Disorders, 26*(6), 1022–1031.

Weintraub, D., Mavandadi, S., Mamikonyan, E., Siderowf, A. D., Duda, J. E., Hurtig, H. I., . . . Stern, M. B. (2010). Atomoxetine for depression and other neuropsychiatric symptoms in Parkinson disease. *Neurology, 75*(5), 448–455.

Weintraub, D., Moberg, P. J., Duda, J. E., Katz, I. R., & Stern, M. B. (2003). Recognition and treatment of depression in Parkinson's disease. *J Geriatr Psychiatry Neurol, 16*(3), 178–183.

Weintraub, D., Newberg, A. B., Cary, M. S., Siderowf, A. D., Moberg, P. J., Kleiner-Fisman, G., . . . Katz, I. R. (2005). Striatal dopamine transporter imaging correlates with anxiety and depression symptoms in Parkinson's disease.. *Journal of Nuclear Medicine, 46*(2), 227–232.

Weintraub, D., Taraborelli, D., Morales, K. H., Duda, J. E., Katz, I. R., & Stern, M. B. (2006). Escitalopram for major depression in Parkinson's disease: an open-label, flexible-dosage study. *Journal of Neuropsychiatry and Clinical Neuroscience, 18*(3), 377–383.

Weisskopf, M. G., Chen, H., Schwarzschild, M. A., Kawachi, I., & Ascherio, A. (2003). Prospective study of phobic anxiety and risk of Parkinson's disease. *Movement Disorders, 18*(6), 646–651.

Williams,.W. E. S., Jr., Anderson, K., Bush, A. L., Goldstein, S. R., Grill, S., Lehmann, S., . . . Marsh, L. (2012). A comparison of nine scales to detect depression in Parkinson disease: Which scale to use? *Neurology, 78*(13), 998–1006.

Witjas, T., Kaphan, E., Azulay, J. P., Blin, O., Ceccaldi, M., Pouget, J., . . . Cherif, A. A. (2002). Nonmotor fluctuations in Parkinson's disease: frequent and disabling. *Neurology, 59*(3), 408–413.

11 Impulse Control Disorders, Apathy, and Psychosis

Daniel Weintraub and Jennifer G. Goldman

IMPULSE CONTROL DISORDERS

Introduction

Impulse control disorders (ICDs) typically involve pleasurable behaviors that are performed repetitively, excessively, and compulsively, and to an extent that interferes in major areas of life functioning. ICDs have been conceptualized as "behavioral" addictions (Dagher & Robbins, 2009; Holden, 2001), due to extensive overlap between ICDs and disorders of addiction in terms of risk factors, clinical presentation, cognitive aspects, neurobiology, and treatment.

Phenomenology

There is increasing evidence and awareness that ICDs, including compulsive or pathological gambling (PG), and buying, sexual, and eating behaviors can occur as behavioral complications of Parkinson's disease (PD) (Voon & Fox, 2007). Of these disorders, only PG is included as an ICD in the *Diagnostic and Statistical Manual of Mental Disorders* (*DSM-IV-TR*) (2000), but, for convenience, the term ICD has been broadly applied to cover all four of the major ICDs that have been reported to occur in PD patients.

Epidemiology

One of the earliest ICD case series in PD came from Driver-Dunckley et al. (Driver-Dunckley, Samanta, & Stacy, 2003), who identified nine patients (0.5% of the sample) with clinical record documentation of PG. Initial cross-sectional prevalence estimates for ICDs in PD patients from larger formal assessment studies ranged from 1.7% to 7.0% for compulsive gambling, from 2.0 to 4.0% for compulsive sexual behavior, and from 0.4 to 3.0% for compulsive buying (Grosset et al., 2006; Lu, Bharmal, & Suchowersky, 2006; Pontone, Williams, Bassett, & Marsh, 2006; Voon & Fox, 2007; Weintraub, 2008). Compulsive or binge eating was also reported in PD, but its prevalence was not reported initially (Giovannoni, O'Sullivan, Turner, Manson, & Lees, 2000; Nirenberg & Waters, 2006).

Weintraub and co-investigators (Weintraub, Koester, et al., 2010) used a semistructured interview and formal diagnostic criteria (The Massachusetts Gambling Screen score for current problem or pathological gambling, the Minnesota Impulsive Disorders Interview score for compulsive sexual behavior and buying, and *DSM-IV-TR* research criteria for binge eating [i.e., compulsive eating] disorder) to assess the frequency of the four main aforementioned ICDs in more than 3,090 medicated PD patients from 46 movement disorder centers in the United States and Canada (the *DOMINION* study). One or more ICDs was identified in 13.6% of patients (gambling in 5.0%, compulsive sexual behavior in 3.5%, compulsive buying in 5.7%, and binge-eating disorder in 4.3%), and 3.9% of participants had 2 or more ICDs. Similar prevalence findings have been reported in a large Asian study (Lee et al., 2010). Regarding incidence, a cumulative incidence rate (after starting dopamine replacement therapy [DRT]) of 2.4% was reported for compulsive sexual behavior in PD (Voon et al., 2006).

Early case reporting and cross-sectional studies suggested an association between DRT, particularly dopamine agonist (DA) use, and ICDs in PD. In DOMINION, ICDs were more common in patients treated with a DA (17.1%) than in patients not taking a CA (6.9%). Dopamine agonist treatment in PD was associated with 2- to 3.5-fold increased odds of having an ICD compared to patients not taking DAs, nearly all of whom were taking levodopa as their DRT. The frequency of ICDs was similar for the two most commonly used DAs (i.e., 17.7% for pramipexole and 15.5% for ropinirole). Regarding other PD meds, both levodopa (Weintraub, Koester, et al., 2010), especially higher dosages, and amantadine (used primarily in PD patients to treat dyskinesias) (Weintraub, Sohr, et al., 2010) use were associated with ICDs in this study, although to a lesser extent compared with DA treatment. Interestingly, there was not a dosage effect for DAs in this study.

Additional variables associated with ICDs in different studies are a personal or familial history of alcoholism or gambling, impulsive or novelty-seeking characteristics, younger age, male sex, early onset of PD, being unmarried, and current cigarette smoking (Voon & Fox, 2007); (Weintraub, Koester, et al., 2010). In the DOMINION study, another correlate of having an ICD was living in the United States compared with Canada, suggesting that environmental factors play a role in ICD development in PD. Younger patients are more likely to be treated with a DA, but the age effect remained after controlling for DA exposure. Finally, ICD frequency was similar for men and women, but between-sex differences existed for individual ICDs (i.e., men were both more likely to suffer from compulsive sexual behavior compared with women, and women experienced compulsive buying and binge eating more frequently than men).

Dopamine dysregulation syndrome (i.e., *DDS* or compulsive PD medication use) and other ICD-related disorders in PD have not been as well studied as the aforementioned ICDs. A total of 15 DDS cases were reported in the original description of this syndrome in PD (Giovannoni et al., 2000), but a cross-sectional or cumulative prevalence rate was not reported. Regarding punding (i.e., repetitive, simple, non-goal-directed activity), in one series examining PD patients on higher levodopa equivalent daily dosages (*LEDDs*), 14% met criteria for punding (Evans et al., 2004), but another, larger study of unselected PD patients reported a prevalence rate of only 1.4% (Miyasaki, Hassan, Lang, & Voon, 2007).

There has been limited research examining the frequency of ICDs in de novo, untreated PD patients or in comparison with other populations. One recent study found that the overall prevalence of ICDs in newly diagnosed, drug-naive PD patients was similar to that in the general population (Antonini et al., 2011). The few studies done to date suggest that ICDs may be more common in PD than in the general population (Black, 2007; Coleman, 1992; Lilenfeld, Ringham, Kalarchian, & Marcus, 2008; Pietrzak et al., 2007; Shaffer, Hall, & Vander, 1999; Stucki & Rihs-Middel, 2008; Volberg, Nysse-Carris, & Gerstein, 2006) or in assessed healthy control (*HC*) subjects (Avanzi et al., 2006; Giladi, Weitzman, Schreiber, Shabtai, & Peretz, 2007), although one recent study suggested otherwise (de Chazeron et al., 2011). In a study comparing PD patients with restless legs syndrome (RLS) patients treated with a DA, the frequency of ICDs was higher in PD patients, but not after controlling for DA dosage (Ondo & Lai, 2008). Finally, an on-line survey found that ICDs were significantly more common in PD patients compared with amyotrophic lateral sclerosis (ALS) patients (Wicks & MacPhee, 2009).

Diagnosis and Evaluation

Clinical features, diagnostic criteria, and assessment of the aforementioned ICDs in PD have been widely reviewed and documented (Ceravolo, Frosini, Rossi, & Bonuccelli, 2009; Evans, Strafella, Weintraub, & Stacy, 2009; Giovannoni et al., 2000; Pontone et al., 2006; Voon, 2004; Voon & Fox, 2007; Voon et al., 2009; Weintraub, 2008; Weintraub et al., 2009). ICDs in PD may lead to significant impairments in psychosocial functioning, interpersonal relationships, physical health, and quality of life. Patients may not report such behaviors to a treating physician, perhaps due to embarrassment, not suspecting an association with PD treatment, or ambivalence regarding ceasing the behavior. Hence, there is evidence that ICDs are under-recognized in clinical practice (Weintraub et al., 2006). The apparent under-recognition of ICDs in PD can be addressed by reviewing possible risk factors and through patient education prior to initiating DRT treatment, and by ongoing monitoring for ICD and related behaviors.

Diagnostic criteria for compulsive gambling (DSM-IV-TR, 2000), buying (Lejoyeux, Tassain, Solomon, & Adès, 1997), sexual behavior (Voon et al., 2006), and eating (DSM-IV-TR, 2000), all developed for use in the general population and sometimes adapted, have been applied to PD patients. Compulsive gambling often includes those patients with either problem or pathological gambling based on recommended cut-off points (Fisher, 1996). The *DSM-IV-TR* research criteria for binge-eating disorder have been modified to include general overeating in addition to discrete binge-eating episodes, to better match the eating symptoms that PD patients commonly report.

One general screening instrument for ICDs is the Minnesota Impulsive Disorders Interview (MIDI) (Christenson, Faber, & deZwaan, 1994), which queries for some of the ICDs reported to occur in PD. Recently, a screening instrument, the Questionnaire for Impulsive-Compulsive Disorders in Parkinson's Disease (QUIP) was developed and validated to assess ICDs, other compulsive behaviors (punding, hobbyism, and walkabout), and DDS in PD (Weintraub et al., 2009). In addition, the Dopamine Dysregulation Syndrome–Patient and Caregiver Inventory (DDS-PC) was developed as a screening questionnaire to assess the presence of a range of impulsive-compulsive behaviors in PD (Cabrini et al., 2009). Finally, the Movement Disorder Society–Unified Parkinson's Disease Rating Scale (MDS-UPDRS) includes a single item for dopamine dysregulation syndrome, which cover excessive gambling, sexual behaviors, hobbyism, punding, and DDS (Goetz et al., 2008).

In the validation of the QUIP, agreement between patient and informant reporting of ICD symptoms was fair overall, suggesting that it is important to consider the source of information when assessing ICD symptoms in PD patients (Papay et al., 2011). A general recommendation is to include, when possible, both the patient and a reliable informant in the interview process when inquiring about the presence of ICD symptoms in PD patients.

Cognitive Performance of PD Patients with ICDs

Regarding neurotransmitters, dopamine function, particularly within the mesocorticolimbic pathways, is critical in the mediation of reward and reinforcement behaviors. The brain regions most implicated in ICDs include the ventromedial and orbitofrontal regions of the prefrontal cortex, which are involved in planning and judgment, the ventral striatum (particularly the nucleus accumbens [*NAc*]), which is crucial for the reward system, and the amygdala, known to be involved in emotions and conditioned response. Alterations in cortico-striato-thalamo-cortical circuitry contribute to ICD behaviors, with projections involving the more ventral component of the striatum (including the NAc) more, implicated in urges and impulsive aspects, and those engaging the dorsal striatum more, implicated in motor habits and compulsive aspects (Ceravolo et al., 2009; Steeves et al., 2009; Weintraub, 2008).

There are several plausible explanations for a possible association between ICDs in PD and DRT, especially DAs. First, PD leads to a loss of dopaminergic neurons in the substantia nigra, resulting in a pronounced depletion of dopamine in the nigrostriatal pathway (Bjarkam & Sørensen, 2004). Second, PD patients commonly display a range of impairment in executive abilities (Green et al., 2002; Levin & Katzen, 1995), including response inhibition, which has been linked to degeneration in the frontal-striatal tracts secondary to cell loss within the substantia nigra (Brand et al., 2004; Dubois & Pillon, 1997).

Third, de novo, untreated PD patients demonstrated intact punishment learning and impaired reward learning compared with HCs, and acute DA treatment leads to improved reward learning and impaired punishment learning (Bodi et al., 2009), a pattern similar to that demonstrated by established PD patients (Frank, Samanta, Moustafa, & Sherman, 2007; Frank, Seeberger LC, & O'Reilly RC, 2004). Such executive and reward-learning abilities in PD may also be dependent on genetic (e.g., val^{158}met polymorphism of the *COMT* gene) and medication status (being on versus off DRT) (Brusa et al., 2003; Rowe et al., 2008; Williams-Gray, Hampshire, Barker, & Owen, 2008) . On a computerized gambling task of theoretical relevance to ICD behaviors, PD patients were significantly more impaired than controls in performance (both number of disadvantageous choices and ability to use negative feedback for a decision-shift to an advantageous alternative), and task impairment correlated with impairment on other executive measures (Brand et al., 2004). In a study using an intertemporal choice task (i.e., delayed discounting task [DDT]), PD patients without an ICD showed an increase in impulsive decision making, regardless of medication status, compared with HCs (Milenkova et al., 2011). In a recent study that involved administration of computerized decision-making tasks to PD patients on and off DRT (Frank et al., 2007), the medicated group showed impairment in the ability to learn from negative decision outcomes.

Fourth, most of the first-line DAs, compared with levodopa, have significantly higher D_3: D_2 and D_3: D_1 striatal dopamine receptor activation ratios (Gerlach et al., 2003). D_1 and D_2 receptors are located in the dorsal striatum, and their activation by different PD pharmacotherapies is associated primarily with the medications' motor effects. In contrast, the D_3 receptor is concentrated in limbic areas of the brain, including the ventral striatum, and may mediate psychiatric manifestations of dopamine receptor stimulation (Sokoloff, Giros, Martres, Bouthenet, & Schwartz, 1990).

Recent cognitive neuroscience studies in PD have focused on differential neurodegeneration of the striatum in early or mild PD, with the dorsal striatum being more affected than the ventral striatum (Cools, 2006; Cools, Altamirano, & D'Esposito, 2006). It has been proposed that, in mild PD, DRT stimulation of the relatively intact ventral striatal receptors is associated with impairment on cognitive tasks that depend on ventral striatal activation (i.e., dopaminergic "overdose" hypothesis in PD). Of note, the cognitive tasks that rely on ventral striatal activation include stimulus-outcome tasks, which involve the ability to modify behaviors on the basis of outcomes, an ability that is impaired at a clinical level in PD patients with ICDs. Thus, one hypothesis is that excessive, targeted dopamine stimulation of intact ventral striatal receptors in early or mild PD leads to an "overdose" of ventral striatal-cortical circuitry that can manifest itself in the clinical phenomenon of impulsive-compulsive behaviors, including ICDs. These behaviors, similar to addictive disorders, initially may be maintained due to the pleasure feelings induced by the activities, but eventually they are experienced as nonpleasurable, yet uncontrollable (Evans et al., 2006).

Using standard neuropsychological tests, PD patients with ICDs, compared with non-ICD PD patients, have been shown to be impaired on a range of cognitive domains, although not invariably. Specifically, PG patients have been found to demonstrate impairment on bedside tests of frontal lobe abilities compared with non-ICD patients (Santangelo et al., 2009) (Table 11-1). In another study, ICD patients demonstrated impaired spatial planning and set shifting compared with a matched group of non-ICD patients (Vitale et al., 2011). In contrast to the findings mentioned earlier, one study reported no between-group differences on the Stroop Test on or off dopaminergic mediation (Djamshidian, O'Sullivan, Lees, & Averbeck, 2011).

In an early study, PD patients with PG compared with PD controls had higher novelty seeking personality traits and impaired planning characteristics (Voon et al., 2007). In a study using a experiential discounting task (EDT), PD patients with an ICD showed increased impulsive choice and working-memory deficits when exposed to a DA compared with PD control patients (Voon et al., 2010b). In an fMRI study that used a probabilistic gain-and-loss learning task, PD ICD patients responded to DA exposure with increased rate of learning for gain outcomes compared with PD control patients (Voon et al., 2010a). In a recent study of PD patients with and without an ICD, ICD patients demonstrated intact stimulus-reinforcement learning, but had a strong preference for immediate over future rewards using the DDT (Housden, O'Sullivan, Joyce, Lees, & Roiser, 2010). In a study using the Iowa Gambling Task (IGT), PD patients with PG demonstrated worse decision making compared with PD control patients (Rossi et al., 2010). Another study of PD ICD and non-ICD patients that were tested on an off DA treatment reported that only ICD patients demonstrated increased risk taking on the Balloon Analogue Risk Task (*BART*) with DA exposure (Claassen et al., 2011). Finally, in a series of manuscripts based on the same study population, PD patients with a range of ICDs and related disorders had poorer working memory performance and a pattern of altered reward-punishment learning on DRT that differed from PD patients without an ICD (Djamshidian et al., 2010), as well as increased novelty seeking regardless of medication status (Djamshidian, O'Sullivan, Wittmann, et al., 2011).

Pathophysiology and Neural Substrates

There have been several brain PET studies of ICDs in PD using ^{11}C raclopride, which binds to the D2 and D3 receptors (Table 11-2). In the first study, involving PD patients with PG and PD controls, the PG patients demonstrated decreased D2/D3 binding potential at baseline and a relatively greater decrease in binding potential during performance of a gambling task (Steeves et al., 2009). The next study used a levodopa challenge and rewarding visual cues and found that

Table 11-1 Neuropsychology of impulse control disorders

Reference	*Population*	*Methodology*	*Study design*	*Findings*
Voon et al., 2007	PD-PG, PD-C	Case-control study	BIS and TPQ	PD-ICD>PD-C: ↑ novelty seeking and impaired planning
Santangelo et al., 2009	PG-PG, PD-C	Matched	FAB, fluency, Trails	PD-PG>PD-C: ↑ impairment on FAB
Djamshidian et al., 2010	PD-ICD, PD-C, HC	_	Working memory, learning, and gambling task on/off meds	PD-ICDs>PD-C: ↑ worse working memory, ↑ positive feedback learning in OFF state
Voon et al., 2010b	PD-ICD, PD-C, HC	_	Experiential discounting task (EDT) on/off DA	PD-ICDs>PD-C: on DA ↑ impulsive choice, altered reaction time, ↑ working memory impairments
Voon et al., 2010a	PD-ICD, PD-C, HC	Neuropsychology + BOLD fMRI	Scanned on/off DA using gain-loss task	PD-ICD>PD-C: ↑ gain learning on DA
Housden et al., 2010	PD-ICD, PD-C, HC	_	Delayed discounting task and salience attribution task	PD-ICDs>PD-C: ↑ delay discounting, ↑ stimulus-reward learning
Rossi et al., 2010	PD-PG, PD-C	Matched	IGT, Game of Dice, Investment Task	PD-PG>PD-C: ↑ impairment on IGT
Vitale et al., 2011	PD-ICD, PD-C	Matched on age and education	Neuropsychiatric and neuropsychological features	ICD patients impaired on spatial-planning and set-shifting tasks
Djamshidian et al., 2011	PD-ICB, PD-C, HC	HCs age matched	Stroop test on/off dopaminergic medication	No difference between ICB and non-ICB PD patients
Claassen et al., 2011	PD-ICD, PD-C		BART on/off DA	DA increased risk taking in ICD patients only

PD-PG: PD patients with pathological gambling

PD-C: PD controls

PD-ICD: PD patients with one or more impulse control disorders

HD: Healthy controls

PD-ICB: PD patients with a range of impulse control behaviors

Table 11-2 Neurobiology of impulse control disorders

Manuscript	*Population*	*Methodology*	*Study design*	*Findings*
Cilia et al., 2008	PD-PG, PD-C, HC	SPECT resting perfusion	-	PD-PG>PD-C: ↑ perfusion diffusely, including OFC and VS
Lee et al., 2009	PD-ICD, PD-C, HC	Genetics	During medication use	PD-ICDs>PD-C: DRD3 and GRIN2B variants
Steeves et al., 2009	PD-PG, PD-C	^{11}C raclopride imaging	After PD meds WD	PD-PG>PD-C: ↓ VS D2/D3 availability at baseline and during gambling task
Cilia et al., 2010	PD-PG, PD-C, HC	DAT imaging	After PD meds WD	PD-PG>PD-C: ↓ DAT binding
Voon et al., 2010a	PD-ICD, PD-C, HC	BOLD fMRI	Scanned on/off DA using gain-loss task	PD-ICD>PD-C: ↑ VS activity to positive RPE
Van Eimeren et al., 2010	PD-PG, PD-C	PET perfusion during card game	On/off DA	PD-PG>PD-C: ↓ DA-induced perfusion in OFC, cingulate, amygdala, pallidum
Rao et al., 2010	PD-ICD, PD-C	ASL and BOLD fMRI during BART	On meds	PD-PG>PD-C: ↓ VS baseline perfusion and activity to ↑ risk
Frosini et al., 2010	PD-PG, PD-C	BOLD fMRI with visual cues	After PD meds WD	PD-PG>PD-C: ↑ cingulate, prefrontal cortex, precuneus, inferior parietal, VS
Wu et al., 2010	PD-ICD, PD-C	^{11}C raclopride imaging with visual cues	Levodopa challenge	PD-ICDs>PD-C: ↓ VS D2/D3 availability with rewarding vs. neutral visual cues
Rodriguez-Oroz et al., 2011	PD-ICD, PD-C	Field potentials in STN DBS patients	On/off meds	PD-ICDs>PD-C: theta-alpha activity in ventral STN in ON state and cortico-thalamic coherence in frontal regions
Cilia et al., 2011	PD-PG, PD-C	SPECT resting perfusion	Correlation with SOGS	- Gambling severity associated with dysfunction of network involving VLPFC, ACC, PCC, MPFC, insula and striatum - PD-PG with disconnection between the ACC and striatum
Djamshidian et al., 2011	PD-ICB, PD-C, HC	Salivary cortisol levels	Correlation with risk preference on risk task	Increased cortisol levels correlated with increased risk taking in PD-ICB patients

(continued)

Table 11-2 Continued

Manuscript	*Population*	*Methodology*	*Study design*	*Findings*
O'Sullivan et al., 2011	PD-ICB, PD-C	^{11}C raclopride imaging	Exposure to neutral and reward-related cues	PD-ICB patients had decrease in VS D2/D3 availability following reward-related cue exposure with levodopa exposure
Voon et al., 2011	PD-ICD, PD-C	fMRI	Risk taking task	DA exposure in ICD patients associated with enhanced sensitivity to risk along with decreased ventral striatal activity

PD-PG: PD patients with pathological gambling
PD-C: PD controls
PD-ICD: PD patients with one or more impulse control disorders
HD: Healthy controls
PD-ICB: PD patients with a range of impulse control behaviors
SPECT: Single photon emission computed tomography
DAT: Dopamine transporter imaging
BOLD fMRI: Blood oxygen level dependent functional magnetic resonance imaging
PET: Positron emission tomography
ASL: Arterial spin labeled
OFC: Orbitofrontal cortex
VS: Ventral striatum
DRD3: Dopamine receptor D3
GRIN2B: NMDAR2B subunit
D2/D3: Dopamine 2 and dopamine 3 receptors
RPE: Reward prediction error
VLPFC: Ventrolateral prefrontal cortex
ACC: Anterior cingulate cortex
PCC: Posterior cingulate cortex
MPFC: Medial prefrontal cortex

PD patients with an ICD had decreased ventral striatal D2/D3 binding potential with rewarding versus neutral visual cues compared with PD control patients (Wu et al., 2010). The third study reported that PD patients with a range of impulse control behaviors had decreased ventral striatal D2/D3 binding following reward-related cue exposure with levodopa challenge compared with PD control patients (O'Sullivan et al., 2011). Examining a different component of the dopamine system, PD patients with PG, compared with PD controls, had diminished dopamine transporter (DAT) availability in the ventral striatum, which the authors hypothesized was due to lower membrane DAT expression on presynaptic terminals leading to increased dopamine levels in the ventral striatum in PD gamblers (Cilia et al., 2010).

A SPECT study examining brain perfusion in PD patients with PG showed increased brain perfusion in multiple right hemisphere regions linked with impulse control, including the orbitofrontal cortex, hippocampus, parahippocampal gyrus, amygdala, globus pallidus, and nucleus accumbens, as well as the left insula and bilateral precuneus (Cilia et al., 2008). In a follow-up study by the same research group, gambling severity was associated with dysfunction of a network involving multiple prefrontal cortex and striatal regions, and PD patients with PG demonstrated a disconnection between the anterior cingulate cortex and the striatum (Cilia et al., 2011). In another PET study, PD patients with PG compared with PD controls demonstrated decreased cerebral blood flow in the prefrontal cortex, cingulate, amygdala, and pallidum (Van Eimeren et al., 2010).

In an fMRI study using a probabilistic gain and loss learning task, PD patients with an ICD responded to DA exposure with increased striatal reward prediction error (RPE) activity compared with PD controls (Voon et al., 2010a). In a recent study that used both arterial spin labeling (ASL) perfusion and blood oxygenation level dependent (BOLD) fMRI to measure neural responses to risk taking during performance on the BART, PD patients with an ICD demonstrated diminished resting cerebral blood flow and BOLD activity during risk taking in the right ventral striatum compared with PD controls (Rao et al., 2010). Another fMRI study in PD patients with PG reported increased activation, compared with PD controls, on exposure to gambling-related visual cues in several brain regions, including the cingulate cortex and the ventral striatum (Frosini et al., 2010). Finally, in another fMRI study PD-ICD patients on DA treatment had enhanced sensitivity to risk along with decreased ventral striatal activity compared with PD controls on DA treatment (Voon et al., 2011).

In a study of PD patients undergoing subthalamic nucleus (STN) deep brain stimulation (DBS) surgery, oscillatory activity in the theta-alpha band (4-10 Hz) in the ventral-intermediate portion of the STN with cortico–thalamic coherence in the prefrontal cortex was demonstrated in patients with an ICD but not in non-ICD patients (Rodriguez-Oroz et al., 2011), leading excessive DRT leads either to psychiatric complications through its effects on the ventral portion of the STN or to motor complications (e.g., dyskinesias) through its effects on the dorsal portion of the STN.

One study has reported a genetic association for ICDs in PD, specifically the AA genotype of *DRD3 p.S9G* (a D3 receptor subtype) and the CC genotype of *GRIN2B c.366C>g* (a NMDA receptor subtype) (Lee et al., 2009). Another study reported PD patients with a range of impulse control behaviors had increased salivary cortisol levels with increased risk taking, whereas PD controls did not (Djamshidian, O'Sullivan, Papadopoulos, et al., 2011).

Management

Case reporting and anecdotal experience suggest that ICD behaviors often resolve after reducing the dose of the existing DA, switching to a different DA, discontinuing DA treatment entirely, or receiving counseling (Dodd et al., 2005; Driver-Dunckley et al., 2003). In one retrospective case series, the authors documented the long-term clinical outcomes of 15 ICD patients, 80% of whom discontinued or significantly decreased treatment with DA, and all of them experienced full or partial remission of ICD symptoms by self-report (Mamikonyan et al., 2008). A more recent case series reported similar findings in PD patients with only PG (MacPhee & Copeland, 2009). These clinical results suggest that many ICD patients can be adequately managed by making changes to their PD pharmacotherapy regimen. However, many patients do not want or tolerate DA discontinuation, and a DA withdrawal syndrome (DAWS) was recently described in some ICD patients discontinuing DA treatment, characterized by anxiety, dysphoria, autonomic changes, and medication craving (Rabinak & Nirenberg, 2010).

The relationship between DBS surgery and ICDs appears complex. On the one hand, chronic STN DBS has been associated with improvement in ICD symptoms in a small case series, perhaps secondary to significant reductions in DRT that occurred postsurgery (Ardouin et al., 2006). However, there is also anecdotal evidence that ICDs may begin or worsen transiently immediately after STN DBS surgery (Smeding et al., 2007), and a cognitive neuroscience study of PD DBS patients without an ICD found that patients were more impulsive in their decision making when their stimulators were turned on (Frank et al., 2007).

Although used clinically, there is no clinical trial data to support the use of psychiatric drugs for the treatment of ICDs in PD (Ceravolo et al., 2009). A range of psychiatric treatments, most commonly selective serotonin reuptake inhibitors (SSRIs), has been used in the treatment of ICDs in PD. A case series of 15 PD ICD patients reported good treatment effects for zonisamide, an anticonvulsant (Bermejo, Ruiz-Huete, & Anciones, 2010). There are also case reports of successful treatment of ICDs in PD with antipsychotics, including risperidone (Dodd et al., 2005), quetiapine (Sevincok, Akoglu, & Akyol, 2007), and clozapine (Rotondo, Bosco, Plastino, Consoli, & Bosco, 2010). In addition, valproate, lithium, and bupropion have been reported to help individual patients with ICDs (Klos, Bower, Josephs, Matsumoto, & Ahlskog, 2005; Benincasa, Pellicano, Fanciulli, & Pontieri, 2011). In non-PD patients, recent research suggests that nalmefene and naltrexone, both opioid antagonists, are efficacious in the treatment of PG (Grant et al., 2006; Kim, Grant, Adson, & Shin, 2001). A recent small placebo-controlled study reported benefit for amantadine as a treatment for PG in PD (Thomas, Bonnani, Gambi, Di Iorio, & Onofrj, 2010), although amantadine has also been associated with ICDs in DOMINION study (Weintraub, Sohr, et al., 2010b). Behavioral treatments (e.g., cognitive behavioral therapy, motivational interviewing, and Gamblers Anonymous attendance) appear effective in specific groups of patients with PG (Hodgins & Petry, 2004), but their efficacy has not been examined in individuals with PD.

Conclusion

Mounting data, including from prospective studies, suggest that PD medications, especially dopamine agonists, are associated with the development of a variety of ICDs in a subset of PD patients, particularly those with certain demographic or clinical characteristics, whereas higher dosages of levodopa and short-acting DAs may be associated with DDS and punding. A range of cognitive deficits relevant to ICDs have also been reported in PD patients with ICDs, PD patients in general, and PD patients without ICDs who are exposed to dopaminergic therapy, but studies to date have not been able to disentangle state from trait effects.

Given the potential substantial impact of ICDs and related disorders on personal, familial, social, and financial well-being, clinicians should educate PD patients about and closely monitor them for the occurrence of these disorders. Prevention and treatment strategies involve appropriate patient education, clinical assessment, careful DA dosing, and ICD symptom monitoring throughout treatment. Existing data suggest that clinical management of clinically significant ICDs should involve serious consideration of a prompt discontinuation or decrease in DA treatment. In addition, empirically validated treatments are emerging for ICDs and should be considered for patients with co-occurring PD and ICDs.

APATHY

Introduction

Apathy is gaining increasing recognition as an important clinical syndrome that occurs in the context of many psychiatric, neurological, and neurodegenerative diseases, including PD. However, it is a controversial syndrome, in part due to the lack of self-awareness that hampers assessment, as well as to the significant overlap between apathy and both depression and cognitive impairment. In addition, although great strides have been made in the epidemiology and assessment of apathy, relatively little is known about its pathophysiology and how best to treat it.

Phenomenology

Although apathy is reported to occur in numerous neuropsychiatric disorders and neurodegenerative diseases (Chase, 2011; Onyike et al., 2007), including Alzheimer's disease (AD) (Starkstein, Petracca, Chemerinski, & Kremer, 2001), current psychiatric classifications systems do not provide a clear definition. In general, apathy is succinctly defined as a lack of motivation, manifested as a decrease goal-directed behavior, verbalization, and emotional expression.

It has been proposed that motor fluctuations, characterized by dyskinesias, and ICDs may represent two sides of the same coin (i.e., the motor and nonmotor complications induced by chronic DRT) (Voon et al., 2009). In addition, it has also been proposed that nonmotor behaviors in PD can be roughly characterized as being hypodopaminergic (e.g., apathy and depression) or hyperdopaminergic (e.g., ICDs and DDS; Thobois et al., 2010). For patients who experience motor fluctuations, alternating between "on" (peak dopamine levels) and "off" (trough dopamine levels) periods, it is increasingly recognized that a range of concurrent nonmotor fluctuations (NMFs) can occur as well (Witjas et al., 2002). Apathy has been reported to be a common NMF during "off" periods (Witjas et al., 2002), often improving during "on" periods, even to the extent of experiencing elation or euphoria (Fox & Lang, 2008).

Epidemiology

With the introduction of levodopa in the mid-1960s, an "awakening" effect was reported (Yahr, Duvoisin, Schear, Barrett, & Hoehn, 1969), suggesting that dopaminergic therapy in de novo PD patients can lead to decreased apathy. However, in spite of wide availability and near universal use of dopaminergic therapies, apathy is still reported to be present in approximately 20–50% of PD patients assessed cross-sectionally (Butterfield, Cimino, Oelke, Hauser, & Sanchez-Ramos, 2010; Dujardin et al., 2007; Isella et al., 2002; Kirsch-Darrow, Fernandez, Marsiske, Okun, & Bowers, 2006; Starkstein et al., 1992; Starkstein et al., 2009), but it is less common when comorbid depression and dementia are excluded (Pedersen, Larsen, Alves, & Aarsland, 2009). Due to the significant overlap between apathy, depression, cognitive impairment, and even the motor symptoms of PD (e.g., masked facies and slowness of movement), some have argued that it is difficult to conclude that apathy is an independent clinical syndrome in PD (Bogart, 2011).

However, although there is significant overlap between apathy, depression, and dementia (Pedersen, Alves, Aarsland, & Larsen, 2009; Starkstein et al., 2009), apathy also occurs independently of these syndromes in a subset of patients (Dujardin et al., 2007; Kirsch-Darrow et al., 2006; Reijnders et al., 2010; Starkstein et al., 1992; Varanese, Perfetti, Ghilardi, & Di Rocco, 2011). Similar to depression, apathy is associated with impaired function (Isella et al., 2002) and also has a bidirectional relationship with cognitive decline (Dujardin, Sockeel, Delliaux, Destee, & Defebvre, 2009; Pedersen et al., 2009). The relationship between apathy and motor severity is not clear; in general, there is not a strong association between apathy severity and measures of overall motor impairment (Dujardin et al., 2007; Isella et al., 2002; Pedersen et al., 2009; Reijnders et al., 2010), but specific motor features (e.g., axial impairment) may predict long-term development of apathy (Pedersen et al., 2009).

Diagnosis and Evaluation

Apathy usually is accompanied by diminished self-awareness, so changes typically are noticed and brought to the attention of clinicians by caregivers or informed others. A common assumption is that the patient is depressed, although a lack of endorsement of sad mood and the typical cognitive changes seen in depression (e.g., guilt, helplessness, suicide ideation, and hopelessness) suggest a diagnosis of apathy instead. One of the *DSM-IV-TR* gateway symptoms for major depressive disorder is "diminished interest *or* pleasure in activities," and, to help distinguish apathy from depression, proposed depression criteria for both AD (Olin et al., 2002) and PD (Marsh et al., 2006) have suggested differentiating diminished interest (which is thought to be more specific to apathy) from diminished pleasure (anhedonia is thought to be more specific to depression). It is also important to distinguish between apathy and PD-induced cognitive and motor slowness.

Recently, formal *DSM-IV*-style diagnostic criteria for apathy in PD were proposed, with a focus on impairment in three domains: (1) diminished goal directed behavior, (2) diminished goal directed cognition, and (3) diminished concomitants of goal directed behavior (Starkstein et al., 2009; Starkstein & Leentjens, 2008). In a subsequent study, the acceptability and internal consistency of the criteria were good, and the Lille Apathy Rating Scale (LARS) and the apathy section of the Neuropsychiatric Inventory (NPI) demonstrated good concurrent validity (Drijgers, Dujardin, Reijnders, Defebvre, & Leentjens, 2010). For the use of rating scales to assess apathy, a Movement Disorder Society Task Force recommended the use of the Apathy Scale (Leentjens et al., 2008), although, since this recommendation was published, the LARS has also undergone validation.

Cognitive Performance of PD Patients with Apathy

Most studies using global measures of cognitive abilities (e.g., the Dementia Rating Scale) have shown a strong association between worse global cognition, including presence of dementia, and higher levels of apathy (Dujardin et al., 2007). In addition, presence of apathy at baseline in nondemented PD patients is associated with greater long-term cognitive decline, particular executive impairment, and conversion to dementia (Dujardin et al., 2009). Using specific, detailed neuropsychological tests, associations between apathy and executive deficits, memory impairment, and bradyphrenia have been reported (Starkstein et al., 1992; Isella et al., 2002; Pluck & Brown, 2002; Varanese et al., 2011). In one small study that included both PD patients and HCs, increasing severity of apathy in PD patients was associated with worse performance on executive measures (i.e., category verbal fluency and the Executive Interview [EXIT]), but not on memory measures (Isella et al., 2002). Another recent study also demonstrated an association between increasing severity of apathy, but not depression, and worse executive functioning (Butterfield et al., 2010). Interestingly, both apathy and depression were associated with worse memory performance in this study.

Pathophysiology and Neural Substrates

In general, dysfunction of the limbic cortico–basal ganglia-thalamo–cortical loop is thought to be the common neural substrate of apathy in different disease states (Duffy, 1997; Levy & Dubois, 2006;). Regarding neurotransmitters, goal-directed behavior is associated with both dopaminergic and noradrenergic function (Duffy, 1997). Connections between apathy and the dopaminergic system are also supported by studies and models of drug addiction, in which downregulation of the dopaminergic system is associated with apathy during periods of abstinence, and administration of stimulants, which induce dopamine release, are associated with feelings of euphoria and increased motivation (Volkow, Fowler, Wang, Baler, & Telang, 2009).

Given the high prevalence and adverse impact of apathy symptoms in PD, it is surprising that there have been relatively few neuroimaging studies examining its neural correlates (Kostic & Filippi, 2011). In one recent study, high apathy scores were correlated with low gray matter density values in number of brain regions, including the precentral gyrus, inferior parietal gyrus, inferior frontal gyrus, insula, cingulate gyrus, and precuneus (Reijnders et al., 2010). However, not all imaging studies have reported associations between apathy and brain morphometric changes (Isella et al., 2002), perhaps related to methodological issues (Kostic & Filippi, 2011).

In a PET study examining cerebral metabolism in PD patients who had undergone STN DBS, higher apathy scores were correlated with decreased glucose metabolism in posterior cingulate gyrus, a region thought to be important to the encoding of emotional significance of stimuli (Le Jeune et al., 2009).

With the increasing use of DBS, particularly STN DBS, as a treatment for advanced or severe PD, the relationship between apathy and surgical intervention has undergone increasing scrutiny. Apathy has been reported to occur in a subset of PD patients post-DBS surgery, both in the early postoperative period and on long-term follow-up (Krack et al., 2003). Preliminary research suggested that development of apathy post-DBS might be related to dopaminergic medication withdrawal, and was responsive to administration of dopamine agonist treatment (Czernecki et al., 2008). However, the situation is complex, because no correlation has been found between the decrease in dopaminergic medication and the occurrence of apathy postoperatively (Drapier et al., 2006), and it has been argued that STN stimulation may directly induce apathy through limbic system stimulation (Le Jeune et al., 2009). In a recent prospective study of PD undergoing STN DBS, DA treatment was immediately discontinued postoperatively, and was introduced if patients developed either apathy or depression (Thobois et al., 2010). Overall, total DRT (i.e., DA + levodopa dosage) was reduced by 82%. Approximately 50% of patients developed apathy postoperatively, and 50% of those patients experienced improvement in apathy symptoms with reintroduction of DA treatment. A subset of apathetic and nonapathetic patients underwent brain PET scanning with ^{11}C raclopride, which binds to D2/D3 receptors, pre- and posttreatment with oral methylphenidate, a stimulant that enhances brain dopamine function. In this substudy, apathetic patients demonstrated greater D2/D3 receptor density (or reduced synaptic dopamine levels) in diffuse brain regions, as well as decreased ability to release dopamine in response to methylphenidate challenge. The authors concluded that apathy post-DBS is related to a delayed dopamine withdrawal syndrome, and is associated with mesolimbic dopaminergic denervation.

Management

There have been no controlled treatment studies for apathy, neither in PD nor in the context of any other disease state (Chase, 2011). Treatable co-morbid psychiatric conditions (e.g., depression) should be addressed initially. Anecdotally, psychostimulants (e.g., methylphenidate and dextroamphetamine) and stimulant-related compounds (e.g., modafinil and bupropion) are used in clinical practice, but their effectiveness for this condition is not known beyond case reporting (Chatterjee & Fahn, 2002). Based on the proposed neuropathophysiology of apathy, antidepressants and other medications that increase dopamine or norepinephrine activity (e.g., DAs, tricyclic antidepressants [TCAs], dual reuptake inhibitor antidepressants, bupropion, and atomoxetine) may be beneficial (Marin, Fogel, Hawkins, Duffy, & Krupp, 1995), and there is case reporting that suggests benefit with cholinesterase inhibitor treatment in AD patients (Chase, 2011). As mentioned previously, apathy in the context of DRT withdrawal post-DBS surgery is reported to be responsive to reintroduction of DA treatment (Czernecki et al., 2008; Thobois et al., 2010). In addition to pharmacologic treatment, it is important to educate patients and families on the distinction between apathy and depression and to encourage steps that overcome patient inertia and may lead to improved functioning and quality of life (Shulman, 2000).

Conclusion

Apathy is a common and little-understood nonmotor complication in PD. It is associated with significant impairments in functioning and quality of life, and also leads to caregiver distress. Although the overlap with depression and cognitive impairment is significant, apathy can occur independently of both. Studies of apathy in PD have reported associations with executive deficits, verbal-memory impairment, and bradyphrenia, and the strongest neural correlates are with decreased cingulate and inferior frontal gyri brain volumes. Remarkably, there have been no treatment studies for apathy in PD, but preliminary clinical experience suggests that, in some patients, it may be responsive to dopaminergic therapy. Clearly, a better understanding of neurobiology and improved management strategies are needed for apathy in PD.

PSYCHOSIS

Introduction

PD psychosis is frequent, affecting about one-third of patients treated with chronic dopaminergic therapy (Fenelon & Alves, 2010), and is often associated with increased morbidity, mortality (Factor et al., 2003), nursing-home placement (Goetz & Stebbins, 1995), caregiver stress (Stella, Banzato, Quagliato, Viana, & Christofoletti, 2009), and worsened quality of life (McKinlay et al., 2008). Psychosis is intricately linked to cognitive function in PD. Impaired cognitive status is a risk factor for the development of PD psychosis (Fenelon, Mahieux, Huon,

& Ziegler, 2000); compared to nonhallucinating PD patients, PD hallucinators exhibit greater cognitive deficits, particularly in domains of attention, executive function, and visuospatial abilities. Moreover, recent studies have explored the potential of cholinesterase inhibitors in the treatment of demented PD patients with hallucinations. Medications such as cholinesterase inhibitors could provide alternative pharmacological strategies for the treatment of PD psychosis, which can be especially challenging since antipsychotic medications with dopamine blocking properties can worsen motor symptoms of PD.

Phenomenology

Psychosis in PD manifests predominantly as hallucinations and delusions (Diederich, Goetz, & Stebbins, 2005; Fenelon et al., 2000; Graham, Grunewald, & Sager, 1997; Papapetropoulos & Mash, 2005; Sanchez-Ramos, Ortoll, & Paulson, 1996). Recently revised criteria, however, extend the clinical spectrum of PD psychosis to include illusions, a false sense of presence, hallucinations, and delusions (Ravina et al., 2007). On the milder end of the spectrum are "minor" hallucinations including illusions, presence hallucinations, and passage hallucinations. Illusions or misperceptions of real stimuli include the interpretation of inanimate objects as living beings (e.g., a chair mistaken for a dog, a lamppost mistaken for a tree). "Presence" hallucinations evoke the sense that someone is nearby when no one is really there, whereas "passage" hallucinations involve the sensation of a person or animal passing in the person's peripheral visual field. These "minor" hallucinations are usually not troublesome for the patient or caregiver and, thus, may not necessitate treatment interventions with antipsychotics.

Hallucinations in PD are defined by the sensory modality affected and classified as simple or complex. Most hallucinations in PD are visual, although they also can occur in auditory, tactile, olfactory, and gustatory modalities (Fenelon, Thobois, Bonnet, Broussolle, & Tison, 2002; Tousi & Frankel, 2004). In general, hallucinations in nonvisual modalities are frequently accompanied by visual hallucinations and occur in more advanced PD (Fenelon et al., 2000; Goetz, Stebbins, & Ouyang, 2011). In a longitudinal study, the presence of hallucinations in both visual and nonvisual modalities increased over time, occurring in 26% of PD hallucinators at 4-year follow up and in 60% at 10-year follow up; once hallucinations occurred in multiple sensory modalities, the risk of continuing to have multimodal hallucinations was high (odds ratio 3.67, confidence interval 1.13–11.96) (Goetz et al., 2011). Auditory hallucinations in PD are often vague and, in contrast to schizophrenia, are less common and less likely to be threatening or directly interact with the patient (Diederich et al., 2005). Simple hallucinations in PD lack form (e.g., photopsias, flashes of light or color). Complex hallucinations include clearly defined or formed visions that may take the shape of animals, humans, or other objects (Barnes & David, 2001; Friedman et al., 2011). In PD, common complex visual hallucinations include mice scurrying on the floor; children playing in the house; or sometimes distorted, grotesque, or bizarre figures.

Hallucinations in PD tend to be nonthreatening, consist of familiar humans or animals, and occur with a clear sensorium (Goetz, Tanner, & Klawans, 1982; Graham et al., 1997). They are typically brief (lasting seconds to minutes) and may increase at night or in instances of compromised or low vision (Marsh, 2005). Some hallucinations are "benign," but others can be quite elaborate or frightening. Some seemingly benign hallucinations, however, may evolve into "malignant" hallucinations, particularly in the setting of advanced PD, clouded sensorium, diminished insight or cognitive function, or when accompanied by delusions (Goetz, Ouyang, Negron, & Stebbins, 2010; Papapetropoulos & Mash, 2005).

Delusions are less common than hallucinations in PD psychosis and affect about 5–10% of drug-treated PD patients (Fenelon & Alves, 2010). In PD, delusions often focus on a single theme such as jealousy, spousal infidelity, paranoia, abandonment, or somatic illnesses (Marsh, 2005). Although persecutory delusions are common in both PD and schizophrenia, delusions in schizophrenia more frequently encompass themes of grandiosity, reference, and bizarre beliefs (Black & Boffeli, 1989). Systematized paranoid delusions were more common than nonspecific paranoid ideation (56% versus 44%) in a small cohort of PD patients with psychosis (Marsh, 2004). Misidentification syndromes are specific types of delusions and are frequently associated with PD dementia. Two common misidentification syndromes include: Capgras syndrome, in which the patient thinks that his recognizable spouse is an imposter (Aarsland, Marsh, & Schrag, 2009), and Fregoli syndrome, in which the patient believes that familiar people are, often malevolently, disguised as strangers (Stewart, 2008). These misidentification syndromes can lead to difficult interpersonal situations for the patient and caregiver. In a prospective study of demented PD patients, delusional misidentification syndromes occurred in 16.7% (Pagonabarraga et al., 2008). Case reports describe misidentification syndromes in patients with parkinsonism and dementia (Roane, Rogers, Robinson, & Feinberg, 1998), and in one report of a PD patient with Fregoli syndrome, the misidentification syndrome resolved with reduction in levodopa dose (Stewart, 2008).

Epidemiology

Prevalence estimates of PD psychosis range from approximately 20–60% but vary greatly due to methodological differences among studies (Aarsland, Larsen, Cummings, & Laake, 1999; Fenelon & Alves, 2010; Graham et al., 1997; Holroyd, Currie, & Wooten, 2001; Sanchez-Ramos et al., 1996). Studies differ regarding the population source (community versus clinic based), design (retrospective versus prospective), types of prevalence values (point, period, or lifetime), symptoms included (illusions, hallucinations and/or delusions), and measurements or rating scales used. Further, reliance on the subjective accounts of the patient and/or caregiver makes identifying and rating psychosis challenging. Clinic-based and cross-sectional studies provide point prevalence rates in PD patients on dopaminergic treatment, whereas others provide frequency estimates of developing hallucination (Fenelon & Alves, 2010). In a longitudinal study, 60% of PD patients developed hallucinations or delusions at 12-year follow-up; 42% of the cohort developed new psychosis during the study, at a mean of 13 years after motor symptom onset (Forsaa et al., 2010). In a long-term follow-up study of PD patients without hallucinations at baseline, 93% of the original 60 nonhallucinating PD patients had hallucinations on at least one interview at 10-year follow-up. The prevalence of hallucinations increased from 33% at baseline to 63% at 10 years, and the odds of having hallucinations increased annually by a factor of 1.26 (Goetz et al., 2010). In the Sydney Multicenter Study, which followed a cohort of initially levodopa-naïve PD patients, 50% of patients had formed visual hallucinations at 15-year follow-up, with a mean time to onset of hallucinations of 10.7 years (Hely, Morris, Reid, & Trafficante, 2005). Among the survivors of the same cohort, 74% experienced visual hallucinations at 20-year follow-up, requiring reduction of dopaminergic medication in all and initiation of an atypical antipsychotic in 10 patients (Hely, Reid, Adena, Halliday, & Morris, 2008).

Recently, a National Institutes of Health NINDS-NIMH sponsored working group reviewed and proposed diagnostic criteria for PD psychosis (Ravina et al., 2007). Prevalence estimates of PD psychosis depend, in part, on operational definitions used, and uniform diagnostic criteria may help to reduce variability in frequency estimates. According to the NINDS-NIMH criteria, the diagnosis of PD psychosis requires at least one of the following: illusions, false sense of presence, hallucinations, or delusions. These features should occur after the onset of PD and be present for at least one month, either as recurrent or continuous symptoms; other medical, neurological, or psychiatric causes and acute delirium should be excluded. Associated features for assessment include the presence or absence of insight, dementia, or treatment for PD. When NINDS-NIMH criteria were applied to a cross-sectional PD cohort, the prevalence of PD psychosis was 60%, compared to 43% when defined by only the presence of hallucinations and/or delusions (Fenelon, Soulas, Zenasni, & de Langavant, 2010). Minor psychotic phenomena and nonvisual hallucinations, features not often included in older epidemiological studies, represent an important part of the PD psychosis spectrum.

Diagnosis and evaluation

In the clinical setting, the diagnosis of PD psychosis is largely based on the historical report obtained from the patient, caregiver, or other informant. Hallucinations and delusions, by virtue of their potentially bizarre nature, are frequently underreported. PD patients may be reluctant to spontaneously report illusions, hallucinations, or delusions. In many cases, caregivers are often unaware of them until the psychosis becomes problematic. Thus, the physician or other medical professional needs to ask about these phenomena at clinic visits, regularly and in a nonjudgmental manner.

Several rating scales for PD psychosis have been developed for research or clinical purposes, but most have been borrowed or adapted from assessment tools used in other psychotic disorders such as schizophrenia. Since psychosis in schizophrenia and PD, however, differ phenomenologically, rating scales that specifically address hallucinations, delusions, and other psychotic phenomena in PD are needed. Furthermore, psychotic symptoms in PD are inherently difficult to rate since the symptoms are subjective in nature and may not occur in the presence of physicians or at the time of the clinic visit. To address some of these issues, the Movement Disorder Society Task Force on Rating Scales for PD systematically critiqued scales used for assessing PD psychosis (Fernandez et al., 2008). The Task Force designated scales as Recommended, if they had been used specifically in PD, used by multiple authors or groups other than the people who developed the scale, and had clinimetric testing of the scale. A total of 12 psychosis scales or questionnaires were reviewed, and 4 scales met the Recommended criteria: the Neuropsychiatric Inventory (NPI), Brief Psychiatric Rating Scale (BPRS), Positive and Negative Syndrome Scale (PANSS), and Scale for Assessment of Positive Symptoms (SAPS). Each scale has different advantages and disadvantages. Some have a more structured format and standardized method of administration; others include questions on other behavioral or motor features. None of these scales, however, was considered by the Task Force to be a definitive rating tool for assessing PD psychosis; efforts to develop a new scale for PD psychosis are currently ongoing (Goetz, 2009).

Dopaminergic medications have been well recognized to induce psychosis in PD by stimulating or inducing hypersensitivity of mesocorticolimbic dopamine receptors. Virtually all classes of antiparkinsonian medications may produce psychosis in PD. Some studies suggest particular susceptibility with dopamine agonists with D2 or D3 receptor agonism compared to levodopa (Biglan, Holloway, McDermott, & Richard, 2007; LeWitt, Lyons, Pahwa, & SP 650 Study, 2007; Rascol et al., 2000) and with anticholinergics, especially in elderly PD patients (de Smet et al., 1982). Although dopaminergic and anticholinergic medications can contribute to PD psychosis, other extrinsic factors (e.g., infections, medical illnesses) or PD-related complications (e.g., visual, sleep, mood, or cognitive disturbances) may play a role in acute or chronic psychosis and may necessitate further evaluation.

Acute psychosis in PD, particularly when accompanied by delirium, should prompt an evaluation for other medical and neurological conditions besides PD and a review of the patient's medication regimen. Although acute psychosis in PD with or without delirium may be due to effects of dopaminergic medications, other causes such as toxic-metabolic encephalopathy, urinary or pulmonary infections, stroke, subdural hematoma, or medication interaction (Klein, Prokhorov, Miniovitz, Dobronevsky, & Rabey, 2009) should be excluded. When delirium is present, confusion, agitation, and myoclonus may accompany the psychosis. Evaluations may require basic laboratory studies, work-up for infection, toxicology screens, and neuroimaging. It is important to determine if there have been recent changes in medications for PD or other disorders (e.g., bladder dysfunction, pain, sleep, etc.), adjustments in medication doses, or any interactions between medications. The initial evaluation for acute PD psychosis frequently occurs in the emergency department or outpatient clinic setting, and psychotic PD patients may require hospital admission for management. Of all PD patient admissions to a community hospital during a 6-year period, 24% were due to psychosis, and drug-induced psychosis was the cause of repeated and prolonged admissions in 29% of patients (Klein et al., 2009). In addition, it is useful to ascertain if the patient has previously experienced similar presentations, particularly in the context of urinary tract infections or noncompliance with medications. Other features such as sensory deficits (i.e., visual or hearing impairment or loss) may contribute to PD psychosis.

Cognitive Performance of PD Patients with Psychosis

PD psychosis is closely tied to cognitive functions including visual processing, attention, executive function, and memory. Several studies suggest that PD hallucinators exhibit distinct neuropsychological deficits. Visual hallucinations are common in demented PD patients, occurring in about 40–87% (Fenelon & Alves, 2010). The presence of cognitive impairment and dementia in PD is associated with higher risk of developing psychosis. PD patients with psychosis, particularly minor visual hallucinations, may or may not retain cognitive insight. Hallucinations, however, also occur in nondemented PD patients, with prevalence estimates ranging from 5–17% (Fenelon & Alves, 2010; Kulisevsky et al., 2008). This section will review cognitive features of nondemented and demented PD patients with hallucinations.

Several studies examining cognitive deficits in nondemented PD hallucinators suggest that on neuropsychological testing, these patients have worse attentional, executive, and visuospatial function (Table 11-3). Nondemented PD hallucinators (defined by Mini-Mental State Examination (MMSE) scores > 23) exhibited significantly worse performance on tasks of verbal learning—immediate recall (Rey auditory 15-word learning test [RAVLT]), semantic fluency (production of words belonging to 4 semantic categories each within 2 minutes) and phonological fluency (words beginning with the letters F, A, and S within 1 minute), compared to nondemented PD without hallucinations (Grossi et al., 2005); performance on delayed free recall or the Raven's 47 Colored Progressive Matrices, however, was not significantly different between patient groups. In a follow-up study of 36 PD patients from this cohort, 21 PD patients had hallucinations at 2 years (Santangelo et al., 2007), including 9 patients who had hallucinations at baseline. Comparison of those PD patients with hallucinations at baseline and follow-up, only at follow-up, and at neither time point (nonhallucinators) revealed group differences in semantic fluency, phonological fluency, and immediate free recall, due to worse scores in those with hallucinations. Ramirez-Ruiz et al. examined PD patients with and without hallucinations, who were considered nondemented by the *DSM-IV-TR* criteria for dementia, and healthy controls, using a neuropsychological battery that tested general intellectual ability, language, verbal memory, visual memory, executive function, and visuoperceptive function (Ramirez-Ruiz, Junque, Marti,

Table 11–3 Cognitive performance in non-demented PD hallucinators

Reference	*PD-H (n)*	*PD-NH (n)*	*Worse performance in PD-H*
Barnes et al., 2003	17	20	• Visual object perception • Facial recognition memory
Grossi et al., 2005	14	34	• Verbal learning—immediate recall (RAVLT) • Semantic/phonological fluency
Ramirez-Ruiz, et al., 2006	24	21	• RAVLT learning • Benton facial recognition (controlling for MMSE, Hoehn &Yahr stage, Hamilton depression) • BNT, Token test • Semantic fluency • Visual form discrimination
Barnes et al., 2008	17	20	• Stroop, Go-No-Go • Verbal fluency • 2-back test (false alarms)
Llebaria et al., 2010	29	28	• Verbal fluency • PD-CRS posterior cortical score, clock copy task

Abbreviations:

PD-H: PD hallucinators, PD-NH: PD non-hallucinators; RAVLT: Raven's Auditory Verbal Learning Test; MMSE: Mini-mental state examination; PD-CRS: PD-Cognitive Rating Scale

Valldeoriola, & Tolosa, 2006). Hallucinating PD patients had significantly worse performance on all neuropsychological tests except for the recognition task of the RAVLT, compared to healthy controls and significantly worse scores on language (Token Test, Boston Naming Test), verbal learning (RAVLT), semantic fluency (animal names produced within 1 minute), and visuoperceptive function (Benton Facial Recognition, Visual Form Discrimination), compared to nonhallucinators; these differences were independent of general cognitive status, disease severity, and depression. These authors also followed a cohort of PD hallucinators, PD nonhallucinators, and healthy controls over 1 year, reporting that about 70% of the nondemented PD hallucinators had impairment on multiple cognitive domains, with 45% meeting dementia criteria at follow-up (Ramirez-Ruiz et al., 2007). Another study of PD patients with and without hallucinations and age-matched controls found greater impairment on tests of inhibitory ability (Stroop, Go-no-go, and verbal fluency) in the hallucinator group (Barnes & Boubert, 2008). In a prospective study of hallucinating PD patients matched for age, education, medications, and disease duration to nonhallucinating PD patients, those PD patients with minor visual hallucinations did not differ significantly in any cognitive domain from the nonhallucinators.

PD patients with major visual hallucinations and retained insight, however, exhibited executive dysfunction (worse verbal fluency) suggesting frontal–subcortical impairment, and those hallucinators lacking insight had impairment in cognitive tasks reflecting posterior cortical dysfunction (Llebaria et al., 2010). Although these studies have small sample sizes (ranging from 14–29 PD hallucinators) and differ in definitions of PD dementia and neuropsychological test batteries used, they suggest that not only frontal–striatal cognitive deficits, but also more widespread cortical dysfunction occurs in hallucinating PD patients, particularly those who convert to dementia.

Psychotic phenomena in PD, particularly "minor visual hallucinations" (illusions, presence hallucinations, and passage hallucinations) may reflect aberrant visual cognitive processes. Misinterpretation or false recognition of very brief, minor perceptual cues due to impairment in visual cognitive processing and perceptual representations may lead to visual hallucinations (Fenelon et al., 2000). PD hallucinators may exhibit impaired source monitoring such that there is confusion between internal representations of events and real events (Barnes, Boubert, Harris, Lee, & David, 2003). Barnes et al. studied visual cognitive function in PD patients with and without visual hallucinations and age-matched controls, using tests of visual imagery (mental imagery questions, vividness of visual imagery questionnaire), visual perception (Visual Object and Space Perception Test), and visual memory (facial recognition test, word and picture memory). Hallucinating PD patients had intact visual imagery processes and spatial perception but impaired facial recognition memory and object perception as well as misidentification of stimuli sources (word or image), compared to the nonhallucinating PD and healthy controls. PD hallucinators demonstrated impaired identification of silhouettes of common objects and animals, termed "visual silhouette agnosia," suggestive of a conflict of higher and lower-order perceptual processes. Visual hallucinations in PD have been hypothesized to be the behavioral consequences of abnormally processed externally derived and internally generated visual information, due to factors including dopaminergic/cholinergic imbalances, impaired contrast and color discrimination, visual memory deficits, and disruptions of attention and sleep cycles (Diederich et al., 2005).

Few studies have examined neuropsychological profiles in large groups of demented PD patients. In a subanalysis of PDD patients who participated in a large, double-blind, placebo-controlled trial of rivastigmine (Emre et al., 2004), cognitive profiles of 86 PDD patients with hallucinations were compared to 86 PDD patients without hallucinations, who were matched for age, education, sex, and levodopa equivalent doses (Bronnick, Emre, Tekin, Haugen, & Aarsland, 2011). In logistic regression models, worse choice reaction time was the only independent predictor of hallucinations in demented PD, thereby suggesting a possible association between impaired top-down attentional control processes and hallucinations in PDD.

Pathophysiology and Neural Substrates

PD psychosis may be caused by extrinsic (i.e., pharmacological treatment with dopaminergics) and/or intrinsic (i.e., disease-related) factors. Intrinsic or PD-related factors that may contribute to psychosis include abnormalities in the visual, sleep, mood, and cognitive processes. Other intrinsic factors associated with increased risk of developing psychosis include older age, greater axial rigidity, advanced disease, and potentially genetic susceptibilities (Factor et al., 2011; Fenelon et al., 2000; Sanchez-Ramos et al., 1996). The pathophysiology of PD psychosis has focused on three main neurotransmitter systems, dopamine, acetylcholine, and serotonin and on three primary neuroanatomical areas, the visual system, brainstem function and cortex. These neurotransmitter systems and neuroanatomical regions underlie the clinical manifestations of psychosis and associated nonmotor features of visual disturbances, sleep disturbances, mood disorders, or cognitive impairment. PD psychosis may result from interactions between behavioral and cognitive phenomena and abnormalities in "top-down" and/or "bottom-up" processing. This section will briefly review the pathophysiology of PD psychosis, with special emphasis on the relationship between cognitive impairment and psychosis.

Visual dysfunction has been hypothesized to play a role in PD psychosis and ranges from ocular pathology and retinal dopamine loss, impaired visual acuity and color or contrast discrimination, to disturbed attentional and visuospatial processing and abnormal cortical activation patterns (Diederich et al., 1998; Diederich et al., 2005; Holroyd et al., 2001; Holroyd & Wooten, 2006; Pieri, Diederich, Raman, & Goetz, 2000; Stebbins et al., 2004). Retinal dopaminergic dysfunction in PD may reduce the input of meaningful information for central visual processing (Djamgoz, Hankins, Hirano, & Archer, 1997). Moreover, PD hallucinators have impaired visual acuity, contrast sensitivity, and color discrimination, compared to nonhallucinators (Diederich et al., 1998; Pieri et al., 2000).

Hallucinations may be the consequence of altered brainstem function, as manifested by sleep dysfunction. Sleep disturbances are frequent in PD patients, including those with hallucinations. PD hallucinations may be related to sleep fragmentation and altered dream phenomena, but whether this represents a stepwise pattern or "continuum" (Arnulf I et al., 2000), distinct but related factors (Goetz, Wuu, Curgian, & Leurgans, 2005), or predictors of future hallucinations (Forsaa et al., 2010; Goetz et al., 2005) is uncertain. Visual hallucinations in PD may represent intrusions of rapid-eye movement (REM) sleep into wakefulness, and the hypothesis of visual hallucinations as overflow dream phenomenon has been supported by several studies (Arnulf et al., 2000; Comella, Tanner, & Ristanovic, 1993). Compared to PD patients without hallucinations, hallucinators have decreased sleep efficiency, total REM sleep time and REM sleep percentage on polysomnography (Comella et al., 1993; Arnulf et al., 2000; Manni et al., 2002; Nomura et al., 2003), and altered circadian rest-activity rhythms on actigraphy (Whitehead, Davies, Playfer, & Turnbill, 2008). In addition, REM sleep behavior disorder (RBD) significantly correlates with hallucinations independent of age, gender, PD duration, or PD stage (Onofrj et al., 2006). These disturbances in sleep architecture, REM sleep, and circadian patterns suggest involvement of brainstem and hypothalamic sleep centers with interactions among neurotransmitters such as acetylcholine, serotonin, noradrenaline, histamine, GABA, hypocretin, and dopamine.

Cognitive impairment and dementia have been associated with PD psychosis in many studies, suggesting both subcortical and cortical dysfunction (Aarsland et al., 2007; Barnes & Boubert, 2008; Fenelon et al., 2000). Hallucinations are significant predictors of dementia in PD, and cognitive decline is faster in hallucinating PD patients (Aarsland, Andersen, Larsen, Lolk, & Kragh-Sørensen, 2003; Aarsland et al., 2004). As previously discussed, PD hallucinators exhibit poor executive, attentional, and visuospatial abilities. Posterior cortical dysfunction in PD may be a risk factor for both dementia (Williams-Gray, Foltynie, Brayne, Robbins, & Barker, 2007) and hallucinations (Boecker et al., 2007; Llebaria et al., 2010).

Neuroimaging studies demonstrating distinct structural, functional, and metabolic abnormalities in PD hallucinators support clinical links between hallucinations and cognitive impairment in PD. Structural magnetic resonance imaging (MRI) studies comparing hallucinating and nonhallucinating PD patients demonstrate greater gray matter volume loss in limbic, temporal, and parietal regions in PD hallucinators (Ibarretxe-Bilbao et al., 2008; Ramirez-Ruiz et al., 2007), regions also implicated in PD dementia. Moreover, postmortem studies reveal Lewy body pathology in temporal and limbic regions, areas associated with memory function, in PD hallucinators (Harding, Broe, & Halliday, 2002; Papapetropoulos, McCorquodale, Gonzalez, Jean-Gilles, & Mash, 2006). Functional MRI (fMRI) studies in PD patients with hallucinations demonstrate altered cortical activation patterns compared to PD nonhallucinators. Findings include increased activation in the visual association cortex and deficits in the primary visual cortex (Holroyd & Wooten, 2006) or greater frontal and subcortical activation and less posterior cortical activation to stroboscopic and kinematic stimuli (Stebbins et al., 2004); others, however, have demonstrated decreased activation in frontal regions and anterior cingulate gyrus in response to complex visual stimuli (face recognition task) (Ramirez-Ruiz et al., 2008) or reduced activation of the lateral occipital cortex and extrastriate temporal visual cortices several seconds prior to an image recognition task (Meppelink et al., 2009). These findings suggest disruptions between anterior (e.g., frontal) and posterior (e.g., parietal, temporal, occipital) regions that are important in processing visual stimuli. Thus, PD hallucinators have difficulty distinguishing relevant from irrelevant visual information. Decreased perfusion or glucose metabolism in predominantly posterior brain regions (temporal, parietal, and/or occipital lobes) has been reported in PD hallucinators using single photon emission computed tomography (SPECT) (Okada, Suyama, Oguro, Yamaguchi, & Kobayashi, 1999) or positron emission tomography (PET) (Boecker et al., 2007; Nagano-Saito et al., 2004) modalities. Overall, these neuroimaging studies in different modalities emphasize the relationships between frontal and posterior brain regions and visual and cognitive processing in the pathogenesis of PD hallucinations.

Management

Treatments for PD psychosis include pharmacological and nonpharmacological strategies. Factors such as temporal course (acute versus chronic), patient age, presence of dementia, mood or sleep disturbances, and motor severity may influence treatment decisions. Acutely psychotic patients who are very agitated may require cautious, short-term use of low-dose benzodiazepines (intramuscular or oral) (Marsh, 2005). Specific medical reasons (e.g., infection or metabolic abnormality) contributing to the acute psychosis should be addressed appropriately. Non-PD medications with centrally acting properties (e.g., anticholinergics for bladder hyperactivity, tricyclics for depression, benzodiazepines for anxiety or sleep, hypnotics for sleep, and opioids for pain) should be reduced or stopped. Dopaminergic medications for PD may need to be reduced or discontinued, in some cases. PD medications with the highest risk-to-benefit ratio should be tapered and stopped first, while monitoring for worsened motor function; one schema proposes to reduce or discontinue anticholinergics first, followed by amantadine, selegiline, dopamine agonists, dopaminergic-enzyme inhibitors, and then levodopa (Olanow, Watts, & Koller, 2001). Antipsychotic medications may be required, particularly if dopaminergic medications cannot be reduced without exacerbating parkinsonism. Doses of antipsychotics used to treat PD psychosis typically are lower than those used for schizophrenia or other psychiatric disorders. Once antipsychotic therapy is initiated, continued treatment may be necessary to maintain control of psychosis. Atypical antipsychotics, such as clozapine and quetiapine, which have greater serotonergic antagonism than dopamine receptor blockade are preferred in the treatment of PD psychosis. Atypical and typical antipsychotics with dopamine-blocking properties are generally contraindicated in PD due to the increased risk of worsened parkinsonism and other extrapyramidal syndromes. Antipsychotic use also carries a recent "black box" warning by the FDA due to an increased risk of death in elderly, demented patients treated with antipsychotics. In the management of chronic psychosis, there may be a role for nonpharmacological strategies such as use of night-lights, reassurance, and other cognitive and visual coping techniques (Diederich, Pieri, & Goetz, 2003), alone or in conjunction with pharmacological interventions.

To date, there have been few randomized, double blind, placebo-controlled trials of the atypical antipsychotics in PD. Treatment trials of PD psychosis have been the focus of evidence-based medical reviews by the Movement Disorder Society (MDS) (Goetz, Koller, Poewe, Rascol, & Sampaio, 2002; Seppi et al., 2011) and American Academy of Neurology (AAN; Miyasaki et al., 2006). According to the MDS evidence-based medical reviews, clozapine was considered "Efficacious, with acceptable safety with need for specialized monitoring, and clinical useful." Quetiapine was deemed as having "insufficient data, with acceptable safety without specialized monitoring, but investigational in clinical practice," and olanzapine as "Not efficacious, with unacceptable risk, and not clinically useful." Similarly, the AAN practice parameter on treatment of PD psychosis (Miyasaki, 2006) recommended that clozapine should be considered (Level B), quetiapine may be considered (Level C), and olanzapine should not be considered (Level B). Although clozapine remains the gold standard atypical antipsychotic for PD psychosis, with the majority of double blind, placebo-controlled trials demonstrating improvement in psychosis with minimal motor worsening (The French Clozapine Parkinson Study Group, 1999; The Parkinson Study Group, 1999; Wolters, Hurwitz, Mak, et al., 1990), its use is tempered by the risk of agranulocytosis and need for blood-count monitoring, side effects of sedation or hypotension, and the "black box" warning for antipsychotic use in elderly patients with dementia. Quetiapine demonstrates comparable efficacy to clozapine in comparison studies, frequent and easy administration, and a relatively low-risk side effect profile. However, quetiapine has yet to demonstrate robust findings of psychosis reduction in its double-blind, placebo-controlled randomized trials (Kurlan, Cummings, Raman, Thal, & the ADCS, 2007; Ondo, Tintner, Voung, Lai, & Ringholz, 2005; Rabey, Prokhorov, Miniovitz, Dobronevsky, & Klein, 2007; Shotbolt, Samuel, Fox, & David, 2009). Atypical antipsychotic agents with novel pharmacological profiles have been studied recently, including aripiprazole, which exhibits partial agonism (agonism/antagonism) at D2 and 5-HT1A receptors and antagonism at 5-HT2 receptors (Fernandez, Trieschmann, & Friedman, 2004; Friedman et al., 2006), but has demonstrated motor worsening and pimavanserin, a 5HT-2A receptor inverse agonist (Friedman et al., 2010; Meltzer et al., 2010; Cummings et al., 2014), which may have promise in recent trials without worsened motor outcomes.

In clinical practice, however, quetiapine was prescribed in about two-thirds of patients in an outpatient United States Veterans Affairs population. High-potency antipsychotics were used in about one-third and few were treated with clozapine; despite recent evidence-based medicine reviews, prescriptions for quetiapine and aripiprazole grew in recent years (Weintraub, Chen, Ignacio, Mamikonyan, & Kales, 2011). Physician specialty may be an important determinant of antipsychotic choice; in a Taiwanese cohort based on National Health Insurance data, internal-medicine specialists were 10.6 times more likely to prescribe typical antipsychotics than neurologists (Wang et al., 2011).

Clinical trials in PD dementia and dementia with Lewy bodies have demonstrated positive effects of cholinesterase inhibitors on psychosis. A subanalysis of 188 PD hallucinators from a large, multicenter, double-blind, placebo-controlled trial of rivastigmine in mild to moderate PD dementia was conducted (Burn et al., 2006; Emre et al., 2004). Rivastigmine-placebo differences for several measures (i.e., AD Assessment Scale–cognitive subscale, AD Cooperative Study—Clinician's Global Impression of Change, and NPI-10) were found to be significantly larger in the hallucinators than in the nonhallucinators. Greater therapeutic benefit could be potentially derived from the use of cholinesterase inhibitors in select PD patients with dementia and hallucinations. Although cholinesterase inhibitors may benefit demented PD patients with psychosis, these medications are not useful in acute psychosis or in the emergency setting, as they take longer to work than antipsychotics. At present, there is not enough evidence to suggest cholinesterase inhibitors for psychosis in nondemented PD. Although the trials described were primarily focused on the safety and efficacy of the antipsychotic agent tested, these studies vary regarding a number of factors including the definitions of PD psychosis used (some exclude patients with minor hallucinations), inclusion/exclusion of demented PD patients, definitions of dementia used, as well as trial duration and psychosis rating scales used. Furthermore, very few antipsychotic trials have included neuropsychological tests as secondary/tertiary outcome measures. Overall, improved, safe and effective antipsychotic medications that treat psychotic symptoms in both nondemented and demented PD patients, across the broad psychotic symptom spectrum, and without compromising motor function, are greatly needed.

Conclusion

Psychosis represents an important nonmotor complication of PD, which increases with advanced disease, is associated with poor outcomes, and lacks optimal, effective antipsychotic treatments. In addition to dopamine, neurotransmitters such as acetylcholine and serotonin among others underlie the pathophysiology of PD psychosis and also may explain the relationship of psychosis to visual impairment, sleep disturbances, and cognitive dysfunction in PD. There is a need for improved recognition of the broad psychosis spectrum on the part of physicians, increased reporting by patients and caregivers, and more effective antipsychotic therapies that do not aggravate motor parkinsonism.

REFERENCES

American Psychiatric Association. (2000). *Diagnostic and Statistical Manual of Mental Disorders, Fourth Edition, Text Revision*. Washington, DC: American Psychiatric Association.

Aarsland, D., Andersen, K., Larsen, J. P., Lolk, A., & Kragh-Sørensen, P. (2003). Prevalence and characteristics of dementia in Parkinson disease: an 8-year prospective study. *Archives of Neurology, 60*, 387–392.

Aarsland, D., Andersen, K., Larsen, J. P., Perry, R., Wentzel-Larsen, T., Lolk, A., & Kragh-Sørensen, P. (2004). The rate of cognitive decline in Parkinson disease. *Archives of Neurology, 61*, 1906–1911.

Aarsland, D., Brønnick, K., Ehrt, U., De Deyn, P. P., Tekin, S., Emre, M., & Cummings, J. L. (2007). Neuropsychiatric symptoms in patients with Parkinson's disease and dementia: frequency, profile and associated caregiver stress. *Journal of Neurology, Neurosurgery and Psychiatry, 78*, 36–42.

Aarsland, D., Larsen, J. P., Cummings, J. L., & Laake, K. (1999). Prevalence and clinical correlates of psychotic symptoms in Parkinson disease: a community-based study. *Archives of Neurology, 56*, 595–601.

Aarsland, D., Marsh, L., & Schrag, A. (2009). Neuropsychiatric symptoms in Parkinson's disease. *Movement Disorders, 24*, 2175–2186.

Antonini, A., Siri, C., Santangelo, G., Cilia, R., Poletti, M., Canesi, M., ... Barone, P. (2011). Impulsivity and compulsivity in drug-naive patients with Parkinson's disease. *Movement Disorders, 26*, 464–468.

Ardouin, C., Voon, V., Worbe, Y., Abouazar, N., Czernecki, V., Hosseini, H., ... Krack, P. (2006). Pathological gambling in Parkinson's disease improves on chronic subthalamic nucleus stimulation. *Movement Disorders, 21,* 1941–1946.

Arnulf, I., Bonnet, A.-M., Damier, P., Bejjani, B.-P., Seilhean, D., Derenne, J.-P., & Agid, Y. (2000). Hallucinations, REM sleep, and Parkinson's disease: a medical hypothesis. *Neurology, 55,* 281–288.

Avanzi, M, Baratti, M., Cabrini, S., Uber, E., Brighetti, G., & Bonfà, F. (2006). Prevalence of pathological gambling in patients with Parkinson's disease. *Movement Disorders, 21,* 2068–2072.

Barnes, J. & Boubert, L. (2008). Executive functions are impaired in patients with Parkinson's disease with visual hallucinations. *Journal of Neurology, Neurosurgery and Psychiatry, 79,* 190–192.

Barnes, J., Boubert, L., Harris, J., Lee, A., & David, A. S. (2003). Reality monitoring and visual hallucinations in Parkinson's disease. *Neuropsychologia, 41,* 565–574.

Barnes, J., & David, A. S. (2001). Visual hallucinations in Parkinson's disease: a review and phenomenological survey. *Journal of Neurology, Neurosurgery and Psychiatry, 70,* 727–733.

Benincasa, D., Pellicano, C., Fanciulli, A., & Pontieri, F. E. (2011). Bupropion abates dopamine agonist-mediated compulsive behaviors in Parkinson's disease. *Movement Disorders, 26,* 355–356.

Bermejo, P. E., Ruiz-Huete, C., & Anciones, B. (2010). Zonisamide in managing impulse control disorders in Parkinson's disease. *Journal of Neurology, 257,* 5603–5607.

Biglan, K. M., Holloway, R. G. J., McDermott, M. P., & Richard, I. (2007). Risk factors for somnolence, edema, and hallucinations in early Parkinson disease. *Neurology, 69,* 187–195.

Bjarkam, C. R., & Sørensen, J. C. (2004). Therapeutic strategies for neurodegenerative disorders: emerging clues from Parkinson's disease. *Biological Psychiatry, 56,* 213–216.

Black, D. W. (2007). A review of compulsive buying disorder. *World Psychiatry, 6,* 14–18.

Black, D. W., & Boffeli, T. (1989). Simple schizophrenia: past, present, and future. *American Journal of Psychiatry, 146,* 1267–1273.

Bodi, N., Keri, S., Nagy, H., Moustafa, A., Myers, C. E., Daw, N., ... Gluck, M. (2009). Reward-learning and the novelty-seeking personality: a between- and within-subjects study of the effects of dopamine agonists on young Parkinson's patients. *Brain, 132,* 2385–2395.

Boecker, H., Ceballos-Baumann, A. O., Volk, D., Conrad, B., Forstl, H., & Haussermann, P. (2007). Metabolic alterations in patients with Parkinson disease and visual hallucinations. *Archives of Neurology, 64,* 984–988.

Bogart, K. R. (2011). Is apathy a valid and meaningful symptom or syndrome in Parkinson's disease? A critical review. *Health Psychology, 30,* 386–400.

Brand, M., Labudda, K., Kalbe, E., Hilker, R., Emmans, D., Fuchs, G., . . . Markowitsch, H. J. (2004). Decision-making impairments in patients with Parkinson's disease. *Behavioural Neurology, 15,* 77–85.

Bronnick, K., Emre, M., Tekin, S., Haugen, S. B., & Aarsland, D. (2011). Cognitive correlates of visual hallucinations in dementia associated with Parkinson's disease. *Movement Disorders, 26,* 824–829.

Brusa L, Bassi A, Stefani A, Pierantozzi M, Peppe A, Caramia MD, . . . Stanzione P (2003). Pramipexole in comparison to l-dopa: a neuropsychological study. *Journal of Neural Transmission, 110,* 373–380.

Burn, D., Emre, M., McKeith, I., De Deyn, P. P., Aarsland, D., Hsu, C., & Lane, R. (2006). Effects of rivastigmine in patients with and without visual hallucinations in dementia associated with Parkinson's disease. *Movement Disorders, 21*, 1899–1907.

Butterfield, L. C., Cimino, C. R., Oelke, L. E., Hauser, R. A., & Sanchez-Ramos, J. (2010). The independent influence of apathy and depression on cognitive functioning in Parkinson's disease. *Movement Disorders, 24*, 721–730.

Cabrini, S., Baratti, M., Bonfa, F., Cabri, G., Uber, E., & Avanzi, M. (2009). Preliminary evaluation of the DDS-PC inventory: a new tool to assess impulsive-compulsive behaviours associated to dopamine replacement therapy in Parkinson's disease. *Neurological Sciences, 30*, 307–313.

Ceravolo, R., Frosini, D., Rossi, C., & Bonuccelli, U. (2009). Impulse control disorders in Parkinson's disease: definition, epidemiology, risk factors, neurobiology and management. *Parkinsonism and Related Disorders, 15S*, S111–S115.

Chase, T. N. (2011). Apathy in neuropsychiatric disease: diagnosis, pathophysiology, and treatment. *Neurotoxicity Research, 19*, 266--278.

Chatterjee, A. & Fahn, S. (2002). Methylphenidate treats apathy in Parkinson's disease. *Journal of Neuropsychiatry and Clinical Neurosciences, 14*, 461–462.

Christenson, G. A., Faber, R. J., & deZwaan, M. (1994). Compulsive buying: descriptive characteristics and psychiatric comorbidity. *Journal of Clinical Psychiatry, 55*, 5–11.

Cilia, R., Cho, S. S., Van Eimeren, T., Marotta, G., Siri, C., Ko, J. H., . . . Strafella, A. P. (2011). Pathological gambling in patients with Parkinson's disease is associated with fronto-striatal disconnection: a path modeling analysis. *Movement Disorders, 26*, 225–233.

Cilia, R., Ko, J. H., Cho, S. S., Van Eimeren, T., Marotta, G., Pellecchia, G., . . . Strafella, A. P. (2010). Reduced dopamine transporter density in the ventral striatum of patients with Parkinson's disease and pathological gambling. *Neurobiology of Disease, 39*, 98–104.

Cilia, R., Siri, C., Marotta, G., Isaias, I. U., De Gaspari, D., Canesi, M., ... Antonini, A. (2008). Functional abnormalities underlying pathological gambling in Parkinson disease. *Archives of Neurology, 65*, 1604–1611.

Claassen, D. O., van den Wildenberg, W. P. M., Ridderinkhof, K. R., Jessup, C. K., Harrison, M. B., Wooten, G. F., & Wylie, S. A. (2011). The risky business of dopamine agonists in Parkinson's disease and impulse control disorders. *Behavioral Neuroscience,125*(4), 492–500.

Coleman, E. (1992). Is your patient suffering from compulsive sexual behavior? *Psychiatric Annals, 22*, 320–325.

Comella, C. L., Tanner, C. M., & Ristanovic, R. K. (1993). Polysomnographic sleep measures in Parkinson's disease patients with treatment-induced hallucinations. *Annals of Neurology, 34*, 710–714.

Cools, R. (2006). Dopaminergic modulation of cognitive function—implications for L-DOPA treatment in Parkinson's disease. *Neuroscience and Biobehavioral Reviews, 30*, 1–23.

Cools, R., Altamirano, L., & D'Esposito, M. (2006). Reversal learning in Parkinson's disease depends on medication status and outcome valence. *Neuropsychologia, 44*, 1663–1673.

Cummings, J., Isaacson, S., Mills, R., Williams, H., Chi-Burris, K., Corbett, A, . . . Ballard, C. (2014). Pimavanserin for patients with Parkinson's disease psychosis: a randomised, placebo-controlled phase 3 trial. *Lancet* 2014;383(9916):533–540.

Czernecki, V., Schupbach, M., Yaici, S., Levy, R., Bardinet, E., Yelnik, J., . . . Agid, Y. (2008). Apathy following subthalamic stimulation in Parkinson disease: a dopamine responsive symptom. *Movement Disorders, 23,* 964–969.

Dagher, A., & Robbins, T. W. (2009). Personality, addiction, dopamine: insights from Parkinson's disease. *Neuron, 61,* 502–510.

de Chazeron, I., Llorca, P.-M., Chereau-Boudet, I., Blanc, O., Perriot, J., Ouchchane, L., ... Durif, F. (2011). Hypersexuality and pathological gambling in Parkinson's disease: a cross-sectional case-control study. *Movement Disorders,* 26(11), 2127–2130.

de Smet, Y., Ruberg, M., Serdaru, M., Dubois, B., Lhermitte, F., & Agid, Y. (1982). Confusion, dementia and anticholinergics in Parkinson's disease. *Journal of Neurology, Neurosurgery and Psychiatry, 45,* 1161–1164.

Diederich, N. J., Goetz, C. G., Raman, R., Pappert, E. J., Leurgans, S., & Piery, V. (1998). Poor visual discrimination and visual hallucinations in Parkinson's disease. *Clinical Neuropharmacology, 21,* 289–295.

Diederich, N. J., Goetz, C. G., & Stebbins. G. T. (2005). Repeated visual hallucinations in Parkinson's disease as disturbed external/internal perceptions: focused review and a new integrative model. *Movement Disorders, 20,* 130–140.

Diederich, N. J., Pieri, V., & Goetz, C. G. (2003). Coping strategies for visual hallucinations in Parkinson's disease. *Movement Disorders, 18,* 831–832.

Djamgoz, M. B., Hankins, M. W., Hirano, J., & Archer, S. N. (1997). Neurobiology of retinal dopamine in relation to degenerative states of the tissue. *Vision Research, 37,* 3509–3529.

Djamshidian, A., Jha, A., O'Sullivan, S. S., Silveira-Moriyama, L., Jacobson, C., Brown, P., . . . Averbeck, B. B. (2010). Risk and learning in impulsive and nonimpulsive patients with Parkinson's disease. *Movement Disorders,* 25(13), 2203–2210.

Djamshidian, A., O'Sullivan, S. S., Lees, A., & Averbeck, B. B. (2011). Stroop test performance in impulsive and non impulsive patients with Parkinson's disease. *Parkinsonism and Related Disorders, 17,* 212–214.

Djamshidian, A., O'Sullivan, S. S., Papadopoulos, A., Bassett, P., Shaw, K., Averbeck, B. B., . . . Lees, A. (2011). Salivary cortisol levels in Parkinson's disease and its correlation to risk behaviour. *Journal of Neurology, Neurosurgery and Psychiatry, 10.1136/jnnp.2011.245746.*

Djamshidian, A., O'Sullivan, S. S., Wittmann, B. C., Lees, A. J., & Averbeck, B. B. (2011). Novelty seeking behaviour in Parkinson's disease. *Neuropsychologia, 49,* 2483–2488.

Dodd, M. L., Klos, K. J., Bower, J. H., Geda, Y. E., Josephs, K. A., & Ahlskog, J. E. (2005). Pathological gambling caused by drugs used to treat Parkinson disease. *Archives of Neurology,* 62(9), 1377–1381.

Drapier, D., Drapier, S., Sauleau, P., Haegelen, C., Raoul, S., Biseul, I., . . . Millet, B. (2006). Does subthalamic nucleus stimulation induce apathy in Parkinson's disease? *Journal of Neurology, 8,* 1083–1091.

Drijgers, R. L., Dujardin, K., Reijnders, J. S. A. M., Defebvre, L., & Leentjens, A. F. G. (2010). Validation of diagnostic criteria for apathy in Parkinson's disease. *Parkinsonism and Related Disorders, 16,* 656–660.

Driver-Dunckley, E., Samanta, J., & Stacy, M. (2003). Pathological gambling associated with dopamine agonist therapy in Parkinson's disease. *Neurology, 61,* 422–423.

Dubois, B. & Pillon, B. (1997). Cognitive deficits in Parkinson's disease. *Journal of Neurology, 244,* 2–8.

Duffy, J. D. (1997). The neural substrates of motivation. *Psychiatric Annals, 27,* 39–43.

Dujardin, K., Sockeel, P., Delliaux, M., Destee, A., & Defebvre, L. (2009). Apathy may herald cognitive decline and dementia in Parkinson's disease. *Movement Disorders, 24*, 2391–2397.

Dujardin, K., Sockeel,, P., Devos, D., Delliaux, M., Krystkowiak, P., Destee, A., & Defebvre, L. (2007). Characteristics of apathy in Parkinson's disease. *Movement Disorders, 22*, 778–784.

Emre, M., Aarsland, D., Albanese, A., Byrne, E. J., Deuschl, G., De Deyn, P. P., . . . Lane, R. (2004). Rivastigmine for dementia associated with Parkinson's disease. *New England Journal of Medicine, 351*, 2509–2518.

Evans, A. H., Katzenschlager, R., Paviour, D., O'Sullivan, J. D., Appel, S., Lawrence, A. D., & Lees, A. J. (2004). Punding in Parkinson's disease: its relation to the dopamine dysregulation syndrome. *Movement Disorders, 19*, 397–405.

Evans, A. H, Pavese, N., Lawrence, A. D., Tai, Y. F., Appel, S., Doder, M., . . . Piccini, P. (2006). Compulsive drug use linked to sensitized ventral striatal dopamine transmission. *Annals of Neurology, 59*, 852–858.

Evans, A. H., Strafella, A. P., Weintraub, D., & Stacy, M. (2009). Impulsive and compulsive behaviors in Parkinson's disease. *Movement Disorders, 24*, 1561–1570.

Factor, S. A., Feustel, P. J., Freidman, J. H., Comella, C. L., Goetz, C. G., Kurlan, R., . . . Parkinson Study Group. (2003). Longitudinal outcome of Parkinson's disease patients with psychosis. *Neurology, 60*, 1756–1761.

Factor, S. A., Steenland, N. K., Higgins, D. S., Molho, E. S., Kay, D. M., Montimurro, J., . . . Payami, H. (2011). Disease-related and genetic correlates of psychotic symptoms in Parkinson's disease. *Movement Disorders, 26*, 2190–2195.

Fenelon, G., & Alves, G. (2010). Epidemiology of psychosis in Parkinson's disease. *Journal of Neurological Sciences, 289*, 12–17.

Fenelon, G., Mahieux, F., Huon, R., & Ziegler, M. (2000). Hallucinations in Parkison's disease: prevalence, phenomenology and risk factors. *Brain, 123 (Pt 4)*, 733–745.

Fenelon, G., Soulas, T., Zenasni, F., & de Langavant, L. C. (2010). The changing face of Parkinson's disease-associated psychosis: a cross-sectional study based on the new NINDS-NIMH criteria. *Movement Disorders, 25*, 763–766.

Fenelon, G., Thobois, S., Bonnet, A. M., Broussolle, E., & Tison, F. (2002). Tactile hallucinations in Parkinson's disease. *Journal of Neurology, 249*, 1699–1703.

Fernandez, H. H., Aarsland, D., Fénelon, G., Friedman, J. H., Marsh, L., Tröster, A. I., . . . Goetz, C. G. (2008). Scales to assess psychosis in Parkinson's disease: critique and recommendations. *Movement Disorders, 23*, 484–500.

Fernandez, H. H, Trieschmann, M. E., & Friedman, J. H. (2004). Aripiprazole for drug-induced psyhcosis in Parkinson's disease: preliminary experience. *Clinical Neuropharmacology, 27*, 4–5.

Fisher, S. E. (1996). *Gambling and Problem Gambling Among Casino Patrons* (Rep. No. Report to the British Casino Industry Consortium).

Forsaa, E. B., Larsen, J. P., Wentzel-Larsen, T., Goetz, C. G., Stebbins, G. T., Aarsland, D., . . . Alves, G. (2010). A 12-year population-based study of psychosis in Parkinson disease. *Archives of Neurology, 67*, 996–1001.

Fox, S. H. & Lang, A. E. (2008). Levodopa-related motor complications-phenomenology. *Movement Disorders, 23*(Suppl 3), S509–S514.

Frank, M. J., Samanta, J., Moustafa, A. A., & Sherman, S. J. (2007). Hold your horses: impulsivity, deep brain stimulation, and medication in parkinsonism. *Science, 318*, 1309–1312.

Frank, M. J., Seeberger, L. C., & O'Reilly, R. C. (2004). By carrot or by stick: cognitive reinforcement learning in Parkinsonism. *Science, 306*, 1940–1943.

The French Clozapine Parkinson Study Group (1999). Clozapine in drug-induced psychosis in Parkinson's disease. *Lancet, 353*, 2041–2042.

Friedman, J. H., Agarwal, P., Alcalay, R., Black, K. J., Chou, K. L., Cote, L., . . . Zesiewich, T. (2011). Clinical vignettes in Parkinson's disease: a collection of unusual medication-induced hallucinations, delusions, and compulsive behaviors. *International Journal of Neuroscience, 121*, 472–476.

Friedman, J. H., Berman, R. M., Goetz, C. G., Factor, S. A., Ondo, W. G., et al. (2010). A multicenter, placebo controlled, double blind trial to examine the safety and efficacy of pimavanserin in the treatment of psychosis in Parkinson's disease. *Neurology, 74*, A299.

Friedman, J. H., Berman, R. M., Goetz, C. G., Factor, S. A., Ondo, W. G., Wojcieszek, J., . . . Marcus, R. N. (2006). Open-label flexible-dose pilot study to evaluate the safety and tolerability of aripiprazole in patients with psychosis associated with Parkinson's disease. *Movement Disorders, 21*, 2078–2081.

Frosini, D., Pesaresi, I., Cosottini, M., Belmonte, G., Rossi, C., Dell'Osso, L., ... Ceravolo, R. (2010). Parkinson's disease and pathological gambling: results from a functional MRI study. *Movement Disorders, 25*, 2449–2453.

Gerlach, M., Double, K., Arzberger, T., Leblhuber, F., Tatschner, T., & Riederer, P. (2003). Dopamine receptor agonists in current clinical use: comparative dopamine receptor binding profiles defined in the human striatum. *Journal of Neural Transmission, 110*, 1119–1127.

Giladi, N., Weitzman, N., Schreiber, S., Shabtai, H., & Peretz, C. (2007). New onset heightened interest or drive for gambling, shopping, eating or sexual activity in patients with Parkinson's disease: the role of dopamine agonist treatment and age at motor symptoms onset. *Journal of Psychopharmacology, 21*, 501–506.

Giovannoni, G., O'Sullivan, J. D., Turner, K., Manson, A. J., & Lees, A. J. L. (2000). Hedonistic homeostatic dysregulation in patients with Parkinson's disease on dopamine replacement therapies. *Journal of Neurology, Neurosurgery and Psychiatry, 68*, 423–428.

Goetz, C. G. (2009). Scales to evaluate psychosis in Parkinson's disease. *Parkinsonism and Related Disorders, 15(Suppl 3)*, S38-S41.

Goetz, C. G., Koller, W. C., Poewe, W., Rascol, O., & Sampaio, C. (2002). Management of Parkinson's disease: an evidence based review. *Movement Disorders, 17*, s120–s127.

Goetz, C. G., Ouyang, B., Negron, A., & Stebbins, G. T. (2010). Hallucinations and sleep disorders in PD: ten-year prospective longitudinal study. *Neurology, 75*, 1773–1779.

Goetz, C. G. & Stebbins, G. T. (1995). Mortality and hallucinations in nursing home patients with advanced Parkinson's disease. *Neurology, 45*, 669–671.

Goetz, C. G., Stebbins, G. T., & Ouyang, B. (2011). Visual plus nonvisual hallucinations in Parkinson's disease: development and evolution over 10 years. *Movement Disorders, 26*, 2196–2200.

Goetz, C. G., Tanner, C. M., & Klawans, H. L. (1982). Pharmacology of hallucinations induced by long-term drug therapy. *American Journal of Psychiatry, 139*, 494–497.

Goetz, C. G., Tilley, B. C., Shaftman, S. R., Stebbins, G. T., Fahn, S., Martinez-Martin, P., . . . LaPelle, N.; Movement Disorder Society UPDRS Revision Task Force (2008). Movement Disorder Society-sponsored revision of the Unified Parkinson's Disease Rating Scale (MDS-UPDRS): Scale presentation and climimetric testing results. *Movement Disorders, 23*, 2129–2170.

Goetz, C. G., Wuu, J., Curgian, L. M., & Leurgans, S. (2005). Hallucinations and sleep disorders in PD: six-year prospective longitudinal study. *Neurology, 64,* 81–86.

Graham, J., Grunewald, R., & Sager, H. (1997). Hallucinosis in idiopathic Parkinson's disease. *Journal of Neurology, Neurosurgery and Psychiatry, 63,* 434–440.

Grant, J. E., Potenza, M. N., Hollander, E., Cunningham-Williams, R., Nurminen, T., Smits, G., . . . Kallio, A. (2006). Multicenter investigation of the opioid antagonist nalmefene in the treatment of pathological gambling. *American Journal of Psychiatry, 163,* 303–312.

Green, J., McDonald, W. M., Vitek, J. L., Evatt, M., Freeman, A., Haber, M., . . . DeLong, M. R. (2002). Cognitive impairments in advanced PD without dementia. *Neurology, 59,* 1320–1324.

Grosset, K. A., Macphee, G., Pal, G., Stewart, D., Watt, A., Davie, J., & Grosset, D. G. (2006). Problematic gambling on dopamine agonists: not such a rarity. *Movement Disorders, 21,* 2206–2208.

Grossi, D., Trojano, L., Pellecchia, M. T., Amboni, M., Fragassi, N. A., & Barone, P. (2005). Frontal dysfunction contributes to the genesis of hallucinations in non-demented Parkinsonian patients. *International Journal of Geriatric Psychiatry, 20,* 668–673.

Harding, A. J., Broe, G. A., & Halliday, G. M. (2002). Visual hallucinations in Lewy body disease relate to Lewy bodies in the temporal lobe. *Brain, 125,* 391–403.

Hely, M. A., Morris, J. G., Reid, W. G., & Trafficante, R. (2005). Sydney Multicenter Study of Parkinson's disease: non-L-dopa-responsiveness problems dominate at 15 years. *Movement Disorders, 23,* 190–199.

Hely, M. A., Reid, W. G. J., Adena, M. A., Halliday, G. M., & Morris, J. G. L. (2008). The Sydney multicenter study of Parkinson's disease: the inevitability of dementia at 20 years. *Movement Disorders, 23,* 837–844.

Hodgins, D. C. & Petry, N. M. (2004). Cognitive and behavioral treatments. In Grant JE & Potenza MN (Eds.), *Pathological Gambling: A Clinical Guide to Treatment* (pp. 169–188). Washington DC: American Psychiatric Press.

Holden, C. (2001). 'Behavioral' addictions: do they exist? *Science, 294,* 980–982.

Holroyd, S., Currie, L., & Wooten, G. F. (2001). Prospective study of hallucinations and delusions in Parkinson's disease. *Journal of Neurology, Neurosurgery and Psychiatry, 70,* 734–738.

Holroyd, S., & Wooten, G. F. (2006). Preliminary fMRI evidence of visual system dysfunction in Parkinson's disease patients with visual hallucinations. *Journal of Neuropsychiatry and Clinical Neurosciences, 18,* 402–404.

Housden, C. R., O'Sullivan, S. S., Joyce, E. M., Lees, A. J., & Roiser, J. P. (2010). Intact reward learning but elevated delay discounting in Parkinson's disease patients with impulsive-compulsive spectrum behaviors. *Neuropsychopharmacology, 10.1038/npp.2010.84.*

Ibarretxe-Bilbao, N., Ramírez-Ruiz, B., Tolosa, E., Martí, M. J., Valldeoriola, F., Bargalló, N., & Junqué, C. (2008). Hippocampal head atrophy predominance in Parkinson's disease with hallucinations and with dementia. *Journal of Neurology, 255,* 1324–1331.

Isella, V., Melzi, P., Grimaldi, M., Iurlaro, S., Piolti, R., Ferrarese, C., . . . Appollonio, I. (2002). Clinical, neuropsychological, and morphometric correlates of apathy in Parkinson's disease. *Movement Disorders, 17,* 366–371.

Kim, S. W., Grant, J. E., Adson, D. E., & Shin, Y. C. (2001). Double-blind naltrexone and placebo comparison study in the treatment of pathological gambling. *Biological Psychiatry, 49,* 914–921.

Kirsch-Darrow, L., Fernandez, H. F., Marsiske, M., Okun, M. S., & Bowers, D. (2006). Dissociating apathy and depression in Parkinson disease. *Neurology, 67,* 33–38.

Klein, C., Prokhorov, T., Miniovitz, A., Dobronevsky, E., & Rabey, J. M. (2009). Admission of Parkinsonian patients to a neurological ward in a community hospital. *Journal of Neural Transmission, 116,* 1509–1512.

Klos, K. J., Bower, J. H., Josephs, K. A., Matsumoto, J. Y., & Ahlskog, J. E. (2005). Pathological hypersexuality predominantly linked to adjuvant dopamine agonist therapy in Parkinson's disease and multiple system atrophy. *Parkinsonism and Related Disorders, 11,* 381–386.

Kostic, V. S. & Filippi, M. (2011). Neuroanatomical correlates of depression and apathy in Parkinson's disease: magnetic resonance imaging studies. *Journal of Neurological Science, 310,* 61–63.

Krack, P., Batir, A., Van Blercom, N., Chabardes, S., Fraiz, V., Aldouin, C., . . . Pollack, P. (2003). Five-year follow-up of bilateral stimulation of the subthalamic nucleus in advanced Parkinson's disease. *New England Journal of Medicine, 13,* 1925–1934.

Kulisevsky, J., Pagonabarraga, J., Pascual-Sedano, B., García-Sánchez, C., Gironell, A, & The Trapecio Group Study (2008). Prevalence and correlates of neuropsychiatric symptoms in Parkinson's disease without dementia. *Movement Disorders, 23,* 1889–1896.

Kurlan, R., Cummings, J., Raman, R., Thal, L., & the ADCS (2007). Quetiapine for agitation or psychosis in patients with dementia and parkinsonsim. *Neurology, 68,* 1356–1363.

Lee, J.-Y., Kim, J.-M., Kim, J. W., Cho, J., Lee, W. Y., Kim, H.-J., & Jeon, B. S. (2010). Association between the dose of dopaminergic medication and the behavioral disturbances in Parkinson disease. *Parkinsonism and Related Disorders, 16,* 202–207.

Lee, J.-Y., Lee, E. K., Park, S. S., Lim, J.-Y., Kim, H. J., Kim, J. S., & Jeon, B. S. (2009). Association of *DRD3* and *GRIN2B* with impulse control and related behaviors in Parkinsoon's disease. *Movement Disorders, 24,* 1803–1810.

Leentjens, A. F., Dujardin, K., Marsh, L., Martinez-Martin, P., Richard, I. H., Starkstein, S. E., . . . Goet z, C. G. (2008). Apathy and anhedonia rating scales in Parkinson's disease: critique and recommendations. *Movement Disorders, 23,* 2015–2025.

Le Jeune, F., Drapier, D., Bourguignon, A., Peron, J., Mesbah, H., Drapier, S., . . . Vérin, M. (2009). Subthalamic nucleus stimulation in Parkinson disease induces apathy: a PET study. *Neurology, 73,* 1746–1751.

Lejoyeux, M., Tassain, V., Solomon, J., & Adès, J. (1997). Study of compulsive buying in depressed patients. *Journal of Clinical Psychiatry, 58,* 169–173.

Levin, B. E., & Katzen, H. L. (1995). Early cognitive changes and nondementing behavioral abnormalities in Parkinson's disease. In Weiner WJ & Lang AE (Eds.), *Behavioral Neurology of Movement Disorders* (pp. 85–95). New York: Raven Press, Ltd.

Levy, R., & Dubois, B. (2006). Apathy and the functional anatomy of the prefrontal cortex-basal ganglia circuits. *Cerebral Cortex, 16,* 916–928.

LeWitt, P. A., Lyons, K. E., Pahwa, R., & S. P. 650 Study (2007). Advanced Parkinson disease paitents treated with rotigotine transdermal system: PREFER Study. *Neurology, 68,* 1262–1267.

Lilenfeld, L. R. R., Ringham, R., Kalarchian, M. A., & Marcus, M. D. (2008). A family history study of binge-eating disorder. *Comprehensive Psychiatry, 49,* 247–254.

Llebaria, G., Pagonabarraga, J., Martinez-Corral, M., García-Sánchez, C., Pascual-Sedano, B., Gironell, A., & Kulisevsky, J. (2010). Neuropsychological correlates of mild to severe hallucinations in Parkinon's disease. *Movement Disorders, 25,* 2785–2791.

Lu, C., Bharmal, A., & Suchowersky, O. (2006). Gambling and Parkinson's disease. *Archives of Neurology, 63,* 298.

MacPhee, G. J. A., & Copeland, C. (2009). Clinical follow up of pathological gambling in Parkinson's disease in the West Scotland study. *Movement Disorders, 24,* 2430–2431.

Mamikonyan, E., Siderowf, A. D., Duda, J. E., Potenza, M. N., Horn, S., Stern, M. B., & Weintraub, D. (2008). Long-term follow-up of impulse control disorders in Parkinson's disease. *Movement Disorders, 23,* 75–80.

Manni, R., Pacchetti, C., Terzaghi, M., Sartori, I., Mancini, F., & Nappi, G. (2002). Hallucinations and sleep-wake cycle in PD: a continuous polysomnographic study. *Neurology, 59,* 1979–1981.

Marin, R. S., Fogel, B. S., Hawkins, J., Duffy, J., & Krupp, B. (1995). Apathy: a treatable syndrome. *Journal of Neuropsychiatry and Clinical Neurosciences, 7,* 23–30.

Marsh, L. (2004). Psychosis in Parkinson's disease. *Current Treatment Options in Neurology, 6,* 181–189.

Marsh, L. (2005). Psychosis in Parkinson's disease. *Primary Psychiatry, 12,* 56–62.

Marsh, L., McDonald, W. M., Cummings, J. L., Ravina, B.; NINDS/NIMH Work Group on Depression and Parkinson's Disease. (2006). Provisional diagnostic criteria for depression in Parkinson's disease: report of an NINDS/NIMH work group. *Movement Disorders, 21,* 148–158.

McKinlay, A., Grace, R. C., Dalrymple-Alford, J. C., Anderson, T., Fink, J., & Roger, D. (2008). A profile of neuropsychiatric problems and their relationship to quality of life for Parkinson's disease patients without dementia. *Parkinsonism and Related Disorders, 14,* 37–42.

Meltzer, H. Y., Mills, R., Revell, S., Williams, H., Johnson, A., Bahr, D., . . . Friedman, J. H. (2010). Pimavanserin, a serotonin2A receptor inverse agonist, for the treatment of Parkinson's disease psychosis. *Neuropsychopharmacology, 35,* 881–892.

Meppelink, A. M., de Jong, B. M., Renken, R., Leenders, K. L., Cornelissen, F. W., & van Laar, T. (2009). Impaired visual processing preceding image recognition in Parkinson's disease patients with visual hallucinations. *Brain, 132,* 2980–2993.

Milenkova, M., Mohammadi, B., Kollewe, K., Schrader, C., Fellbrich, A., Wittfoth, M., . . . Münte, T. F. (2011). Intertemporal choice in Parkinson's disease. *Movement Disorders, 26,* 2004–2010.

Miyasaki, J., Hassan, K. L., Lang, A. E., & Voon, V. (2007). Punding prevalence in Parkinson's disease. *Movement Disorders, 22,* 1179–1181.

Miyasaki, J. M., Shannon, K., Voon, V., Ravina, B., Kleiner-Fisman, G., Anderson, K., . . . Weiner, W. J.. (2006). Practice parameter: Evaluation and treatment of depression, psychosis, and dementia in Parkinson disease (an evidence-based review). Report of the Quality Standards Subcommittee of the American Academy of Neurology. *Neurology, 66,* 996–1002.

Nagano-Saito, A., Washimi, Y., Arahata, Y., Iwai, K., Kawatsu, S., Ito, K., . . . Kachi, T. (2004). Visual hallucination in Parkinson's disease with FDG PET. *Movement Disorders, 19,* 801–806.

Nirenberg, M. J., & Waters, C. (2006). Compulsive eating and weight gain related to dopamine agonist use. *Movement Disorders, 21,* 524–529.

Nomura, T., Inoue, Y., Mitani, H., Kawahara, R., Miyake, M., & Nakashima, K. (2003). Visual hallucinations as REM sleep behavior disorders in patients with Parkinson's disease. *Movement Disorders, 18,* 812–817.

Okada. K., Suyama, N., Oguro, H., Yamaguchi, S., & Kobayashi, S. (1999). Medication-induced hallucinations and cerebral blood flow in Parkinson's disease. *Journal of Neurology, 246*, 365–368.

Olanow, C. W., Watts, R. L., & Koller, W. C. (2001). An algorithm (decision tree) for the management of Parkinson's disease (2001): treatment guidelines. *Neurology, 56 (Suppl 5)*, S1-S88.

Olin, J. T., Schneider, L. S., Katz, I. R., Meyers, B. S., Alexopoulos, G. S., . . . Breitner, J. C., (2002). Provisional diagnostic criteria for depression of Alzheimer disease. *American Journal of Geriatric Psychiatry, 10*, 125–128.

Ondo, W. G., & Lai, D. (2008). Predictors of impulsivity and reward seeking behavior with dopamine agonists. *Parkinsonism and Related Disorders, 14*, 28–32.

Ondo, W. G., Tintner, R., Voung, K. D., Lai, D., & Ringholz G (2005). Double-blind, placebo-controlled, unforced titration parallel trial of quetiapine for dopaminergic-induced hallucinations in Parkinson's disease. *Movement Disorders, 20*, 958–963.

Onofrj, M., Bonanni, L., Albani, G., Mauro, A., Bulla, D., & Thomas, A. (2006). Visual hallucinations in Parkinson's disease: clues to separate origins. *Journal of the Neurological Sciences, 248*, 143–150.

Onyike, C. U., Sheppard, J.-M. E., Tschanz, J. T., Norton, M. C., Green, R. C., Steinberg, M., . . . Lyketsos. C. G. (2007). Epidemiology of apathy in older adults: The Cache County Study. *American Journal of Geriatric Psychiatry, 15*, 365–375.

O'Sullivan, S. S., Wu, K., Politis, M., Lawrence, A. D., Evans, A. H., Bose, S. K., . . . Piccini, P. (2011). Cue-induced striatal dopamine release in Parkinson's disease-associated impulsive-compulsive behaviours. *Brain, 134*, 969–978.

Pagonabarraga, J., Llebaria, G., García-Sánchez, C., Pascual-Sedano, B., Gironell, A., & Kulisevsky, J. (2008). A prospective study of delusional misidentification in Parkinson's disease with dementia. *Movement Disorders, 15*, 443–448.

Papapetropoulos, S. & Mash, D. C. (2005). Psychotic symptoms in Parkinson's disease. From description to etiology. *Journal of Neurology, 252*, 753–764.

Papapetropoulos, S., McCorquodale, D. S., Gonzalez, J., Jean-Gilles, L., & Mash, D. C. (2006). Cortical and amygdalar Lewy body burden in Parkinson's disease patients with visual hallucinations. *Parkinsonism and Related Disorders, 12*, 253–256.

Papay, K., Mamikonyan, E., Siderowf, A. D., Duda, J. E., Lyons, K. E., Pahwa, R.. . . Weintraub, D. (2011). Patient versus informant reporting of ICD symptoms in Parkinson's disease using the QUIP: Validity and variability. *Parkinsonism and Related Disorders, 17*, 153–155.

The Parkinson Study Group (1999). Low-dose clozapine for the treatment of drug-induced psychosis in Parkinson's disease. *New England Journal of Medicine, 340*, 757–763.

Pedersen, K. F., Alves G, Aarsland D, & Larsen JP (2009). Occurrence and risk factors for apathy in Parkinson disease: a 4-year prospective longitudinal study. *Journal of Neurology, Neurosurgery and Psychiatry, 80*, 1279–1282.

Pedersen, K. F., Larsen JP, Alves G, & Aarsland D (2009). Prevalence and clinical correlates of apathy in Parkinson's disease: a community-based study. *Parkinsonism and Related Disorders, 15*, 295–299.

Pieri, V., Diederich, N. J., Raman, R., & Goetz, C. G. (2000). Decreased color discrimination and contrast sensitivity in Parkinson's disease. *Journal of the Neurological Sciences, 172*, 7–11.

Pietrzak, R. H., Morasco, B. J., Blanco, C., Grant, B. F., & Petry, N. M. (2007). Gambling level and psychiatric and medical disorders in older adults: results from the National

Epidemiologic Survey on Alcohol and Related Conditions. *American Journal of Geriatric Psychiatry, 15*, 301–313.

Pluck, G. C., & Brown, R. G. (2002). Apathy in Parkinson's disease. *Journal of Neurology, Neurosurgery and Psychiatry, 73*, 636–642.

Pontone, G., Williams, J. R., Bassett, S. S., & Marsh, L. (2006). Clinical features associated with impulse control disorders in Parkinson disease. *Neurology, 67*, 1258–1261.

Rabey, J. M., Prokhorov, T., Miniovitz, A., Dobronevsky, E., & Klein, C. (2007). Effect of quetiapine in psychotic Parkinson's disease patients: a double-blind labeled study of 3 months' duration. *Movement Disorders, 22*, 313–318.

Rabinak, C. A. & Nirenberg, M. J. (2010). Dopamine agonist withdrawal syndrome in Parkinson disease. *Archives of Neurology, 67*, 58–63.

Ramirez-Ruiz, B., Junque, C., Marti, M.-J., Valldeoriola, F., & Tolosa, E. (2006). Neuropsychological deficits in Parkinson's disease patients with visual hallucinations. *Movement Disorders, 21*, 1483–1487.

Ramirez-Ruiz, B., Marti, M.-J., Tolosa, E., Gimenez, M., Bargallo, N., Valldeoriola, F. & Jun (2007). Cerebral atrophy in Parkinson's disease patients with visual hallucinations. *European Journal of Neurology, 14*, 750–756.

Ramirez-Ruiz, B., Martí, M. J., Tolosa, E., Falcón, C., Bargalló, N., Valldeoriola, F. & Junqué, C. (2008). Brain response to complex visual stimuli in Parkinson's patients with hallucinations: a functional magnetic resonance imaging study. *Movement Disorders, 23*, 2335–2343.

Rao, H., Mamikonyan, E., Detre, J. A., Siderowf, A. D., Stern, M. B., Potenza, M. N., & Weintraub, D. (2010). Decreased ventral striatal activity with impulse control disorders in Parkinson's disease. *Movement Disorders, 10.1002/mds.23147.*

Rascol, O., Brooks, D. J., Korczyn, A. D., De Deyn, P. P., Clarke, C. E., & Lang, A. E. (2000). A five-year study of the incidence of dyskinesia in patients with early Parkinson's disease who were treated with ropinirole or levodopa. *New England Journal of Medicine, 342*, 1484–1491.

Ravina, B., Marder, K., Fernandez, H. H., Friedman, J. H., McDonald, W., Murphy, D., . . . Goetz, C. (2007). Diagnostic criteria for psychosis in Parkinson's disease: report of an NINDS, NIMH work group. *Movement Disorders, 22*, 1061–1068.

Reijnders, J. S. A. M., Scholtissen, B., Weber, W. E. J., Aalten, P., Verhety, F. R. J., & Leentjens, A. F. G. (2010). Neuroanatomical correlates of apathy in Parkinson's disease: a magnetic resonance imaging study using voxel-based morphometry. *Movement Disorders, 25*, 2318–2325.

Roane, D. M., Rogers, J. D., Robinson, J. H., & Feinberg, T. E. (1998). Delusional misidentification in association with parkinsonism. *Journal of Neuropsychiatry and Clinical Neurosciences, 10*, 194–198.

Rodriguez-Oroz, M. C., Lopez-Azcarate, J., Garcia-Garcia, D., Alegre, M., Toledo, J., Valencia, M., . . . Obeso, J. A. (2011). Involvement of the subthalamic nucleus in impulse control disorders associated with Parkinson's disease. *Brain, 134*, 36–49.

Rossi, M., Gerschovich, E. R., de Achaval, D., Perez-Lloret, S., Cerquetti, D., Cammarota, A., . . . Leiguarda, R. (2010). Decision-making in Parkinson's disease patients with and without pathological gambling. *European Journal of Neurology, 17*, 97–102.

Rotondo, A., Bosco, D., Plastino, M., Consoli, A., & Bosco, F. (2010). Clozapine for medication-related pathological gambling in Parkinson disease [Letter to the Editor]. *Movement Disorders, 25*, 1994–1995.

Rowe, J. B., Hughes, L., Ghosh, B. C. P., Eckstein, D., Williams-Gray, C. H., Fallon, S., . . . Owen, A. M. (2008). Parkinson's disease and dopaminergic therapy-differential effects on movement, reward and cognition. *Brain, 131*, 2094–2105.

Sanchez-Ramos, J. R., Ortoll, R., & Paulson, G. W. (1996). Visual hallucinations associated with Parkinson disease. *Archives of Neurology, 53*, 1265–1268.

Santangelo, G., Vitale, C., Trojano, L., Verde, F., Grossi, D., & Barone, P. (2009). Cognitive dysfunctions and pathological gambling in patients with Parkinson's disease. *Movement Disorders, 24*, 899–905.

Santangelo, G., Trojano, L., Vitale, C., Ianniciello, M., Amboni, M., Grossi, D., & Barone, P. (2007). A neuropsychological longitudinal study in Parkinson's patients with and without hallucinations. *Movement Disorders, 22*, 2418–2425.

Seppi, K., Weintraub, D., Coelho, M., Perez-Lloret, S., Fox, S. H., Katzenschlager, R., . . . Sampaio, C. (2011). The Movement Disorders Society Evidence-Based Medicine Review Update: Treatments for the non-motor symptoms of Parkinson's disease. *Movement Disorders, 26 (Suppl 3)*, S42–S80.

Sevincok, L., Akoglu, A., & Akyol, A. (2007). Quetiapine in a case with Parkinson disease and pathological gambling [letter]. *Journal of Clinical Psychopharmacology, 27*, 107–108.

Shaffer, H. J., Hall, M. N., & Vander, J. (1999). Estimating the prevalence of disordered gambling behavior in the United States and Canada: a research synthesis. *American Journal of Public Health, 89*, 1369–1376.

Shotbolt, P., Samuel, M., Fox, C., & David, A. S. (2009). A randomized controlled trial of quetiapine for psychosis in Parkinson's disease. *Neuropsychiatric Disease and Treatment, 5*, 327–332.

Shulman, L. M. (2000). Apathy in patients with Parkinson's disease. *International Review of Psychiatry, 12*, 298–306.

Smeding, H. M. M., Goudriaan, A. E., Foncke, E. M. J., Schuurman, P. R., Speelman, J. D., & Schmand, B. (2007). Pathological gambling after bilateral subthalamic nucleus stimulation in Parkinson disease. *Journal of Neurology, Neurosurgery and Psychiatry, 78*, 517–519.

Sokoloff, P., Giros, B., Martres, M. P., Bouthenet, M. L., & Schwartz, J. C. (1990). Molecular cloning and characterization of a novel dopamine receptor (D3) as a target for neuroleptics. *Nature, 347*, 146–151.

Starkstein, S. E., Petracca, G., Chemerinski, E., & Kremer, J. (2001). Syndromic validity of apathy in Alzheimer's disease. *American Journal of Psychiatry, 158*, 872–877.

Starkstein, S. E. & Leentjens, A. F. G. (2008). The nosological position of apathy in clinical practice. *Journal of Neurology, Neurosurgery and Psychiatry, 79*, 10.1136/jnnp.2007.136895.

Starkstein, S. E., Mayberg, H. S., Preziosi, T. J., Andrezejewski, P., Leiguarda, R., & Robinson, R. G. (1992). Reliability, validity, and clinical correlates of apathy in Parkinson's disease. *Journal of Neuropsychiatry and Clinical Neurosciences, 4*, 134–139.

Starkstein, S. E., Merello, M., Jorge, R., Brockman, S., Bruce, D., & Power, B. (2009). The syndromic validity and nosological position of apathy in Parkinson's disease. *Movement Disorders, 24*, 1211–1216.

Stebbins, G. T., Goetz, C. G., Carrillo, M. C., Bangen, K. J., Turner, D. A., Glover, G. H., & Gabriele, J. D. (2004). Altered cortical visual processing in PD with hallucinations: an fMRI study. *Neurology, 63*, 1409–1416.

Steeves, T. D. L., Miyasaki, J., Zurowski, M., Lang, A. E., Pellecchia, G., Van Eimeren, T., . . . Strafella, A. P. (2009). Increased striatal dopamine release in parkinsonian patients with pathological gambling: a 11C raclopride PET study. *Brain, 132,* 1376–1385.

Stella, F., Banzato, C. E., Quagliato, E. M., Viana, M. A., & Christofoletti, G. (2009). Psychopathological features in patients with Parkinson's disease and related caregivers' burden. *International Journal of Geriatric Psychiatry, 24,* 1158–1165.

Stewart, J. T. (2008). Fregoli syndrome associated with levodopa treatment. *Movement Disorders, 23,* 308–309.

Stucki, S., & Rihs-Middel, M. (2008). Prevalence of adult problem and pathological gambling between 2000 and 2005: an update. *Journal of Gambling Studies, 23,* 245–257.

Thobois, S., Ardouin, C., Lhommée, E., Klinger, H., Lagrange, C., Xie, J., . . . Krack, P. (2010). Non-motor dopamine withdrawal syndrome after surgery for Parkinson's disease: predictors and underlying mesolimbic denervation. *Brain, 133,* 1111–1127.

Thomas, A., Bonnani, L., Gambi, F., Di Iorio, A., & Onofrj, M. (2010). Pathological gambling in Parkinson disease is reduced by amantadine. *Annals of Neurology, 68,* 400–404.

Tousi, B., & Frankel, M.(2004). Olfactory and visual hallucinations in Parkinson's disease. *Parkinsonism and Related Disorders, 10,* 253–254.

Van Eimeren, T., Pellecchia, G., Cilia, R., Ballanger, B., Steeves, T. D. L., Houle, S., . . . Strafella, A. P. (2010). Drug-induced deactivation of inhibitory networks predicts pathological gambling in PD. *Neurology, 75,* 1711–1716.

Varanese, S., Perfetti, B., Ghilardi, M. F., & Di Rocco, A. (2011). Apathy, but not depression, reflects inefficient cognitive strategies in Parkinson's disease. *PLoS ONE, 6,* e17846.

Vitale, C., Santangelo, G., Trojano, L,. Verde, F., Rocco, M., Grossi, D., & Barone, P. (2011). Comparative neuropsychological profile of pathological gambling, hypersexuality, and compulsive eating in Parkinson's disease. *Movement Disorders, 26,* 830–836.

Volberg, R. A., Nysse-Carris, K. L., & Gerstein, D. R. (2006). *2006 California Problem Gambling Prevalence Survey* National Opinion Research Center at the University of Chicago.

Volkow, N. D., Fowler, J. S., Wang, G. J., Baler, R., & Telang, F. (2009). Imaging dopamine's role in drug abuse and addiction. *Neuropharmacology, 56 (Suppl. 1),* 3–8.

Voon, V. (2004). Repetition, repetition, and repetition: compulsive and punding behaviors in Parkinson's disease. *Movement Disorders, 19,* 367–370.

Voon, V., Fernagut, P.-O., Baunez, C., Rodriguez, M., Pavon, N., Juncos, J. L., . . . Bezard, E. (2009). Chronic dopaminergic stimulation in Parkinson's disease: from dyskinesias to impulse control disorders. *Lancet Neurology, 8,* 1140–1149.

Voon, V. & Fox, S. H. (2007). Medication-related impulse control and repetitive behaviors in Parkinson disease. *Archives of Neurology, 64,* 1089–1096.

Voon, V., Gao, J., Brezing, Z., Symmonds, M., Ekanayake, V., Fernandez, H., . . . Hallett, M. (2011). Dopamine agonists and risk: impulse control disorders in Parkinson's disease. *Brain, 134,* 1438–1446.

Voon, V., Hassan, K., Zurowski, M., de Souza, M., Thomsen, T., Fox, S., . . . Miyasaki, J. (2006). Prevalence of repetitive and reward-seeking behaviors in Parkinson disease. *Neurology, 67,* 1254–1257.

Voon, V., Pessiglione, M., Brezing, C., Gallea, C., Fernandez, H. H., Dolan, R. J., ... Hallett, M. (2010a). Mechanisms underlying dopamine-mediated reward bias in compulsive behaviors. *Neuron, 65,* 135–142.

Voon, V, Reynolds, B., Brezing, C., Gallea C., Skaljic, M., Ekanayake, V., ... Hallett, M. (2010b). Impulsive choice and response in dopamine agonist-related impulse control behaviors. *Psychopharmacology, 207,* 645–659.

Voon, V, Thomsen, T., Miyasaki, J. M., de Souza, M., Shafro, A., Fox, S. H., . . . Zurowski, M. (2007). Factors associated with dopaminergic drug-related pathological gambling in Parkinson disease. *Archives of Neurology, 64*, 212–216.

Wang, M.-T., Lian, P.-W., Yeh, C.-B., Yen, C.-H., Ma, K.-H., & Chan, A. L. F. (2011). Incidence, prescription patterns, and determinants of antipsychotic use in patients with Parkinson's disease. *Movement Disorders, 10.1002/mds.23719.*

Weintraub, D. (2008). Dopamine and impulse control disorders in Parkinson's disease. *Annals of Neurology, 64 (suppl.)*, S93-S100.

Weintraub, D., Chen, P., Ignacio, R. V., Mamikonyan, E., & Kales, H. C. (2011). Patterns and trends in antipsychotic prescribing for Parkinson disease psychosis. *Archives of Neurology, 68*, 899–904.

Weintraub, D., Koester, J., Potenza, M. N., Siderowf, A. D., Stacy, M. A., Voon, V., . . . Lang, A. E. (2010a). Impulse control disorders in Parkinson disease: A cross-sectional study of 3090 patients. *Archives of Neurology, 67*, 589–595.

Weintraub, D., Siderowf, A. D., Potenza, M. N., Goveas, J., Morales, K. H., Duda, J. E., . . . Stern, M. B. (2006). Association of dopamine agonist use with impulse control disorders in Parkinson disease. *Archives of Neurology, 63*, 969–973.

Weintraub, D., Sohr, M., Potenza, M. N., Siegal, A., Stacy, M., Voon, V., . . . Lang, A. E. (2010b). Amantadine use associated with impulse control disorders in Parkinson disease in cross-sectional study. *Annals of Neurology, 68*, 963–968.

Weintraub, D.., Stewart, S., Shea, J. A., Lyons, K. E., Pahwa, R., Driver-Dunckley, E. D., . . . Voon, V. (2009). Validation of the Questionnaire for Impulsive-Compulsive Behaviors in Parkinson's Disease (QUIP). *Movement Disorders, 24*, 1461–1467.

Whitehead, D. L., Davies, A. D., Playfer, J. R., & Turnbill, C. J. (2008). Circadian rest-activity rhythm is altered in Parkinson's disease patients with hallucinations. *Movement Disorders, 23*, 1137–1145.

Wicks, P., & MacPhee, G. J. A. (2009). Pathological gambling amongst Parkinson's disease and ALS patients in an online community (PatientsLikeMe.com). *Movement Disorders, 24*, 1085–1088.

Williams-Gray, C. H., Foltynie, T., Brayne, C. E. G., Robbins, T. W., & Barker, R. A. (2007). Evolution of cognitive dysfunction in an incident Parkinson's disease cohort. *Brain, 130*, 1787–1798.

Williams-Gray, C. H., Hampshire, A., Barker, R. A., & Owen, A. M. (2008). Attentional control in Parkinson's disease is dependent on COMT val158met genotype. *Brain, 131*, 397–408.

Witjas, T., Kaphan, E., Azulay, J. P., Blin, O., Ceccaldi, M., Pouget, J., . . . Chérif, A. A. (2002). Nonmotor fluctuations in Parkinson's disease: frequent and disabling. *Neurology, 59*, 408–413.

Wolters, E. C., Hurwitz, T. A., Mak, E., Teal, P., Peppard, F. R., Remick, R., . . . Calne, D. B. (1990). Clozapine in the treatment of parkinsonian patients with dopaminomimetic psychosis. *Neurology, 40*, 832–834.

Wu, K., O'Sullivan, S., Politis, M., Bose, S., Lees, A., & Piccini, P. (2010). Rewarding visual cues increase dopamine neurotransmission in Parkinson's patients with impulse control disorders: a PET study. *Journal of Neurology, Neurosurgery and Psychiatry, 81*, e29-e30.

Yahr, M. D., Duvoisin, R. C., Schear, M. J., Barrett, E., & Hoehn, M. M. (1969). Treatment of parkinsonism with levodopa. *Archives of Neurology, 21*, 343–354.

12 Effects of Deep Brain Stimulation in Movement Disorders on Cognition and Behavior

Julie A. Fields

INTRODUCTION

Although modern-day techniques are often deemed "relatively safe" from a cognitive and behavioral standpoint, evidence suggests that nonmotor adverse events occur in approximately 10% of deep brain stimulation (DBS) patients (Tröster, 2009a). Therefore, the question remains as to whether the surgical treatment is truly "safe."

Optimal cognitive and behavioral outcomes depend on appropriate selection of surgical candidates, informed by detailed pre- and postoperative assessment of cognitive and psychiatric status. Currently, an expert consensus panel recommends dementia and significant psychiatric comorbidity should be exclusionary criteria for DBS (Bronstein et al., 2011). However, in the absence of frank dementia and psychiatric symptoms, there are no guidelines to help determine at what level cognitive or psychiatric compromise elevates risk for poor neurobehavioral outcomes following DBS. Evidence suggests that preoperative depression, hypomania, "frontal lobe behaviors," and suicide ideation/attempts engender greater risk of post-DBS psychiatric disturbance (Appleby, Dugan, Regenberg, & Rabins, 2007; Voon, Kuba, Krack, Houeto, & Tröster, 2006). Additionally, evidence of prominent preoperative executive dysfunction or a diagnosis of mild cognitive impairment (MCI) confers greater risk of postoperative dementia (Levy et al., 2002; Woods & Tröster, 2003). Yet, the degree to which DBS contributes to cognitive or behavioral decline, time to conversion to dementia, and the impact on quality of life remains elusive.

PRESURGICAL ASSESSMENT

Thorough baseline testing can delineate existing difficulties, such as predementia syndromes and prominent psychiatric or behavioral phenomena that are harbingers of further decline and poor neurobehavioral outcomes postsurgically. In cases of significant preexisting impairment, surgical decision making can become an ethical dilemma. Quite often, patients are so focused on their debilitating motor dysfunction that they are unaware of or assign less importance to coexisting nonmotor symptoms. In some circumstances, they do not have the mental capacity to understand the consequences. Neuropsychological assessment prior to DBS provides patients, families, caregivers, and health-care providers with necessary information regarding an individual's cognitive and emotional status that is used to:

- Determine the presence and pattern of deficits that warrant caution.
- Assess the ability to comply with pre-, peri-, and postoperative treatment demands.
- Assess the risk of postoperative confusion (e.g., association with executive deficits; Pilitsis et al., 2005) and future decline.
- Evaluate surgical candidacy in the context of providing input to a multidisciplinary DBS team.
- Provide the patient and family with as much information as possible to make an informed decision regarding surgery.
- Delineate strengths and weaknesses to help guide the patient and family in making appropriate accommodations to work, home, and social environment pre- and postsurgically.
- Gain insight into patient's capacity for important decision making and consent to treatment.
- Establish a baseline prior to intervention that allows the measurement of treatment outcomes.

A comprehensive battery should measure a variety of abilities in each cognitive domain. See Table 12-1 for commonly used neuropsychological tests.

INDICATIONS AND TARGETS FOR DBS

DBS has become the treatment of choice for a variety of movement and psychiatric disorders (Miocinovic, Somayajula, Chitnis, & Vitek, 2013). Surgical target selection is usually based on motor symptom profile (Thevathasan & Gregory, 2010) and nonmotor factors (Follett et al., 2010). See Table 12-2 for indications and DBS targets in movement disorders. Choosing the optimal target involves weighing the benefits against the costs. For instance, a large, multicenter, prospective study that randomized patients to either subthalamic nucleus (STN) or pallidal (GPi) stimulation for Parkinson's disease (PD) found at 24-month follow-up that there was no difference in motor function or number of serious adverse events, but visuomotor processing speed declined and depression

Table 12-1 Commonly used neuropsychological tests by cognitive domain assessed

Premorbid estimates	Barona Demographic Equations; North American Adult Reading Test (NAART); Wechsler Test of Adult Reading (WTAR); Wide Range Achievement Test (WRAT)
Neuropsychological screening	Mattis Dementia Rating Scale (DRS); Mini-Mental State Examination (MMSE); Repeatable Battery for the Assessment of Neuropsychological Status (RBANS)
Intelligence	Kaufman Brief Intelligence Test (KBIT); Raven's Progressive Matrices; Wechsler Abbreviated Scale of Intelligence (WASI); Wechsler Adult Intelligence Scale (WAIS)
Attention and working memory	Auditory Consonant Trigrams (ACT); Brief Test of Attention (BTA); Continuous Performance Tests (CPT); Digit and Visual Span subtests (Wechsler Memory Scale); Paced Auditory Serial Addition Test (PSAT); Stroop test*
Executive function	Cognitive Estimation Test (CET); Delis-Kaplan Executive Function Scale (DKEFS); Halstead Category Test; Trail Making Test (TMT)*; Wisconsin Card Sorting Test (WCST); Tower of Toronto; Tower of London; DKEFS Tower Test*
Memory	Benton Visual Retention Test (BVRT-R); California Verbal Learning Test (CVLT); Rey Auditory Verbal Learning Test (RAVLT); Selective Reminding Test; Rey Complex Figure Test (RCFT)*; Wechsler Memory Scale (WMS)*; Hopkins Verbal Learning Test (HVLT)
Language	Boston Naming Test (BNT); Controlled Oral Word Association Test (COWAT); Sentence Repetition; Token Test; Complex Ideational Material
Visuoperception	Benton Facial Recognition Test; Benton Judgment of Line Orientation (JLO); Hooper Visual Organization Test (HVOT)
Motor and sensory perception	Finger Tapping*; Grooved Pegboard*; Hand Dynamometer*; Sensory-Perceptual Examination (SPE)
Mood state and personality	Beck Anxiety Inventory (BAI); State-Trait Anxiety Inventory (STAI); Hospital Anxiety and Depression Scale (HDAS); Beck Depression Inventory (BDI); Hamilton Depression Rating Scale (HDRS); Patient Health Questionnaire (PDQ-9); Mood Disorder Questionnaire (MDQ); Montgomery-Asberg Depression Rating Scale; Profile of Mood States (POMS); Starkstein Apathy Scale; Maudsley Obsessional-Compulsive Inventory; Yale-Brown Obsessive Compulsive Scale; Neuropsychiatric Inventory (NPI); Minnesota Multiphasic Personality Inventory (MMPI); Personality Assessment Inventory (PAI)
Quality of life, coping and stressors	Parkinson's Disease Questionnaire (PDQ); Medical Outcomes Study 26-item short form (SF-36); Sickness Impact Profile (SIP); Linear Analog Self Assessment (LASA); Coping Responses Inventory (CRI); Ways of Coping Questionnaire; Life Stressors and Social Resources Inventory (LISRES)

* Note: Test may not be appropriate for patients with marked speech and/or motor impairment.

Adapted from Tröster and Fields (2013). Reprinted with permission from Psychology Press © 2008.

Table 12-2 DBS indications and targets

	PD (Smith, Wichmann, Factor, & DeLong, 2012; Thevathasan & Gregory, 2010)	*ET (Thevathasan & Gregory, 2010)*	*DT (Andrews, Aviles-Olmos, Hariz, & Foltynie, 2010; Thevathasan & Gregory, 2010)*	*TS (Piedad, Rickards, & Cavanna, 2012; Viswanathan, Jimenez-Shahed, Baizabal Carvallo, & Jankovic, 2012)*
Target				
cZi	X (tremor)	X		
CM/Spv/Voi				X
CM/Pf	X (gait, tremor, dyskinesia)			X
VIM	X (tremor)	X		
VIM/Vop/Voa			X (marked tremor)	
STN	X (bradykinesia, rigidity, tremor, reduction in Rx)		X	X
GPi	X (motor fluctuations, dyskinesia)		X	X
GPe				X
PPN	X (gait, freezing)			
ALIC/NA				X

PD, Parkinson's disease; ET, essential tremor; DT, dystonia; TS, Tourette syndrome; cZi, caudal zone incerta; CM/Spv/Voi, centromedian nucleus/substantia periventricularis/ventralis oralis internus; CM/Pf, centromedian-parafascicular nuclei complex; VIM, ventral intermediate nucleus; VIM/Vop/Voa, ventral intermediate nucleus/ventralis oralis posterior/ventralis oralis anterior; STN, subthalamic nucleus; GPi, globus pallidus internus; GPe, globus pallidus externus; PPN, pedunculopontine nucleus; GPe, globus pallidus externus; ALIC/NA, anterior limb of the internal capsule/nucleus accumbens; Rx, medication.

worsened more after STN stimulation than after GPi, and in fact depression symptoms improved with GPi stimulation (Follett et al., 2010). However, this study also showed that those undergoing STN stimulation required less dopaminergic medication following surgery than did those receiving GPi stimulation, which is a desire expressed frequently by patients prior to surgery. Another large, randomized study also found dopaminergic medications to be more reduced after STN than GPi stimulation, but rates of neurobehavioral adverse events (e.g., cognitive decline, depression, loss of job or relationship) were comparable after STN and GPi DBS (Odekerken et al., 2013).

CONSIDERATIONS IN DATA INTERPRETATION

Methodological limitations and procedural differences hinder interpretation of existing studies and their clinical significance. Patient characteristics (e.g., age, preoperative cognition, mood, and psychiatric variables), selection criteria, small sample sizes, lack of appropriate control groups, ill-defined impairment cutoffs, and statistical methods for assessing change are all issues that contribute to discordant findings across studies and prevent generalizable conclusions. Multiple assessments can produce practice effects that may falsely suggest improvement or mask decline. In addition, disease progression or fluctuations, measurement error, and regression to the mean can cloud interpretation. Surgical targets and procedures, as well as "on" and "off" stimulation, medication dosing, and stimulation parameters must also be considered when drawing conclusions.

PARKINSON'S DISEASE

Mechanisms of Nonmotor Changes Following DBS

The mechanisms responsible for the nonmotor features induced or exacerbated by DBS are not clearly understood, but potentially include the spread of stimulation to nonmotor circuits and dopamine dysregulation. PD is associated primarily with dysfunction of the basal ganglia and frontostriatal circuits. The complex interactions of dorsolateral, orbitofrontal, and cingulate circuits are particularly important in the regulation of cognition, affect, and motivation, respectively (Middleton & Strick, 2000), and are probably responsible for the neurobehavioral changes in PD (Zgaljardic, Borod, Foldi, & Mattis, 2003). In the later stages of PD, the amygdala, hippocampi, and frontal and temporoparietal association cortices are involved (Braak et al., 2003). Thus, dementia in PD probably evolves from the progressive involvement of structural and neurochemical changes.

Selection Criteria

An expert consensus panel recently reviewed the key issues in DBS for PD and determined that "patients with PD without significant active or psychiatric problems who have medically intractable motor fluctuations, intractable tremor, or intolerance of medication adverse effects are good candidates for DBS" (Bronstein et al., 2011). More specifically, they recommended that there should be no or very mild cognitive impairment and there should be the absence of or well-controlled psychiatric disease.

DBS in MCI and Dementia

In unoperated samples, recent studies utilizing new consensus criteria for diagnosing PD-MCI (Litvan et al., 2012) have found conversion rates from baseline

Table 12-3 Risk factors associated with dementia in Parkinson's disease

Risk factors
Demographic Variables
Older age
Later age of PD onset
Disease Variables
Severity of motor symptoms
Longer duration of PD symptoms
Akinetic-dominant type
Axial impairment
Presence of ApoE2 and ApoE4 alleles
Neurobehavioral Variables
Presence of hallucinations or psychosis
Depression
Lower MMSE at baseline
Declines in cognitive test performance:
Executive/attention
Verbal fluency
Visuoperceptual
List learning

Adapted from Fields and Tröster (2013). Reprinted with permission from Taylor & Francis © 2013.

MCI to dementia of 27.8% at 1-year follow-up (Pedersen, Larsen, Tysnes, & Alves, 2013) and 19.4% (Broeders et al., 2013) to 45.5% (Pedersen et al., 2013) by 3-year follow-up. DBS outcomes have not been systematically examined in PD patients with MCI, and it is unknown whether DBS exacerbates MCI or psychiatric morbidity in this population. However, it has been shown that the improvements in quality of life that have been associated with improvements in motor functioning following DBS do not appear to hold in patients with poor baseline cognition despite improved motor functioning (Witt et al., 2011). There are no guidelines for determining the level of baseline neurobehavioral dysfunction or dementia risks (Table 12-3) that would contraindicate DBS. A subjective determination may result in individuals who might benefit from DBS being excluded based on borderline cognitive performance or psychiatric symptoms, or conversely, inclusion of similar patients who may not fare so well. It has been suggested that cases with preexisting dementia be evaluated on an individual basis, with pros and cons weighed, in terms of caregiving and quality of life, and all potential risks outlined for the patient and caregivers before a decision is made (Lang et al., 2006).

Cognitive Outcomes Following DBS in Parkinson's Disease

Table 12-4 delineates cognitive and behavioral findings from controlled and randomized studies, of which the key findings are summarized in the following sections.

Table 12-4 Controlled and randomized (when so indicated under Study Design) studies of cognition and behavior following DBS for Parkinson's disease

Investigator	*Study Design*	*Follow-up (mos.)*	*Med/Stim status*	*Domains assessed*	*Improvement*	*Decline*
Deuschl et al. (2006)	78 B-STN 78 BMT Controls; randomized	6	On med, On stim	GCF, quality of life	Quality of life in DBS vs. no change in BMT	DBS 1 suicide, BMT 1 psychosis
Smeding et al. (2006)	99 B-STN 36 BMT Controls	6	On med, On stim	A/Ex, L, V/S, M, mood, quality of life	Tension and quality of life in STN	STN: phonemic and semantic fluency, alternating fluency, Stroop color, Stroop color-word interference, verbal memory; STN: 1 suicide attempt, 9% w/psychiatric symptoms (psychosis, voyeurism, pathologic gambling, aggressiveness) Controls: 1 patient depression
Rothlind et al. (2007)	19 U/15 B-STN (13L, 6R); 23 U/14 B GPI (14L, 9R) (staged); randomized	6 after unilat 15 after bilat	On med, On stim	A/Ex, L, M	Depression in unilateral GPi	Unilateral: STN-Digit Symbol; all DBS-Digit Span back, Stroop word, phonemic and semantic fluency, supermarket fluency Bilateral: STN-Digit Symbol; GPi-Digit Span back; all DBS-phonemic and semantic fluency, arithmetic
York et al. (2008)	23 B-STN 28 BMT Controls	6	Not noted	GCF, A/Ex, L, V/S, M, mood	–	STN: greater decline in delayed verbal recall; using Reliable Change Index, STN more frequent declines in verbal fluency, Stroop color-word; 1 DBS, 0 Controls progressed to dementia; 1 suicide and 1 suicidal ideation in STN
Witt et al. (2008)	60 B-STN 63 BMT Controls; randomized	6	On med, On stim	GCF, A/Ex, L, V/S, M, mood, quality of life	Quality of life, depression, and anxiety in STN	DBS vs. BMT change from baseline: DRS Initiation/Perseveration subtest, phonemic and semantic fluency, Stroop word reading errors, Stroop color naming time and errors, Stroop color-word interference time STN: 1 suicide, 4 depression (transient), 4 psychosis, 1 apathy BMT: 1 death in psychotic episode, 7 psychosis

Okun et al. (2009)	22 U-STN 23 U-GPi; randomized	7	Off med, On stim (optimal, dorsal, ventral locations), Off stim	L, mood	–	STN only: phonemic fluency in all stim conditions (including off) STN more anxiety, confusion, irritability, aggressiveness, obsessive-compulsiveness, mania, and decreased motivation than GPi.
Weaver et al. (2009)[79]	60 B-STN 61 B-GPi, 134 BMT Controls; randomized	6	On med, On stim	GCF, A/Ex, L, V/M, M, mood, quality of life	DBS greater improvement in quality of life than BMT	DBS vs. BMT, change relative to baseline: DBS worsening in working memory index, processing speed index, phonemic fluency, visual memory; 11 DBS vs. 2 BMT psychiatric adverse events
Zahodne et al. (2009)	10 U-STN (7L, 3R) 12 U-GPi (7L, 5R) 19 BMT Controls	12	On med, On stim	A/Ex, L, mood	–	DBS significant declines in phonemic and semantic fluency relative to baseline vs. no pre-post change in Controls; Reliable Change Index: DBS greater declines than Controls on 1 or both fluencies; semantic fluency declines more likely after left-sided surgery
Zangaglia et al. (2009)	32 B-STN 33 BMT Controls	1, 6, 12, 24, 36	On med, On stim	GCF, A/Ex, L, M	–	STN: worsening in phonemic fluency (transient), WCST, Raven's Matrices (6 mos.), MMSE (36 mos.) Controls: MMSE, WCST (36 mos.) STN vs. Controls: phonemic fluency (36 mos.)
Castelli et al. (2010)	27 B-STN 31 BMT Controls	12	On med, On stim	A/Ex, L, M	–	STN decline in phonemic fluency compared to Controls

(continued)

Table 12-4 Continued

Investigator	*Study Design*	*Follow-up (mos.)*	*Med/Stim status*	*Domains assessed*	*Improvement*	*Decline*
Daniels et al. (2010)	60 B-STN 63 BMT Controls; randomized	6	On med, On stim	A/Ex, L, M	–	STN vs. Controls: STN decline in executive function domain score (incl. phonemic and semantic fluency and Stroop interference)
Follett et al. (2010)	147 B-STN 152 B-GPi; randomized	24	On med, On stim	GCF, A/Ex, L, M, mood, quality of life	Quality of life improved in both groups in 6 of 8 subscales of PDQ; depression improved in GPi	STN vs. GPi: STN greater decline in processing speed; within-group change over time not noted; depression worsened in STN; GPi 1 suicide, STN 2 suicide attempts and 1 suicidal ideation
Mikos et al. (2010)	11 U-STN (8L, 3R) 13 U-GPi (8L, 5R) 19 BMT Controls	16	On med, On stim	A/Ex, V/M, V/S, M	DBS > Controls (Reliable Change Index): JLO	DBS vs. Controls: DBS Trails A; Reliable Change Index: DBS word-list recall and processing speed
Smeding et al. (2011)	105 B-STN 40 BMT Controls	12	On med, On stim	GCF, A/Ex, L, M, mood, quality of life	Quality of life in STN	STN vs. Controls: STN greater change from baseline in phonemic and semantic fluency, alternating fluency, DRS total score, AVLT immediate and delayed recall, Stroop color, Stroop word, and Stroop color-word

Williams et al. (2011)	19 B-STN 18 BMT Controls	24	Not stated	GCF, A/Ex, L, V/S, M	–	STN vs. Controls: STN impairments in nonverbal recall, oral Symbol Digit Modalities Test (SDMT), phonemic and semantic fluency; Reliable Change Index: STN greater declines in nonverbal memory, SDMT, phonemic fluency; STN and Controls semantic fluency; progression to dementia 32% STN, 16% Controls (not significant)
Saez-Zea et al. (2012)	9 B-STN 12 BMT Controls	6	On med, On stim	A/Ex, L, M, praxis, quality of life	Quality of life in STN	STN and Controls: phonemic fluency, Trails B, Digit Symbol, Stroop color naming STN vs. Controls: no significant difference; quality of life in Controls
Weaver et al. (2012)	70 B-STN 89 B-GPi; randomized	36	On med, On stim	GCF, A/Ex, L, V/M, M, mood, quality of life	–	DBS relative to baseline: DRS, processing speed index, working memory index, phonemic and semantic fluency, perseverative responses, verbal learning and memory, visuospatial memory; STN vs. GPi: STN greater decline on DRS, verbal learning and memory; initial gains in quality of life at 6 mos. lost at 36 mos.
Zangaglia et al. (2012)	30 B-STN 17 BMT Controls	96 (8 yrs.)	On med, On stim	GCF, A/Ex, L, V/S, M	–	DBS vs. Controls: phonemic fluency DBS and Controls: MMSE Controls: Ravens Progressive Matrices; DBS and Controls progressed to dementia at similar rates (16.7% vs. 17.6%)

(continued)

Table 12-4 Continued

Investigator	*Study Design*	*Follow-up (mos.)*	*Med/Stim status*	*Domains assessed*	*Improvement*	*Decline*
Merola et al. (2013)	19 B-STN 16 BMT Controls; retrospective	72 (6 yrs. avg.)	On med, On stim	A/Ex, L, M, mood	–	STN vs. Controls: STN worse phonemic fluency over time STN: Raven Colour Matrices, word repetition, Trails B, Nelson Modified Card Sorting Test categories and perseverations, phonemic and semantic fluency Controls: Nelson Modified Card Sorting Test perseverations; STN and Controls progressed to dementia at same rates (21% vs. 25%)
Odekerken et al. (2013)	63 B-STN 65 B-GPi; randomized	12	On med, On stim	Cognition, mood and behavior composite score, quality of life	–	–

A/Ex, Attention/Executive Functioning; AVLT, Auditory Verbal Learning Test; B-GPi, bilateral globus pallidus internus; BMT, best medical therapy; B-STN, bilateral subthalamic nucleus; DBS, deep brain stimulation; DRS, Mattis Dementia Rating Scale; FLF, Frontal Lobe Functioning; GCF, global cognitive functioning; JLO, Judgment of Line Orientation; L, language; M, memory; MMSE, Mini-Mental State Examination; PDQ, Parkinson's Disease Questionnaire; quality of life, quality of life; U-GPi, unilateral globus pallidus internus; U-STN, unilateral subthalamic nucleus; V/M, visuomotor; V/S, visuospatial; WCST, Wisconsin Card Sorting Test

Thalamic Stimulation

There are few studies assessing cognition following ventral intermediate (VIM) nucleus of the thalamus DBS for PD, but studies have generally reported no change in overall level of cognitive functioning (Hugdahl & Wester, 2000; Tröster, Fields, Wilkinson, Busenbark, et al., 1997). Fluency declines following thalamic DBS in PD are uncommon, but when noted are more likely to be associated with left-sided VIM stimulation (Schuurman, Bruins, Merkus, Bosch, & Speelman, 2002). Improvements on tasks of problem solving, verbal fluency, naming, and delayed recall have been observed up to 12 months postsurgery (Tröster, Fields, Wilkinson, Pahwa, et al., 1997; Caparros-Lefebvre, Blond, Pecheux, Pasquier, & Petit, 1992; Woods et al., 2001).

The interpretation of cognitive changes following VIM DBS surgery is challenging. In addition to medication and practice effects, neurocognitive changes may reflect a microthalamotomy effect. For example, Tröster and colleagues (Tröster, Wilkinson, Fields, Miyawaki, & Koller, 1998) assessed cognitive functioning postsurgically in a PD patient on and off medication and on and off stimulation and observed that an initial verbal fluency decrement was improved with stimulation regardless of medication condition, suggesting that stimulation may alleviate potential cognitive sequelae associated with the microthalamotomy effect. There is also evidence to suggest that stimulation parameters (polarity, amplitude, frequency, pulse width) could play a role in cognitive outcome (Woods, Fields, Lyons, Pahwa, & Tröster, 2003). In fact, intraoperative studies have shown lower frequencies (i.e., 60 Hz) to be more predictive of memory impairment following thalamotomy than the higher frequencies (i.e., 200 Hz) that are typically utilized in chronic VIM DBS (Hugdahl & Wester, 2000).

Pallidal Stimulation

Overall, pallidal DBS does not appear to increase the risk of cognitive decline (Fields, Tröster, Wilkinson, Pahwa, & Koller, 1999; Trepanier, Kumar, Lozano, Lang, & Saint-Cyr,2000; Vingerhoets, van der Linden, et al., 1999). Specifically, several studies have found no significant changes in overall level of cognitive functioning 3 months after unilateral pallidal DBS (Vingerhoets, van der Linden, et al., 1999; Merello et al., 1999; Tröster, Fields, Wilkinson, Busenbark, et al., 1997). Postoperative declines that have been observed in visuoconstructional ability and semantic verbal fluency are usually not clinically significant (Tröster, Fields, Wilkinson, Busenbark, et al., 1997; Volkmann, 2004) and go unnoticed by the patient. Patients who experience some level of cognitive decrement tend to be older and taking higher medication dosages prior to surgery than patients showing no change or improvement (Vingerhoets et al., 1999).

There are a few studies examining cognitive outcomes following bilateral GPi, but they are usually in small samples and follow-up is short term. However, it appears that the results are comparable to those observed with unilateral GPi stimulation. That is, no significant cognitive morbidity has been observed in small samples of patients at 3 (Ghika et al., 1998), 6 (Ardouin et al., 1999), or 12 (Pillon et al., 2000) months postsurgically. Earlier findings demonstrated that staged bilateral GPi DBS electrode implantation did not appear to pose any significant risk of cognitive decline either (Fields et al., 1999). Conversely, there are studies that suggest stimulation has a negative impact on cognition. A study of 42 patients randomly assigned to staged bilateral GPi or STN DBS revealed declines in verbal fluency and working memory 6 months after unilateral and 15 months after bilateral procedures regardless of surgical target (Rothlind, Cockshott, Starr, & Marks, 2007). The verbal fluency declines were significant only after left-sided surgery and were not associated with age. Executive functioning was disrupted in a single case study after bilateral GPi DBS, but was partially reversed when the stimulators were turned off (Dujardin, Krystkowiak, Defebvre, Blond, & Destee, 2000).

GPi stimulation appears to carry less risk of cognitive and behavioral decline than STN stimulation (see below). Some researchers have proposed that bilateral GPi DBS is a safe and effective treatment for PD patients for whom STN DBS is contraindicated, such as those with preexisting cognitive impairment or psychiatric disturbance (Rouaud et al., 2010), but this requires further investigation.

Subthalamic Nucleus Stimulation

Most recent studies regarding neurobehavioral side effects of DBS have focused on the STN (Voon et al., 2006), as it is currently the target of choice due to its success in relieving most of the cardinal symptoms of PD as well as greatly reducing the amount of medication required postsurgery (Follett et al., 2010; Moro et al., 2010).

Despite improvement from a motor standpoint, its effect on neuropsychological and neurobehavioral functioning, however, remains highly debated (Castelli et al., 2010; Tröster, 2009b), with evidence from many studies supporting no significant cognitive morbidity (Ardouin et al., 1999; Pillon et al., 2000; Alegret et al., 2001; Krack et al., 2003; Heo et al., 2008; Frarccio, Ptito, Sadikot, Panisset, & Dagher, 2008), especially if cases are carefully selected (Parsons, Rogers, Braaten, Woods, & Tröster, 2006). However, others find decrements (York et al., 2008; Smeding et al., 2005), and some have estimated that approximately 40% of bilateral STN DBS patients experience postsurgical cognitive problems (Temel et al., 2006). Older age, moderate levels of baseline cognitive impairment, and longer disease duration have been associated with more frequent adverse cognitive and psychiatric events (Trepanier et al., 2000; Alegret et al., 2001; Hariz, Rehncrona, Quinn, Speelman, & Wensing, 2008; Houeto et al., 2002) and are more common following STN than GPi stimulation.

Declines in phonemic (Ardouin et al., 1999; Castelli et al., 2010; Alegret et al., 2001; Parsons et al., 2006; York et al., 2008; Contarino et al., 2007; Daniele et al., 2003; Daniels et al., 2010; Fasano et al., 2010; Merola et al., 2013; Okun et al., 2009; Saez-Zea, Escamilla-Sevilla, Katati, & Minguez-Castellanos, 2012; Smeding et al., 2006; Smeding, Speelman, Huizenga, Schuurman, & Schmand,

2011; Williams et al., 2011; Witt et al., 2008; Yamanaka et al., 2012; Zangaglia et al., 2009; Zibetti et al., 2011) and semantic (Alegret et al., 2001; Parsons et al., 2006; Daniels et al., 2010; Merola et al., 2013; Smeding et al., 2006; Smeding et al., 2011; Williams et al., 2011; Witt et al., 2008; Yamanaka et al., 2012; Zibetti et al., 2011; Funkiewiez et al., 2004; Moretti et al., 2003) verbal fluency are undisputedly the most frequently documented changes following STN DBS. However, studies over the past decade have also shown declines in other cognitive domains, including verbal memory (Trepanier et al., 2000; Alegret et al., 2001; Heo et al., 2008; Daniele et al., 2003; Fasano et al., 2010; Smeding et al., 2006; Smeding et al., 2011; Aybek et al., 2007; Morrison et al., 2004; Weaver et al., 2012), spatial memory (Trepanier et al., 2000; Alegret et al., 2001; Williams et al., 2011; Weaver et al., 2012), visual attention (Saez-Zea et al., 2012; Smeding et al., 2006; Witt et al., 2008), selective attention (Smeding et al., 2006), processing speed (Follett et al., 2010; Weaver et al., 2012), and "frontal"/executive functioning (Trepanier et al., 2000; Daniels et al., 2010; Fasano et al., 2010; Merola et al., 2013; Smeding et al., 2011; Witt et al., 2008; Yamanaka, et al., 2012; Zangaglia et al., 2009; Zibetti et al., 2011; Aybek et al., 2007; Weaver et al., 2012; Merola et al., 2011; Schupbach et al., 2005). Others have reported improvements in mental flexibility (Alegret et al., 2001; Zibetti et al., 2011; Castelli et al., 2006; Jahanshahi et al., 2000; Lhomme et al., 2012), working memory (Jahanshahi et al., 2000), visuomotor sequencing (Ardouin etal., 1999; Pillon et al., 2000; Daniele et al., 2003; Jahanshahi, et al., 2000), conceptual reasoning (Daniele et al., 2003; Jahanshahi, 2000), and overall cognitive functioning (Daniele et al., 2003). Although STN DBS is most commonly performed bilaterally, cognitive outcomes of unilateral STN DBS are similar to those observed following bilateral stimulation, that is, frontal executive functioning, phonemic and semantic fluency, processing speed, and word list recall (Mikos, Zahodne, Okun, Foote, & Bowers, 2010; Zahodne, Okun, Foote, Fernandez, Rodriguez, Kirsch-Darrow, et al., 2009).

Controlled studies have reported greater declines across a wide range of cognitive measures, including attention, processing speed, executive functioning, verbal fluency, and aspects of verbal and visuospatial memory, following bilateral STN DBS as compared to non-surgical PD controls (i.e., best medical treatment [BMT]; Castelli et al., 2010; York et al., 2008; Merola et al., 2013; Saez-Zea et al., 2012; Smeding et al., 2006; Smeding et al., 2011; Williams et al., 2011; Witt et al., 2008; Zangaglia et al., 2009; Mikos et al., 2010; Zahodne, Okun, Foote, Fernandez, Rodriguez, Kirsch-Darrow, et al., 2009; Zangaglia et al., 2012).

When patients are randomized to treatment, results are quite similar from a cognitive perspective. Several groups have examined cognitive performance following randomization to bilateral STN DBS or BMT. Deuschl et al. (2006) reported no significant changes in global cognitive functioning at 6-month follow-up. However, cognitive functioning in specific domains was not assessed. Studies by Witt et al. (2008) and Daniels et al. (2010) utilizing a broader range of measures demonstrated declines in phonemic and semantic fluency as well as declines in executive functioning 6 months following randomization as compared to controls.

A multicenter, randomized, controlled trial of bilateral STN and GPi DBS versus BMT found that DBS patients experienced small decrements on measures of working memory, processing speed, phonemic fluency, and visual delayed recall, whereas the BMT group showed slight (but not statistically significant) improvements on these measures (Weaver et al., 2009) at 6-month follow-up. These same investigators reported 3-year follow-up in their group of patients randomized to STN or GPi (Weaver et al., 2012). DBS patients as a whole demonstrated a wider range of declines relative to baseline, including global cognitive functioning, working memory, phonemic and semantic fluency, cognitive flexibility, and visuospatial and verbal memory. When cognitive performance in STN was compared to that of those undergoing GPi stimulation, STN DBS patients showed greater declines in global cognitive functioning as well as verbal learning and memory. Follett et al. (2010) assessed performance in a larger number of patients (some overlap with Weaver et al. (2009 and 2012) studies) randomized to STN or GPi DBS 2 years after surgery. Both groups showed similarly slight decrements in most cognitive domains, but there was significantly greater decline in processing speed for STN versus GPi.

Rothlind et al. (2007) examined the effects of staged STN or GPi DBS 6 months after randomization to unilateral implantation and 15 months following bilateral implantation. Following unilateral DBS, declines in processing speed were observed in those randomized to STN surgery. Additionally, both groups evidenced declines in working memory, visual attention, and phonemic, semantic, and supermarket fluency. STN patients still showed similar declines following bilateral surgery, with the exception of working memory decline that was observed only in the GPi group. Both groups showed persistent declines in phonemic and semantic fluency. Okun et al. (2009) examined language 7 months after randomization to unilateral STN or GPi in off medication and on and off stimulation conditions. Phonemic fluency declined in all stimulation conditions, but only in STN.

Long-term outcomes (3 to 9 years) show that the greatest declines over time are in frontal/executive functioning and verbal fluency, followed by reasoning and memory (Krack et al., 2003; Contarino, 2007; Fasano et al., 2010; Zibetti et al., 2011; Funkiewiez et al., 2004; Aybek et al., 2007; Weaver et al., 2012; Merola et al., 2011; Schupbach et al., 2005; Kishore et al., 2010). Further, evidence from recent controlled studies indicates that patients undergoing STN DBS progress to dementia at similar rates as BMT controls (Merola et al., 2013; Williams et al., 2011; Zibetti et al., 2011; Zangaglia et al., 2012).

It is unclear whether neurobehavioral declines are due to surgery (i.e., "microsubthalamotomy effect"), stimulation, or a combination of factors. Morrison et al. (2004) examined the cognitive effects in 17 STN DBS with PD in both on- and off-stimulation conditions, 3 months following implantation, as compared to 11 matched nonsurgical PD controls. The STN DBS group showed a mild decline on indices of attention and language as compared to controls, with no differences between on and off conditions in the DBS group except for one individual, suggesting these changes were related to the procedure and not stimulation per se.

Similarly, Okun et al. (2009) compared 45 subjects randomized to either STN or GPi DBS, and at 7 months postsurgery found no differences between the groups on measures of language at optimal stimulation settings. The STN group, however, exhibited a larger decline in phonemic fluency than GPi when compared to baseline, with an even larger deterioration observed when stimulators were turned off. The authors concluded that declines were related to surgical rather than stimulation-induced effects. Pillon et al. (2000), too, found evidence of a lesioning effect. They compared 48 STN DBS patients with 8 GPi DBS patients after surgery in on- and off-stimulation conditions (most patients without levodopa for 12 hours) and found no overall differences between STN and GPi stimulation, but the STN group showed a greater postoperative decline in category fluency that persisted 12 months after surgery, both with and without stimulation. On the other hand, others have found reduced working memory and response inhibition under challenging conditions during stimulation (Hershey et al., 2004), while another group found that stimulation improved patients' ability to shift cognitive sets (Page & Jahanshahi, 2007).

Some investigators have posited that the neurobehavioral consequences of STN DBS are related to lead positioning, particularly the anterior ventral region, and connectivity with the limbic circuitry (Lambert et al., 2012; Tsai et al., 2007). Further, data from a subset of patients who had been randomized to either STN DBS (n = 31) or BMT (n = 31) revealed that lead trajectory predicted cognitive decline 6 months postsurgery (Witt et al., 2013). In addition, some studies have suggested that the cognitive and psychiatric sequelae of STN stimulation are related to a reduction in dopaminergic medication (Krach, Fraix, Mendes, Benabid, & Pollak, 2002), although others have found evidence of improvement in these non-motor symptoms with medication reduction (Lhomme et al., 2012; Castrioto et al., 2013). Lastly, it is postulated that DBS settings (i.e., pulse width, amplitude, and frequency) may play a role in cognitive outcomes and therefore may explain some of the disparate findings across studies. Schoenberg, Mash, Bharucha, Francel, and Scott (2008) evaluated 20 patients 5 months following STN DBS and found declines in verbal fluency and improvements in visuoconstructional skills that were significantly correlated with amplitude and pulse width. Wojtecki et al. (2006) examined verbal fluency performance in 12 patients in high-frequency, low-frequency, and no-stimulation conditions and found that verbal fluency was facilitated at low frequencies whereas high frequencies disrupted word generation. A meta-analysis of 28 DBS studies, however, failed to find a relationship between postoperative decline in verbal fluency and differences in stimulation parameters (Parsons et al., 2006).

In summary, cognitive declines are frequently observed following DBS. Based on limited data from the small number of studies following VIM and GPi stimulation, they appear to be associated with less cognitive morbidity than STN DBS. Declines in verbal fluency are more frequently reported, but frontal/executive functioning is also often diminished following stimulation. There is less consistency with regard to verbal and visuospatial memory. However, despite the observed declines, patients treated with DBS do not appear to progress to dementia more rapidly than BMT controls. The mechanisms underlying postsurgical cognitive changes remain elusive and are probably multifactorial, but likely suspects include stimulation parameters, lead positioning, microlesioning effects, and changes in levels of dopamine replacement.

Behavioral Outcomes Following DBS in Parkinson's Disease

Thalamic Stimulation

There are very few studies that have reported mood and quality of life outcomes following thalamic stimulation for PD. Some of the literature to date suggests that VIM DBS may lead to fewer reported symptoms of depression and anxiety (Caparros-Lefevbre et al., 1992; Woods et al., 2001, yet others have found no significant reduction in depressive symptoms (Straits-Tröster et al., 2000). The relationship between VIM DBS and quality of life remains unclear as well. It is likely that small sample sizes and the instruments used to assess mood and quality of life play a role in discrepant findings. Straits-Tröster et al. (2000) failed to detect changes in quality of life at 3 months post VIM DBS surgery. Utilizing a disease-specific measure of quality of life, Woods et al. (2001) found that patients reported significant improvements in depression, anxiety, and quality of life that were maintained at 12 months post unilateral VIM DBS surgery. Psychiatric adverse events are rare. Hariz et al. (2008) reported, in a 6-year follow-up, multicenter study of 38 patients treated with VIM DBS, only one case of hallucinations among all centers.

Pallidal Stimulation

Small but significant improvements in self-reported anxiety and vigor (Fields et al., 1999; Tröster, Fields, Wilkinson, Pahwa, et al., 1997; Straits-Tröster et al., 2000) have been reported following unilateral GPi stimulation, but most studies do not find similar improvements in depressive symptoms (Ghika et al., 1998; Pillon et al., 2000; Straits-Tröster et al., 2000; Pahwa et al., 2001). Rothlind et al. (2007), however, did find in a group of patients randomized to staged GPi or STN stimulation that there was a decrease in self-reported depression in the GPi group 6 months after unilateral implantation and a trend toward improvement 15 months after bilateral implantation. Contrary to what others have shown, there was no change in symptoms of anxiety at either time point. Improvement in both depression and anxiety scores has been documented with bilateral GPi stimulation (Follett et al., 2010; Ardouin et al., 1999; Higginson, Fields, & Tröster, 2001; Volkmann et al., 2001), but there has been report of suicide in a randomized trial (Follett et al., 2010).

Behavioral changes are infrequently reported following GPi DBS, but when they occur they appear to be related to bilateral surgery. Miyawaki, Perlmutter, Tröster, Videen, and Koller, (2000) described a single patient who underwent bilateral staged GPi DBS surgery and developed transient manic episodes after his second (right GPi) surgery that subsided with a reduction in his levodopa dosage.

Similarly, a case of hypersexuality (Roane, Yu, Feinberg, & Rogers, 2002) has been reported following left GPi DBS subsequent to previous right pallidotomy.

Both unilateral and bilateral GPi DBS have been associated with significant improvements in quality of life. Vingerhoets, Lannoo, et al. (1999) reported significant improvements in physical, psychosocial, and overall functioning 3 months following unilateral GPi DBS. Similarly, unilateral GPi DBS patients who completed a disease-specific quality of life measure 3 months after surgery noted improved mobility and ability to perform activities of daily living as well as decreased stigma (Straits-Tröster et al., 2000). Rodrigues, Walters, Watson, Stell, and Mastaglia (2007) reported that, in a sample of 11 patients (4 unilateral, 7 bilateral) 8 months after surgery, there were significant improvements in mobility, activities of daily living, bodily discomfort, emotional well-being, communication, and cognition subscales on a PD quality of life questionnaire and that these changes were not the effect of motor improvement. More recently, two randomized trials of bilateral GPi and STN stimulation have reported improvements on disease-specific measures of quality of life 6 months (Weaver et al., 2009) to 2 years (Follett et al., 2010) following implantation, and improvements were significantly greater as compared to controls.

Subthalamic Nucleus Stimulation

Mood and psychiatric complications following STN DBS have been widely reported and are believed to occur more frequently than following stimulation to other surgical sites (Woods et al., 2001; Okun et al., 2009; Anderson, Burchiel, Hogarth, Favre, & Hammerstad, 2005; Rodriguez-Oroz et al., 2005). There are mixed findings with regard to these nonmotor symptoms following STN DBS, with some investigators showing declines postsurgically (Follett et al., 2010; Fasano et al., 2010; Witt et al., 2008), some showing no significant change (York et al., 2008; Zibetti et al., 2011), and others showing improvement (Ardouin et al.,1999; Witt et al., 2008; Funkiewiez et al., 2004; Castelli et al., 2006; Lhomme et al., 2012; Volkmann et al., 2001). Despite vast research in this area, it remains unknown to what extent non-motor symptoms are due to the effects of stimulation, postsurgical reduction of dopaminergic medication, preexisting mood and psychiatric comorbidities, physical symptoms, psychosocial factors, or an interaction among any or all of these variables. What does seem clear, however, is that nonmotor symptoms have a negative impact on overall quality of life (Anderson & Mullins, 2003; Kleiner-Fisman et al., 2006).

Estimates of postsurgical depression with STN stimulation vary from 1.5% to 25% (Appleby et al., 2007; Follett et al., 2010; Krack et al., 2003; Rodriguez-Oroz et al., 2005; Martinez-Martin et al., 2002). Okun et al. (2009) reported that stimulation of either STN or GPi targets resulted in less happy and less energetic behavior. Benabid et al. (2001) observed depression in approximately 12% of their STN DBS patients, and similarly, Tir et al. (2007) observed depression in 18% of their patients 12 months after STN DBS, 72% of whom in the latter study had a past history of depression. There were 2 suicide attempts among their depressed cohort, with 1 suicide completion. Volkmann et al. (2001) and Follett et al. (2010) found that depression occurred more frequently in patients receiving STN than GPi DBS, and Gervais-Bernard et al. (2009) and Schupbach et al. (2005) observed that depression persisted up to 5 years postsurgery in approximately 22% to 40% of their STN DBS patients.

Other studies have reported improvement in depression (Ardouin et al., 1999; Pillon et al., 2000; Daniele et al., 2003; Funkiewiez et al., 2004; Dujardin, Defebvre, Krystkowiak, Blond, & Destee, 2001) and anxiety (Witt et al., 2008) following STN DBS. Witt et al. (2008) found that STN DBS had a slight positive effect on depression and a significant positive effect on anxiety as compared to patients receiving BMT. One patient in the STN group committed suicide, and 1 patient in the BMT group died in a psychotic episode. Still others have shown no effect of STN DBS on mood symptoms (Heo et al., 2008; York et al., 2008; Zibetti et al., 2011). Montel and Bungener (2009) found no significant change in depression or anxiety 12 months following surgery in 40 STN DBS patients as compared to 40 dopamine therapy patients. Morrison et al. (2004) found no effects on depression scores in 17 STN DBS patients 3 months after implantation, and similarly, York et al. (2008) observed no changes in depression, anxiety, or psychological distress scores in 23 patients 6 months after surgery. Zibetti et al. (2011) reported no changes in mood in patients followed for up to 9 years. Worsening of preexisting anxiety has been reported (Rodriguez-Oroz et al., 2005), but more commonly there are reports of improvement (Daniele et al., 2003; Schupbach et al., 2007) or stability (York et al., 2008), even as far as 8 years out from surgery (Fasano et al., 2010).

Of growing concern are the reports of suicidal tendencies in some patients with PD STN DBS, especially in the first postoperative year (Soulas et al., 2008; Voon et al., 2008). Baseline PD suicide rates range from equal to 10 times *lower* than in the general population (Juurlink, Herrmann, Szalai, Kopp, & Redelmeier, 2004; Myslobodsky, Lalonde, & Hicks, 2001). Suicide attempts and/or completions, however, have been reported in from 0.5% to 4% of STN DBS cases (Krack et al., 2003; Houeto et al., 2002; Voon, Moro, Saint-Cyr, Lozano, & Lang, 2005; Doshi, Chhaya, & Bhatt, 2002; Burkhard et al., 2004). Burkhard et al. (2004) reported a suicide rate of 4.3% in a series of 140 STN DBS patients. All but one of the patients who committed suicide had a preoperative history of major depression as well as prior suicide attempts or suicidal ideation. A retrospective study of 200 STN DBS patients conducted by Soulas et al. (2008) noted that 2 patients (1%) committed suicide and 4 (2%) attempted suicide. There were no differences between the suicidal and nonsuicidal patients with regard to age, disease duration, preoperative depression, or cognitive status. They did find, however, that suicidal behavior was associated with postoperative depression and/or impulsivity. In a multicenter study (55 centers) on suicide outcomes following STN DBS, the completed suicide rate was 0.45% and the attempted suicide rate was 0.90% (Voon et al., 2008). Identified factors included postoperative depression, being single, a history of impulse control disorders, and compulsive medication use. Younger age, younger age at PD onset, and preoperative suicide attempts were also weakly associated, but gender and preoperative depression were not. In contrast to what the preceding studies have shown, a recent randomized, controlled trial of 255 patients followed for 6 months found that not only was suicidal ideation rare, it was no different than that observed in a BMT group (1.9% for DBS and 0.9% for the BMT group) nor were there differences between the STN and GPi stimulation groups (Weintraub et al., 2013).

An increase in apathy has frequently been observed following STN DBS (Contarino et al., 2007; Funkiewiez et al., 2004; Schupbach et al., 2005; Czernecki et al., 2008; Kirsch-Darrow et al., 2011; LeJeune et al., 2009; Porat, Cohen, Schwartz, & Hassin-Baer, 2009; Thobois et al., 2010, whereas some studies have shown no postsurgical change (Castelli et al., 2006, 2007). Studies report that apathy persists in up to 25% of patients at 3-year follow-up (Funkiewiez et al., 2004) and up to 12% of cases at 5-year follow-up (Krack et al., 2003). Interestingly, in the latter study, 80% of the patients with postoperative apathy also developed incident dementia. In a large study of 238 STN DBS patients, Romito and Albanese (2010) found persistent apathy 5 years later. Kirsch-Darrow et al. (2011) examined the trajectory of apathy in 48 patients randomized to unilateral STN or GPi DBS and 48 matched controls at baseline and 2, 4, and 6 months postsurgery. They found a linear increase in apathy in the DBS group in comparison to the control group, which showed no change, but there was no difference between STN and GPi. Further, although there was an association between apathy and depression at baseline, depression was not associated with change in apathy. Those age 65 or less had a steeper trajectory than those older than age 65. Since STN stimulation generally results in a reduction in dopaminergic medication (Moro et al., 1999), some have suggested that the depression and apathy observed following STN DBS may actually be the result of dopamine withdrawal (Volkmann et al., 2001) but Kirsch-Darrow et al. (2011) did not find an association between apathy trajectory and dopamine reduction.

Impulse control disorders (ICDs), such as pathological gambling, hypersexuality, and compulsive eating, are present in up to 13.6% of patients with PD (Weintraub et al., 2010). Dopamine agonists have been correlated with ICDs (Antonini et al., 2011; Lee et al., 2010), and hence it is hypothesized that with the reduction in dopamine that most often accompanies STN DBS, there may be a reduction in ICDs (Wolters, van der Werf, & van den Heuvel, 2008). Some studies do in fact report improvement or abatement of ICDs with STN stimulation (Ardouin et al., 2006; Witjas et al., 2005. However, others report new onset or worsening (Contarino et al., 2007; Funkiewiez et al., 2004; Halbig et al., 2009; Lim et al., 2009; Smeding et al., 2007; Zahodne et al., 2011). More recently, Kim et al. (Kim et al., 2013) evaluated ICDs in 89 patients before and after bilateral STN DBS and found improvement in 65% of those with pre-existing ICDs (with complete resolution in 6 of the 13 patients that improved), and new-onset ICDs in 10% of the patients postoperatively. There was no association with levodopa equivalent daily doses, but ICDs were more severe in older patients and were more likely to worsen when depression scores decreased. The investigators postulate that different mechanisms, for example, risk factors, may underlie the different outcomes. New onset or worsening of punding (stereotyped behavior characterized by fascination with complex, excessive, repetitive activities) can occur following STN DBS surgery even with reductions in dopamine replacement therapy (Fasano, Ricciardi, Pettorruso, & Bentivoglio, 2011; Lim & Lang, 2010). Transient confusion (Herzog et al., 2003; Molinuevo et al., 2000; Tamma et al., 2003) and hallucinations and delusions have been observed immediately following surgery (Zibetti et al., 2011; Romito & Albanese, 2010), but there may also be a decrease in preexisting hallucinations following STN DBS after a reduction in dopaminergic medication (Umemura, Oka, Okita, Matsukawa, & Yamada, 2011; Yoshida et al., 2009). Cases of mania/hypomania (Krack et al., 2003; Daniele et al., 2003; Funkiewiez et al., 2004; Schupbach et al., 2005; Romito & Albanese, 2010, Herzog et al., 2003) and pathological laughter and euphoria (Benabid et al., 2001; Benjani et al., 1999; Houeto et al., 2000; Kumar, Lozano, Sime, Halket, & Lang, 1999) are also among the psychiatric symptoms reported following STN DBS. Witt et al. (2004), in contrast, found that severe psychiatric adverse events following STN DBS were only slightly higher than in patients receiving BMT.

Improvements in quality of life ratings are generally reported after STN DBS (Follett et al., 2010; Saez-Zea et al., 2012; Smeding et al., 2006; Smeding et al., 2011; Witt et al., 2008; Kishore et al., 2010; Diamond & Jankovic, 2005; Erola et al., 2005; Lezcano et al., 2004), but not in all cases are they sustained over time (Weaver et al., 2012; Volkmann et al., 2009). Capus et al. (2001) reported up to 50% improvement in disease-specific quality of life in 7 patients at 14.5 months following surgery. A large randomized, controlled, multicenter study of 156 patients with advanced PD that compared 78 STN DBS patients to 78 medication-only PD controls 6 months after surgery reported improvement in mobility, activities of daily living, emotional well-being, stigma, and bodily discomfort in the stimulation group (Deuschl et al., 2006). In another randomized, controlled trial, quality of life was improved after 18 months in the surgical versus nonsurgical PD control group (Schupbach et al., 2007). In studies randomizing patients to STN or GPi DBS, Follett et al. (2010) found that 2 years following bilateral stimulation, both STN and GPi reported improved quality of life, and Zahodne, Okun, Foote, Fernandez, Rodriguez, Wu, et al. (2009) found improved quality of life in both unilateral GPi and STN 6 months postsurgically, with the GPi showing greater improvement than STN. Although several studies have shown that improvements in quality of life are maintained even longer, that is, up to 3 to 5 years postsurgery (Krack et al., 2003; Schupbach et al., 2005; Volkmann et al., 2009), Volkmann et al. (2009) reported that many of the initial STN DBS benefits in quality of life were lost after 3 years. Ferrara et al. (2010) found improvements in quality of life related to movement and general health (e.g., energy level/enjoyment of life, controllability/fluidity of movement) but no change in quality of life items related to general life issues (e.g., occupational function, interpersonal relationships, leisure activities). A study by Derost et al. (2007) suggests that changes in quality of life following STN DBS may be age-dependent, with younger (age<65) but not older (age 65+) patients reporting improvement in quality of life in spite of equal improvement in motor function. In contrast, Tykocki,

Szalecki, Koziara, Nauman, and Mandat (2013) observed that improvements in quality of life and motor functioning reported at 6 months deteriorated proportionately at 24 months, suggesting that quality of life is related to motor functioning. Improvements in depression were sustained. Maier et al. (2013) evaluated quality of life 3 months following STN DBS in 30 patients and found that, despite significant improvements in motor functioning, 8 patients perceived surgical outcome as negative. Further investigation showed that negative outcomes were characterized by unrealistic expectations, and that presurgical depression and apathy were significant predictors of perceived negative outcomes.

The explanation for disparate findings regarding postsurgical neurobehavioral changes is probably related to the complex interplay of physiological and psychological variables. In addition to a potential stimulation-medication interaction, coping strategies and expectations may play an important role in behavioral outcomes.

NEUROBEHAVIORAL OUTCOMES IN OTHER MOVEMENT DISORDERS

DBS has been used effectively to treat a variety of neurologic disorders other than PD, such as essential tremor (ET) and dystonia, and in the last decade has been applied experimentally to treatment-refractory psychiatric disorders such as Tourette syndrome (TS), depression, and obsessive-compulsive disorder as well. Depression and obsessive-compulsive disorder are beyond the scope of this chapter, but TS will be subsumed under the umbrella of movement disorders given its prominent motor presentation.

Essential Tremor

Essential tremor (ET) is one of the most, if not the most, common movement disorders among adults (Louis & Ferreira, 2010). The neuropathology of ET is uncertain, but it is widely believed that the abnormal rhythmic motor unit entrainment emerges from abnormal oscillation within the cerebello-thalamo-cortical pathway (Elble, 2006). It can affect either the proximal or distal musculature and occurs when maintaining limb position or posture (postural tremor), during active movement (action tremor), or when a limb is approaching a target (intention tremor; Plaha et al., 2011). Traditionally ET has been regarded as a neurologic condition without other motor features than tremor and without nonmotor features, but numerous studies have now shown that indeed there are cognitive deficits common to ET (Higginson et al., 2008). In fact, recently Benito-Leon, Louis, Mitchell, and Bermejo-Pareja (2011) examined the association between MCI and ET and found that after adjusting for age, education, gender, and other potential confounding factors, ET cases were 28% more likely to have MCI than non-ET subjects and that this percentage increased to 57% in those with tremor onset after age 65. Moreover, in a population-based study of people age 65 or older, nondemented ET cases and controls were followed prospectively and during the 3-year follow-up period, it was shown that not only were baseline global cognition scores in ET lower than controls, their scores declined 7 times faster than those of controls (Louis, Benito-Leon, Vega-Quiroga, & Bermejo-Parejo, 2010). Similar findings have been reported by Thawani, Schupf, and Louis (2009), who showed that ET was associated with increased odds of prevalent dementia as well as increased risk of incident dementia. Whether there is a characteristic pattern of cognitive dysfunction in ET has not been clearly determined, but there is a large body of evidence indicating that deficits are similar to those seen in PD, that is, frontal subcortical dysfunction (Higginson et al., 2008; Gasparini et al., 2001; Lacritz, Dewey, Giller, & Cullum, 2002). Others have posited that cerebello-thalamo-cortical pathophysiology is responsible for the cognitive deficits observed in ET (Sahin et al., 2006; Tröster et al., 2002).

Despite the mounting evidence that ET is not benign from a cognitive standpoint and that DBS is not without cognitive and behavioral consequences, only a handful of studies have evaluated (or at least reported) mood and cognition in DBS candidates prior to or following surgery. Tröster et al. (1999) examined cognitive performance, mood, and quality of life in 40 patients undergoing unilateral (38 left) thalamic stimulation and found that, 3 months postsurgery, as a group they improved in visuomotor coordination, visual attention, visuoperceptual and constructional abilities, word-list recognition, and verbal recall. In addition, patients reported feeling less anxious and had a better quality of life. However, decrements in verbal fluency were noted. Fields et al. (2003) followed this same group and reported that 1 year following stimulation there were no group-wise declines, but on an individual basis, more patients showed declines than improvements on language and visualmemory tasks. In particular, semantic fluency declines were persistent, with 10% of the patients (versus 7.5% at 3 months) showing decline relative to baseline. It was observed that all the patients showing persistent verbal fluency declines had diminished verbal fluency at baseline. Anxiety and quality of life remained improved. In contrast, a case study by Lucas, Rippeth, Uitti, Shuster, and Wharen (2000) showed improvements in verbal fluency and verbal memory on stimulation. They evaluated cognition and mood in an 80-year-old patient 3 months post bilateral thalamic stimulation with stimulators on and off. Cognitive performance was similar in the on and off conditions for attention, mental tracking, visuospatial perception, verbal learning, and verbal recognition. In the off stimulation condition, there were declines in verbal fluency and verbal memory, but an improvement in Stroop Color-Word performance, suggesting that stimulation differentially impacts cognitive abilities, facilitating some aspects of processing while simultaneously inhibiting others. The patient also reported a higher level of distress, especially anxiety, when off stimulation.

The mechanisms leading to cognitive declines and conflicting findings following thalamic stimulation are not clear, but there has been some suggestion that it is related to stimulation parameters. In order to elucidate this theory, Woods et al. (2003) assessed cognition functioning before and 3 months after unilateral thalamic stimulation in 49 patients with ET. They found that 55% of the patients showed decline from baseline of at least 1 standard deviation on one or more tests in two domains of cognitive functioning. When the "decliners" (n = 27) were compared to the "cognitively stable" (n = 22), higher pulse width settings and disease onset greater than age 37 were the best predictors of postsurgical cognitive decline.

There is a paucity of reported long-term outcomes following DBS in ET. The study with the longest follow-up period was recently conducted by Heber et al. (2013), who examined 9 ET patients 1 year following left unilateral thalamic stimulation as well as at 6 years postsurgery, with 5 of those having undergone bilateral implantation by that time point. Patients were assessed on and off stimulation, and no cognitive or mood changes on a wide range of tests were observed in either condition, with one exception. Simple reaction time was slower when off stimulation (unilateral) but was restored when on stimulation. The authors interpreted this as evidence of a lesion effect attributable to disruption of cerebello-thalamo-cortical pathways rather than an effect of stimulation.

Although the VIM has been the surgical target of choice for suppression of tremor in ET, some investigators have performed bilateral stimulation of the caudal or motor portion of the zona inerta nucleus (cZi; Plaha et al., 2011) and achieved satisfactory motor results, with benefit maintained over a follow-up period of 1 to 7 years in 15 patients. They did not report cognitive effects of stimulation, but they did report improved quality of life on both physical and mental components of the SF-36 in those patients who were followed up to 4 years.

Sandvik, Hariz, and Blomstedt (2012) also evaluated quality of life in 16 ET patients who had undergone DBS of the cZi. In addition to the generic SF-36, they utilized a disease-specific instrument, the QUEST (Quality of Life in Essential Tremor Questionnaire; Tröster, Pahwa, Fields, Tanner, & Lyons, 2005). Results showed statistically significant improvements in psychosocial and ADL subscores of the QUEST, but there were no significant changes on the SF-36 despite good tremor reduction. Hariz, Lindberg, and Bergenheim (2002) evaluated the impact of DBS on quality of life in 27 patients undergoing thalamic DBS (4 previously underwent thalamotomy, with 2 ipsilateral to current DBS) and found improvement in health-related quality of life and disability.

In summary, ET is a disabling action tremor that appears to have associated cognitive deficits consistent with cerebello-thalamo-cortical (i.e., frontal) circuit dysfunction. In particular, declines in attention, executive functioning, fluency, and aspects of memory are most commonly reported and resemble the pattern of impairment in PD. Verbal fluency declines are the most consistent finding after thalamic DBS in ET and can persist, especially if already present at baseline. Further, dementia in late-onset ET is more common than in the general population. Regardless of pattern or pathophysiology, it appears that executive dysfunction and neuropsychiatric symptoms, that is, apathy and depression, are important predictors of self-perceived health status in ET (Woods, Scoot, Fields, Poquette, & Tröster, 2008). Careful consideration should be given to presurgical candidates, and contraindications to DBS should include dementia, significant frontal lobe dysfunction, advanced age, significant depression or anxiety, and poor coping skills.

Dystonia

Dystonia is a common movement disorder with multiple etiologies and subtypes. Reports of surgical outcomes are diverse, owing in large part to the differing etiologies and the phenomenology. An international committee of experts recently convened and developed consensus criteria for defining and classifying dystonia (Albanese et al., 2013). They define dystonia as a movement disorder characterized by sustained or intermittent muscle contractions causing abnormal, often repetitive, movements, postures or both. The dystonic movements are typically patterned, twisting, and may be tremulous, and are often initiated or worsened by voluntary action and associated with overflow of muscle activation. Further, they propose that dystonia be classified according to clinical characteristics, such as age at onset, body distribution, temporal pattern and other associated neurological features, and etiology, including nervous system pathology and inheritance. Primary (i.e., no other neurologic conditions and no abnormalities in brain structure or metabolism) and secondary (i.e., resulting from other causes, such as brain injury, drugs/toxins, postencephalitis) dystonias will be the focus of this section, because they have been the most thoroughly investigated from a cognitive perspective.

Preoperative declines in cognition are not characteristic of primary dystonia (see Jahanshahi, Czernecki, & Zurowski, 2011 for review), although some studies have inconsistently shown mild decrements in visuospatial functioning, semantic verbal fluency, and aspects of frontal lobe functioning. Baseline cognition in secondary dystonia has been less systematically investigated but appears to be heterogeneous in pattern and severity.

Two studies (same patients) evaluated a wide range of cognitive abilities in addition to mood and quality of life in 22 patients with primary generalized dystonia 1 year (Pillon et al., 2006) and 3 years (Vidailhet et al., 2007) following bilateral GPi stimulation. One year postsurgically there were small but significant improvements in verbal recall and some aspects of executive functioning. Mood was unchanged at 1- and 3-year assessments, but quality of life was improved at both time points. Cognitive changes observed at 1 year were maintained, with further slight improvements in frontal executive functions.

In a randomized, controlled study, Kupsch et al. (2006) randomized 40 patients with primary segmental or generalized dystonia to receive neurostimulation or sham stimulation of the GPi for 3 months, after which all patients received open-label neurostimulation. Global cognitive functioning (Mattis Dementia Rating Scale), mood, and quality of life were assessed. There was no change in cognition between those who had and had not received stimulation. At the 3-month assessment, sham differed from stimulation only on the physical component of a quality of life measure, but at 6 months combined analyses of both groups revealed improvement in depression and quality of life.

Gruber et al. (2010) treated 10 patients with myoclonic dystonia with bilateral DBS of either the GPi ($n = 1$), the VIM ($n = 1$), or a combination of both GPi and VIM ($n = 8$) and utilized a comprehensive battery to assess cognition, mood, and quality of life. For those patients receiving GPi and VIM, cognition was measured in four conditions of stimulation: off, on GPi, on VIM, and on both. Mean time of assessment was 25.6 months, with a range of 6–72 months. Mood and cognition did not change postsurgically regardless of stimulation condition with the exception of worse simple reaction time in the GPi versus VIM condition, but there was significant improvement in quality of life.

Three studies have examined cognitive and behavioral changes following DBS for cervical dystonia, one following bilateral STN (Kleiner-Fisman et al., 2007) and the others following bilateral GPi (Hung et al., 2007; Valldeoriola et al., 2010). Kleiner-Fisman et al. (2007) found a wide range of variability in cognitive functioning in their 4 patients 12 month after STN stimulation but determined the changes were not clinically significant overall. Hung et al. (2007) did not report any psychiatric or neuropsychological changes in his 10 patients following bilateral GPi stimulation for cervical dystonia. Similarly, Valldeoriola et al. (2010) found no change in global cognitive functioning in 22 patients following bilateral GPi for primary generalized and segmental cervical dystonia 1 year post surgery. Mood and certain aspects of quality of life, primarily related to physical functioning, improved significantly.

Halbig et al. (2005) comprehensively assessed cognitive abilities, mood, and quality of life in 15 consecutive patients with different forms of dystonia (13 primary and 2 tardive dystonia) following bilateral GPi stimulation. No group deteriorations were noted. There were mild but significant improvements in visuomotor attention (Trails A) and depression, and significant improvements in quality of life.

There are a few studies of secondary dystonia in smaller samples. In general, there has been no reported change in cognition with either bilateral GPi (Damier et al., 2007; Gruber et al., 2009; Vidailhet et al., 2009) or bilateral thalamic (ventralis oralis anterior) stimulation (Ghika et al., 2002). Vidailhet et al. (2009) found no worsening of cognition or mood in 13 patients with dystonia-choreoathetosis cerebral palsy 12 months after GPi stimulation, and mental health-related quality of life improved. In Damier et al.'s (2007) 10 patients with tardive dyskinesia, no cognitive changes were noted 6 months post GPi stimulation, but depression improved in 1 patient and worsened in 3. Gruber et al. (2009) administered a battery of tests to 9 patients with tardive dystonia before and 18–80 months following GPi implantation and also found no change in cognition, whereas mood and physical quality of life improved significantly. Ghika et al. (2002) evaluated a patient with generalized postanoxic dystonia with preexisting depression, 3 suicide attempts, and minimal to mild deficits in executive functioning and verbal memory, respectively. The patient initially underwent bilateral GPi implantation, but because of marginal clinical benefit, 6 weeks postoperatively the electrodes were relocated to the ventralis oralis anterior (Voa). Three months later, there was dramatic improvement in motor functioning and cognition was stable. Despite this, the patient committed suicide one month later.

In summary, neither pallidal or thalamic stimulation appears to have a significant negative impact on cognition in dystonia, regardless of classification type.

Improvements in mood and quality of life are consistently reported and frequently parallel improvements in physical functioning. One caveat to this interpretation, however, is that often dystonia patients are treated with anticholineregic medications that are reduced or withdrawn postsurgery. It is possible that the stability or lack of decline is actually a reflection of withdrawal of medications known to negatively impact cognition, thereby masking true decline.

Tourette Syndrome

TS is a complex neuropsychiatric disorder, defined by 1) multiple motor tics and one or more vocal tics that occur often throughout the day, either simultaneously or at different periods throughout the illness, and 2) recur for a period of more than 1 year, 3) with no tic-free period of more than 3 months (APA, 2000). Tics consist of sudden, repetitive, stereotyped movements, sounds and verbal utterances. Motor symptoms usually precede vocal symptoms, beginning on average around age 3 and persisting until approximately the second decade of life, when symptoms generally diminish (Leckman, 2002; Robertson, 2000). However, TS persists into adulthood in a significant number of patients (Pappert, Goetz, Louis, Blasucci, & Leurgans, 2003) and can result in functional impairment (Leckman, 2006) and poor quality of life (Eddy et al., 2011). The international prevalence of TS in young people is estimated to be 0.4% to 3.8% (Robertson, 2008), and boys are more commonly affected than girls (Muller-Vahl et al., 2011). Frequently tics are accompanied by other psychiatric comorbidities (Cavanna, Servo, Monaco, & Robertson, 2009), often attention-deficit/hyperactivity disorder and obsessive-compulsive behavior.

Previously thought of as psychogenic, it is now recognized that there are biologic abnormalities in TS cortical and subcortical brain regions primarily involving the basal ganglia (Richards, 2009; Steeves & Fox, 2008). Evidence from pharmacological (Singer, Butler, Tune, Seifert, & Coyle, 1982) and neuroimaging (Singer et al., 2002) studies suggests that the pathogenesis of TS is related to aberrant dopamine signaling in the striatum, resulting in reduced inhibitory output from the basal ganglia and subsequent disinhibition of cortico-striato-thalamo-cortical circuits (Visser-Vandewalle, 2007). Serotongeric and adrenergic neurotransmitters and their corresponding circuits are also implicated, although the precise relationship is unclear (Leckman et al., 1991; Wong et al., 2008).

A considerable proportion of patients with TS does not respond to pharmacotherapy and/or behavioral approaches (e.g., habit reversal, exposure and response inhibition; Mukhida, Bishop, Hong, & Mendes, 2008; Temel & Visser-Vandewalle, 2004). In intractable cases such as these, surgical intervention represents an alternative treatment. Although several groups of experts have published guidelines regarding the selection of TS patients for DBS (Muller-Vahl, 2013), there are no standard agreed-upon criteria. Most experts agree that the tics/TS (not always differentiated) must be treatment-resistant, yet several different definitions for "treatment-resistance" have been proposed, including failure to benefit from multiple pharmacotherapies in the same or different classes, lack of response to behavioral interventions, or a combination of the two. Next, experts agree that patients should be "severely affected," although again there is no agreement as to what constitutes "severe." Most guidelines stipulate a cut-off score of > 35 (0–50) on the Yale Global Tic Severity Scale (Leckman et al., 1989). Lastly, published guidelines recommend DBS in adult patients only. This is based on the fact that the vast majority of young patients improve spontaneously with age, and there is no way to reliably predict which patients will not.

DBS for TS was introduced in 1997 (Vandewalle, van der Linden, Groenewegen, & Caemaert, 1999) and has since been performed in a number of centers (Saleh et al. for review; Piedad, Rickards, & Cavanna, 2012; Saleh, Gonzalez, & Cif, 2012) but few studies have reported on the cognitive effects of DBS in TS. Six studies have investigated changes in cognition and behavior following thalamic stimulation. Porta et al. (2009) reports in the largest sample studied to date (*n* = 15) no change in global cognition, frontal/executive functions, visuospatial organization, or verbal fluency after 24 months of thalamic stimulation but improvements in symptoms of obsessive-compulsivity, anxiety, and depression as well as significant improvement in quality of life. Similarly, in Ackermans and colleagues' (2011) double-blind clinical trial of 6 patients with TS followed for 12 months there was decline on a measure of selective attention and response inhibition but otherwise cognition, mood, and behavior were relatively unchanged. No changes in cognition were found in two other studies (Kaido et al., 2011; Maciunas et al., 2007) following small groups of patients from 1 to 12 months, whereas quality of life improved in the short term in one of these studies (Maciunas et al., 2007). These results should be interpreted with caution, however, as the test batteries administered were often selective and did not measure cognition in all domains. Schoenberg et al. (2007) did observe a decline in verbal memory 24 months following thalamic implantation in their case study. In a long-term study, 1 of 2 patients followed by Ackermans et al. (Ackermans et al., 2010) for 6 and 10 years, respectively, showed a decline in verbal memory and verbal fluency as well as increased anger, aggression, and difficulties with social adaptation. No cognitive or behavioral changes were noted in the patient with 10-year follow-up.

Welter et al. (2008) conducted a controlled, double-blind, randomized crossover design study after 8 months in 3 patients with stimulating electrodes implanted in the centromedian-parafascicular nuclei complex (Cm-Pf) and GPi and found no changes in memory, attention, or executive functioning, nor were there adverse psychiatric sequelae. Dehning, Mehrkens, Muller, and Botzel (2008) did not observe a change in cognition in their patient 12 months after GPi implantation, although there were reports that the patient suffered from depression related to social adjustment issues. In contrast, the single case of Shahed, Poysky, Kenney, Simpson, and Jankovic (2007) improved in psychomotor functioning, cognitive flexibility, visuospatial functioning, mood, behavior, and quality of life 6 months post GPi.

In summary, there are mixed findings with regard to cognitive and quality of life outcomes following DBS in TS. Sample sizes are too small to draw definitive conclusions. The largest study to date suggests that there are no cognitive consequences and there are improvements in mood and quality of life. This is supported by a few other studies, but there is also evidence of decline in verbal memory and verbal fluency in individual cases.

CONCLUSION

The functional impact of movement disorders is significant, including physical, occupational, and social functioning as well as negatively impacting performance of activities of daily living, mood, and quality of life. DBS has effectively ameliorated motor symptoms, and by and large without serious cognitive and behavioral consequences. STN DBS, although alleviating a wider range of motor symptoms and allowing for substantial medication reduction, appears to carry a greater risk of cognitive and behavioral decline than other DBS targets. However, this is not a uniform finding, and it remains to be determined what treatment works best for whom and at what cost. There is a multitude of factors that can impact outcomes, including demographic and disease variables, baseline cognition, baseline mood/behavioral characteristics, environmental variables (e.g., social support, geographical constraints, financial limitations), motivation for surgery, expectations, surgical factors, and stimulation parameters. The ability to develop reliable guidelines for clinical decision making will depend on the accumulation of data from larger, well-controlled, randomized trials. Only then will we be able to predict cognitive and behavioral outcomes following surgery in order to provide optimal care and enhance quality of life.

FUTURE DIRECTIONS

Novel surgical sites show promise for improvement of cognitive dysfunction but studies are few and preliminary. There is a small amount of evidence that pedunculopontine nucleus (PPN) stimulation may improve gait and postural instability to some degree, although not to the magnitude experienced with STN stimulation. However, from a cognitive standpoint, there have been reports of significant improvements in executive functioning, working memory, phonemic fluency and delayed recall in patients implanted in the STN plus PPN (Alessandro et al., 2010; Stefani et al., 2013).

Historically DBS has been reserved for late-stage PD when pharmacotherapy has failed. The EARLYSTIM trial is currently underway to investigate whether STN stimulation can be recommended at an earlier stage of PD, potentially offering a longer period free of debilitating motor, cognitive, and behavioral symptoms (Deuschl et al., 2013).

Lastly, some patients are currently denied DBS secondary to cognitive dysfunction and psychiatric manifestations. Studies examining the trajectory of patients with pre-existing mild cognitive impairment and behavioral symptoms following DBS are needed in order to more clearly define who is a "safe" surgical candidate.

REFERENCES

Ackermans, L., Duits, A., Temel, Y., Winogrodzka, A., Peeters, F., Beuls, E. A., & Visser-Vandewalle, V. (2010). Long-term outcome of thalamic deep brain stimulation in two patients with Tourette syndrome. *Journal of Neurology, Neurosurgery and Psychiatry, 81*(10), 1068–1072.

Ackermans, L., Duits, A., van der Linden, C., Tijssen, M., Schruers, K., Temel, Y., ... Visser-Vandewalle, V. (2011). Double-blind clinical trial of thalamic stimulation in patients with Tourette syndrome. *Brain, 134*(Pt 3), 832–844.

Albanese, A., Bhatia, K., Bressman, S. B., Delong, M. R., Fahn, S., Fung, V. S., ... Teller, J. K. (2013). Phenomenology and classification of dystonia: A consensus update. *Movement Disorders, 28*(7), 863–873.

Alegret, M., Junque, C., Valldeoriola, F., Vendrell, P., Pilleri, M., Rumia, J., & Tolosa, E. (2001). Effects of bilateral subthalamic stimulation on cognitive function in Parkinson disease. *Archives of Neurology, 58*(8), 1223–1227.

Alessandro, S., Ceravolo, R., Brusa, L., Pierantozzi, M., Costa, A., Galati, S., ... Peppe, A. (2010). Non-motor functions in parkinsonian patients implanted in the pedunculopontine nucleus: focus on sleep and cognitive domains. *Journal of Neurological Science,* 289(1–2), 44–48.

American Psychiatric Association. (2000). *Diagnostic and Statistical Manual of Mental Disorders-IV-TR*. Washington, DC, Author.

Anderson, K. E., & Mullins, J. (2003). Behavioral changes associated with deep brain stimulation surgery for Parkinson's disease. *Current Neurology & Neuroscience Report,* 3(4), 306–313.

Anderson, V. C., Burchiel, K. J., Hogarth, P., Favre, J., Hammerstad, J. P. (2005). Pallidal vs subthalamic nucleus deep brain stimulation in Parkinson disease. *Archives of Neurology, 62*(4), 554–560.

Andrews, C., Aviles-Olmos, I., Hariz, M., & Foltynie, T. (2010). Which patients with dystonia benefit from deep brain stimulation? A metaregression of individual patient outcomes. *Journal of Neurology, Neurosurgery and Psychiatry, 81*(12), 1383–1389.

Antonini, A., Siri, C., Santangelo, G., Cilia, R., Poletti, M., Canesi, M., ... Barone, P. (2011). Impulsivity and compulsivity in drug-naive patients with Parkinson's disease. *Movement Disorders, 26*(3), 464–468.

Appleby, B. S., Duggan, P. S., Regenberg, A., & Rabins, P. V. (2007). Psychiatric and neuropsychiatric adverse events associated with deep brain stimulation: A meta-analysis of ten years' experience. *Movement Disorders,* 22(12), 1722–1728.

Ardouin, C., Pillon, B., Peiffer, E., Bejjani, P., Limousin, P., Damier, P., ... Pollak, P. (1999). Bilateral subthalamic or pallidal stimulation for Parkinson's disease affects neither memory nor executive functions: a consecutive series of 62 patients. *Annals of Neurology, 46*(2), 217–223.

Ardouin, C., Voon, V., Worbe, Y., Abouazar, N., Czernecki, V., Hosseini, H., ... Krack, P. (2006). Pathological gambling in Parkinson's disease improves on chronic subthalamic nucleus stimulation. *Movement Disorders,* 21(11), 1941–1946.

Aybek, S., Gronchi-Perrin, A., Berney, A., ChiuvÃ¨, S. C., Villemure, J. G., Burkhard, P. R., & Vingerhoets, F. J. G. (2007). Long-term cognitive profile and incidence of dementia after STN-DBS in Parkinson's disease. *Movement Disorder, 22*(7), 974–981.

Bejjani, B. P., Damier, P., Arnulf, I., Thivard, L., Bonnet, A. M., Dormont, D., ... Agid, Y. (1999). Transient acute depression induced by high-frequency deep-brain stimulation. *New England Journal of Medicine, 340*(19), 1476–1480.

Benabid, A. L., Koudsie, A., Benazzouz, A., Vercueil, L., Fraix, V., Chabardes, S., . . . Pollak, P. (2001). Deep brain stimulation of the corpus luysi (subthalamic nucleus) and other targets in Parkinson's disease. Extension to new indications such as dystonia and epilepsy. *Journal of Neurology, 248*(Suppl 3), III37–47.

Benito-Leon, J., Louis, E. D., Mitchell, A. J., & Bermejo-Pareja, F. (2011). Elderly-onset essential tremor and mild cognitive impairment: A population-based study (NEDICES). *Journal of Alzheimers Disease, 23*(4), 727–735.

Braak, H., Del Tredici, K., Rub, U., de Vos, R. A., Jansen Steur, E. N., & Braak, E. (2003). Staging of brain pathology related to sporadic Parkinson's disease. *Neurobiology and Aging, 24*(2), 197–211.

Broeders, M., de Bie, R. M., Velseboer, D. C., Speelman, J. D., Muslimovic, D., & Schmand, B. (2013). Evolution of mild cognitive impairment in Parkinson disease. *Neurology, 81*(4), 346–352.

Bronstein, J. M., Tagliati, M., Alterman, R. L., Lozano, A. M., Volkmann, J., Stefani, A., . . . DeLong, M. R. (2011). Deep brain stimulation for Parkinson disease: an expert consensus and review of key issues. *Archives of Neurology, 68*(2), 165.

Burkhard, P. R., Vingerhoets, F. J., Berney, A., Bogousslavsky, J., Villemure, J. G., & Ghika, J. (2004). Suicide after successful deep brain stimulation for movement disorders. *Neurology, 63*(11), 2170–2172.

Caparros-Lefebvre, D., Blond, S., Pecheux, N., Pasquier, F., & Petit, H. (1992). Evaluation neuropsychologique avant et apres stimulation thalamique chez 9 parkinsoniens. *Revue Neurologique, 148*,117–122.

Capus, L., Melatini, A., Zorzon, M., Torre, P., Carraro, N., Moretti, D., . . . Marsala, S. Z. (2001). Chronic bilateral electrical stimulation of the subthalamic nucleus for the treatment of advanced Parkinson's disease. *Neurological Sciences, 22*(1), 57–58.

Castelli, L., Lanotte, M., Zibetti, M., Caglio, M., Rizzi, L., Ducati, A., . . . Lopiano, L.Castelli, L., Lanotte, M., Zibetti, M., et al. (2007). Apathy and verbal fluency in STN-stimulated PD patients: An observational follow-up study. *Journal of Neurology, 254*(9), 1238–1243.

Castelli, L., Perozzo, P., Zibetti, M., Crivelli, B., Morabito, U., Lanotte, M., . . . Lopiano, L. (2006). Chronic deep brain stimulation of the subthalamic nucleus for Parkinson's disease: Effects on cognition, mood, anxiety and personality traits. *European Neurology, 55*(3),136–144.

Castelli, L., Rizzi, L., Zibetti, M., Angrisano, S., Lanotte, M., & Lopiano, L. (2010). Neuropsychological changes 1-year after subthalamic DBS in PD patients: A prospective controlled study. *Parkinsonism & Related Disorders, 16*(2), 115–118.

Castrioto, A., Kistner, A., Klinger, H., Lhommee, E., Schmitt, E., Fraix, V., . . . Krack, P. (2013). Psychostimulant effect of levodopa: reversing sensitisation is possible. *Journal of Neurology, Neurosurgery and Psychiatry, 84*(1),18–22.

Cavanna, A. E., Servo, S., Monaco, F., & Robertson, M. M. (2009). The behavioral spectrum of Gilles de la Tourette syndrome. *Journal of Neuropsychiatry & Clinical Neuroscience, 21*(1), 13–23.

Contarino, M. F., Daniele, A., Sibilia, A. H., Romito, L. M. A., Bentivoglio, A. R., Gainotti, G., & Albanese, A. (2007). Cognitive outcome 5 years after bilateral chronic stimulation of subthalamic nucleus in patients with Parkinson's disease, *Journal of Neurology, Neurosurgery and Psychiatry, 78*(3), 248–252.Czernecki, V., Schüpbach, M., Yaici, S., Lévy, R., Bardinet, E., Yelnik, J., . . . Agid, Y. (2008). Apathy following subthalamic stimulation in parkinson disease: A dopamine responsive symptom. *Movement Disorders, 23*(7), 964–969.

Damier, P., Thobois, S., Witjas, T., Cuny, E., Derost, P., Raoul, S.,...Rascol, O. (2007). Bilateral deep brain stimulation of the globus pallidus to treat tardive dyskinesia. *Archives of General Psychiatry, 64*(2), 170–176.

Daniele, A., Albanese, A., Contarino, M. F., Zinzi, P., Barbier, A., Gasparini, F.,...Scerrati, M. (2003). Cognitive and behavioural effects of chronic stimulation of the subthalamic nucleus in patients with Parkinson's disease. *Journal of Neurology, Neurosurgery and Psychiatry, 74*(2), 175–182.

Daniels, C., Krack, P., Volkmann, J., Pinsker, M. O., Krause, M., Tronnier, V.,...Witt, K. (2010). Risk factors for executive dysfunction after subthalamic nucleus stimulation in Parkinson's disease. *Movement Disorders, 25*(11), 1583–1589.

Dehning, S., Mehrkens, J. H., Muller, N., & Botzel, K. (2008). Therapy-refractory Tourette syndrome: beneficial outcome with globus pallidus internus deep brain stimulation. *Movement Disorders, 23*(9), 1300–1302.

Derost, P. P., Ouchchane, L., Morand, D., Ulla, M., Llorca, P. M., Barget, M.,...Durif, F. (2007). Is DBS-STN appropriate to treat severe Parkinson disease in an elderly population? *Neurology, 68*(17), 1345–1355.

Deuschl, G., Schade-Brittinger, C., Krack, P., Volkmann, J., Schäfer, H., Bötzel, K.,...Voges, J. (2006). A randomized trial of deep-brain stimulation for Parkinson's disease. *New England Journal of Medicine. 355*(9), 896–908.

Deuschl, G., Schupbach, M., Knudsen, K., Pinsker, M. O., Cornu, P., Rau, J.,...Schade-Brittinger, C. (2013). Stimulation of the subthalamic nucleus at an earlier disease stage of Parkinson's disease: concept and standards of the EARLYSTIM-study. *Parkinsonism & Related Disorders, 19*(1), 56–61.

Diamond, A., & Jankovic, J. (2005). The effect of deep brain stimulation on quality of life in movement disorders. *Journal of Neurology, Neurosurgery and Psychiatry, 76*(9), 1188–1193.

Doshi, P. K., Chhaya, N., & Bhatt, M. H. (2002). Depression leading to attempted suicide after bilateral subthalamic nucleus stimulation for Parkinson's disease. *Movement Disorders, 17*(5), 1084–1085.

Dujardin, K., Defebvre, L., Krystkowiak, P., Blond, S., & Destee, A. (2001). Influence of chronic bilateral stimulation of the subthalamic nucleus on cognitive function in Parkinson's disease. *Journal of Neurology, 248*(7), 603–611.

Dujardin, K., Krystkowiak, P., Defebvre, L., Blond, S., & Destee, A. (2000). A case of severe dysexecutive syndrome consecutive to chronic bilateral pallidal stimulation. *Neuropsychologia, 38*(9), 1305–1315.

Eddy, C. M., Rizzo, R., Gulisano, M., Agodi, A., Barchitta, M., Cali, P.,...Cavanna, A. E. (2011). Quality of life in young people with Tourette syndrome: a controlled study. *Journal of Neurology, 258*(2), 291–301.

Elble, R. J. (2006). Report from a U.S. conference on essential tremor. *Movement Disorders, 21*(12), 2052–2061.

Erola, T., Karinen, P., Heikkinen, E., Tuominen, J., Haapaniemi, T., Koivukangas, J., & Myllylä, V. (2005). Bilateral subthalamic nucleus stimulation improves health-related quality of life in Parkinsonian patients. *Parkinsonism & Related Disorders, 11*(2), 89–94.

Fasano, A., Ricciardi, L., Pettorruso, M., & Bentivoglio, A. R. (2011). Management of punding in Parkinson's disease: an open-label prospective study. *Journal of Neurology, 258*(4), 656–660.

Fasano, A., Romito, L. M., Daniele, A., Piano, C., Zinno, M., Bentivoglio, A. R., & Albanese, A. (2010). Motor and cognitive outcome in patients with Parkinson's disease 8 years after subthalamic implants. *Brain, 133*(9), 2664–2676.

Ferrara, J., Diamond, A., Hunter, C., Davidson, A., Almaguer, M., & Jankovic, J. (2010). Impact of STN-DBS on life and health satisfaction in patients with Parkinson's disease. *Journal of Neurology, Neurosurgery and Psychiatry, 81*(3), 315–319.

Fields, J. A., & Tröster, A. I. (2013). Neuropsychological aspects. In R. Pahwa and K. E. Lyons (Eds.), *Handbook of Parkinson's disease* (5th ed., pp. 144–170). Boca Raton, FL: Taylor & Francis.

Fields, J. A., Tröster, A. I., Wilkinson, S. B., Pahwa, R., & Koller, W. C. (1999). Cognitive outcome following staged bilateral pallidal stimulation for the treatment of Parkinson's disease. *Clinical Neurology and Neurosurgery, 101*(3), 182–188.

Fields, J. A., Tröster, A. I., Woods, S. P., Higginson, C. I., Wilkinson, S. B., Lyons, K. E.,... Pahwa, R. (2003). Neuropsychological and quality of life outcomes 12 months after unilateral thalamic stimulation for essential tremor. *Journal of Neurology, Neurosurgery and Psychiatry, 74*(3), 305–311.

Follett, K. A., Weaver, F. M., Stern, M., Hur, K., Harris, C. L., Luo, P.,... Reda, D. J. (2010). Pallidal versus subthalamic deep-brain stimulation for Parkinson's disease. *New England Journal of Medicine, 362*(22), 2077–2091.

Fraraccio, M., Ptito, A., Sadikot, A., Panisset, M., & Dagher, A. (2008). Absence of cognitive deficits following deep brain stimulation of the subthalamic nucleus for the treatment of Parkinson's disease. *Archives of Clinical Neuropsychology, 23*(4), 399–408.

Funkiewiez, A., Ardouin, C., Caputo, E., Krack, P., Fraix, V., Klinger, H.,... Pollak, P. (2004). Long term effects of bilateral subthalamic nucleus stimulation on cognitive function, mood, and behaviour in Parkinson's disease. *Journal of Neurology, Neurosurgery and Psychiatry, 75*(6), 834–839.

Gasparini, M., Bonifati, V., Fabrizio, E., Fabbrini, G., Brusa, L., Lenzi, G. L., & Meco, G. (2001). Frontal lobe dysfunction in essential tremor: a preliminary study. *Journal of Neurology, 248*(5), 399–402.

Gervais-Bernard, H., Xie-Brustolin, J., Mertens, P., Polo, G., Klinger, H., Adamec, D.,... Thobois, S. (2009). Bilateral subthalamic nucleus stimulation in advanced Parkinson's disease: Five year follow-up. *Journal of Neurology, 256*(2), 225–233

Ghika, J., Villemure, J. G., Fankhauser, H., Favre, J., Assal, G., & Ghika-Schmid, F. (1998). Efficiency and safety of bilateral contemporaneous pallidal stimulation (deep brain stimulation) in levodopa-responsive patients with Parkinson's disease with severe motor fluctuations: a 2-year follow-up review. *Journal of Neurosurgery, 89*(5), 713–718.

Ghika, J., Villemure, J. G., Miklossy, J., Temperli, P., Pralong, E., Christen-Zaech, S.,... Vingerhoets, F. (2002). Postanoxic generalized dystonia improved by bilateral Voa thalamic deep brain stimulation. *Neurology, 58*(2), 311–313.

Gruber, D., Kuhn, A. A., Schoenecker, T., Kivi, A., Trottenberg, T., Hoffmann, K. T.,... Kupsch, A. (2010). Pallidal and thalamic deep brain stimulation in myoclonus-dystonia. *Movement Disorders, 25*(11), 1733–1743.

Gruber, D., Trottenberg, T., Kivi, A., Schoenecker, T., Kopp, U. A., Hoffmann, K. T.,... Kupsch, A. (2009). Long-term effects of pallidal deep brain stimulation in tardive dystonia. *Neurology, 73*(1), 53–58.

Halbig, T. D., Gruber, D., Kopp, U. A., Schneider, G. H., Trottenberg, T., & Kupsch, A. (2005). Pallidal stimulation in dystonia: Effects on cognition, mood, and quality of life. *Journal of Neurology, Neurosurgery and Psychiatry, 76*(12), 1713–1716.

Halbig, T. D., Tse, W., Frisina, P. G., Baker, B. R., Hollander, E., Shapiro, H.,... Olanow, C. W. (2009). Subthalamic deep brain stimulation and impulse control in Parkinson's disease. *European Journal of Neurology, 16*(4), 493–497.

Hariz, G. M., Lindberg, M., & Bergenheim, A. T. (2002). Impact of thalamic deep brain stimulation on disability and health-related quality of life in patients with essential tremor. *Journal of Neurology, Neurosurgery and Psychiatry, 72*(1), 47–52.

Hariz, M. I., Rehncrona, S., Quinn, N. P., Speelman, J. D., & Wensing, C. (2008). Multicenter study on deep brain stimulation in Parkinson's disease: An independent assessment of reported adverse events at 4 years. *Movement Disorders, 23*(3), 416–421.

Heber, I. A., Coenen, V. A., Reetz, K., Schulz, J. B., Hoellig, A., Fimm, B., & Kronenbuerger, M. (2013). Cognitive effects of deep brain stimulation for essential tremor: evaluation at 1 and 6 years. *Journal of Neural Transmission, 120*(11), 1569–1577.

Heo, J. H., Lee, K. M., Paek, S. H., Kim, M. J., Lee, J. Y., Kim, J. Y., . . . Jeon, B. S. (2008). The effects of bilateral Subthalamic Nucleus Deep Brain Stimulation (STN DBS) on cognition in Parkinson disease. *Journal of Neurological Science, 273*(1–2), 19–24.

Hershey, T., Revilla, F. J., Wernle, A., Gibson, P. S., Dowling, J. L., & Perlmutter, J. S. (2004). Stimulation of STN impairs aspects of cognitive control in PD. *Neurology. 62*(7), 1110–1114.

Herzog, J., Reiff, J., Krack, P., Witt, K., Schrader, B., Müller, D., & Deuschl, G. (2003). Manic episode with psychotic symptoms induced by subthalamic nucleus stimulation in a patient with Parkinson's disease. *Movement Disorders, 18*(11), 1382–1384.

Herzog, J., Volkmann, J., Krack, P., Kopper, F., Potter, M., Lorenz, D., . . . Deuschl, G. (2003). Two-year follow-up of subthalamic deep brain stimulation in Parkinson's disease. *Movement Disorders, 18*(11), 1332–1337.

Higginson, C. I., Fields, J. A., & Tröster, A. I. (2001). Which symptoms of anxiety diminish after surgical interventions for Parkinson disease? *Neuropsychiatry, Neuropsychology and Behavioral Neurology*, 14(2), 117–121.

Higginson, C. I., Wheelock, V. L., Levine, D., King, D. S., Pappas, C. T., & Sigvardt, K. A. (2008). Cognitive deficits in essential tremor consistent with frontosubcortical dysfunction. *Journal of Clinical and Experimental Neuropsychology, 30*(7), 760–765.

Houeto, J. L., Damier, P., Bejjani, P. B., Staedler, C., Bonnet, A. M., Arnulf, I., . . . Agid, Y. (2000). Subthalamic stimulation in Parkinson disease: a multidisciplinary approach. *Archives of Neurology*, 57(4), 461–465.

Houeto, J. L., Mesnage, V., Mallet, L., Pillon, B., Gargiulo, M., du Moncel, S. T., . . . Agid, Y. (2002). Behavioural disorders, Parkinson's disease and subthalamic stimulation. *Journal of Neurology, Neurosurgery and Psychiatry*, 72(6), 701–707.

Hugdahl, K., & Wester, K. (2000). Neurocognitive correlates of stereotactic thalamotomy and thalamic stimulation in Parkinsonian patients. *Brain and Cognition, 42*(2), 231–252.

Hung, S. W., Hamani, C., Lozano, A. M., Poon, Y. Y., Piboolnurak, P., Miyasaki, J. M., . . . Moro, E. (2007). Long-term outcome of bilateral pallidal deep brain stimulation for primary cervical dystonia. *Neurology, 68*(6), 457–459.

Jahanshahi, M., Ardouin, C. M., Brown, R. G., Rothwell, J. C., Obeso, J., Albanese, A., . . . Limousin-Dowsey, P. (2000). The impact of deep brain stimulation on executive function in Parkinson's disease. *Brain, 123*(Pt 6), 1142–1154.

Jahanshahi, M., Czernecki, V., & Zurowski, A. M. (2011). Neuropsychological, neuropsychiatric, and quality of life issues in DBS for dystonia. *Movement Disorders,* 26(Suppl 1), S63–78.

Juurlink, D. N., Herrmann, N., Szalai, J. P., & Kopp, A., (2004). Redelmeier, D. A. Medical illness and the risk of suicide in the elderly. *Archives of Internal Medicine, 164*(11), 1179–1184.

Kaido, T., Otsuki, T., Kaneko, Y., Takahashi, A., Omori, M., & Okamoto, T. (2011). Deep brain stimulation for Tourette syndrome: a prospective pilot study in Japan. *Neuromodulation, 14*(2), 123–128; discussion 129.

Kim, Y. E., Kim, H. J., Lee, J. Y., Yun, J. Y., Kim, J. Y., Paek, S. H., & Jeon, B. S. (2013). Impulse control and related behaviors after bilateral subthalamic stimulation in patients with Parkinson's disease. *Journal of Clinical Neuroscience, 20*(7), 964–969.

Kirsch-Darrow, L., Zahodne, L. B., Marsiske, M., Okun, M. S., Foote, K. D., & Bowers, D. (2011). The trajectory of apathy after deep brain stimulation: from pre-surgery to 6 months post-surgery in Parkinson's disease. *Parkinsonism & Related Disorders, 17*(3), 182–188.

Kishore, A., Rao, R., Krishnan, S., Panikar, D., Sarma, G., Sivasanakaran, M. P., & Sarma, S. (2010). Long-term stability of effects of subthalamic stimulation in Parkinson's disease: Indian Experience. *Movement Disorders 25*(14), 2438–2444.

Kleiner-Fisman, G., Herzog, J., Fisman, D. N., Tamma, F., Lyons, K. E., Pahwa, R., ... Deuschl, G. (2006). Subthalamic nucleus deep brain stimulation: Summary and meta-analysis of outcomes. *Movement Disorders, 21*(Suppl. 14), S290–304.

Kleiner-Fisman, G., Liang, G. S., Moberg, P. J., Ruocco, A. C., Hurtig, H. I., Baltuch, G. H., ... Stern, M. B. (2007). Subthalamic nucleus deep brain stimulation for severe idiopathic dystonia: impact on severity, neuropsychological status, and quality of life. *Journal of Neurosurgery, 107*(1), 29–36.

Krack, P., Batir, A., Van Blercom, N., Chabardes, S., Fraix, V., Ardouin, C., ... Pollak, P. (2003). Five-year follow-up of bilateral stimulation of the subthalamic nucleus in advanced Parkinson's disease. *New England Journal of Medicine, 349*(20),1925–1934.

Krack, P., Fraix, V., Mendes, A., Benabid, A. L., & Pollak, P. (2002). Postoperative management of subthalamic nucleus stimulation for Parkinson's disease. *Movement Disorders, 17*(Suppl 3), S188–197.

Kumar, R., Lozano, A. M., Sime, E., Halket, E., Lang, & A. E. (1999). Comparative effects of unilateral and bilateral subthalamic nucleus deep brain stimulation. *Neurology, 53*(3), 561–566.

Kupsch, A., Benecke, R., Muller, J., Trottenberg, T., Schneider, G. H., Poewe, W., ... Volkmann, J. (2006). Pallidal deep-brain stimulation in primary generalized or segmental dystonia. *New England Journal of Medicine, 355*(19), 1978–1990.

Lacritz, L. H., Dewey, R., Jr., Giller, C., & Cullum, C. M. (2002). Cognitive functioning in individuals with "benign" essential tremor. *Journal of the International Neuropsychological Society, 8*(1), 125–129.

Lambert, C., Zrinzo, L., Nagy, Z., Lutti, A., Hariz, M., Foltynie, T., ... Frackowiak, R. (2012). Confirmation of functional zones within the human subthalamic nucleus: patterns of connectivity and sub-parcellation using diffusion weighted imaging. *Neuroimage, 60*(1), 83–94.

Lang, A. E., Houeto, J. L., Krack, P., Kubu, C., Lyons, K. E., Moro, E., ... Voon, V. (2006). Deep brain stimulation: Preoperative issues. *Movement Disorders, 21*(Suppl. 14), S171–196.

Leckman, J. F. (2002). Tourette's syndrome. *Lancet, 360*(9345), 1577–1586.

Leckman, J. F., Bloch, M. H., Scahill, L., & King, R. A. (2006). Tourette syndrome: The self under siege. *Journal of Child Neurology, 21*(8), 642–649.

Leckman, J. F., Hardin, M. T., Riddle, M. A., Stevenson, J., Ort, S. I., & Cohen, D. J. (1991). Clonidine treatment of Gilles de la Tourette's syndrome. *Archives of General Psychiatry, 48*(4), 324–328.

Leckman, J. F., Riddle, M. A., Hardin, M. T., Ort, S. I., Swartz, K. L., Stevenson, J., & Cohen, D. J. (1989). The Yale Global Tic Severity Scale: initial testing of a clinician-rated scale of tic severity. *Journal of the American Academy of Child and Adolescent Psychiatry, 28*(4), 566–573.

Lee, J. Y., Kim, J. M., Kim, J. W., Cho, J., Lee, W. Y., Kim, H. J., & Jeon, B. S. (2010). Association between the dose of dopaminergic medication and the behavioral disturbances in Parkinson disease. *Parkinsonism & Related Disorders 16*(3), 202–207.

Le Jeune, F., Drapier, D., Bourguignon, A., Péron, J., Mesbah, H., Drapier, S., . . . Vérin, M. (2009). Subthalamic nucleus stimulation in Parkinson disease induces apathy: A PET study. *Neurology, 73*(21), 1746–1751.

Levy, G., Jacobs, D. M., Tang, M. X., Cote, L. J., Louis, E. D., Alfaro, B., . . . Marder, K. (2002). Memory and executive function impairment predict dementia in Parkinson's disease. *Movement Disorders, 17*(6), 1221–1226.

Lezcano, E., Gómez-Esteban, J. C., Zarranz, J. J., et al. (2004). Improvement in quality of life in patients with advanced Parkinson's disease following bilateral deep-brain stimulation in subthalamic nucleus. *European Journal of Neurology, 11*(7), 451–454.

Lhommee, E., Klinger, H., Thobois, S., Schmitt, E., Ardouin, C., Bichon, A., . . . Krack, P. (2012). Subthalamic stimulation in Parkinson's disease: restoring the balance of motivated behaviours. *Brain, 135*(Pt 5), 1463–1477.

Lim, S. Y., & Lang, A. E. (2010). The nonmotor symptoms of Parkinson's disease—an overview. *Movement Disorders, 25*(Suppl 1), S123–130.

Lim, S. Y., O'Sullivan, S. S., Kotschet, K., Gallagher, D. A., Lacey, C., Lawrence, A. D., . . . Evans, A. H. (2009). Dopamine dysregulation syndrome, impulse control disorders and punding after deep brain stimulation surgery for Parkinson's disease. *Journal of Clinical Neuroscience, 16*(9), 1148–1152.

Litvan, I., Goldman, J. G., Tröster, A. I., Schmand, B. A., Weintraub, D., Petersen, R. C., . . . Emre, M. (2012). Diagnostic criteria for mild cognitive impairment in Parkinson's disease: Movement Disorder Society Task Force guidelines. *Movement Disorders, 27*(3), 349–356.

Louis, E. D., Benito-Leon, J., Vega-Quiroga, S., & Bermejo-Pareja, F. (2010). Faster rate of cognitive decline in essential tremor cases than controls: a prospective study. *European Journal of Neurology, 17*(10), 1291–1297.

Louis, E. D., & Ferreira, J. J. (2010). How common is the most common adult movement disorder? Update on the worldwide prevalence of essential tremor. *Movement Disorders, 25*(5), 534–541.

Lucas, J. A., Rippeth, J. D., Uitti, R. J., Shuster, E. A., & Wharen, R. E. (2000). Neuropsychological functioning in a patient with essential tremor with and without bilateral VIM stimulation. *Brain and Cognition, 42*(2), 253–267.

Maciunas, R. J., Maddux, B. N., Riley, D. E., Whitney, C. M., Schoenberg, M. R., Ogrocki, P. J., . . . Gould, D. J. (2007). Prospective randomized double-blind trial of bilateral thalamic deep brain stimulation in adults with Tourette syndrome. *Journal of Neurosurgery, 107*(5), 1004–1014.

Maier, F., Lewis, C. J., Horstkoetter, N., Eggers, C., Kalbe, E., Maarouf, M., . . . Timmermann, L. (2013). Patients' expectations of deep brain stimulation, and subjective perceived outcome related to clinical measures in Parkinson's disease: a mixed-method approach. *Journal of Neurology, Neurosurgery and Psychiatry, 84*(11), 1273–1281.

Martinez-Martin, P., Valldeoriola, F., Tolosa, E., Pilleri, M., Molinuevo, J. L., Rumia, J., & Ferrer, E. (2002). Bilateral subthalamic nucleus stimulation and quality of life in advanced Parkinson's disease. *Movement Disorders, 17*(2), 372–377.

Merello, M., Nouzeilles, M. I., Kuzis, G., Cammarota, A., Sabe, L., Betti, O.,... Leiguarda, R. (1999). Unilateral radiofrequency lesion versus electrostimulation of posteroventral pallidum: a prospective randomized comparison. *Movement Disorders, 14*(1), 50–56.

Merola, A., Rizzi, L., Zibetti, M., Artusi, C. A., Montanaro, E., Angrisano, S.,... Lopiano, L. (2013). Medical therapy and subthalamic deep brain stimulation in advanced Parkinson's disease: a different long-term outcome? *Journal of Neurology, Neurosurgery and Psychiatry,* doi: 10.1136/jnnp-2013-305271.

Merola, A., Zibetti, M., Angrisano, S., et al. (2011). Parkinson's disease progression at 30 years: a study of subthalamic deep brain-stimulated patients. *Brain,* 134(Pt 7), 2074–2084.

Middleton, F. A., & Strick, P. L. (2000). Basal ganglia output and cognition: evidence from anatomical, behavioral, and clinical studies. *Brain Cognition, 42*(2), 183–200.

Mikos, A., Zahodne, L., Okun, M. S., Foote, K., & Bowers, D. (2010). Cognitive declines after unilateral deep brain stimulation surgery in Parkinson's disease: a controlled study using Reliable Change, part II. *Clinical Neuropsychology, 24*(2), 235–245.

Miocinovic, S., Somayajula, S., Chitnis, S., & Vitek, J. L. (2013). History, applications, and mechanisms of deep brain stimulation. *JAMA Neurology, 70*(2), 163–171.

Miyawaki, E., Perlmutter, J. S., Tröster, A. I., Videen, T. O., & Koller, W. C. (2000). The behavioral complications of pallidal stimulation: a case report. *Brain and Cognition 42*(3), 417–434.

Molinuevo, J. L., Valldeoriola, F., Tolosa, E., Rumia, J., Valls-Sole, J., Roldan, H., & Ferrer, E. (2000). Levodopa withdrawal after bilateral subthalamic nucleus stimulation in advanced Parkinson disease. *Archives of Neurology,* 57(7), 983–988.

Montel, S. R., & Bungener, C. (2009). Coping and quality of life of patients with Parkinson disease who have undergone deep brain stimulation of the subthalamic nucleus. *Surgical Neurology,* 72(2), 105–110.

Moretti, R., Torre, P., Antonello, R. M., Capus, L., Marsala, S. Z., Cattaruzza, T.,... Bava, A. (2003). Neuropsychological changes after subthalamic nucleus stimulation: A 12 month follow-up in nine patients with Parkinson's disease. *Parkinsonism & Related Disorders, 10*(2), 73–79.

Moro, E., Lozano, A. M., Pollak, P., Agid, Y., Rehncrona, S., Volkmann, J.,... Lang, A. E. (2010). Long-term results of a multicenter study on subthalamic and pallidal stimulation in Parkinson's disease. *Movement Disorders, 25*(5), 578–586.

Moro, E., Scerrati, M., Romito, L. M., Roselli, R., Tonali, P., & Albanese, A. (1999). Chronic subthalamic nucleus stimulation reduces medication requirements in Parkinson's disease. *Neurology, 53*(1), 85–90.

Morrison, C. E., Borod, J. C., Perrine, K., Beric, A., Brin, M. F., Rezai, A.,... Olanow, C. W. (2004). Neuropsychological functioning following bilateral subthalamic nucleus stimulation in Parkinson's disease. *Archives of Clinical Neuropsychology, 19*(2), 165–181.

Mukhida, K., Bishop, M., Hong, M., & Mendez, I. (2008). Neurosurgical strategies for Gilles de la Tourette's syndrome. *Neuropsychiatric Disease & Treatment 4*(6), 1111–1128.

Muller-Vahl, K. R. (2013). Surgical treatment of Tourette syndrome. *Neuroscience & Biobehavioral Reviews,* 37(6), 1178–1185.

Muller-Vahl, K. R., Cath, D. C., Cavanna, A. E., Dehning, S., Porta, M., Robertson, M. M., & Visser-Vandewalle, V. (2011). European clinical guidelines for Tourette syndrome and other tic disorders. Part IV: Deep brain stimulation. *European Child & Adolescent Psychiatry, 20*(4), 209–217.

Myslobodsky, M., Lalonde, F. M., & Hicks, L. (2001). Are patients with Parkinson's disease suicidal? *Journal of Geriatric Psychiatry and Neurology, 14*(3), 120–124.

Odekerken, V. J., van Laar, T., Staal, M. J., Mosch, A., Hoffmann, C. F., Nijssen, P. C., ... de Bie, R. M. (2013). Subthalamic nucleus versus globus pallidus bilateral deep brain stimulation for advanced Parkinson's disease (NSTAPS study): a randomised controlled trial. *Lancet Neurology, 12*(1), 37–44.

Okun, M. S., Fernandez, H. H., Wu, S. S., Kirsch-Darrow, L., Bowers, D., Bova, F., ... Foote, K. D. (2009). Cognition and mood in Parkinson's disease in subthalamic nucleus versus globus pallidus interna deep brain stimulation: The COMPARE trial. *Annals of Neurology, 65*(5), 586–595.

Page, D., & Jahanshahi, M. (2007). Deep brain stimulation of the subthalamic nucleus improves set shifting but does not affect dual task performance in Parkinson's disease. *IEEE Transactions on Neural Systems and Rehabilitation Engineering.* 15(2), 198–206.

Pahwa, R., Lyons, K. E., Wilkinson, S. B., Tröster, A. I., Overman, J., Kieltyka, J., & Koller, W. C. (2001). Comparison of thalamotomy to deep brain stimulation of the thalamus in essential tremor. *Movement Disorders, 16*(1), 140–143.

Pappert, E. J., Goetz, C. G., Louis, E. D., Blasucci, L., & Leurgans, S. (2003). Objective assessments of longitudinal outcome in Gilles de la Tourette's syndrome. *Neurology. 61*(7), 936–940.

Parsons, T. D., Rogers, S. A., Braaten, A. J., Woods, S. P., & Tröster, A. I. (2006). Cognitive sequelae of subthalamic nucleus deep brain stimulation in Parkinson's disease: a meta-analysis. *Lancet Neurology, 5*(7), 578–588.

Pedersen, K. F., Larsen, J. P., Tysnes, O. B., & Alves, G. (2013). Prognosis of mild cognitive impairment in early Parkinson disease: The Norwegian ParkWest study. *JAMA Neurology, 70*(5), 580–586.

Piedad, J. C., Rickards, H. E., & Cavanna, A. E. (2012). What patients with gilles de la tourette syndrome should be treated with deep brain stimulation and what is the best target? *Neurosurgery, 71*(1), 173–192.

Pilitsis, J. G., Rezai, A. R., Boulis, N. M., Henderson, J. M., Busch, R. M., & Kubu, C. S. (2005). A preliminary study of transient confusional states following bilateral subthalamic stimulation for Parkinson's disease. *Stereotactic and Functtional Neurosurgery, 83*(2–3), 67–70.

Pillon, B., Ardouin, C., Damier, P., Krack, P., Houeto, J. L., Klinger, H., ... Agid, Y. (2000). Neuropsychological changes between "off" and "on" STN or GPi stimulation in Parkinson's disease. *Neurology, 55*(3), 411–418.

Pillon, B., Ardouin, C., Dujardin, K., Vittini, P., Pelissolo, A., Cottencin, O., ... Vidailhet, M. (2006). Preservation of cognitive function in dystonia treated by pallidal stimulation. *Neurology, 66*(10), 1556–1558.

Plaha, P., Javed, S., Agombar, D., G, O. F., Khan, S., Whone, A., & Gill, S. (2011). Bilateral caudal zona incerta nucleus stimulation for essential tremor: outcome and quality of life. *Journal of Neurology, Neurosurgery and Psychiatry, 82*(8), 899–904.

Porat, O., Cohen, O. S., Schwartz, R., & Hassin-Baer, S. (2009). Association of preoperative symptom profile with psychiatric symptoms following subthalamic nucleus stimulation in patients with Parkinson's disease. *Journal of Neuropsychiatry and Clinical Neurosciences, 21*(4), 398–405.

Porta, M., Brambilla, A., Cavanna, A. E., Servello, D., Sassi, M., Rickards, H., & Robertson, M. M. (2009). Thalamic deep brain stimulation for treatment-refractory Tourette syndrome: Two-year outcome. *Neurology, 73*(17), 1375–1380.

Rickards, H. (2009). Functional neuroimaging in Tourette syndrome. *Journal of Psychosomatic Research, 67*(6), 575–584.

Roane, D. M., Yu, M., Feinberg, T. E., & Rogers, J. D. (2002). Hypersexuality after pallidal surgery in Parkinson disease. *Neuropsychiatry, Neuropsychology and Behavioral Neurology, 15*(4), 247–251.

Robertson, M. M. (2000). Tourette syndrome, associated conditions and the complexities of treatment. *Brain,123*(Pt 3), 425–462.

Robertson, M. M. (2008). The prevalence and epidemiology of Gilles de la Tourette syndrome. Part 1: the epidemiological and prevalence studies. *Journal of Psychosomatic Research, 65*(5), 461–472.

Rodrigues, J. P., Walters, S. E., Watson, P., Stell, R., & Mastaglia, F. L. (2007). Globus pallidus stimulation improves both motor and nonmotor aspects of quality of life in advanced Parkinson's disease. *Movement Disorders, 22*(13), 1866–187

Rodriguez-Oroz, M. C., Obeso, J. A., Lang, A. E., Houeto, J. L., Pollak, P., Rehncrona, S.,... Van Blercom, N. (2005). Bilateral deep brain stimulation in Parkinson's disease: A multicentre study with 4 years follow-up. *Brain, 128*(10), 2240–2249.

Romito, L. M., & Albanese, A. (2010). Dopaminergic therapy and subthalamic stimulation in Parkinson's disease: a review of 5-year reports. *Journal of Neurology, 257*(Suppl 2), S298–304.

Rothlind, J. C., Cockshott, R. W., Starr, P. A., & Marks, Jr, W. J. (2007). Neuropsychological performance following staged bilateral pallidal or subthalamic nucleus deep brain stimulation for Parkinson's disease. *Journal of the International Neuropsychological Society*, 13(1), 68–79.

Rouaud, T., Dondaine, T., Drapier, S., Haegelen, C., Lallement, F., Peron, J.,... Verin, M. (2010). Pallidal stimulation in advanced Parkinson's patients with contraindications for subthalamic stimulation. *Movement Disorder, 25*(12), 1839–1846.

Saez-Zea, C., Escamilla-Sevilla, F., Katati, M. J., & Minguez-Castellanos, A. (2012). Cognitive effects of subthalamic nucleus stimulation in Parkinson's disease: a controlled study. *European Neurology, 68*(6), 361–366.

Sahin, H. A., Terzi, M., Ucak, S., Yapici, O., Basoglu, T., & Onar, M. (2006). Frontal functions in young patients with essential tremor: A case comparison study. *Journal of Neuropsychiatry and Clinical Neuroscience, 18*(1), 64–72.

Saleh, C., Gonzalez, V., Cif, L., & Coubes, P. (2012). Deep brain stimulation of the globus pallidus internus and Gilles de la Tourette syndrome: Toward multiple networks modulation. *Surgical Neurology International*, 3(Suppl 2), S127–142.

Sandvik, U., Hariz, G. M., & Blomstedt, P. (2012). Quality of life following DBS in the caudal zona incerta in patients with essential tremor. *Acta Neurochirurgica, 154*(3), 495–499.

Schoenberg, M. R., Grocki, P., Maciunas, R. J., Maddux, B. N., Riley, D., & Gould, D. (2007). A case of refractory Tourette's syndrome in adulthood: neuropsychological pre—and post-operative outcome from deep brain stimulation (DBS) surgical treatment. *Archives of Clinical Neuropsychology,* 22(7), 794–795.

Schoenberg, M. R., Mash, K. M., Bharucha, K. J., Francel, P. C., & Scott, J. G. (2008). Deep brain stimulation parameters associated with neuropsychological changes in subthalamic nucleus stimulation for refractory Parkinson's disease. *Stereotactic and Functional Neurosurgery, 86*(6), 337–344.

Schüpbach, W. M. M., Chastan, N., Welter, M. L., Houeto, J. L., Mesnage, V., Bonnet, A. M.,... Agid, Y. (2005). Stimulation of the subthalamic nucleus in Parkinson's disease: A 5 year follow up. *Journal of Neurology, Neurosurgery and Psychiatry, 76*(12), 1640–1644.

Schüpbach, W. M. M., Maltete, D., Houeto, J. L., Du Montcel, S. T., Mallet, L., Welter, M. L.,... Agid, Y. (2007). Neurosurgery at an earlier stage of Parkinson disease: A randomized, controlled trial. *Neurology, 68*(4), 267–271.

Schuurman, P. R., Bruins, J., Merkus, M. P., Bosch, D. A., & Speelman, J. D. (2002). A comparison of neuropsychological effects of thalamotomy and thalamic stimulation. *Neurology, 59*(8), 1232–1239.

Shahed, J., Poysky, J., Kenney, C., Simpson, R., & Jankovic, J. (2007). GPi deep brain stimulation for Tourette syndrome improves tics and psychiatric comorbidities. *Neurology, 68*(2), 159–160.

Singer, H. S., Butler, I. J., Tune, L. E., Seifert, W. E., Jr., & Coyle, J. T. (1982). Dopaminergic dsyfunction in Tourette syndrome. *Annals of Neurology, 12*(4), 361–366.

Singer, H. S., Szymanski, S., Giuliano, J., Yokoi, F., Dogan, A. S., Brasic, J. R.,... Wong, D. F. (2002). Elevated intrasynaptic dopamine release in Tourette's syndrome measured by PET. *American Journal of Psychiatry, 159*(8), 1329–1336.

Smeding, H. M., Esselink, R. A., Schmand, B., Koning-Haanstra, M., Nijhuis, I., Wijnalda, E. M., & Speelman, J. D. (2005). Unilateral pallidotomy versus bilateral subthalamic nucleus stimulation in PD—a comparison of neuropsychological effects. *Journal of Neurology, 252*(2), 176–182.

Smeding, H. M. M., Goudriaan, A. E., Foncke, E. M. J., Schuurman, P. R., Speelman, J. D., & Schmand, B. (2007). Pathological gambling after bilateral subthalamic nucleus stimulation in Parkinson disease. *Journal of Neurology, Neurosurgery and Psychiatry. 78*(5), 517–519.

Smeding, H. M., Speelman, J. D., Huizenga, H. M., Schuurman, P. R., & Schmand, B. (2011). Predictors of cognitive and psychosocial outcome after STN DBS in Parkinson's Disease. *Journal of Neurology, Neurosurgery and Psychiatry, 82*(7), 754–760.

Smeding, H. M. M., Goudriaan, A. E., Foncke, E. M. J., Schuurman, P. R., Speelman, J. D., & Schmand, B. (2006). Neuropsychological effects of bilateral STN stimulation in Parkinson disease: A controlled study. *Neurology, 66*(12), 1830–1836.

Smith, Y., Wichmann, T., Factor, S. A., & DeLong, M. R. (2012). Parkinson's disease therapeutics: new developments and challenges since the introduction of levodopa. *Neuropsychopharmacology, 37*(1), 213–246

Soulas, T., Gurruchaga, J. M., Palfi, S., Cesaro, P., Nguyen, J. P., & Fénelon, G. (2008). Attempted and completed suicides after subthalamic nucleus stimulation for Parkinson's disease. *Journal of Neurology, Neurosurgery and Psychiatry, 79*(8), 952–954.

Steeves, T. D., & Fox, S. H. (2008). Neurobiological basis of serotonin-dopamine antagonists in the treatment of Gilles de la Tourette syndrome. *Progress in Brain Research, 172*, 495–513.

Stefani, A., Peppe, A., Galati, S., Bassi, M. S., D'Angelo, V., & Pierantozzi, M. (2013). The serendipity case of the pedunculopontine nucleus low-frequency brain stimulation: chasing a gait response, finding sleep, and cognition improvement. *Frontiers in Neurology, 4*, 68.

Straits-Tröster, K., Fields, J. A., Wilkinson, S. B., Pahwa, R., Lyons, K. E., Koller, W. C., & Tröster, A. I. (2000). Health-related quality of life in Parkinson's disease after pallidotomy and deep brain stimulation. *Brain Cognition, 42*(3), 399–416.

Tamma, F., Rampini, P., Egidi, M., Caputo, E., Locatelli, M., Pesenti, A.,... Priori, A. (2003). Deep brain stimulation for Parkinson's disease: the experience of the Policlinico-San Paolo Group in Milan. *Neurological Sciences, 24*(Suppl 1), S41–42.

Temel, Y., Blokland, A., Ackermans, L., Boon, P., Van Kranen-Mastenbroek, V. H. J. M., Beuls, E. A. M.,... Visser-Vandewalle, V. (2006). Differential effects of subthalamic nucleus stimulation in advanced Parkinson disease on reaction time performance. *Experimental Brain Research, 169*(3), 389–399.

Temel, Y., & Visser-Vandewalle, V. (2004). Surgery in Tourette syndrome. *Movement Disorders, 19*(1), 3–14.

Thawani, S. P., Schupf, N., & Louis, E. D. (2009). Essential tremor is associated with dementia: prospective population-based study in New York. *Neurology, 73*(8), 621–625.

Thevathasan, W., & Gregory, R. (2010). Deep brain stimulation for movement disorders. *Practical Neurology,* 10(1), 16–26.

Thobois, S., Ardouin, C., Lhommée, E., Klinger, H., Lagrange, C., Xie, J.,...Krack, P. (2010). Non-motor dopamine withdrawal syndrome after surgery for Parkinson's disease: predictors and underlying mesolimbic denervation. *Brain, 133*(Pt 4), 1111–1127.

Tir, M., Devos, D., Blond, S., Touzet, G., Reyns, N., Duhamel, A.,...Krystkowiak, P. (2007). Exhaustive, one-year follow-up of subthalamic nucleus deep brain stimulation in a large, single-center cohort of parkinsonian patients. *Neurosurgery, 61*(2), 297–304; discussion 304–295.

Trépanier, L. L., Kumar, R., Lozano, A. M., Lang, A. E., & Saint-Cyr, J. A. (2000). Neuropsychological outcome of GPi pallidotomy and GPi or STN deep brain stimulation in Parkinson's disease. *Brain and Cognition, 42*(3), 324–347.

Tröster, A. I. (2009a). Cognitive and mood effects of subthalamic deep brain stimulation in Parkinson's disease. *Minerva Psichiatrica, 50*(1), 79–92.

Tröster, A. I. (2009b). Neuropsychology of deep brain stimulation in neurology and psychiatry. *Frontiers in Bioscience, 14,* 1857–1879.

Tröster, A. I., & Fields, J. A. (2008). Parkinson's disease, progressive supranuclear palsy, corticobasal degeneration and related disorders of the frontostriatal system. In J. E. Morgan and J. H. Ricker (Eds.), *Textbook of Clinical Neuropsychology* (pp. 536–577). New York, NY: Psychology Press.

Tröster, A. I., Woods, S. P., Fields, J. A., Lyons, K. E., Pahwa, R., Higginson, C. I., & Koller, W. C. (2002). Neuropsychological deficits in essential tremor: an expression of cerebello-thalamo-cortical pathophysiology? *European Journal of Neurology, 9*(2), 143–151.

Tröster, A. I., Fields, J. A., Pahwa, R., Wilkinson, S. B., Strait-Tröster, K. A., Lyons, K.,...Koller, W. C. (1999). Neuropsychological and quality of life outcome after thalamic stimulation for essential tremor. *Neurology, 53*(8), 1774–1780.

Tröster, A. I., Fields, J. A., Wilkinson, S. B., Pahwa, R., Miyawaki, E., Lyons, K. E., & Koller, W. C. (1997). Unilateral pallidal stimulation for Parkinson's disease: neurobehavioral functioning before and 3 months after electrode implantation. *Neurology, 49*(4), 1078–1083.

Tröster, A. I., Fields, J. A., Wilkinson, S. B., Busenbark, K., Miyawaki, E., Overman, J.,...Koller, W. C. (1997). Neuropsychological functioning before and after unilateral thalamic stimulating electrode implantation in Parkinson's disease [electronic manuscript]. *Neurosurgical Focus, 2*(3), 1–6.

Tröster, A. I., Pahwa, R., Fields, J. A., Tanner, C. M., & Lyons, K. E. (2005). Quality of life in Essential Tremor Questionnaire (QUEST): development and initial validation. *Parkinsonism & Related Disorders, 11*(6), 367–373.

Tröster, A. I., Wilkinson, S. B., Fields, J. A., Miyawaki, K., & Koller, W. C. (1998). Chronic electrical stimulation of the left ventrointermediate (Vim) thalamic nucleus for the treatment of pharmacotherapy-resistant Parkinson's disease: a differential impact on access to semantic and episodic memory? *Brain and Cognition, 38*(2), 125–149.

Tsai, S. T., Lin, S. H., Lin, S. Z., Chen, J. Y., Lee, C. W., & Chen, S. Y. (2007). Neuropsychological effects after chronic subthalamic stimulation and the topography of the nucleus in Parkinson's disease. *Neurosurgery. 61*(5), E1024–1029..

Tykocki, T.,Szalecki, K., Koziara, H., Nauman, P., & Mandat, T. (2013). Quality of life and depression symptoms in Parkinson's disease after subthalmic deep brain stimulation: A 2-year follow-up study. *Turkish Neurosurgery, 23*(3), 379–384.

Umemura, A., Oka, Y., Okita, K., Matsukawa, N., & Yamada, K. (2011). Subthalamic nucleus stimulation for Parkinson disease with severe medication-induced hallucinations or delusions. *Journal of Neurosurgery, 114*(6), 1701–1705.

Valldeoriola, F., Regidor, I., Minguez-Castellanos, A., Lezcano, E., Garcia-Ruiz, P., Rojo, A.,... Tolosa, E. (2010). Efficacy and safety of pallidal stimulation in primary dystonia: results of the Spanish multicentric study. *Journal of Neurology, Neurosurgery and Psychiatry, 81*(1), 65–69.

Vandewalle, V., van der Linden, C., Groenewegen, H. J., & Caemaert, J. (1999). Stereotactic treatment of Gilles de la Tourette syndrome by high frequency stimulation of thalamus. *Lancet, 353*(9154), 724.

Vidailhet, M., Vercueil, L., Houeto, J. L., Krystkowiak, P., Lagrange, C., Yelnik, J.,... Pollak, P. (2007). Bilateral, pallidal, deep-brain stimulation in primary generalised dystonia: a prospective 3 year follow-up study. *Lancet Neurology, 6*(3), 223–229.

Vidailhet, M., Yelnik, J., Lagrange, C., Fraix, V., Grabli, D., Thobois, S.,... Pollak, P. (2009). Bilateral pallidal deep brain stimulation for the treatment of patients with dystonia-choreoathetosis cerebral palsy: A prospective pilot study. *Lancet Neurology, 8*(8), 709–717.

Vingerhoets, G., Lannoo, E., van der Linden, C., Caemaert, J., Vandewalle, V., van den Abbeele, D., & Wolters, M. (1999). Changes in quality of life following unilateral pallidal stimulation in Parkinson's disease. *Journal of Psychosomatic Research, 46*(3), 247–255.

Vingerhoets, G., van der Linden, C., Lannoo, E., Vandewalle, V., Caemaert, J., Wolters, M., & Van den Abbeele, D. (1999). Cognitive outcome after unilateral pallidal stimulation in Parkinson's disease. *Journal of Neurology, Neurosurgery and Psychiatry, 66*(3), 297–304.

Visser-Vandewalle, V. (2007). DBS in tourette syndrome: rationale, current status and future prospects. *Acta Neurochirurgica Supplement, 97*(Pt 2), 215–222.

Viswanathan, A., Jimenez-Shahed, J., Baizabal Carvallo, J. F., & Jankovic, J. (2012). Deep brain stimulation for Tourette syndrome: target selection. *Stereotactic and Functional Neurosurgery, 90*(4), 213–224. doi: 10.1159/000337776

Volkmann, J. (2004). Deep brain stimulation for the treatment of Parkinson's disease. *Journal of Clinical Neurophysiology, 21*(1), 6–17.

Volkmann, J., Albanese, A., Kulisevsky, J., Tornqvist, A. L., Houeto, J. L., Pidoux, B.,... Agid, Y. (2009). Long-term effects of pallidal or subthalamic deep brain stimulation on quality of life in Parkinson's disease. *Movement Disorders, 24*(8), 1154–1161.

Volkmann, J., Allert, N., Voges, J., Weiss, P. H., Freund, H. J., & Sturm, V. (2001). Safety and efficacy of pallidal or subthalamic nucleus stimulation in advanced PD. *Neurology, 56*(4), 548–551.

Voon, V., Krack, P., Lang, A. E., Lozano, A. M., Dujardin, K., Schüpbach, M.,... Moro, E. (2008). A multicentre study on suicide outcomes following subthalamic stimulation for Parkinson's disease. *Brain, 131*(10), 2720–2728.

Voon, V., Kubu, C., Krack, P., Houeto, J. L., & Tröster, A. I. (2006). Deep brain stimulation: Neuropsychological and neuropsychiatric issues. *Movement Disorders, 21*(Suppl. 14), S305–327.

Voon, V., Moro, E., Saint-Cyr, J. A., Lozano, A. M., & Lang, A. E. (2005). Psychiatric symptoms following surgery for Parkinson's disease with an emphasis on subthalamic stimulation. *Advances in Neurology, 96*, 130–147.

Weaver, F. M., Follett, K., Stern, M., Hur, K., Harris, C., Marks Jr, W. J., . . . Huang, G. D. (2009). Bilateral deep brain stimulation vs best medical therapy for patients with advanced parkinson disease: A randomized controlled trial. *JAMA,.301*(1), 63–73.

Weaver, F. M., Follett, K. A., Stern, M., Luo, P., Harris, C. L., Hur, K., . . . Reda, D. J. (2012). Randomized trial of deep brain stimulation for Parkinson disease: thirty-six-month outcomes. *Neurology, 79*(1), 55–65.

Weintraub, D., Duda, J. E., Carlson, K., Luo, P., Sagher, O., Stern, M., . . . Weaver, F. M. (2013). Suicide ideation and behaviours after STN and GPi DBS surgery for Parkinson's disease: Results from a randomised, controlled trial. *Journal of Neurology, Neurosurgery and Psychiatry.*

Weintraub, D., Koester, J., Potenza, M. N., Siderowf, A. D., Stacy, M., Voon, V., . . . Lang, A. E. (2010). Impulse control disorders in Parkinson disease: a cross-sectional study of 3090 patients. *Archives of Neurology, 67*(5), 589–595.

Welter, M. L., Mallet, L., Houeto, J. L., Karachi, C., Czernecki, V., Cornu, P., . . . Agid, Y. (2008). Internal pallidal and thalamic stimulation in patients with Tourette syndrome. *Archives of Neurology, 65*(7), 952–957.

Williams, A. E., Arzola, G. M., Strutt, A. M., Simpson, R., Jankovic, J., & York, M. K. (2011). Cognitive outcome and reliable change indices two years following bilateral subthalamic nucleus deep brain stimulation. *Parkinsonism & Related Disorders, 17*(5), 321–327.

Witjas, T., Baunez, C., Henry, J. M., Delfini, M., Regis, J., Cherif, A. A., . . . Azulay, J. P. (2005). Addiction in Parkinson's disease: Impact of subthalamic nucleus deep brain stimulation. *Movement Disorders, 20*(8), 1052–1055.

Witt, K., Daniels, C., Krack, P., Volkmann, J., Pinsker, M. O., Kloss, M., . . . Deuschl, G. (2011). Negative impact of borderline global cognitive scores on quality of life after subthalamic nucleus stimulation in Parkinson's disease. *Journal of Neurological Sciences,310*(1–2), 261–266.

Witt, K., Daniels, C., Reiff, J., Krack, P., Volkmann, J., Pinsker, M. O., . . . Deuschl, G. (2008). Neuropsychological and psychiatric changes after deep brain stimulation for Parkinson's disease: a randomised, multicentre study. *Lancet Neurology, 7*(7), 605–614.

Witt, K., Granert, O., Daniels, C., Volkmann, J., Falk, D., van Eimeren, T., & Deuschl, G. (2013). Relation of lead trajectory and electrode position to neuropsychological outcomes of subthalamic neurostimulation in Parkinson's disease: results from a randomized trial. *Brain, 136*(Pt 7), 2109–2119.

Witt, K., Pulkowski, U., Herzog, J., Lorenz, D., Hamel, W., Deuschl, G., & Krack, P. (2004). Deep brain stimulation ofsubthalamic nucleus improves cognitive flexibility but impairs response inhibition in Parkinson disease. *Archives of Neurology, 61*(5), 697–700.

Wojtecki, L., Timmermann, L., Jörgens, S., Südmeyer, M., Maarouf, M., Treuer, H., . . . Schnitzler, A. (2006). Frequency-dependent reciprocal modulation of verbal fluency and motor functions in subthalamic deep brain stimulation. *Archives of Neurology, 63*(9), 1273–1276.

Wolters, E., van der Werf, Y. D., & van den Heuvel, O. A. (2008). Parkinson's disease-related disorders in the impulsive-compulsive spectrum. *Journal of Neurology, 255*(Suppl 5), 48–56.

Wong, D. F., Brasic, J. R., Singer, H. S., Schretlen, D. J., Kuwabara, H., Zhou, Y., . . . Grace, A. (2008). Mechanisms of dopaminergic and serotonergic neurotransmission in Tourette syndrome: Clues from an in vivo neurochemistry study with PET. *Neuropsychopharmacology, 33*(6), 1239–1251.

Woods, S. P., Fields, J. A., Lyons, K. E., Koller, W. C., Wilkinson, S. B., Pahwa, R., & Tröster, A. I. (2001). Neuropsychological and quality of life changes following unilateral thalamic deep brain stimulation in Parkinson's disease: a one-year follow-up. *Acta Neurochirurgica (Wien), 143*(12), 1273–1277; discussion 1278.

Woods, S. P., Fields, J. A., Lyons, K. E., Pahwa, R., & Tröster, A. I. (2003). Pulse width is associated with cognitive decline after thalamic stimulation for essential tremor. *Parkinsonism & Related Disorders, 9*(5), 295–300.

Woods, S. P., Scott, J. C., Fields, J. A., Poquette, A., & Tröster, A. I. (2008). Executive dysfunction and neuropsychiatric symptoms predict lower health status in essential tremor. *Cognitive and Behavioral Neurology, 21*(1), 28–33.

Woods, S. P., & Tröster, A. I. (2003). Prodromal frontal/executive dysfunction predicts incident dementia in Parkinson's disease. *Journal of the International Neuropsychological Society, 9*(1), 17–24.

Yamanaka, T., Ishii, F., Umemura, A., Miyata, M., Horiba, M., Oka, Y.,... Ojika, K. (2012). Temporary deterioration of executive function after subthalamic deep brain stimulation in Parkinson's disease. *Clinical Neurology & Neurosurgery, 114*(4), 347–351.

York, M. K., Dulay, M., Macias, A., Levin, H. S., Grossman, R., Simpson, R., & Jankovic, J. (2008). Cognitive declines following bilateral subthalamic nucleus deep brain stimulation for the treatment of Parkinson's disease. *Journal of Neurology, Neurosurgery and Psychiatry, 79*(7), 789–795.

Yoshida, F., Miyagi, Y., Kishimoto, J., Morioka, T., Murakami, N., Hashiguchi, K.,... Sasaki, T. (2009). Subthalamic nucleus stimulation does not cause deterioration of preexisting hallucinations in Parkinson's disease patients. *Stereotactic and Functional Neurosurgery, 87*(1), 45–49.

Zahodne, L. B., Okun, M. S., Foote, K. D., Fernandez, H. H., Rodriguez, R. L., Kirsch-Darrow, L., & Bowers, D. (2009) Cognitive declines one year after unilateral deep brain stimulation surgery in parkinson's disease: A controlled study using reliable change. *Clinical Neuropsychologist, 23*(3), 385–405.

Zahodne, L. B., Okun, M. S., Foote, K. D., Fernandez, H. H., Rodriguez, R. L., Wu, S. S.,... Bowers, D. (2009). Greater improvement in quality of life following unilateral deep brain stimulation surgery in the globus pallidus as compared to the subthalamic nucleus. *Journal of Neurology, 256*(8), 1321–1329.

Zahodne, L. B., Susatia, F., Bowers, D., Ong, T. L., Jacobson, C. E. t., Okun, M. S.,... Fernandez, H. H. (2011). Binge eating in Parkinson's disease: prevalence, correlates and the contribution of deep brain stimulation. *Journal of Neuropsychiatry and Clinical Neuroscience, 23*(1), 56–62.

Zangaglia, R., Pacchetti, C., Pasotti, C., Mancini, F., Servello, D., Sinforiani, E.,... Nappi, G. (2009). Deep brain stimulation and cognitive functions in Parkinson's disease: A three-year controlled study. *Movement Disorder, 24*(11), 1621–1628.

Zangaglia, R., Pasotti, C., Mancini, F., Servello, D., Sinforiani, E., & Pacchetti, C. (2012). Deep brain stimulation and cognition in Parkinson's disease: an eight-year follow-up study. *Movement Disorders, 27*(9), 1192–1194.

Zgaljardic, D. J., Borod, J. C., Foldi, N. S., & Mattis, P. (2003). A review of the cognitive and behavioral sequelae of Parkinson's disease: Relationship to frontostriatal circuitry. *Cognitive & Behavioral Neurology, 16*(4), 193–210.

Zibetti, M., Merola, A., Rizzi, L., Ricchi, V., Angrisano, S., Azzaro, C.,... Lopiano, L. (2011). Beyond nine years of continuous subthalamic nucleus deep brain stimulation in Parkinson's disease. *Movement Disorders, 26*(13), 2327–2334.

PART THREE
OTHER MOVEMENT DISORDERS

13 Huntington's Disease

Arshia Sadreddin and Ioan Stroescu

INTRODUCTION

Huntington's disease (HD) is a hereditary, progressive neurodegenerative disorder that was recognized in Europe in the middle ages as the "dancing mania." It was described in Norway by the district physician in Setesdal, Johan Christian Lund as early as 1859. However, this work was not translated into English until 1959. Across the Atlantic, in Long Island, New York, Dr. George Huntington, a general practitioner who first as a child observed the afflicted patients with his father and grandfather in their family-run clinic, described the disease by a graphic portrayal of the involuntary movements. In 1872, his essay "on Chorea" was published. He described involuntary dancelike movements seen in multiple generations of patients followed by his grandfather, father, and then himself. The eponym Huntington's Chorea was adapted in literature to draw attention to chorea *(derived from Latin choreus, meaning "dance")*. However, the term Huntington's disease (HD) is now considered a more appropriate name since many other manifestations of the disease exist and chorea may not even be present (Penny & Young 1998; Jankovic & Fahn, 2007).

EPIDEMIOLOGY

HD occurs worldwide with a higher prevalence in Europe, North America, and Australia and lower prevalence in Asia. A meta-analysis and review (Pringsheim et al., 2012) showed an incidence of 0.38 per 100,000 per year. The worldwide prevalence in HD based on meta-analysis was 2.71 per 100,000. Prevalence in Europe, North America, and Australia was 5.70 per 100,000 population, whereas in Asia, prevalence was 0.40 per 100,000. The difference in prevalence of HD can be largely explained by huntingtin gene haplotypes. The largest known concentration of HD is in the state of Zulia in Venezuela, where now more than 10,000 individuals are thought to be descendants from a progenitor who lived by Lake

Maracaibo 200 years ago. In the United States, approximately 25,000 individuals have symptoms of HD and another 125,000 people are at risk (Watts & Koller, 2004).

CLINICAL FEATURES

Huntington's disease is a disorder with a phenotype consisting of the triad of motor, psychiatric, and cognitive symptoms starting mainly in adulthood with mean age of onset of symptoms usually in the late 30s or early 40s. Approximately 10% of patients become symptomatic before age 20 and are described as having juvenile Huntington's disease or the Westphal variant. About 10% develop symptoms after age 60. The disease course progresses with gradual decline in function and independence as motor symptoms lead to significant involuntary movements, and gait, balance, speech, and swallowing impairment. Psychiatric symptoms along with worsening cognitive challenges and eventually dementia often lead to institutionalization. Patients usually die 10–30 years after onset of motor symptoms (see Table 13-1).

MOTOR SYMPTOMS

Chorea is the most common motor feature of Huntington's disease. The phenomenology is best described as involuntary, jerky movements that flow from one body part to another in an unpredictable fashion. The movements usually involve the face, neck, trunk, and upper and lower extremities. The chorea often starts in distal limbs such as toes and fingers and, with disease progression, it involves more proximal muscle groups. The movements will lead to motor impersistence and inability to sustain a specific posture and result in difficulty in

Table 13-1 Cognitive deficits in Huntington's disease

Common motor, psychiatric and motor symptoms	*Psychiatric*	*Cognitive*
Chorea	Depression	Executive function
Dystonia	Apathy	Organization, sequencing tasks
Myoclonus	Anxiety	Working memory
Tics	OCD	Time management
Parkinsonism	Agitation	Facial expression recognition
Tremor	Paranoia	Distance perception
Dysarthria	Psychosis	Lack of insight into disease limitations
Abnormal eye Movements		
Gait impairment/Ataxia		

handling utensils, tools, and performing tasks requiring precision. The choreiform movements, especially early on, can be small in amplitude and sometimes give the appearance of "restlessness or fidgetiness" and can even be incorporated into normal movements (parakinesias). When mild, the chorea may not be recognized by the patient. Patients may also lack insight into severity of their chorea. With disease progression, the movements are more likely to be high amplitude, ballistic, flailing movements of an arm or a leg or a sudden, high amplitude flexion or extension of the trunk. The movements usually increase in frequency and intensity with anxiety, stress, or excitement. Chorea distribution and intensity increases with advancing disease especially in the middle stage of HD. However, in the majority of patients, in the latter stages of the disease, the chorea diminishes and is replaced with increased rigidity and dystonia.

Eye movement abnormalities are one of the earliest motor signs of HD and may include delayed or slowed and uncoordinated voluntary initiation of ocular saccades in the horizontal and vertical directions. There is also a component of oculomotor apraxia. Patients often find it difficult to suppress head movements, and often blink in order to break a fixation and generate a saccadic burst (Patel, 2012; Watts & Koller, 2004). Also, abnormalities of antisaccade and memory-guided saccade impairment have been reported (Ha & Fung, 2012). With disease progression and gait and balance impairment, eye movement abnormalities contribute to falls. Other abnormal movements include dystonia, which is an involuntary co-contraction of an agonist and its antagonist muscle leading to twisting and abnormal posturing of limbs and trunk. A combination of chorea and dystonia at a joint leads to athetoid movements. Myoclonus, a rapid, shock like, sudden movement, tics, rigidity, and parkinsonism are also seen in Huntington's disease. Juvenile HD or the Westphal variant usually presents with significant rigidity along with myoclonus and sometimes with seizures. Gait and balance also are progressively affected by advancing disease leading to falls and eventually to profound disability. Dysarthria limits communication as HD progresses. Dysphagia also progresses and may lead to feeding tube placement, and ultimately to aspiration and death.

NONMOTOR SYMPTOMS

Nonmotor symptoms of HD are just as disabling as motor symptoms and might alter the quality of life of the patient and produce significant challenges for caregivers. In fact, nonmotor symptoms are more strongly associated than are motor symptoms with functional decline, caregiver burden, and institutionalization. Several behavioral symptoms can predate the motor symptoms by several years: depression, apathy, anxiety, obsessive compulsive tendencies, agitation, psychotic behavior. Data from the European Huntington's Disease Network's REGISTRY (2010) revealed a life-time history of behavioral symptoms with approximately 20% of their HD participants having severe psychiatric problems, such as suicidal ideation or attempts, aggression, and psychosis being less common. Mood, impulse control, and other behavioral challenges often hinder family relationships and dynamics and may lead to substance abuse and trouble with the law. Sleep disturbances and fragmentation also contributes to cognitive and mood changes.

Cognitive deficits progressively manifest themselves with executive dysfunction, and difficulties with attention, visuospatial, and construction deficits often seen as the earliest cognitive alterations. Over the course HD, job performance and maintenance of employment become more challenging. As dementia develops and evolves, the performance of most if not all domains of daily living become compromised and, ultimately, most patients have to be placed in long-term-care facilities.

STAGES OF HUNTINGTON'S DISEASE

Huntington's disease can best be divided into 3 stages (although a 5-stage scale is sometimes used) based on functional capacity. These include the early, middle and late stages.

Early Stage: Patients are independent, usually still working, still driving, handle money, and live independently. Their neurological symptoms may include mild involuntary movements, subtle balance, and coordination changes. Cognitively, they may have difficulty with complex problem solving. Psychiatric symptoms include mild depression, anxiety, irritability, and disinhibition.

Middle Stage: Individuals become more dependent as they have more difficulty with activities of daily living (ADLs). They also lose the ability to work or drive. They may not be able to manage their own finances and take care of their household chores. They can feed, dress, and attend to their personal hygiene with some assistance. Chorea becomes prominent in this stage, and patients will have more difficulty with voluntary motor tasks. During this stage, balance becomes progressively worse and falls occur. Speech and swallowing become more of a challenge and weight loss is more prominent. Cognitive challenges worsen as problem solving becomes more difficult and individuals have difficulty managing their time. Individual relationships also suffer as a result of depression, agitation, obsessive-compulsive behavior, paranoia, and other psychotic behaviors.

Late Stage: In this stage, individuals with HD will need assistance in all their activities of daily living. There is now significant disability due to inability to communicate, walk without falling, and perform any purposeful activity without either severe chorea or dystonic rigidity and bradykinesia. Patients continue to comprehend until the very late stages. However, the inability to speak makes it extremely difficult to recognize concerns and address psychiatric symptoms. This last stage may last several years. Due to enormous challenges of caring for patients with late-stage HD, individuals are often unable to be cared for at home and need to be placed in a long-term-care facility. Aspiration followed by cardiovascular causes are the leading causes of death. Other causes of death include falls and suicide.

GENETICS

Huntington's disease is an autosomal dominant disorder, inherited in a Mendelian fashion. Men and women are equally affected, and individuals have a 50:50 chance of inheriting the disease gene if they have one parent with the disease. HD results from an unstable expanded CAG triplet repeat in the huntingtin gene (HTT), leading to an expanded polyglutamine stretch in the huntingtin protein (Htt) (Ha & Fung, 2012). The abnormally elongated protein is unable to be processed normally within the cells and its fragments lead to accumulation of intranuclear inclusions. Normal huntingtin genes contain 10–26 CAG repeats. Those with 27–35 repeats are considered intermediate. Repeat sizes of 36–39 are abnormal but have reduced penetrance. Those who have 40 or greater CAG repeats in one of their huntingtin genes will develop HD in their lifetime. There is evidence that there is some degree of motor, cognitive, and behavioral abnormalities in individuals with intermediate CAG repeats. This suggests the presence of subtle, but relevant disease manifestations in patients with intermediate CAG repeats (Killoran, 2013; Squitieri, 2012). These results have important implications for the pathogenesis of disease and genetic counseling (Jankovic & Fahn, 2007). Normal CAG repeat numbers tend not to change much during meiosis in the egg and sperm. However, due to "meiotic instability" in Huntington's disease, there is tendency for CAG repeat numbers in the abnormal range to change as they pass through the meiosis. CAG repeats usually increase, but they can decrease as well from one generation to the next. Thus, a child who inherits an abnormal HD gene from an affected parent can have a CAG repeat different from the affected parent. There is a relationship between the CAG repeat number and the age of onset of HD symptoms. Approximately 60–70% of the variation in onset age is determined by the length of the repeat gene. Longer CAG repeat is generally associated with earlier disease-onset age; thus, the concept of "anticipation," the earlier onset of symptoms with subsequent generations. The interaction between the normal and mutant alleles of the huntingtin gene and their effect on the clinical onset of HD has been examined recently. The number of CAG repeats within the normal allele does not influence the age of onset. Normal allele CAG length, interaction between expanded and normal alleles, and presence of a second expanded allele do not influence age at onset of motor manifestations, indicating that the rate of HD pathogenesis leading to motor diagnosis is determined by a completely dominant action of the longest expanded allele and yet-unidentified genetic or environmental factors (Lee et al., 2012).

PATHOPHYSIOLOGY

Several molecular pathways have been implicated in HD. Some of them are discussed here. The mutant Htt gene is thought to be responsible for disruption of multiple cellular functions including protein clearance, protein-protein interaction, function of mitochondria, axonal transport, gene transcription, N-methyl aspartate (NMDA) receptor activation, and gene posttranslational modification

(Ha &Fung, 2012). One mechanism for neuronal death involves excitotoxicity mediated by glutamate and the NMDA receptor. Another important pathway involves calcium homeostasis and mitochondrial dysfunction. In addition, there is direct toxicity of trinucleotide-repeat-induced aggregates and transcriptional dysregulation (which leads to accumulation of proteins that may be toxic; Sabbagh, & Shill, 2010). The two major pathways for protein degradation and handling of cellular waste in HD are also impaired. Essentially, continued toxic damage along with abnormal clearance of protein aggregates and accumulation of damaged cellular components lead to cell dysfunction and eventually cell death (Young, 1997)

NEUROPATHOLOGY

Striatal atrophy is the neuropathological hallmark of HD. Gross atrophy of caudate and putamen is accompanied by marked neuronal loss, astrogliosis, and reactive microgliosis. The striatal astrogliosis appears to reflect relative astrocyte survival in a shrinking striatum (Watts & Koller, 2004). Although neuroradiological studies have shown caudate atrophy in moderate HD, frequently no caudate atrophy is found early in the illness. Volumetric measurement of putamen is a more sensitive indicator of brain abnormalities in mild HD than measures of caudate atrophy (Harris, 1992). Quantitative microscopic studies have demonstrated selective neuronal degeneration in the neostriatum with relative preservation of large striatal neurons and severe loss of medium-sized striatal neurons. Medium spiny neurons comprise more than 80% of striatal neurons and are inhibitory projection neurons with gamma-amino butyric acid (GABA) as their primary neurotransmitter. Chorea seems to be related to the loss of medium spiny neurons projecting to the lateral pallidum (GPe).

NEUROIMAGING

Several neuroimaging methodologies have been implemented in understanding brain changes that occur in Huntington's disease. These include MRI, magnetic resonance spectroscopy (MRS), single-photon emission computed tomography, and positron emission tomography (PET). Although a significant body of research has focused on striatum (caudate and putamen), the brain region most severely affected in HD, more recent work using new available techniques has demonstrated measurable changes globally in the brain, even in presymptomatic and early stage HD. Regional cortical thinning has been shown in frontal, parietal, posterior temporal, parahippocampal, and occipital lobe. Regional thinning is variable in individuals with HD, which may explain some of the variability of the clinical symptoms and the phenotypes. More extensive loss of volumes of other brain structures such as the hippocampus, amygdala, hypothalamus, globus pallidus and brainstem have been demonstrated in individuals in early and middle stages of HD. Caudate atrophy (see Figure 13-1) has traditionally been used as an index of striatal atrophy in Huntington's disease and has been demonstrated to correlate well with the degree of cognitive impairment in early HD (Bamford,

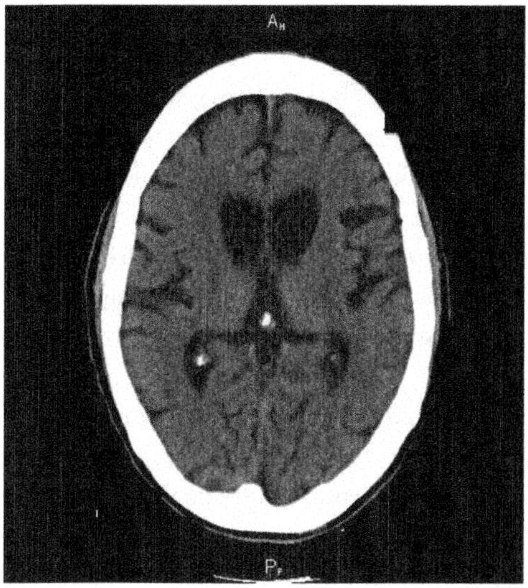

FIGURE 13-1
Global volume loss and atrophy of caudate nuclei evident on a computed tomography (CT) scan of the brain in Huntington's disease.

Caine, Kido, Cox, & Shoulson, 1995). However, subsequent studies have suggested that the putamen is either underdeveloped in HD or that it is one of the earliest structures to atrophy. The reduction in putaminal volume measured by MRI was a more sensitive index of neurological dysfunction than caudate atrophy (Jankovic & Fahn, 2007). Except for atrophy, MRI is unremarkable, although patients with the akinetic-rigid form are more likely to show striatal hyperintensity on T2- weighted MRI than are patients with the choreic form of HD. Other techniques such as real-time sonography showed abnormalities in caudate and substantia nigra in those with HD. Many MRI volumetric and single photon emission computed tomography blood flow studies have shown reduced basal ganglia volume and blood flow even in presymptomatic HD patients. PET scans of 18F -2 Fluoro-2 deoxyglucose uptake and single photon emission computed tomography have shown hypometabolism and reduced regional blood flow in the basal ganglia and the cortex. Regional cerebral metabolic rate of glucose consumption has been found to be decreased by 2% in caudate and 56% in the lenticular nucleus, and 17% in the cerebral cortex. MRI morphometry has found significant reduction in the gray matter volume in the left striatum, bilateral insula, dorsal midbrain, and bilateral intraparietal sulcus in the gene carriers as opposed to gene negative controls (Thieben et al., 2002; Jankovic & Fahn, 2007). Using tensor-based morphometry, Kipps Duggins, McCusker, and Calder (2007) were able to demonstrate progression of gray matter atrophy in presymptomatic HD mutation carriers.

NEUROIMAGING AND COGNITION

Regarding structural and functional neuroimaging findings, in a meta analysis of neuroimaging studies, striatal and cortical atrophy were most commonly correlated with deficits in attention, working-memory, and executive function (Montoya, Price, Menear, & Page, 2006). Striatal hypoperfusion and decreased glucose utilization correlated with executive dysfunction, whereas cortical hypometabolism tended to correlate with performance on recognition memory and language and perceptual tasks (Montoya, Price, et al., 2006). Pre- and postsynaptic dopamine action tended to correlate with episodic memory, processing speed, and executive functioning performance (Montoya, Price et al., 2006). Other findings suggest that left caudate head volumes are smaller in participants that were deemed closer to clinical diagnosis relative to controls (Paulsen et al., 2004). No significant differences were observed for the right caudate head or for the right or left caudate body. Reduced striatal volume was found to correlate with greater neurologic impairment (primarily motor), slower mental processing speed, and poorer verbal learning in prodromal individuals (Campodonico et al., 1998). Significant differences in functional activation patterns also emerged for the thalamus, caudate/putamen, and presupplementary motor area/cingulate, with reduced activation in participants close to diagnosis relative to controls (Paulsen et al., 2004). Regarding potential biomarkers for neurodegeneration, other investigators have reported predictive utility using structural (MRI) and functional (fMRI) neuroimaging measures in presymptomatic HD, in particular for a set of volumetric variables from the basal ganglia/lentiform nucleus and striatum, as well as measures from the caudate, corticospinal tract, and functional data from the insular cortex (Rizk-Jackson et al., 2011). Other investigators have found that white matter/subcortical volume loss and cortical glucose hypometabolism (frontal and temporal lobes and striatum) precede gray matter atrophy early in the disease process in asymptomatic individuals (Ciarmiello et al., 2006). These findings are consistent with earlier PET and CT studies suggesting an association between striatal and cortical glucose hypometabolism and volume loss in HD and cognitive impairment and decline early in the disease process; with psychomotor function and decline correlating with striatal changes and frontal and temporal-parietal changes linked to more general cognitive and functional impairment and dementia (Kuwert, Lange, Langen, Herzog, Aulich, & Feinendegen, 1990; Bamford et al., 1995). Regarding potential protective factors, recent findings suggest that cognitive reserve (as assessed by estimated premorbid intellectual functioning, occupational history, and years of education) may be associated with a slower rate of cognitive decline and striatal volume loss (Bonner-Jackson et al., 2013).

NEUROCOGNITIVE AND BEHAVIORAL ASPECTS OF HUNTINGTON'S DISEASE

Neurocognitively, HD is traditionally thought of as manifesting a "subcortical" or frontal–subcortical/frontostriatial pattern of dysfunction and has served as a useful model to elucidate the role of the basal ganglia in cognition and behavior (Cummings, 1986; Paulsen & Mikos, 2008). It has also offered the opportunity to study preclinical/predyskinesia cognitive impairment and decline (Brandt et al., 2008; Paulsen, 2010; Snowden, Craufurd, Thompson, & Neary, 2002; Stout et al.,

2011). Although the cortical versus subcortical distinction probably represents an oversimplified framework, especially as there is widespread cortical involvement in HD (Kuwert et al., 1990; Montoya, Price, et al., 2006; Walker, 2007), it has served as a useful heuristic for describing and understanding degenerative neurocognitive and neuropsychiatric dysfunction and dementia, especially in movement disorders (Cummings, 1993; Salmon & Filoteo, 2007; Savage, 1997; Turner, Moran, & Kopelman, 2002).

In the case of HD, cortical cognitive abnormalities such as aphasia, amnesia, or agnosia are typically missing (Paulsen & Mikos, 2008). Huntington's disease patients evidence progressive impairment in multiple aspects of executive and related functions, most prominently attention, working-memory and dual processing, psychomotor speed and efficiency (with marked cognitive slowing also evident in the absence of motor demands), and inhibitory control (Lezak, Howieson, Bigler, & Tranel, 2012; Paulsen, 2010; Peavy et al., 2010; Stout, Rodwalt, & Siemers, 2011). As the disease progresses, language, memory, and visuospatial functions are eventually also affected (Montoya, Price, et al., 2006; Montoya, Pelletier, et al., 2006; Paulsen et al., 1995; Robins Whalin & Byrne, 2012). Cognitive decline appears to be more closely related to severity of motor dysfunction and CAG expansion than to duration of the disease (Brandt, Strauss, Laurus, Jensen, Folstein, & Folstein, 1984; Paulsen & Mikos, 2008). There is also some evidence that overall clinical severity and degree of functional disability or dementia (as measured by a composite neuropsychological impairment and functional deficits/status) in HD are tied to cortical glucose hypometabolism, whereas chorea severity is associated with lentiform nucleus pathology (Kuwert et al., 1990). Furthermore, cognitive decline appears to be tied to multiple biological/physiological factors in the disease process, including levels of brain-derived neurotrophic factor, insulin-like growth factor I, and multiple dopamine receptor/synaptic actions (Paulsen, 2011).

Given the neurodegenerative/progressive nature of HD, the associated cognitive and behavioral dysfunction broadly conforms to preclinical/prodromal, clinical/manifest, and dementia stages. These stages or phases of the disease are associated with progressive cognitive and behavioral dysfunction and increasing degrees of functional compromise and disability (Paulsen et al., 2008; Robins Whalin & Byrne, 2012). Once clinical signs and symptoms manifest, a common method of assessing, tracking, and staging impairment and decline in HD is the Unified Huntington's Disease Rating Scale (UHDRS; Huntington Study Group, 1996). The UHDRS assesses four domains of clinical performance and capacity: motor function, cognitive function, behavioral abnormalities, and functional capacity.

THE PRODROMAL STAGE

The early or prodromal phase of HD has received a lot of attention, and most studies define prodromal HD as having ≥ 36 CAG expansion (repeats) on genetic testing without manifest motor signs. Given the prominent and early striatal involvement in HD, the most sensitive measures for detecting the prodromal neurocognitive effects of HD tend to involve psychomotor processing speed and attention. Other domains that can be affected in premanifest populations include working-memory, object and space perception, emotion recognition, learning and memory retrieval, and aspects of executive function and individuals with greater CAG expansion tend to show earlier onset, faster progression/decline, and more pronounced cognitive impairment (Lee et al., 2012; Lemiere, Decruyenaere, Evers-Kiebooms, Vandenbussche, & Dom, 2004; Paulsen, Zhao, et al., 2001; Stout et al., 2011; Verny et al., 2007).

Reports suggest that subtle cognitive changes can predate by 2 to 15 years the neurologic or motor signs of the disease; findings across studies vary, in large part due to methodological differences/measures used (Brandt et al., 2008; Lemiere, Decruyenaere, Evers-Kiebooms, Vandenbussche, & Dom, 2004; Paulsen & Mikos, 2008; Solomon et al., 2007; Stout et al., 2011; Verny et al., 2007). Several neuropsychological measures assessing attention and psychomotor speed, including verbal generative fluency, the Symbol Digit Modalities Test (SDMT), and the Stroop Color Word Test (color, reading, and interference) have been shown to detect impairment at least two years prior to onset of manifest motor disease in "at risk" individuals (Paulsen et al., 2001a). In another comparison of premanifest and early HD patients to normal controls, longitudinal change/decline (at 12 and 24 months) in SDMT, Circle Tracing, direct and indirect (a measure of visuomotor integration), and Stroop word-reading performance showed greatest sensitivity in the early HD group, with very little evidence of deterioration in the premanifest group relative to controls (Stout et al., 2012). Asymptomatic huntingtin-mutation carriers who later develop signs of HD demonstrate poorer performance on a test of conceptual-level and novel problem solving (Wisconsin Card Sorting Test; WCST) an average of 8.6 years prior to clinical diagnosis (Brandt et al., 2008). In particular, early converters (who develop manifest signs within 8.6 years of exam) evidence fewer category sorts and commit more errors relative to late converters (after 8.6 years) and individuals who remain asymptomatic.

In a more recent factor analytic study of several neurocognitive domains, motor planning/speed and sensory-perceptual processing predicted time to diagnosis in prodromal HD patients after controlling for CAG repeats and age (CAG–age product score: CAP) and motor signs (Harrington et al., 2012). This was especially true in the high-risk group with an estimated 5 years until clinical diagnosis based on CAP score (Harrington et al., 2012). Overall, this study identified 6 neurocognitive factors that were sensitive to cognitive decline in prodromal HD (and typically more sensitive than performance on individual tests), including speed and inhibition, verbal working memory, motor planning/speed, attention-information integration, sensory-perceptual processing, and verbal learning/memory (see Figure 13-2). Years to diagnosis in HD can also be relatively accurately estimated using fine motor speed, word list learning, and smell/odor identification (Paulsen et al., 2008).

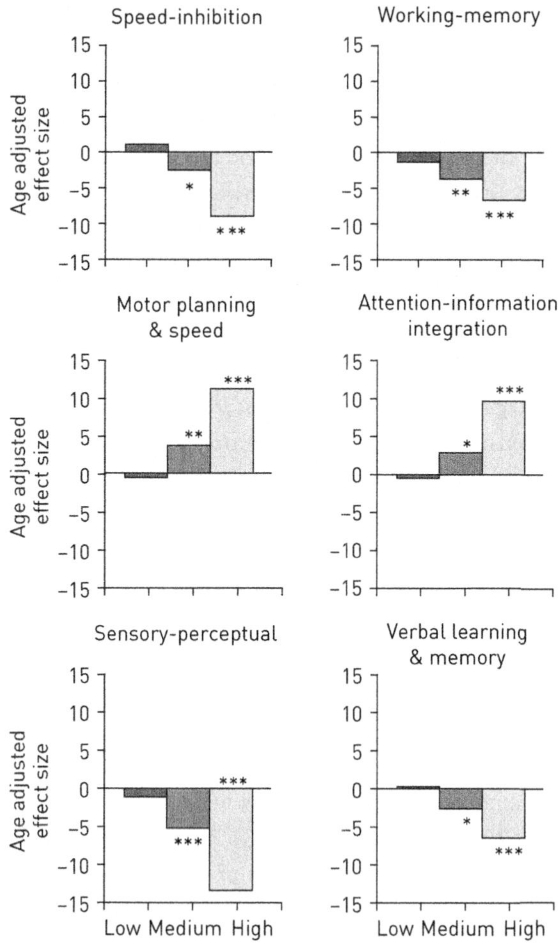

FIGURE 13-2

Age adjusted effect sizes for six factors in the low, medium, and high CAP groups. Standardized effect size = effect size/standard error of effect size. Asterisks denote the significance of pairwise comparisons between the control group and each CAP group where $^*p < 0.02$, $^{**}p < 0.001$, and $^{***}p < 0.0001$. From Harrington et al. (2012). *Journal of Neurology, Neurosurgery and Psychiatry, 83*, 616. © by the British Medical Journal Publishing Group. All rights reserved. Reprinted with permission.

In one study performance on verbal episodic memory tests (e.g., Hopkins Verbal Learning Test—Revised; HVLT-R) was associated with probability of HD diagnosis within 5 years (Solomon et al., 2007). For example, subtle declines in learning/acquisition on the HVLT-R were evident in individuals with minimal motor abnormalities (Solomon et al., 2007). Performance on recognition measures tends to be relatively better than on free-recall measures, suggesting retrieval-based deficits early in the disease process (Montoya, Pelletier, et al., 2006). Other authors have reported impairments in multiple aspects of learning and memory in pre-HD, including semantic clustering, free recall, and recognition discriminability (Lanto, Riege, Mazziotta, Pahl, & Phelps, 1990; Rosenberg, Sorensen, & Christensen, 1995).

In a large study of neurocognitive signs in prediagnosis HD ($N = 738$), psychomotor performance, emotion recognition, and working memory were the most sensitive measures of the prodromal neurocognitive effects of HD and also evidenced a graded/progressive pattern, with larger deficits in individuals within 9 years to diagnosis relative to individuals estimated to be between 9 to 15 years from diagnosis (Stout et al., 2011). Although, significant effects were also detected for more than half of the neurocognitive variables measured in individuals between 9 to 15 years from diagnosis (Stout et al., 2011).

THE CLINICAL STAGE

In the clinical stage of HD (when the motor signs and symptoms manifest), there is continued decline in attention, processing speed, working memory, visual-perceptual abilities, and multiple aspects of executive function (including appropriately maintaining and shifting attentional focus, inhibition, planning and organization, and abstract thinking). Additionally, learning and episodic memory dysfunction and impairment in reasoning/judgment and decision making become more pronounced, whereas semantic memory and language functions remain relatively unaffected (Montoya, Pelletier, et al., 2006; Robins Wahlin, Larsson, Luszcz, & Byrne, 2010; Stout, et al., 2001). Generative cognitive fluency, including phonemic/lexical and semantic fluency can show marked decline at this stage (Verny et al., 2007). It is also typically at this stage that visuoperceptual and constructional deficits become a lot more severe (Robins Whalin & Byrne, 2012; Paulsen et al., 1995). Additionally, impairments in recognition of facial emotion that are typically present in premanifest HD become more global and severe during the clinical stage (Labuschagne et al., 2012). Depending on the severity of cognitive dysfunction, driving and work status typically become issues of clinical concern at this stage and should be evaluated more comprehensively, including neuropsychological assessment and a formal driving evaluation.

THE DEMENTIA STAGE

In the dementia stage of HD, there is a general decline across all neurocognitive domains, including psychometric intellectual functioning (e.g., as measured by the Wechsler scales) and generalized cortical atrophy is commonly observed (Montoya, Price, et al., 2006). The severe cognitive and functional deficits can also be complicated by marked apathy and loss of initiation and substantial bradyphrenia. At this stage, deficits in semantic and language functions also become evident. The cognitive domains of initiation, construction, and memory as assessed by the Dementia Rating Scale (DRS) show marked decline in the advanced or severe stages of HD dementia (Paulsen & Mikos, 2008; Paulsen et al., 1995) and caregiver burden becomes substantial, with patients typically requiring some level of institutional care and assistance, especially as they start to experience significant gait abnormalities, weight loss, speech and swallowing

Table 13-2 General progression of neurobehavioral symptoms in Huntington's disease derived from a survey of 1,238 individuals with a minimum 6-year history of symptomatic HD.

NEUROBEHAVIORAL SYMPTOMS DIVIDED INTO STAGES					
Initial symptom	*Early*	*Early-middle*	*Middle*	*Middle-late*	*Late*
Involuntary Movements	Sadness Depression Difficult to get along with	Avolition Sexual dysfunction Paranoia	Sleeping trouble, Delusions, Cognitive decline, Memory loss	Speech difficulty	Bowel & bladder inconti- nence, Dementia

<1 year → 2–5 years → 6–10 years → >10 years

Based on participating families completion of the Affected Individuals Questionnaire, which includes 19 physical, emotional, and cognitive signs commonly associated with HD disease progression. Adapted from Kirkwood et al., 2001.

difficulties, and loss of bowel and bladder control (Kirkwood, Su, Conneally, & Foroud, 2001; see Table 13-2).

NEUROPSYCHIATRIC FEATURES

Mood and psychiatric symptoms are highly prevalent in HD and can present early in the premanifest stage of the disease before any other signs are present, including cognitive or motor (Paulsen, Ready, Hamilton, Mega, & Cummings, 2001). Like the cognitive and motor signs and symptoms of the disease, the mood and neuropsychiatric features tend to become more pronounced as HD progresses and depression severity can be a contributor to poorer cognitive performance (Smith et al., 2012). Frequently reported neuropsychiatric symptoms are depressed mood, anxiety, irritability, and apathy, with prevalences ranging from 33 to 76%; obsessive-compulsive symptoms and psychosis are also common, with prevalences of 10 to 52% and 3 to 11%, respectively (van Duijn, Kingma, & van der Mast, 2007). Obsessive-compulsive features tend to involve perseveration and becoming "stuck" or fixated on a particular need or topic (Paulsen & Mikos, 2008). Suicidal ideation and risk are also frequently encountered in HD patients, with the frequency of suicidal ideation doubling from 9.1% in at-risk persons with a normal neurological examination to 19.8% in at-risk persons with soft neurological signs and increasing to 23.5% in persons with "possible HD" (Paulsen, Ferneyhough Hoth, Nehl, & Stierman, 2005). In 4,171 individuals with a diagnosis of HD, 16.7% had suicidal ideation in stage 1 (using Total Functional Capacity Scale scores for staging), and 21.6% had suicidal ideation in stage 2, whereas the proportion of HD patients with suicidal ideation diminished thereafter (Paulsen et al., 2005). The first critical period for suicidal ideation in HD appears to be immediately before receiving a formal diagnosis (when soft signs of the disease are present), and the second is in stage 2 of the disease, when independence diminishes and functional deficits become more pronounced (Paulsen et al., 2005). Anger, irritability, hypersexuality, impulsivity and temper control problems represent the other side of the spectrum in neurobehavioral changes in HD patients, and they are not surprising given the frontal–subcortical circuit pathology involved (Paulsen, Pelletier, et al., 2001).

The precise underlying mechanisms of mood dysfunction and suicidal ideation in HD are not fully understood, but functional neuroimaging findings have suggested lower activity in dorsal and ventral sectors of the prefrontal lobe, in the parietal lobe, right thalamus, and the cerebellum in emotional processing and dysphoria in early HD patients relative to healthy controls (Paradiso et al., 2008). In addition, early HD patients showed higher glucose metabolism in the left thalamus, transverse temporal gyrus, hippocampus, and primary and secondary visual cortices (Paradiso et al., 2008). These findings are consistent with the common pattern of functional frontal–subcortical disconnection in HD and also suggest that using functional imaging (fMRI and PET) and affective probes can aid in early/premanifest detection of HD (Paradiso et al., 2008). Most other neuropsychiatric symptoms in HD are also typically related to frontal–subcoritcal circuit dysregulation, including dopaminergic dysfunction, which is also prominently involved in the psychotic symptoms that HD patients experience (including, paranoia, thought disorder, hallucinations, and delusional ideation). The prominent neuropsychiatric and cognitive features of HD play an important role in research and treatment because these aspects tend to place the greatest burden on families of patients and caregivers and are also closely linked to functional decline, disability, quality of life, and need for institutional care (Paulsen, 2011).

TREATMENT

Currently, the mainstay of treatments for HD are symptomatic therapies. These include pharmacotherapy for treatment of involuntary movements and psychiatric symptoms. At this time, tetrabenazine, a dopamine depletor remains the only medication licensed in North America and Europe for treatment of chorea in HD. Exacerbation of depression is a potential side effect. Treatment with tetrabenazine should be individualized and patients should be followed closely to monitor for adverse events including hypersomnolence, insomnia, depression, and parkinsonism, especially with advancing disease when rigidity and dystonia replaces chorea. Neuroleptics remain the preferred treatment for chorea in Europe. In North America and Australia, the use of tetrabenazine and antipsychotic drugs are split almost equally (Ha & Fung, 2012). Amantadine efficacy has mixed results. Deep brain stimulation of the bilateral posteroventral globus pallidus internus (Gpi) has been reported in only a handful of patients (Fasano et al., 2008). Although there have been improvements in chorea, long-term follow-up thus far has shown progressive deterioration in overall function secondary to worsened gait and balance as well as cognitive decline. More studies are needed to better assess utility of DBS in HD.

Treatment of psychiatric symptoms involves management of depression, anxiety, irritability and agitation, impulsivity, obsessive-compulsiveness, paranoia, and psychotic behavior. SSRIs and SNRIs are the main treatments used for depression, and sometimes for irritability and anxiety. Neuroleptics (typical and atypical antipsychotics) are used for psychosis and chorea suppression (Epping & Paulsen 2011). Tardive dyskinesia (especially oro-bucco-lingual dyskinesia) complicating the existing chorea as well rigidity and parkinsonism can be potential side effects. Benzodiazepines are often used for treatment of anxiety and insomnia. Management of cognitive dysfunction in Huntington's disease remains limited. There is insufficient data regarding the benefits of using cholinesterase inhibitors such as donepezil (Armstrong, 2012). There may be a role for use of memantine, a partial glutamate antagonist (Hjermind, Law, Jønch, Stokholm, & Nielsen, 2011).

FUTURE DIRECTIONS

Basic science research is trending toward identifying disease-modifying, neuroprotective therapies (Ha & Fung, 2012; Ross & Tabrizi, 2011). These include altering disease process at the level of transcription and translation where various important proteins and enzyme are being formed (Renna, Jimenez-Sanchez, Sarkar, & Rubinsztein, 2010; Ross & Tabrizi, 2011). Other areas of research involve cellular bioenergetics and methods in which mitochondrial dysfunction can be delayed or prevented (Jiang et al., 2012; Jeong, 2011; Scahill, 2012). These include antioxidants and compounds that reduce excitotoxicity. Accumulation and clearance of mutant Htt as well as cellular waste are also being studied. Potential therapeutic targets include growth factors such as brain derived neurotrophic factor (BDNF), an important neurotrophin involved in striatal neuronal survival and cortical-striatal synapse activity (Xie, Hayden, & Xu, 2010; Martin et al., 2011).

The continued use and development of neurocognitive tests in Huntington's disease research provides meaningful information about the onset, course, and progression of the disease in premanifest individuals who appear healthy, much like the study of mild cognitive impairment and preclinical Alzheimer's dementia. As research is increasingly moving toward the study of potential disease-modifying and neuroprotective therapies, the development and refinement of neurocognitive measures that are sensitive to therapeutic effects are going to become important, especially as cognitive impairment or change represents an early disease indicator that has implications for diagnosis, functional disability, and quality of life. Psychometrically sound, sensitive and specific cognitive tests can play a very important role in combination with other biomarkers, not only in the early detection of HD, but, importantly, in providing a crucial marker for therapeutic efficacy and outcome. Furthermore, studies addressing potential cognitive rehabilitation/remediation interventions that could delay the onset of functional disability due to cognitive impairment are needed.

CONCLUSIONS

Huntington's disease is a complex, devastating hereditary neurodegenerative disorder that manifests itself with significant psychiatric, motor, and cognitive symptoms, ultimately leading to death. Currently the only available treatments are symptomatic and no cure exists. However, with increased awareness of the disease, a growing research is contributing to knowledge of disease pathogenesis, identification of biomarkers, and development of better therapeutic agents, especially neuroprotective and disease-modifying therapies.

REFERENCES

Armstrong, M. (2012). Evidence-based guideline: Pharmacologic treatment of chorea in Huntington disease. *Neurology* 79(6), 597–603.

Bamford, K. A, Caine, E. D., Kido, D. K., Cox, C., & Shoulson, I. (1995). A prospective evaluation of cognitive decline in early Huntington's disease. *Neurology;* 45(10), 1867–1873

Bonner-Jackson, A., Long, J. D., Westervelt, H., Tremont, G., Aylward, E., Paulsen, J. S., & The PREDICT-HD Investigators and Coordinators of the Huntington Study Group. (2013). Cognitive reserve and brain reserve in prodromal Huntington's disease. *Journal of the International Neuropsychological Society, 19,* 739–750.

Brandt, J., Inscore, A. B., Ward, J., Shpritz B., Rosenblatt, A., Margolis, R. L., & Ross, C. A. (2008). Neuropsychological deficits in Huntington's disease gene carries and correlates of early "conversion." *The Journal of Neuropsychiatry and Clinical Neurosciences, 20,* 466–472.

Brandt, J., Strauss, M., Laurus, J., Jensen, B., Folstein, S., & Folstein, M. (1984). Clinical correlates of dementia and disability in Huntington's disease. *Journal of Clinical Neuropsychology, 6,* 401–412.

Campodonico, J., Aylward, E., Codori, A., Young, C., Krafft, L., Magdalinski, M., . . . Brandt, J. (1998). When does Huntington's disease begin? *Journal of International Neuropsychological Society,* 4(5), 467–73.

Ciarmiello, A., Cannella, M., Lastoria, S., Simonelli, M., Frati, L., Rubinsztein, D. C., & Squitieri, F. (2006). Brain white-matter volume loss and glucose hypometabolism precede the clinical symptoms of Huntington's disease. *The Journal of Nuclear Medicine,* 47(2), 215–222.

Cummings, J. L. (1986). Subcortical dementia: Neuropsychology, neuropsychiatry, and pathophysiology. *The British Journal of Psychiatry, 149,* 682–697.

Cummings, J. L. (1993). Frontal-subcortical circuits and human behavior. *Archives of Neurology,* 50(8), 873–880.

Epping, E., & Paulsen, J. (2011). Depression in the early stages of Huntington disease. *Neurodegenerative Disease Management.* 1(5), 407–414.

The European Huntington's Disease Network (2010). F02 Observing Huntington's disease (HD): The European Huntington's disease Nework Registry, *Journal of Neurology, Neurosurgery and Psychiatry, 8,* A23.

Jankovic, J., & Fahn, S., (2007). *Huntington's Disease in Principles and Practice of Movement Disorders* (pp. 369–392). Philadelphia, Churchill Livingstone Elsevier.

Fasano, A., Mazzone, P., Piano, C., Quaranta, D., Soleti, F., & Bentivoglio, A. (2008). GPi-DBS in Huntington's disease: Results on motor function and cognition in a 72-year-old case, *Journal of Movement Disorders* 23(9), 1289–1292.

Ha, A., Beck, C., & Jankovic, J. (2012). Intermediate CAG Repeats in Huntington's Disease: Analysis of COHORT. *Tremor and Other Hyperkinetic Movements, 1*, 1–7.

Ha, A., Fung, V. (2012)..Huntington's disease. *Current Opinion in Neurology, 25*(4), 491–498. doi: 10.1097/WCO.0b013e3283550c97.

Harris, G. J., Pearlson, G. D., Peyser, C. E., Aylward, E. H., Roberts, J., Barta, P. E., . . . Folstein, S. E. (1992). Putamen volume reduction on magnetic resonance imaging exceeds caudate changes in mild Huntington's disease. *Annals of Neurology, 31*(1), 69–75.

Harrington, D. L., Smith, M. M., Zhang, Y., Carlozzi, N. E., Paulsen, J. S., & the PREDICT-HD Investigators of the Huntington Study Group (2012). Cognitive domains that predict time to diagnosis in prodromal Huntington disease. *Journal of Neurology, Neurosurgery and Psychiatry, 83*, 612–619.

Hjermind, L., Law, I., Jønch, A., Stokholm, J., & Nielsen, J. E. (2011) Huntington's disease: effect of memantine on FDG-PET brain metabolism? *Journal of Neuropsychiatry and Clinical Neuroscience, 23*(2), 206–210.

Huntington Study Group. (1996). Unified Huntington's Disease Rating Scale: Reliability and consistency. *Movement Disorders, 11*(2), 136–142.

Jankovic, J., & Fahn, S. (2007). *Huntington's disease in principles and practice of movement disorders* (pp. 369–392). Philadelphia, PA: Churchill Livingstone Elsevier.

Jeong, H., Cohen, D., Cui, L., Supinski, A., Savas, J., Mazzulli, J., . . . Krainc, D. (2011). Sirt1 mediates neuroprotection from mutant huntingtin by activation of the TORC1 and CREB transcriptional pathway. *Nature Medicine*, 18(1),159–165. doi: 10.1038/nm.2559

Jiang, L., Liao, M., Xu, X., Huang, S., Tan, H., Peng, T., . . . Li, H. (2012). GRP78 counteracts cell death and protein aggregation caused by mutant huntingtin proteins. *Journal of Neuroscience Letters, 516*(2),182–187.

Killoran, A., Biglan, K., Jankovic, J., Eberly, S., Kayson, E., Oakes, D., . . . Shoulson, I. (2013). Characterization of the Huntington intermediate CAG repeat expansion phenotype in PHAROS. *Neurology, 80*(22), 2022–2027.

Kipps, C., Duggins, A., McCusker, E., & Calder, A. (2007). Disgust and happiness recognition correlate with anteroventral insula and amygdala volume respectively in preclinical Huntington's disease. *Journal of Cognitive Neuroscience, 19*(7), 1206–1217.

Kirkwood, S. C., Su, J. L., Conneally, P., & Foroud, T. (2001). Progression of symptoms in the early and middle stages of Huntington disease. *Archives of Neurology, 58*(2), 273–278.

Kuwert, T., Lange, H. W., Langen, K. J., Herzog, H., Aulich, A., & Feinendegen, L. E. (1990). Cortical and subcortical glucose consumption measured by PET in patients with Huntington's disease. *Brain, 113*(5), 1405–1423.

Labuschagne, I., Jones, R., Callaghan, J., Whitehead, D., Dumas, E., Say, M., . . . Stout, J. (2012). TRACK-HD Investigators. Emotional face recognition deficits and medication effects in pre-manifest through stage-II Huntington's disease. *Psychiatry Research. 15*, 207(1–2), 118–126.

Lanto, A. B., Riege, W. H., Mazziotta, J. C., Pahl, J. J., & Phelps, M. E. (1990). Increased false alarms in a subset of persons at-risk for Huntington's disease. *Archives of Clinical Neuropsychology, 5*(4), 393–404.

Lee, J., Ramos, E. Lee, J., Gillis, T., Mysore, J., Hayden, M., . . . Jones, R. (2012). CAG repeat expansion in Huntington disease determines age at onset in a fully dominant fashion. *Neurology, 78*(10), 690–695.

Lemiere, J., Decruyenaere, M., Evers-Kiebooms, G., Vandenbussche, E., & Dom, R. (2004). Cognitive changes in patients with Huntington's disease (HD) and asymptomatic carries of the HD mutation. *Journal of Neurology, 251,* 935–942.

Lezak, M. D., Howieson, D. B., Biger, E. D., & Tranel, D. (2012). *Neuropsychological assessment* (5th ed). New York, NY: Oxford University Press.

Martin, E., Betuing, S., Pagès, C., Cambon, K., Auregan, G., Deglon, N., Roze, E., & Caboche J. (2011) Mitogen- and stress-activated protein kinase 1-induced neuroprotection in Huntington's disease: Role on chromatin remodeling at the PGC-1-alpha promoter. *Human Molecular Genetics, 20*(12), 2422–2434.

Montoya, A., Price, B. H., Menear, M., & Lepage, M. (2006). Brain imaging and cognitive dysfunctions in Huntington's disease. *Journal of Psychiatry and Neuroscience, 31*(1), 21–29.

Montoya, A., Pelletier, M., Menear, M., Duplessis, E., Richer, F., & Lepage, M. (2006). Episodic memory impairment in Huntington's disease: A meta-analysis. *Neuropsychologia, 44,* 1984–1994.

Patel, S., Jankovic, J., Hood, A., Jeter, C., & Sereno, A (2012). Reflexive and volitional saccades: Biomarkers of Huntington disease severity and progression. *Journal of Neurological Sciences,* 313(1–2), 35–41.

Paradiso, S., Turner, B. M., Paulsen, J. S., Jorge, R., Boles Ponto, L. L., & Robinson, R. G. (2008). Neural bases of dysphoria in early Huntington's disease. *Psychiatry Research, 162*(1), 73–87.

Paulsen, J. S. (2010). Early detection of Huntington's disease. *Future Neurology, 5*(1), 85–104.

Paulsen, J. S. (2011). Cognitive impairment in Huntington's disease: Diagnosis and treatment. *Current Neurology and Neuroscience Reports, 11*(5), 474–483.

Paulsen, J. S., Butters, N., Sadek, J. R., Johnson, S. A., Salmon, D. P., Swerdlow, N. R., & Swenson, M. R. (1995). Distinct cognitive profiles of cortical and subcortical dementia in advanced illness. *Neurology, 45,* 951–956.

Paulsen, J. S., Ferneyhough Hoth, K., Nehl, C., & Stierman, L. (2005). Critical periods of suicide risk in Huntington's disease. *American Journal of Psychiatry, 162,* 725–731.

Paulsen, J. S., Langbehn, D. R., Stout, J. C., Aylward, E., Ross, C. A., Nance, M.,... Hayden, M. (2008). Detection of Huntington's disease decades before diagnosis: The predict-HD study. *Journal of Neurology, Neurosurgery and Psychiatry, 79,* 874–880.

Paulsen, J. S. & Mikos A. (2008). Huntington's disease. In J. E. Morgan & J. H. Ricker (Eds.), Textbook of clinical neuropsychology (pp. 616–635). New York, NY: Taylor & Francis.

Paulsen, J. S., Ready, R. E., Hamilton, J. M., Mega, M. S., & Cummings, J. L. (2001). Neuropsychiatric aspects of Huntington's disease. *Journal of Neurology, Neurosurgery and Psychiatry, 71,* 310–314.

Paulsen, J. S., Zhao, H., Stout, J. C., Brinkman, R. R., Guttman, M., & Ross, C. A. (2001). Clinical markers of early disease in persons near onset of Huntington's disease. *Neurology, 57*(4), 658–662.

Paulsen, J. S., Zimbelman, J. L., Hinton, S. C., Langbehn, D. R., Leveroni, C. L., Benjamin, M. L.,... Rao, S. M. (2004). fMRI biomarker of early neuronal dysfunction in presymptomatic Huntington's disease. *American Journal of Neuroradiology, 25,* 1715–1721.

Peavy, G. M., Jacobson, M. W., Goldstein, J. L., Hamilton, J. M., Kane, A., Gamst, A. C.,... Corey-Bloom, J. (2010). Cognitive and functional decline in Huntington's disease: Dementia criteria revisited. *Movement Disorders, 25*(9), 1163–1169.

Penny, J., & Young, A. (1998): Huntington's disease. In J. Jankovic and E. Tolosa (Eds.), *Parkinson's disease and movement disorders,* (3rd ed., pp. 341–356). Baltimore, MD: Williams & Wilkins.

Pringsheim, T., Wiltshire, K., Day, L., Dykeman, J., Steves, T., & Jette, N. (2012) The incidence and prevalence of Huntington's disease: A systematic review and meta-analysis. Movement Disorders. *27*(9), 1083–1091.

Renna, M., Jimenez-Sanchez, M., Sarkar, S., & Rubinsztein, D. (2010). Chemical inducers of autophagy that enhance the clearance of mutant proteins in neurodegenerative diseases. *Journal of Biological Chemistry, 285*(15), 11061–11067.

Rizk-Jackson, A., Stoffers, D., Sheldon, S., Kuperman, J., Dale, A., Goldstein, J., . . . Aron, A. R. (2011). Evaluating imaging biomarkers for neurodegeneration in pre-symptomatic Huntington's disease using machine learning techniques. *NeuroImage, 56*(2), 788–796.

Robins Whalin, T. B. & Byrne, G. J. (2012). Cognition in Huntington's disease. In N. E. Tunali (Ed.), *Huntington's disease: Core concepts and current advances* (pp. 175–200). Europe: InTech/Open Access.

Robins Wahlin, T. B., Larsson, M. U., Luszcz, M. A., & Byrne, G. J. (2010). WAIS-R features of preclinical Huntington's disease: Implications for early detection. *Dementia and Geriatric Cognitive Disorders, 29*(4), 342–350.

Rosenberg N. K., Sorensen S. A., & Christensen A. L. (1995). Neuropsychological characteristics of Huntington's disease carriers: A double blind study. *Journal of Medical Genetics, 32*(8), 600–604.

Ross, C., Tabrizi, S.(2011)..Huntington's disease: from molecular pathogenesis to clinical treatment. *Lancet Neurology,* (1), 83–98.

Sabbagh, M.N. & Shill, H.A., (2010). Latrepirdine, a potential novel treatment for Alzheimer's disease and Huntington's chorea. *Current Opinion on Investigational Drugs, 11*(1), 80–91.

Salmon, D. P. & Filoteo, V., (2007). Neuropsychology of cortical versus subcortical dementia syndromes. *Seminars in Neurology, 27*(1), 7–21.

Savage, C. R. (1997). Neuropsychology of subcortical dementias. *Psychiatric Clinics of North America, 20*(4), 911–931.

Snowden, J. S., Craufurd, D., Thompson, J., & Neary, D. (2002). Psychomotor, executive, and memory function in preclinical Huntington's disease. *Journal of Clinical and Experimental Neuropsychology, 24*(2), 133–145.

Solomon, A. C., Stout, J. C., Johnson, S. A., Langbehn, D. R., Aylward, E. H., Brandt, J., . . . Paulsen, J. S. (2007). Verbal episodic memory declines prior to diagnosis in Huntington's disease. *Neuropsychologia, 45*(8), 1767–1776.

Stout, J. C., Jones, R., Labuschagne, I., O'Reagan, A. M., Say, M. J., Dumas, E. M., . . . Frost, C. (2012). Evaluation of longitudinal 12 and 24 month cognitive outcomes in premanifest and early Huntington's disease. *Journal of Neurology, Neurosurgery and Psychiatry, 83,* 687–694.

Stout, J. C., Paulsen, J. S., Queller, S., Solomon, A. C., Whitlock, K. B., Campbell, J. C., . . . Aylward, E. H. (2011). Neurocognitive signs in prodromal Huntington disease. *Neuropsychology, 25*(1), 1–14.

Stout, J. C., Rodawalt, W. C., & Siemers, E. R. (2001). Risky decision making in Huntington's disease. *Journal of the International Neuropsychological Society, 7*(1), 92–101.

Scahill, R., Wild, E., Tabrizi, S. (2012). Biomarkers for Huntington's disease: An update. *Expert Opinion on Medical Diagnostics, 6*(5), 371–375.

Smith, M., Mills, J., Epping, E., Westervelt, H., Paulsen, J. & PREDICT-HD Investigators of the Huntington Study Group. (2012). Depressive symptom severity is related to poorer cognitive performance in prodromal Huntington disease. *Neuropsychology, 26*(5), 664–669.

Squitieri, F., & Jankovic, J. (2012). Huntington's disease: How intermediate are intermediate repeat lengths? *Movement Disorders, 27*(14), 1714–1717.

Thieben, M., Duggins, A. Good, C. Gomes, L., Mahant, N., Richards, F., . . . Frackowiak, R. (2002). The distribution of structural neuropathology in pre-clinical Huntington's disease. *Brain, 125*(Pt 8), 1815–1828.

Turner, M. A., Moran, N. F., & Kopelman, M. D. (2002). Subcortical dementia. *British Journal of Psychiatry, 180*, 148–151.

van Duijn, E., Kingma, E. M., & van der Mast, R. C. (2007). Psychopathology in verified Huntington's disease gene carriers. *Journal of Neuropsychiatry and Clinical Neurosciences, 19*, 441–448.

Verny, C., Allain, P., Prudean, A., Malinge, M. C., Gohier, B., Scherer, C., . . . Le Gall, D. (2007). Cognitive changes in asymptomatic carriers of the Huntington disease mutation gene. *European Journal of Neurology, 14*(12), 1344–1350.

Walker, F. O. (2007). Huntington's disease. *Lancet Neurology, 369*, 218–228.

Watts, R., & Koller, W. (2004). Huntington's Disease, In *movement disorders: Neurologic principles and practice* (2nd ed., pp. 571–627). New York, NY: McGraw-Hill

Xie, Y., Hayden, M., & Xu, B. (2010). BDNF overexpression in the forebrain rescues Huntington's disease phenotypes in YAC128 mice. *Journal of Neuroscience, 30*(44), 14708–14718.

Young, A. (1997). Impairment of energy metabolism and excitotoxic cell death in Huntington disease. *Review Neurology, 153*(8–9), 496–498.

14 Corticobasal Degeneration

Melissa J. Armstrong and Irene Litvan

INTRODUCTION

Corticobasal degeneration (CBD) was first described in 1968 with varying designations over time including "corticodentatonigral degeneration with neuronal achromasia" (Rebeiz, Kolodny, & Richardson, 1968), "corticonigral degeneration with neuronal achromasia" (Case Records of the Massachusetts General Hospital, Case 38-1985, 1985), "corticobasal ganglionic degeneration" (Watts et al., 1985), "cortical–basal ganglionic degeneration" (Riley, et al., 1990), and "corticobasal degeneration" (Gibb, Luthert, & Marsden, 1989). Pick's disease type 2 (Constantinidis, Richard, & Tissot, 1974) was another name for the same condition. In recent years, however, it has become clear that the clinical syndrome described in these papers and the pathological findings of CBD only sometimes overlap. Thus, current terminology uses "corticobasal syndrome" (CBS) to reflect a specific clinical pattern and CBD to identify pathologically confirmed disease. This chapter will highlight the neuropsychological features of both processes.

CBS is diagnosed by the presence of hallmark clinical features including asymmetric parkinsonism, limb dystonia, gait abnormalities, myoclonus, apraxia, alien limb phenomenon, and cortical sensory loss (Case Records of the Massachusetts General Hospital, Case 38-1985, 1985; Gibb, et al., 1989; Rebeiz, Kolodny, & Richardson, 1968; Riley, et al., 1990; Rinne, Lee, Thompson, & Marsden, 1994). Although it was initially thought to be pathognomonic for CBD, postmortem evaluations of patients with CBS have revealed diverse pathological diagnoses including progressive supranuclear palsy (PSP) (Bhatia et al., 2000; Boeve et al., 1999; Josephs, Petersen, et al., 2006; Ling et al., 2010; Maraganore, Boeve, & Parisi, 1996), various forms of frontotemporal lobar degeneration (FTLD) (Bhatia et al., 2000; Boeve et al., 1999; Gass et al., 2006; Grimes, Bergeron, & Lang, 1999; Hughes, Daniel, Ben-Shlomo, & Lees, 2002; Josephs, Petersen, et al., 2006; Lopez et al., 2008; Maraganore et al., 1996; Spina et al., 2007), Alzheimer's disease (AD) (Ball et al., 1993; Boeve et al., 1999; Doran et al., 2003; Hu et al., 2009; Litvan et al., 1997; Shelley, Hodges, Kipps, Xuereb, & Bak, 2009; Wojcieszek, Lang, Jankovic, Greene, & Deck, 1994), Parkinson's disease (PD) (Hughes et al., 2002; Litvan et al., 1997), Creutzfeldt-Jakob disease (CJD) (Anschel, Simon, Llinas, & Joseph, 2002; Avanzino, Marinelli, Buccolieri, Trompetto, & Abbruzzese, 2006; Boeve et al., 1999; Kleiner-Fisman, Bergeron, & Lang, 2004), and other conditions.

In addition to the clinical presentation of CBS, other clinical phenotypes for patients later shown to have CBD include PSP (Forman et al., 2002; Hodges et al., 2004; Hughes et al., 2002; Josephs & Dickson, 2003; Josephs, Petersen, et al., 2006; Ling et al., 2010; Litvan, et al., 1997; Lopez et al., 2008; Murray et al., 2007; Osaki et al., 2004; Wenning, et al., 1998), frontotemporal dementia (FTD) (Forman et al., 2002; Hodges, et al., 2004; Josephs, Petersen, et al., 2006; Ling et al., 2010; Llado et al., 2008; Murray et al., 2007), AD (Boeve, 2005; Forman et al., 2002; Hodges et al., 2004; Ling et al., 2010; Murray et al., 2007), primary progressive aphasia (PPA)/progressive nonfluent aphasia (PNFA) or apraxia of speech (AOS) (B. Boeve, 2005; Josephs, Duffy, et al., 2006; Ling et al., 2010; Llado et al., 2008), and others. Clinicopathological series demonstrate correct clinical diagnosis in only 25 to 56% of CBD cases (B. Boeve, 2005; Grimes, Lang, & Bergeron, 1999; Hughes et al., 2002; Ling et al., 2010; Litvan et al., 1997; Murray et al., 2007).

CBD, a pathologic diagnosis, is characterized by widespread deposition of hyperphosphorylated 4-repeat tau in neurons and glia in specific topographical areas (Dickson et al., 2002; Yoshida, 2006). In CBD, glial tau deposition forms astrocytic plaques (Figure 14-1) that are distinct from the tufted astrocytes seen in PSP (Dickson et al., 2002; Yoshida, 2006). Recent research suggests that

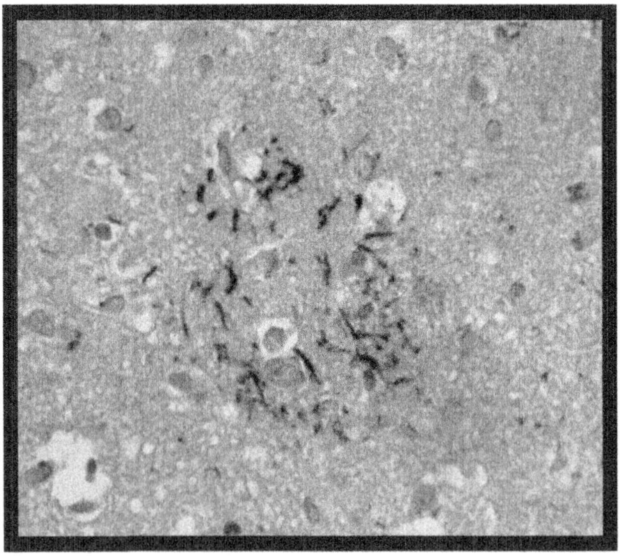

FIGURE 14-1
Example of the astrocytic plaques seen in CBD.

TAR-DNA-binding protein 43 (TDP-43) may be present in some cases of CBD (Uryu et al., 2008).

EPIDEMIOLOGY

Little is known regarding the epidemiology of CBS and CBD. A recent Russian-population-based study of incident parkinsonism over a 2.5-year period found one patient diagnosed with CBS in the Moscow district studied, leading to a crude CBS incidence of 0.03 (95% CI 0.01–0.18) per 100,000 person-years. The age-adjusted incidence was 0.02 (95% CI 0.01–0.12) per 100,000 person-years (Winter et al., 2010). On review of cases in the Queen Square Brain Bank (1989–2009), primarily reflecting movement disorders patients, 21 (1.5%) of autopsied cases presented with CBS and 19 (1.3%) were diagnosed pathologically with CBD (Ling et al., 2010). An earlier series from the same group reported that CBD accounted for four (2.8%) of 143 patients presenting with parkinsonism, but admitted that patients with postmortem studies represented only 8% of patients hospitalized for parkinsonism and 5% of those attending outpatient clinics (Hughes et al., 2002). By estimating that CBD accounts for 1% of patients with parkinsonism at movement disorders clinics, has an 8 year survival, and is sometimes misdiagnosed, the incidence and prevalence of CBD in the United States have been estimated as 0.62–0.92/100,000 and 13,000–20,000, respectively (Togasaki & Tanner, 2000).

PRESENTATION AND CLINICAL COURSE

Although CBS is reported in patients as young as 27 and 28 years-old (Arai et al., 1997; Bugiani et al., 1999), this young age of onset should prompt consideration of genetic or secondary causes of this clinical phenotype rather than classic sporadic CBD. The mean age of onset for sporadic CBD patients is 63.7 (standard deviation [SD] 7.0) years, with a range from 45 to 77.2 years (Josephs, Petersen, et al., 2006; Ling et al., 2010; Murray et al., 2007; Wenning et al., 1998). Men and women are equally affected by CBD (Grimes, Lang, et al., 1999; Josephs, Petersen, et al., 2006; Murray et al., 2007; Wenning, et al., 1998).

CBS typically develops insidiously with prominent lateralized motor findings (e.g., bradykinesia, dystonia) and lateralized higher cortical difficulties (e.g., apraxia, aphasia, cortical sensory loss, and alien limb phenomenon) (Gibb et al., 1989; Riley et al., 1990; Rinne et al., 1994). In one clinical series, CBS presented most frequently with a single akinetic, rigid, and apraxic limb, sometimes associated with dystonia and stimulus-sensitive myoclonus (Rinne et al., 1994). In addition to the classic movement disorder and higher cortical (often, parietal) features described originally in CBS, clinical findings observed in these patients have subsequently included cognitive dysfunction (discussed further later), aphasia (Graham, Bak, Patterson, & Hodges, 2003; Kompoliti et al., 1998), visuospatial neglect (Moretti, Torre, Antonello, Cattaruzza, & Cazzato, 2005; Sato, Nagata, Yokoyama, & Hirata, 1996), oculomotor abnormalities (Garbutt et al., 2008;

Rivaud-Péchoux et al., 2000; Rottach, Riley, DiScenna, Zivotofsky, & Leigh, 1996; Vidailhet & Rivaud-Péchoux, 2000), Balint's syndrome (Mendez, 2000), and visuomotor ataxia (Okuda, Kodama, Tachibana, Sugita, & Tanaka, 2000), among others.

The course of CBS varies according to underlying pathology, but often progresses to a more severe clinical picture. When considered as one presenting phenotype of pathologies grouped under the heading of the "Pick Complex" (Josephs, Petersen, et al., 2006; Kertesz, Martinez-Lage, Davidson, & Munoz, 2000; Kertesz, McMonagle, Blair, Davidson, & Munoz, 2005; Kertesz & Munoz, 2000; McMonagle, Blair, & Kertesz, 2006), CBS is almost always followed by a second clinical syndrome of FTD or progressive aphasia, and it often progresses to display either FTD or progressive aphasia as a third syndrome, as well, regardless of final pathology (Kertesz et al., 2000; Kertesz et al., 2005; McMonagle et al., 2006). In FTD/FTLD clinicopathological studies, most subjects progress to global motor, cognitive/behavioral, and language impairments regardless of presenting symptoms such as CBS (Forman et al., 2006).

Presenting features of over 200 CBD cases were recently compiled during development of new clinical diagnostic criteria for CBD (Armstrong et al., 2013). On review of brain bank data and published series with a minimum of 5 CBD cases, over half of CBD patients present with asymmetric motor presentations, limb rigidity, and/or bradykinesia or clumsy limb. Limb apraxia was also present in almost half of CBD patients at presentation. Other features of classic CBS were less commonly recorded in CBD presentations, including limb dystonia (20%), myoclonus (15%), cortical sensory loss (25%), and alien limb phenomena (22%). Postural instability was described in 41% of CBD patients at presentation, with falls in 36% and abnormal gait in 33%. Most series do not describe the type of gait disturbance or timing of falls, hindering better understanding of their underlying causes. Cognitive and behavioral features, unrecognized in early CBD series, are now well described at presentation. In the literature and brain bank compilation, cognitive impairment in general was described in 52% of CBD patients at presentation, behavioral changes in 46%, and aphasia in 40% (Armstrong et al., 2013). Some recent series that highlight cognitive presentations of CBD have a low rate of parkinsonism at onset (Grimes, Lang, et al., 1999; Lee et al., 2011; Murray et al., 2007). Unsurprisingly, review of the literature suggests that the degree of detail of symptom recording in CBD may depend on the clinician's subspecialty (i.e., movement disorder specialists stress motor disturbances and behavioral neurologists stress cognitive disturbances).

Abnormal eye movements (often poorly characterized) were present in 33% of CBD patients in the CBD case compilation, underscoring the overlap with clinical features of PSP (Armstrong et al., 2013). It is still unclear if the delayed saccadic latency in vertical and horizontal directions described in CBS (i.e., clinically diagnosed CBD) subjects may help differentiate these patients from PSP, in which slowing of vertical saccades is typical (Garbutt et al., 2008; Rivaud-Péchoux, et al., 2000; Rottach et al., 1996; Vidailhet & Rivaud-Péchoux, 2000). Only one study of eye movements includes pathologically proven CBD subjects ($n = 4$); this study showed severely decreased velocity and gain in PSP subjects with similar but milder abnormalities in 1 out of 4 CBD subjects. The other 3 CBD subjects had eye movements indistinguishable from normal controls; increased latency was only observed in AD subjects (Boxer et al., 2011).

Similar to CBS patients, subjects with CBD become globally impaired over time. Almost every presenting feature of CBD becomes more frequent as the disease progresses (Armstrong et al., 2013). Most if not all patients with CBD demonstrate a CBS phenotype at some point in their disease progression, but it may not be until the later stages (Lee et al., 2011; McMonagle et al., 2006).

Time from symptom onset until death in CBD ranges from 2.0–12.5 years (Lee et al., 2011; Murray et al., 2007; Wenning et al., 1998). Bilateral bradykinesia, a frontal syndrome, or the presence of at least two of three extrapyramidal features (tremor, rigidity, or bradykinesia) may predict shorter survival (Wenning et al., 1998). Pneumonia is frequently the cause of death (Wenning et al., 1998).

NEUROPSYCHOLOGICAL/BEHAVIORAL FINDINGS

Corticobasal Syndrome

Neuropsychological and behavioral features are now recognized in CBS both with and without the associated pathological diagnosis of CBD. Many studies referenced here describe clinically diagnosed CBD patients, re-classified here as CBS due to lack of pathological confirmation.

Patients with CBS may exhibit global cognitive impairment on neuropsychological testing consistent with moderate dementia (Pillon et al., 1995). Measures including the Mattis Dementia Rating Scale (Pillon et al., 1995), Raven 47 Colored Progressive Matrices (Pillon et al., 1995), Wechsler Memory Scale (Pillon, et al., 1995), Mini-Mental State Examination (MMSE) (Hirano et al., 2010; Mathew, Bak, & Hodges, 2011; Whitwell et al., 2010) and Addenbrooke's Cognitive Examination-Revised (ACE-R) (Mathew et al., 2011) have all disclosed global cognitive impairments in CBS patients. Although the Montreal Cognitive Assessment—a global cognitive screening tool gaining increased use in PD—has not been formally used in CBS studies, clinical use unsurprisingly demonstrates errors in assessment with this measure as well (Figure 14-2). Even subjects who present with a predominant motor syndrome and have no cognitive complaints at baseline show evidence of global worsening of cognition over 16 months (Moretti et al., 2005).

Most cognitive domains (i.e., frontal/executive, attention, language, visuospatial, and learning/memory) are affected in CBS to varying degrees. Frontal-executive tasks are particularly impaired. Trail-making errors are common in CBS (Graham, Bak, & Hodges, 2003). When compared to controls, CBS patients scored lower on the Wisconsin Card Sorting Test (WCST), phonemic fluency tasks, graphic series, and a global frontal assessment (Pillon, et al., 1995). Phonemic fluency tasks were also worse when CBS patients were compared to clinically diagnosed AD patients (Belfor et al., 2006). CBS patients were more impaired on the Digit Span Backward task when compared to patients with other

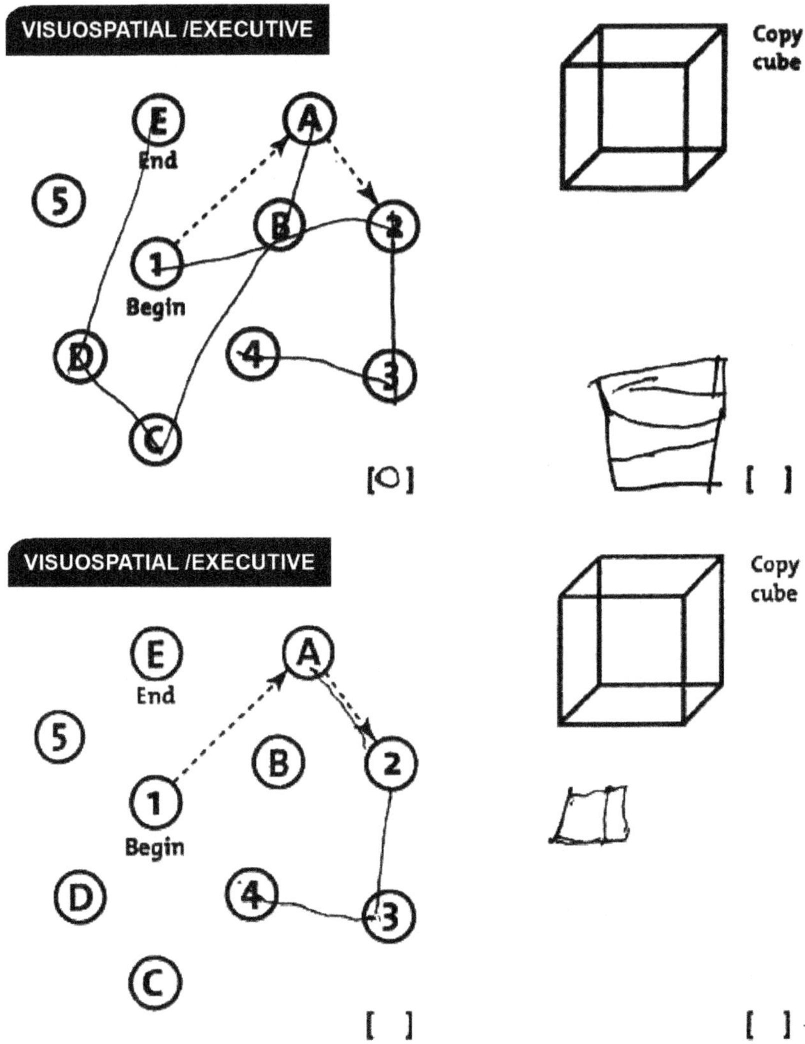

FIGURE 14-2
Examples of errors by CBS subjects on the executive-visuospatial section of the Montreal Cognitive Assessment.

clinically diagnosed neurodegenerative diseases (Libon et al., 2009). The dysexecutive syndrome in CBS is generally similar to that seen in clinically diagnosed PSP (PSP syndrome, or PSPS), but worse than that in clinically diagnosed AD (Pillon, et al., 1995). On longitudinal assessment, CBS and PNFA patients have more executive dysfunction when compared to other clinically diagnosed FTD subtypes and AD (Libon et al., 2009).

In a large study using the Frontal Behavioral Inventory, more than 25% of CBS patients and caregivers reported apathy, aspontaneity, inattention, logopenia, alien hand symptoms, and irritability (Borroni, Alberici, Agosti, Cosseddu, & Padovani, 2009). Compared to PSPS patients, CBS patients had more alien hand and apraxia symptoms (39.7% versus 10.5%, $p=0.001$) but less apathy (33.8% versus 57.9%, $p=0.007$) (Borroni, et al., 2009). Apathy was also present in 40% of CBS patients assessed with the Neuropsychiatric Inventory, though this was still less common than in PSPS subjects (>80%) (Litvan, Cummings, & Mega, 1998). Aspontaneity and irritability were more common in CBS than PSPS on the Frontal Behavioral Inventory, but the difference did not reach statistical significance (Borroni, et al., 2009). On the Neuropsychiatric Inventory, irritability and agitation were each described in 20% of CBS patients. Anxiety, disinhibition, and delusions were uncommon, but 73% of CBS patients had depression (Litvan, et al., 1998). Frontal behaviors such as prehension, imitation, and utilization are also described in CBS patients (Blin, et al., 1992; Pillon, et al., 1995).

Though less commonly reported as a distinct domain, attention and concentration are also impaired in CBS. One study demonstrated this using ACE-R subscores in CBS patients compared to controls (Mathew, et al., 2011).

Initially overshadowed by motor features, the presence of language dysfunction in CBS is increasingly recognized. Although early reports described aphasia in 10–21% of CBS cases (Kompoliti, et al., 1998; Riley, et al., 1990), a later review described aphasia in 31% (Graham, Bak, & Hodges, 2003). Furthermore, language deficits may be subclinical. In the assessment of 10 patients with CBS, most showed some degree of language impairment on formal testing, particularly on spelling and phonologic tests, even though gross language dysfunction was only present in two patients (Graham, Bak, Patterson, et al., 2003). In another study, over half of CBS patients showed evidence of aphasia on Western Aphasia Battery testing (Frattali, Grafman, Patronas, Makhlouf, & Litvan, 2000). Verbal fluency (combining phonemic and category fluency tasks) was the most severely affected cognitive domain in CBS in a study using the ACE-R. Language subscores were impaired to a lesser degree (Mathew, et al., 2011). Abnormal category fluency has been described in CBS cohorts (Pillon, et al., 1995), but in one study CBS patients scored better than clinically diagnosed AD patients on an animal fluency task (Libon, et al., 2009). Confrontation naming as measured by the Boston Naming Test tended to be more impaired in CBS patients than clinically diagnosed AD patients in one study (Belfor, et al., 2006), but was better than in semantic dementia patients in a separate study (Libon, et al., 2009). Action naming may be impaired more than object naming in CBS and other neurodegenerative diseases with frontal impairments (Cotelli, et al., 2006).

Visuospatial impairments are also common in CBS. On the ACE-R, visuospatial was the second-most impaired domain in CBS behind verbal fluency (Mathew, et al., 2011). Visuospatial subscores were the only scores that could differentiate CBS from clinically diagnosed PNFA (Mathew, et al., 2011). CBS patients performed worse on a geometric figure copy test on initial evaluation and longitudinally compared to patients with clinically diagnosed AD and various clinically diagnosed FTD subtypes including PNFA (Libon, et al., 2009). When using the Corsi Block Span and select items of the Wechsler Adult Intelligence Scale Block Design Subtest, CBS patients performed worse on some but not all measures (Pillon, et al., 1995). CBS patients demonstrated more prominent deficits than healthy controls and clinically diagnosed PSP and MSA patients when tested using the Visual Object and Space

Perception Battery. In particular, CBS patients had more difficulty with spatial tasks than object-based tasks (Bak, Caine, Hearn, & Hodges, 2006).

Learning and memory are generally less impaired in CBS than other cognitive domains, though CBS patients scored significantly worse than controls on the memory section of the ACE-R (Mathew et al., 2011). Studies have consistently showed that CBS patients perform better on the California Verbal Learning Test (CVLT) than patients with clinically diagnosed AD (Belfor et al., 2006; Pillon et al., 1995). CVLT scores in CBS patients were lower than in controls, but not to a statistically significant degree. The same was true of scores on the Grober and Buschke test (Pillon et al., 1995). Learning and memory performances were similar between CBS and PSPS patients (Pillon et al., 1995). When present, memory disturbances in CBS (and PSPS) may be more related to frontally mediated retrieval impairments rather than to the memory deficits in AD related to medial temporal structures (Beatty, Scott, Wilson, Prince, & Williamson, 1995; Pillon & Dubois, 2000).

Other cortical features of CBS that can be tested or observed in neuropsychological assessments include apraxia (Leiguarda, Lees, Merello, Starkstein, & Marsden, 1994; Ozsancak, Auzou, Dujardin, Quinn, & Destée, 2004; Soliveri, Piacentini, & Girotti, 2005) and alien limb phenomena (Kompoliti et al., 1998; Rinne et al., 1994). Alien limb phenomena include a variety of behaviors in which one feels dissociated from one's own limb, including enabling synkinesis, intermanual conflict, grasping, impulsive hand groping, magnetic apraxia, and purposeless limb wandering. The exact behaviors sufficient to constitute alien limb are debated (Boeve, Lang, & Litvan, 2003), but consensus suggests that parietal drift and simple levitation are not sufficient (Armstrong, et al., 2013) Additional neuropsychological impairments in CBS include impairments in number knowledge and calculation (Halpern, McMillan, Moore, Dennis, & Grossman, 2003; Koss, et al., 2010).

A critical review of studies of cognitive testing in parkinsonism suggests that select neuropsychological findings may be useful in distinguishing CBS from other parkinsonisms (Lee, Williams, & Storey, 2012). The only cognitive features reliably distinguishing CBS from PD and PSP were more severe orofacial apraxia and ideomotor apraxia, respectively. A number of tests distinguished patients with CBS from MSA, but the clinical implications of this are unclear because these two diagnoses are rarely mistaken for one another (Lee et al., 2012).

The literature referenced earlier investigated CBS patients without established pathology. There is limited data comparing CBS patients found to have different pathologic diagnoses. Two studies compare CBS with AD pathology (CBS/AD) and CBS with CBD pathology (CBS/CBD). Neuropsychological testing showed similar degrees of memory and executive impairment in the two groups in one study (Hu et al., 2009). In the other, however, CBD pathology was predicted by early frontal-behavioral symptoms, nonfluent language impairments, orobuccal apraxia and utilization behavior, whereas early episodic memory concerns and poor performance on combined ACE orientation and memory subtests predicted AD pathology (Shelley et al., 2009). In a separate study, CBS/AD patients scored significantly worse on the Benson figure copy and delayed-recall tasks compared to CBS/CBD, CBS/PSP, and CBS/frontotemporal lobar degeneration with TDP-43 immunoreactive inclusions (FTLD-TDP) subjects (Lee et al., 2011). CBS/AD patients performed more poorly on calculations than CBS/PSP and CBS/FTLD-TDP patients, and CBS/CBD patients performed more poorly on calculations than CBS/FTLD-TDP patients (Lee, et al., 2011). Whether these differences can discriminate between the different pathologies underlying CBS has yet to be established.

Corticobasal Degeneration

Although dementia was formerly an exclusion criterion for CBD (Kumar et al., 1998), the prominence of cognitive and behavioral dysfunction in the disease has become increasingly recognized. Early cognitive-behavioral dysfunction can even be the presenting feature of CBD (Grimes, Lang, et al., 1999; Lee et al., 2011; Murray et al., 2007). Although CBD is now recognized to have distinct clinical phenotypes, the vast majority of the research to date studies CBD patients as a single group rather than subdividing them by phenotype. Only one identified study compared the neuropsychological features of different phenotypes, discussed further later (Lee et al., 2011). Additionally, it should be noted that the cognitive and behavioral features of CBS/CBD, although expected to be largely similar to the profile of CBS patients discussed earlier, may differ somewhat from those patients given the lack of pathological confirmation in most of those studies. Studies comparing the CBS of CBD versus the CBS associated with other pathologies were reviewed earlier.

In terms of global measures, the MMSE is felt to underestimate the degree of cognitive impairment seen in CBD (Murray, et al., 2007), likely given its under-representation of the commonly impaired frontal–executive domain. No studies using newer, broader cognitive screening tools (e.g., the Montreal Cognitive Assessment) were identified.

Similar to CBS, frontal–executive dysfunction is frequently seen in CBD. In one series, over 60% of CBD patients demonstrated impaired planning and mental searching at disease onset, increasing to over 70% of patients prior to death. Perseverative behaviors were present in 40% at onset and inattention and disinhibition were also described in some subjects (Murray, et al., 2007). The presence of frontal–executive decline is also evident on neuropsychological testing. An assessment using forward and reverse digit span, phonemic fluency, and Stroop color-word interference tasks showed that CBD patients had significant difficulty in multiple measures at first assessment with modest progression over time (Murray, et al., 2007). In a separate study, tests for attention/concentration, processing speed, cognitive flexibility, and letter fluency were all impaired in CBD patients compared to controls (Vanvoorst et al., 2008).

The presence of frontal behavioral changes in CBD is underscored by the common clinical diagnosis of behavioral variant FTD (bvFTD) syndrome in patients with CBD on subsequent pathology (Forman et al., 2002; Grimes, Lang, et al.,

1999; Kertesz, et al., 2000; Ling et al., 2010; Llado et al., 2008; McMonagle et al., 2006; Murray et al., 2007). This phenotype is present in 15.5% of CBD patients at presentation and 13.8% later in the disease course (Armstrong et al., 2013). Behavioral changes described in CBD series include apathy, bizarre or antisocial behaviour, personality changes, irritability, disinhibition, excessive eating, and hypersexuality (Forman et al., 2002; Geda et al., 2007; Grimes, Lang, et al., 1999; Ling et al., 2010; Murray et al., 2007). Compulsive behaviors in general are also reported (Geda, et al., 2007). Additionally, over 25% of CBD patients have clinical symptoms of depression at disease onset and over half have depression at some point in their disease course (Armstrong, et al., 2013).

Language complaints and deficits are also common in CBD. In one cohort, over 40% of CBD patients complained of effortful speech at onset and 13% complained of word-finding difficulties (Murray et al., 2007). Despite this, few areas of significant language dysfunction were seen early in the disease in this cohort, who underwent an abbreviated Boston Naming Test, an oral sentence comprehension task, and semantic category tasks. Language comprehension and confrontation worsened over time, though less than in a control population with other neurodegenerative diseases (Murray, et al., 2007). In another study, category fluency tasks were markedly impaired in CBD patients, whereas verbal comprehension, auditory comprehension and category naming were impaired compared to controls, but to a lesser degree (Vanvoorst, et al., 2008).

Language impairment can be a prominent finding in some CBD subjects, underscored by the fact that patients may be diagnosed clinically with PPA, PNFA, or AOS (using historical terminology) before the postmortem diagnosis of CBD (Boeve, 2005; Josephs, Duffy, et al., 2006; Ling et al., 2010; Llado et al., 2008). Aphasia was the presenting phenotype in 14.7% of patients later diagnosed pathologically with CBD; aphasia/AOS was the most prominent phenotype in 4.8% of cases (Armstrong, et al., 2013). Whether AOS represents a language or a speech disorder in CBD remains a matter of some debate.

Visuospatial impairments are seen in CBD to varying degrees. Twenty percent of CBD patients complain of visuospatial difficulties at onset (Murray, et al., 2007) and rare CBD patients present with prominent visuospatial dysfunction and symptoms suggestive of posterior cortical atrophy (PCA) (Lee, et al., 2011; Tang-Wai, et al., 2003). On testing, visuospatial difficulty was seen in 40% of CBD patients at onset when using the constructional praxis portion of the Committee to Establish a Registry for Alzheimer's Disease (CERAD) testing. The difficulties could not be explained by motor deficits alone (Murray et al., 2007). Block design scores were also reported as lower in CBD patients compared to controls (Vanvoorst et al., 2008).

Reported impairments in learning and memory vary across CBD studies. Although one-third of CBD patients complained of memory difficulties at disease onset in one cohort, only 13% showed signs of this on testing. Signs of memory impairment were present in 36% of CBD patients prior to death, but episodic memory tasks even at the last neuropsychological testing showed no impairment in recognition or delayed recall (Murray, et al., 2007). In a separate study, CBD patients showed impairments in learning tasks compared to controls and also had low scaled scores in some immediate and delayed memory tasks (Vanvoorst et al., 2008). The prominence of memory concerns in some CBD patients is underscored by the frequency with which CBD patients are described as clinically misdiagnosed as AD (Boeve, 2005; Forman et al., 2002; Grimes, Lang, et al., 1999; Hodges et al., 2004; Ling et al., 2010; Murray et al., 2007). In the recent compilation of over 200 CBD cases, a diagnosis of AD/dementia was given to 9.3% of CBD cases at presentation and 8.1% of CBD cases later in the disease (Armstrong, et al., 2013). The specific clinical features leading to these clinical misdiagnoses are rarely detailed. As with CBS, it is possible that memory impairments seen in CBD may represent more frontally mediated impairments in encoding and retrieval as opposed to the classic medial temporal memory deficits seen in AD. This is difficult to confirm, however, without further investigation.

Other cognitive and behavioral dysfunctions are also observed in CBD. In one series, over 25% of CBD patients demonstrated acalculia at disease onset (Murray, et al., 2007). Subjects with prominent acalculia may demonstrate difficulties counting objects and performing both oral and written single-digit calculations (Pantelyat, et al., 2011).

Recent evidence unsurprisingly suggests that the neuropsychological features seen in CBD patients will vary according to the presenting phenotype. In a series comparing 18 CBD patients divided into clinical phenotypes of an executive-motor syndrome, PNFA, bvFTD, or PCA, the CBD patients presenting with the bvFTD phenotype performed worse on most cognitive measures, though this was statistically significant only for errors on the Modified Trails task and delayed verbal recall (Lee, et al., 2011). There was also a trend for Neuropsychiatric Inventory scores to be highest in CBD patients presenting with bvFTD and lowest in those presenting with PNFA (Lee, et al., 2011). Neuropsychological differences between subjects with CBS and underlying CBD pathology versus CBS associated with other pathologies were discussed earlier. Recent evidence suggests that there may be neuropsychological differences in subjects with PSPS found to have CBD versus PSP pathology; executive and behavioral abnormalities were significantly more common in PSPS patients with CBD than with PSP (Kouri et al., 2011).

NEUROIMAGING

The neuropsychological findings in CBS reflect its localization as an asymmetrical cortical and subcortical syndrome. Routine magnetic resonance imaging (MRI) in CBS patients usually shows asymmetric cerebral atrophy more severe contralateral to the most prominent clinical symptoms (Figure 14-3). Posterior frontal and parietal atrophy are more prominent than temporal and anterobasal frontal atrophy (Koyama, et al., 2007; Ukmar, et al., 2003). Mild basal ganglia atrophy can sometimes also be appreciated (Ukmar et al., 2003). Voxel-based morphometry (VBM) in CBS patients shows asymmetric atrophy affecting the striatum, bilateral premotor cortex, and superior parietal lobules (Boxer, et al., 2006). Functional MRI shows reduced activation of the more affected supplemental motor

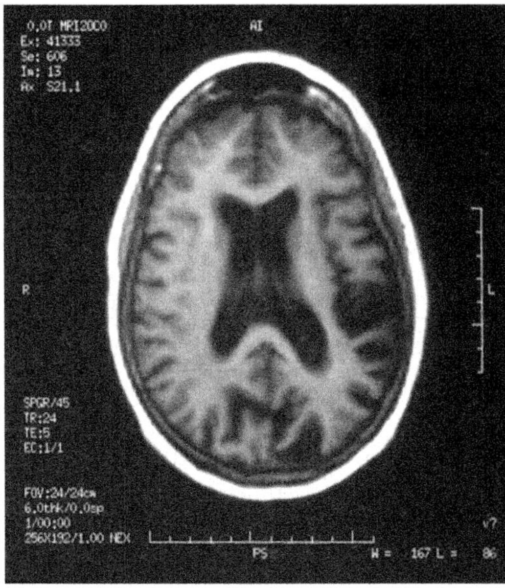

FIGURE 14-3
MRI image of patient with corticobasal syndrome

area (SMA) and rolandic and parietal cortex areas compared to the less affected side. Activation during complex tasks is also abnormal (Ukmar et al., 2003).

Single-photon emission computed tomography (SPECT) demonstrates asymmetric hypoperfusion in the basal ganglia and frontoparietal lobes of CBS patients (Koyama et al., 2007). In one study, [^{18}F]fluorodeoxyglucose (FDG) positron emission tomography (PET) showed decreased glucose metabolism in most cortical and subcortical regions compared to controls. Cortically, the decreased metabolism was most profound in the frontal, temporal, sensorimotor, and parietal associative cortices contralateral to the more affected side. Subcortically, glucose consumption was lower in the caudate nucleus, lenticular nucleus, and thalamus contralateral to the more affected side (Blin, et al., 1992). Similar findings were reported in separate FDG-PET studies. One showed that the primary brain regions involved in CBS patients were the posterior frontal, inferior parietal, and superior temporal regions cortically and the basal ganglia and thalamus subcortically (Coulier, de Vries, & Leenders, 2003). Similar patterns emphasizing involvement of the fronto-parietal areas, caudate, putamen, and thalamus are also shown in other FDG-PET studies (Laureys et al., 1999; Nagasawa et al., 1996). Striatal fluorodopa imaging can also be abnormal (Laureys et al., 1999; Nagasawa et al., 1996). Recently, imaging with [^{11}C] *N*-methylpiperidin-4-yl acetate PET showed decreased acetylcholinesterase activity in CBS subjects in the paracentral region, frontal, parietal, and occipital cortices (Hirano et al., 2010).

Imaging studies displaying prominent fronto–parietal and basal ganglia abnormalities in CBS are consistent with the motor and cognitive-behavioral features. Unfortunately, these imaging findings confirm the localization of the symptoms and signs of CBS without providing insight into the underlying pathology. Recent publications, however, provide early evidence that subtle differences in atrophy patterns in CBS patients may suggest different pathological diagnoses (Lee, et al., 2011; Whitwell, et al., 2010). In one study of 24 patients with CBS and subsequent autopsy, all patients showed atrophy bilaterally in the SMA and unilaterally in the dominant premotor cortex and insula on VBM. At the same time, patients with CBS/AD and CBS/FTLD-TDP showed the most widespread atrophy, with particular temporoparietal loss in CBS/AD and frontotemporal loss in CBS/FTLD-TDP. More focal atrophy particularly involving the premotor cortex and SMA was suggestive of CBS/CBD or CBS/PSP, which were similar on imaging other than more severe loss in CBS/CBD (Whitwell, et al., 2010). Particular symptom patterns in these 24 subjects could not predict pathology, but both behavioral/executive changes and a family history of neurodegenerative disease were most common in the CBS/FTLD-TDP group and vertical supranuclear gaze palsy occurred only in CBS/PSP and CBS/CBD subjects (Whitwell et al., 2010).

In a separate study of 40 CBS subjects with CBD, PSP, AD, FTLD-TDP, and mixed pathologies, MRI VBM also revealed different patterns. CBS/CBD subjects had a frontal–striatal atrophy pattern with gray matter loss in the bilateral frontal cortex including the SMA, dorsolateral prefrontal cortex (DLPFC), pre- and postcentral gyrus, striatum, and brainstem. CBS/PSP subjects had less atrophy. The main areas of atrophy in these patients were the SMA, DLPFC, insula, striatum, and brainstem. Although CBS/AD subjects also had some atrophy of the SMA, insula, and striatum, the temporoparietal and medial parietal cortex demonstrated bilateral atrophy. CBS/FTLD-TDP subjects demonstrated the least amount of atrophy, with abnormalities seen primarily in the inferior frontal gyrus and insula (Lee, et al., 2011). Whether these patterns will have predictive utility in prospective studies has yet to be determined.

There are few studies describing imaging findings in confirmed CBD. The CBS/CBD subjects in the studies mentioned earlier showed premotor cortex and SMA atrophy (Whitwell, et al., 2010) and frontal and striatal atrophy (Lee, et al., 2011). In a separate study, CBD subjects with both extrapyramidal and dementia presentations (versus controls) showed cortical atrophy particularly in the bilateral posterior inferior, middle, and superior frontal lobes, superior premotor cortex, posterior temporal and parietal lobes on VBM. SMA and insular cortex atrophy was also identified. Subcortically, atrophy was present in the globus pallidus, putamen, and caudate head. Small amounts of white matter atrophy were seen (Josephs, et al., 2008). When considering extrapyramidal and dementia presentations of CBD separately, the extrapyramidal group had bilateral grey and white matter atrophy in the superior premotor cortex and posterior superior, middle, and inferior frontal lobes versus controls and grey matter atrophy of the SMA and parietal lobes versus controls. CBD patients presenting with dementia had widespread severe grey matter atrophy particularly involving the lateral superior, middle, and inferior gyri, posterior temporal and parietal lobes and insula. Moderate subcortical loss was seen in the globus pallidus, putamen, and caudate head. These patterns differed slightly from those seen in PSP subjects (Josephs, et al., 2008).

TREATMENT

Current treatments for CBS and CBD remain symptomatic, though potential disease-modifying therapies targeting tauopathies are in development. A pilot study of lithium, a glycogen synthase kinase 3-beta (GSK-3ß) inhibitor, which may decrease kinase activity contributing to tau hyperphosphorylation, has recently been completed in CBS and PSPS subjects (ClinicalTrials.gov indentifier NCT00703677, http://clinicaltrials.gov/ct2/show/NCT00703677?term=NCT00703677&rank=1). Results are not yet available, but the study had to be interrupted in view of significant lithium-related side effects. Although not yet studied in CBS, a double-blind, placebo-controlled study of a different GSK3β inhibitor, NP031112 (tideglusib), has just been completed in PSPS patients and the data are under analysis (ClinicalTrials.gov identifier NCT01049399, http://clinicaltrials.gov/ct2/show/NCT01049399?term=NCT01049399&rank=1). Davunetide (NAPVSIPQ), an octapeptide that interacts with microtubules, reduced tau pathology in an animal model of AD (Matsuoka et al., 2008) and is currently being studied in humans with tau-mediated diseases. A study of intranasal davunetide was underway in CBS and PSPS patients (ClinicalTrials.gov identifier NCT01056965, http://clinicaltrials.gov/ct2/show/NCT01056965?term=NCT01056965&rank=1), but an analysis showed no slowing of disease progression in the larger PSPS group and the study was halted.

Formal studies for pharmacologic options for symptomatic management of CBS and CBD are lacking. Treatment typically consists of symptomatic therapies based on efficacy in other neurodegenerative and parkinsonian conditions. Levodopa is often tried for the parkinsonism commonly seen in CBS, usually with minimal response. Transient mild to moderate benefits have been described in both CBS and CBD, however (Kompoliti et al., 1998; Ling et al., 2010; Riley et al., 1990; Wenning et al., 1998), and dyskinesias may rarely occur even in pathologically confirmed CBD patients (Frucht, Fahn, Chin, Dhawan, & Eidelberg, 2000; Ling et al., 2010). Alternate dopaminergic therapies and other agents such as benzodiazepines and anticholinergics have also been tried, usually without success (Kompoliti et al., 1998). Dystonia may rarely respond to various pharmacologic agents (Kompoliti et al., 1998; Vanek & Jankovic, 2001), but it is usually most successfully treated with targeted botulinum toxin injections (Cordivari, Misra, Catania, & Lees, 2001; Kompoliti, et al., 1998; Vanek & Jankovic, 2001). Benzodiazepines, particularly clonazepam, are generally the most successful therapy for the myoclonus seen in CBS (Boeve, Josephs, & Drubach, 2008; Kompoliti et al., 1998; Riley et al., 1990). Levetiracetam may also be beneficial for myoclonus (Kovács et al., 2009; Rossi et al., 2008), and other agents can be considered (Boeve et al., 2008). Rare reports suggest that there may be a role for specific physical therapies in select CBS patients (Boeve et al., 2008; Steffen, Boeve, Mollinger-Riemann, & Petersen, 2007). Although published reports of CBS patients receiving deep brain stimulation (DBS) are rare—the only case of which we are aware is part of a series of failed DBS attempts (Okun et al., 2005)—unpublished reports suggest that CBS patients do not respond to DBS.

Neuropsychological and behavioral interventions are also symptomatic. Acetylcholinesterase inhibitors (AChEIs) are sometimes tried as a potential therapy for CBS and CBD patients based on anecdotal experience (Boeve, et al., 2008). Recent evidence of a cholinergic deficit in CBS as measured by [^{11}C] *N*-methylpiperdn-4-yl acetate PET may support a potentially beneficial role of AChEIs (Hirano et al., 2010). The role of memantine in CBS and CBD is undefined. Psychostimulants and dopamine agonists are also agents considered for use in CBS and CBD (Boeve et al., 2008), but these are rarely beneficial in our clinical experience.

With regards to the behavioral features of CBS and CBD, the only published literature identified is clinical experience suggesting use of selective serotonin reuptake inhibitors (SSRIs) and/or cognitive behavioral therapy for depression, AChEIs and psychostimulants for apathy, SSRIs for anxiety and obsessive-compulsive features, and atypical neuroleptics or mood-stabilizing agents for problematic inappropriate behavior (Boeve et al., 2008). Of course, atypical neuroleptics must be used cautiously in individuals with parkinsonism. It is possible that the potential disease-modifying agents currently under investigation may have cognitive-behavioral advantages, as well. Lithium has well-established mood-stabilizing properties, but was not well tolerated by CBD subjects in a recent clinical trial. AD mouse models suggest that davunetide may enhance cognitive function (Matsuoka et al., 2008). Cognitive and behavioral scales are secondary endpoints in the ongoing davunetide study in CBS and PSPS (ClinicalTrials.gov identifier NCT01056965, http://clinicaltrials.gov/ct2/show/NCT01056965?term=NCT01056965&rank=1).

CONCLUSIONS

The clinical syndrome of CBS and pathological diagnosis of CBD both have prominent neuropsychological features present in addition to motor findings (or in the case of CBD, even without motor abnormalities). Abnormal behaviors are frequent, and cognitive impairment affects most domains to varying degrees. Frontal/executive impairments are particularly prevalent. Cognitive-behavioral presentations of CBD are now recognized as common and are incorporated into new diagnostic criteria for CBD (Armstrong et al., 2013). Diagnosis, evaluation, and management of CBS and CBD patients are all areas that need further research. In particular, future research should focus on the validation of diagnostic criteria, identification of diagnostic biomarkers, development of appropriate scales to assess the various features of CBD (including the cognitive and behavioral symptoms), and effective therapies targeting both disease-modifying outcomes and symptomatic improvements.

REFERENCES

Anschel, D. J., Simon, D. K., Llinas, R., & Joseph, J. T. (2002). Spongiform encephalopathy mimicking corticobasal degeneration. *Movement Disorders, 17*(3), 606–607.

Arai, H., Morikawa, Y., Higuchi, M., Matsui, T., Clark, C. M., Miura, M.,... Sasaki, H. (1997). Cerebrospinal fluid tau levels in neurodegenerative diseases with distinct tau-related pathology. *Biochemical and Biophysical Research Communications, 236*(2), 262–264.

Armstrong, M. J., Litvan, I., Lang, A. E., Bak T. H., Bhatia, K. P., Borroni, B.,... Weiner, W. J. (2013). Criteria for the diagnosis of corticobasal degeneration. *Neurology, 80*, 496–503.

Avanzino, L., Marinelli, L., Buccolieri, A., Trompetto, C., & Abbruzzese, G. (2006). Creutzfeldt-Jakob disease presenting as corticobasal degeneration: a neurophysiological study. *Neurological Sciences, 27*(2), 118–121.

Bak, T. H., Caine, D., Hearn, V. C., & Hodges, J. R. (2006). Visuospatial functions in atypical parkinsonian syndromes. *Journal of Neurology, Neurosurgery and Psychiatry, 77*(4), 454–456.

Ball, J. A., Lantos, P. L., Jackson, M., Marsden, C. D., Scadding, J. W., & Rossor, M. N. (1993). Alien hand sign in association with Alzheimer's histopathology. *Journal of Neurology, Neurosurgery and Psychiatry, 56*(9), 1020–1023.

Beatty, W. W., Scott, J. G., Wilson, D. A., Prince, J. R., & Williamson, D. J. (1995). Memory deficits in a demented patient with probable corticobasal degeneration. *Journal of Geriatric Psychiatry and Neurology, 8*(2), 132–6.

Belfor, N., Amici, S., Boxer, A. L., Kramer, J. H., Gorno-Tempini, M. L., Rosen, H. J., &Miller, B. L. (2006). Clinical and neuropsychological features of corticobasal degeneration. *Mechanisms of Ageing and Development, 127*(2), 203–207.

Bhatia, K. P., Lee, M. S., Rinne, J. O., Revesz, T., Scaravilli, F., Davies, L., & Marsden, C. D. (2000). Corticobasal degeneration look-alikes. *Advances in Neurology, 82*, 169–182.

Blin, J., Vidailhet, M. J., Pillon, B., Dubois, B., Feve, J. R., & Agid, Y. (1992). Corticobasal degeneration: decreased and asymmetrical glucose consumption as studied with PET. *Movement Disorders, 7*(4), 348–354.

Boeve, B. (2005). Corticobasal degeneration: the syndrome and the disease. In I. Litvan (Ed.), *Atypical Parkinsonian disorders: Clinial and research aspects* (pp. 309–334). Totowa, NJ: Humana Press.

Boeve, B. F., Josephs, K. A., & Drubach, D. A. (2008). Current and future management of the corticobasal syndrome and corticobasal degeneration. *Handbook of Clinical Neurology, 89*, 533–548.

Boeve, B. F., Lang, A. E., Litvan, I. (2003). Corticobasal degeneration and its relationship to progressive supranuclear palsy and frontotemporal dementia. *Annals of Neurology, 54*(Suppl 5), S15–19.

Boeve, B. F., Maraganore, D. M., Parisi, J. E., Ahlskog, J. E., Graff-Radford, N., Caselli, R. J.,... Petersen, R. C. (1999). Pathologic heterogeneity in clinically diagnosed corticobasal degeneration. *Neurology, 53*(4), 795–800.

Borroni, B., Alberici, A., Agosti, C., Cosseddu, M., & Padovani, A. (2009). Pattern of behavioral disturbances in corticobasal degeneration syndrome and progressive supranuclear palsy. *International Psychogeriatrics, 21*(3), 463–468.

Boxer, A. L., Garbutt, S., Seeley, W. W., Jafari, A., Heuer, H. W., Mirsky, J.,... Miller, B. L. (2011). Saccade abnormalities in autopsy-confirmed frontotemporal lobar degeneration and Alzheimer's disease. *Archives of Neurology, 69*(4), 509–517.

Boxer, A. L., Geschwind, M. D., Belfor, N., Gorno-Tempini, M. L., Schauer, G. F., Miller, B. L.,... Rosen, H. J. (2006). Patterns of brain atrophy that differentiate corticobasal degeneration syndrome from progressive supranuclear palsy. *Archives of Neurology, 63*(1), 81–86.

Bugiani, O., Murrell, J. R., Giaccone, G., Hasegawa, M., Ghigo, G., Tabaton, M.,... Ghetti, B. (1999). Frontotemporal dementia and corticobasal degeneration in a family with a P301S mutation in tau. *Journal of Neuropathology and Experimental Neurology, 58*(6), 667–677.

Case Records of the Massachusetts General Hospital, Case 38–1985 (1985). Case records of the Massachusetts General Hospital. *New England Journal of Medicine, 313*, 739–748.

Constantinidis, J., Richard, J., & Tissot, R. (1974). Pick's disease: histological and clinical correlations. *European Neurology, 11*(4), 208–217.

Cordivari, C., Misra, V. P., Catania, S., & Lees, A. J. (2001). Treatment of dystonic clenched fist with botulinum toxin. *Movement Disorders, 16*(5), 907–913.

Cotelli, M., Borroni, B., Manenti, R., Alberici, A., Calabria, M., Agosti, C.,... Cappa, S. F. (2006). Action and object naming in frontotemporal dementia, progressive supranuclear palsy, and corticobasal degeneration. *Neuropsychology, 20*(5), 558–565.

Coulier, I. M. F., de Vries, J. J., & Leenders, K. L. (2003). Is FDG-PET a useful tool in clinical practice for diagnosing corticobasal ganglionic degeneration? *Movement Disorders, 18*(10), 1175–1178.

Dickson, D. W., Bergeron, C., Chin, S. S., Duyckaerts, C., Horoupian, D., Ikeda, K.,... Office of Rare Diseases of the National Institutes of Health (2002). Office of Rare Diseases neuropathologic criteria for corticobasal degeneration. *Journal of Neuropathology and Experimental Neurology, 61*(11), 935–946.

Doran, M., du Plessis, D. G., Enevoldson, T. P., Fletcher, N. A., Ghadiali, E., & Larner, A. J. (2003). Pathological heterogeneity of clinically diagnosed corticobasal degeneration. *Journal of the Neurological Sciences, 216*(1), 127–134.

Forman, M. S., Farmer, J., Johnson, J. K., Clark, C. M., Arnold, S. E., Coslett, H. B.,... Grossman, M. (2006). Frontotemporal dementia: Clinicopathological correlations. *Annals of Neurology, 59*(6), 952–962.

Forman, M. S., Zhukareva, V., Bergeron, C., Chin, S. S., Grossman, M., Clark, C.,... Trojanowski, J. Q. (2002). Signature tau neuropathology in gray and white matter of corticobasal degeneration. *American Journal of Pathology, 160*(6), 2045–2053.

Frattali, C. M., Grafman, J., Patronas, N., Makhlouf, F., & Litvan, I. (2000). Language disturbances in corticobasal degeneration. *Neurology, 54*(4), 990–992.

Frucht, S., Fahn, S., Chin, S., Dhawan, V., & Eidelberg, D. (2000). Levodopa-induced dyskinesias in autopsy-proven cortical-basal ganglionic degeneration. *Movement Disorders, 15*(2), 340–343.

Garbutt, S., Matlin, A., Hellmuth, J., Schenk, A. K., Johnson, J. K., Rosen, H.,... Boxer, A. L. (2008). Oculomotor function in frontotemporal lobar degeneration, related disorders and Alzheimer's disease. *Brain, 131*, 1268–1281.

Gass, J., Cannon, A., Mackenzie, I. R., Boeve, B., Baker, M., Adamson, J.,... Rademakers, R. (2006). Mutations in progranulin are a major cause of ubiquitin-positive frontotemporal lobar degeneration. *Human Molecular Genetics, 15*(20), 2988–3001.

Geda, Y. E., Boeve, B. F., Negash, S., Graff-Radford, N. R., Knopman, D. S., Parisi, J. E.,... Petersen, R. C. (2007). Neuropsychiatric features in 36 pathologically confirmed cases of corticobasal degeneration. *Journal of Neuropsychiatry and Clinical Neurosciences, 19*(1), 77–80.

Gibb, W. R., Luthert, P. J., & Marsden, C. D. (1989). Corticobasal Degeneration. *Brain, 112*, 1171–1192.

Graham, N. L., Bak, T., Patterson, K., & Hodges, J. R. (2003). Language function and dysfunction in corticobasal degeneration. *Neurology, 61*(4), 493–499.

Graham, N. L., Bak, T. H., & Hodges, J. R. (2003). Corticobasal degeneration as a cognitive disorder. *Movement Disorders, 18*(11), 1224–1232.

Grimes, D. A., Bergeron, C. B., & Lang, A. E. (1999). Motor neuron disease-inclusion dementia presenting as cortical-basal ganglionic degeneration. *Movement Disorders, 14*(4), 674–680.

Grimes, D. A., Lang, A. E., & Bergeron, C. B. (1999). Dementia as the most common presentation of cortical-basal ganglionic degeneration. *Neurology, 53*(9), 1969–1974.

Halpern, C., McMillan, C., Moore, P., Dennis, K., & Grossman, M. (2003). Calculation impairment in neurodegenerative diseases. *Journal of the Neurological Sciences, 208*(1–2), 31–38.

Hirano, S., Shinotoh, H., Shimada, H., Aotsuka, A., Tanaka, N., Ota, T.,... Suhara, T. (2010). Cholinergic imaging in corticobasal syndrome, progressive supranuclear palsy and frontotemporal dementia. *Brain, 133*, 2058–2068.

Hodges, J. R., Davies, R. R., Xuereb, J. H., Casey, B., Broe, M., Bak, T. H.,... Halliday, G. M. (2004). Clinicopathological correlates in frontotemporal dementia. *Annals of Neurology, 56*(3), 399–406.

Hu, W. T., Rippon, G. W., Boeve, B. F., Knopman, D. S., Petersen, R. C., Parisi, J. E., & Josephs, K. A. (2009). Alzheimer's disease and corticobasal degeneration presenting as corticobasal syndrome. *Movement Disorders, 24*(9), 1375–1379.

Hughes, A. J., Daniel, S. E., Ben-Shlomo, Y., & Lees, A. J. (2002). The accuracy of diagnosis of parkinsonian syndromes in a specialist movement disorder service. *Brain, 125*, 861–870.

Josephs, K. A., & Dickson, D. W. (2003). Diagnostic accuracy of progressive supranuclear palsy in the Society for Progressive Supranuclear Palsy brain bank. *Movement Disorders, 18*(9), 1018–1026.

Josephs, K. A., Duffy, J. R., Strand, E. A., Whitwell, J. L., Layton, K. F., Parisi, J. E.,... (2006). Clinicopathological and imaging correlates of progressive aphasia and apraxia of speech. *Brain, 129*, 1385–1398.

Josephs, K. A., Petersen, R. C., Knopman, D. S., Boeve, B. F., Whitwell, J. L., Duffy, J. R.,... Petersen, R. C. (2006). Clinicopathologic analysis of frontotemporal and corticobasal degenerations and PSP. *Neurology, 66*(1), 41–48.

Josephs, K. A., Whitwell, J. L., Dickson, D. W., Boeve, B. F., Knopman, D. S., Petersen, R. C.,... Jack, C. R. Jr. (2008). Voxel-based morphometry in autopsy proven PSP and CBD. *Neurobiology of Aging, 29*(2), 280–289.

Kertesz, A., Martinez-Lage, P., Davidson, W., & Munoz, D. G. (2000). The corticobasal degeneration syndrome overlaps progressive aphasia and frontotemporal dementia. *Neurology, 55*(9), 1368–1375.

Kertesz, A., McMonagle, P., Blair, M., Davidson, W., & Munoz, D. G. (2005). The evolution and pathology of frontotemporal dementia. *Brain, 128*, 1996–2005.

Kertesz, A., & Munoz, D. G. (2000). Diagnostic controversies: Is CBD part of the "pick complex"? *Advances in Neurology, 82*, 223–231.

Kleiner-Fisman, G., Bergeron, C., & Lang, A. E. (2004). Presentation of Creutzfeldt-Jakob disease as acute corticobasal degeneration syndrome. *Movement Disorders, 19*(8), 948–949.

Kompoliti, K., Goetz, C. G., Boeve, B. F., Maraganore, D. M., Ahlskog, J. E., Marsden, C. D.,... Riley, D. E.(1998). Clinical presentation and pharmacological therapy in corticobasal degeneration. *Archives of Neurology, 55*(7), 957–961.

Koss, S., Clark, R., Vesely, L., Weinstein, J., Powers, C., Richmond, L.,... Grossman, M. (2010). Numerosity impairment in corticobasal syndrome. *Neuropsychology, 24*(4), 476–492.

Kouri, N., Murray, M. E., Hassan, A., Rademakers, R., Uitti, R. J., Boeve, B. F.,... Dickson, D. W. (2011). Neuropathological features of corticobasal degeneration presenting as corticobasal syndrome or Richardson syndrome. *Brain, 134*, 3264–3275.

Kovács, T., Farsang, M., Vitaszil, E., Barsi, P., Györke, T., Szimai, I., & Kamondi, A. (2009). Levetiracetam reduces myoclonus in corticobasal degeneration: report of two cases. *Journal of Neural Transmission, 116*(12), 1631–1634.

Koyama, M., Yagishita, A., Nakata, Y., Hayashi, M., Bandoh, M., & Mizutani, T. (2007). Imaging of corticobasal degeneration syndrome. *Neuroradiology, 49*(11), 905–912.

Kumar, R., Bergeron, C., Pollanen, M., Lang, A. E. (1998). Cortical-basal ganglionic degeneration. In: J. Jankovic, & E. Tolosa (eds.), *Parkinson's disease & movement disorders* 3rd ed (pp. 297–316). Baltimore, MD: Williams & Wilkins.

Laureys, S., Salmon, E., Garraux, G., Peigneux, P., Lemaire, C., Degueldre, C., & Franck, G. (1999). Fluorodopa uptake and glucose metabolism in early stages of corticobasal degeneration. *Journal of Neurology, 246*(12), 1151–1158.

Lee, S. E., Rabinovici, G. D., Mayo, M. C., Wilson, S. M., Seeley, W. W., DeArmond, S. J.,... Miller, B. L. (2011). Clinicopathological correlations in corticobasal degeneration. *Annals of Neurology, 70*(2), 327–340.

Lee, W., Williams, D. R., & Storey, E. (2012). Cognitive testing in the diagnosis of parkinsonian disorders: A critical appraisal of the literature. *Movement Disorders, 27*(10), 1243–1254.

Leiguarda, R., Lees, A. J., Merello, M., Starkstein, S., & Marsden, C. D. (1994). The nature of apraxia in corticobasal degeneration. *Journal of Neurology, Neurosurgery and Psychiatry, 57*(4), 455–459.

Libon, D. J., Xie, S. X., Wang, X., Massimo, L., Moore, P., Vesely, L.,... Grossman, M. (2009). Neuropsychological decline in frontotemporal lobar degeneration: a longitudinal analysis. *Neuropsychology, 23*(3), 337–346.

Ling, H., O'Sullivan, S. S., Holton, J. L., Revesz, T., Massey, L. A., Williams, D. R.,... Lees, A. J. (2010). Does corticobasal degeneration exist? A clinicopathological re-evaluation. *Brain, 133*, 2045–2057.

Litvan, I., Agid, Y., Goetz, C., Jankovic, J., Wenning, G. K., Brandel, J. P.,... Bartko, J. J. (1997). Accuracy of the clinical diagnosis of corticobasal degeneration: A clinicopathologic study. *Neurology, 48*(1), 119–125.

Litvan, I., Cummings, J. L., & Mega, M. (1998). Neuropsychiatric features of corticobasal degeneration. *Journal of Neurology, Neurosurgery and Psychiatry, 65*(5), 717–721.

Llado, A., Sanchez-Valle, R., Rey, M. J., Ezquerra, M., Tolosa, E., Ferrer, I.,... Catalan collaborative Study Group for FTLD (2008). Clinicopathological and genetic correlates of frontotemporal lobar degeneration and corticobasal degeneration. *Journal of Neurology, 255*(4), 488–494.

López de Munain, A., Alzualde, A., Gorostidi, A., Otaegui, D., Ruiz-Martinez, J., Indakoetxea, B.,... Martí Massó, J. F. (2008). Mutations in progranulin gene: clinical, pathological, and ribonucleic acid expression findings. *Biological Psychiatry, 63*(10), 946–952.

Maraganore, D. M., Boeve, B., & Parisi, J. (1996). Disorders mimicking the "classical" clinical syndrome of cortical-basal ganglionic degeneration [abstract]. *Movement Disorders, 11*, 347.

Mathew, R., Bak, T. H., & Hodges, J. R. (2011). Screening for cognitive dysfunction in corticobasal syndrome: utility of Addenbrooke's cognitive examination. *Dementia and Geriatric Cognitive Disorders, 31*(4), 254–258.

Matsuoka, Y., Jouroukhin, Y., Gray, A. J., Ma, L., Hirata-Fukae, C., Li, H. F., ... Aisen, P. S. (2008). A neuronal microtubule-interacting agent, NAPVSIPQ, reduces tau pathology and enhances cognitive function in a mouse model of Alzheimer's disease. *Journal of Pharmacology and Experimental Therapeutics, 325*(1), 146–153.

McMonagle, P., Blair, M., & Kertesz, A. (2006). Corticobasal degeneration and progressive aphasia. *Neurology, 67*(8), 1444–1451.

Mendez, M. F. (2000). Corticobasal ganglionic degeneration with Balint's syndrome. *Journal of Neuropsychiatry and Clinical Neurosciences, 12*(2), 273–275.

Moretti, R., Torre, P., Antonello, R. M., Cattaruzza, T., & Cazzato, G. (2005). Cognitive impairment in the lateralized phenotype of corticobasal degeneration. *Dementia and Geriatric Cognitive Disorders, 20*(2–3), 158–162.

Murray, R., Neumann, M., Forman, M. S., Farmer, J., Massimo, L., Rice, A., ... Grossman, M. (2007). Cognitive and motor assessment in autopsy-proven corticobasal degeneration. *Neurology, 68*(16), 1274–1283.

Nagasawa, H., Tanji, H., Nomura, H., Saito, H., Itoyama, Y., Kimura, I., ... Ido, T. (1996). PET study of cerebral glucose metabolism and fluorodopa uptake in patients with corticobasal degeneration. *Journal of the Neurological Sciences, 139*(2), 210–217.

Okuda, B., Kodama, N., Tachibana, H., Sugita, M., & Tanaka, H. (2000). Visuomotor ataxia in corticobasal degeneration. *Movement Disorders, 15*(2), 337–340.

Okun, M. S., Tagliati, M., Pourfar, M., Fernandez, H. H., Rodriguez, R. L., Alterman, R. L., Foote, K. D. (2005). Management of referred deep brain stimulation failures—A retrospective analysis from 2 movement disorders centers. *Archives of Neurology, 62*(8), 1250–1255.

Osaki, Y., Ben Shlomo, Y., Lees, A. J., Daniel, S. E., Colosimo, C., Wenning, G. K., Quinn, N. (2004). Accuracy of clinical diagnosis of progressive supranuclear palsy. *Movement Disorders, 19*(2), 181–189.

Ozsancak, C., Auzou, P., Dujardin, K., Quinn, N., Destée, A. (2004). Orofacial apraxia in corticobasal degeneration, progressive supranuclear palsy, multiple system atrophy and Parkinson's disease. *Journal of Neurology, 251*, 1317–1323.

Pantelyat, A., Dreyfuss, M., Moore, P., Gross, R., Schuck, T., Irwin, D., ... (2011). Acalculia in autopsy-proven corticobasal degeneration. *Neurology, 76*, S61-S63.

Pillon, B., Blin, J., Vidailhet, M., Deweer, B., Sirigu, A., Dubois, B., & Agid, Y. (1995). The neuropsychological pattern of corticobasal degeneration: Comparison with progressive supranuclear palsy and Alzheimer's disease. *Neurology, 45*(8), 1477–1483.

Pillon, B., & Dubois, B. (2000). Memory and executive processes in corticobasal degeneration. *Advances in Neurology, 82*, 91–101.

Rebeiz, J. J., Kolodny, E. H., & Richardson, E. P. (1968). Corticodentatonigral degeneration with neuronal achromasia. *Archives of Neurology, 18*(1), 20–33.

Riley, D. E., Lang, A. E., Lewis, A., Resch, L., Ashby, P., Hornykiewicz, O., & Black, S. (1990). Cortical-basal ganglionic degeneration. *Neurology, 40*, 1203–1212.

Rinne, J. O., Lee, M. S., Thompson, P. D., & Marsden, C. D. (1994). Corticobasal degeneration. A clinical study of 36 cases. *Brain, 117*, 1183–1196.

Rivaud-Péchoux, S., Vidailhet, M., Gallouedec, G., Litvan, I., Gaymard, B., & Pierrot-Deseilligny, C. (2000). Longitudinal ocular motor study in corticobasal degeneration and progressive supranuclear palsy. *Neurology, 54*(5), 1029–1032.

Rossi, G., Marelli, C., Farina, L., Laurà, M., Maria Basile, A., Ciano, C.,... Pareyson, D. (2008). The G389R mutation in the MAPT gene presenting as sporadic corticobasal syndrome. *Movement Disorders, 23*(6), 892–895.

Rottach, K. G., Riley, D. E., DiScenna, A. O., Zivotofsky, A. Z., & Leigh, R. J. (1996). Dynamic properties of horizontal and vertical eye movements in parkinsonian syndromes. *Annals of Neurology, 39*(3), 368–377.

Sato, M., Nagata, K., Yokoyama, E., & Hirata, Y. (1996). [Corticobasal degeneration: A combined clinical, PET and pathological study]. *Rinsho Shinkeigaku, 36*(2), 293–299.

Shelley, B. P., Hodges, J. R., Kipps, C. M., Xuereb, J. H., & Bak, T. H. (2009). Is the pathology of corticobasal syndrome predictable in life? *Movement Disorders, 24*(11), 1593–1599.

Soliveri, P., Piacentini, S., & Girotti, F. (2005). Limb apraxia in corticobasal degeneration and progressive supranuclear palsy. *Neurology, 64*(3), 448–453.

Spina, S., Murrell, J. R., Huey, E. D., Wassermann, E. M., Pietrini, P., Grafman, J., & Ghetti, B. (2007). Corticobasal syndrome associated with the A9D Progranulin mutation. *Journal of Neuropathology and Experimental Neurology, 66*(10), 892–900.

Steffen, T. M., Boeve, B. F., Mollinger-Riemann, L. A., & Petersen, C. M. (2007). Long-term locomotor training for gait and balance in a patient with mixed progressive supranuclear palsy and corticobasal degeneration. *Physical Therapy, 87*(8), 1078–1087.

Tang-Wai, D. F., Josephs, K. A., Boeve, B. F., Dickson, D. W., Parisi, J. E., & Petersen, R. C. (2003). Pathologically confirmed corticobasal degeneration presenting with visuospatial dysfunction. *Neurology, 61*(8), 1134–1135.

Togasaki, D. M., & Tanner, C. M. (2000). Epidemiologic aspects. *Advances in Neurology, 82*, 53–59.

Ukmar, M., Moretti, R., Torre, P., Antonello, R. M., Longo, R., & Bava, A. (2003). Corticobasal degeneration: structural and functional MRI and single-photon emission computed tomography. *Neuroradiology, 45*(10), 708–712.

Uryu, K., Nakashima-Yasuda, H., Forman, M. S., Kwong, L. K., Clark, C. M., Grossman, M.,... Neumann, M. (2008). Concomitant TAR-DNA-binding protein 43 pathology is present in Alzheimer disease and corticobasal degeneration but not in other tauopathies. *Journal of Neuropathology and Experimental Neurology, 67*(6), 555–564.

Vanek, Z., & Jankovic, J. (2001). Dystonia in corticobasal degeneration. *Movement Disorders, 16*(2), 252–257.

Vanvoorst, W. A., Greenaway, M. C., Boeve, B. F., Ivnik, R. J., Parisi, J. E., Ahlskog, J. E.,... Josephs, K. A. (2008). Neuropsychological findings in clinically atypical autopsy confirmed corticobasal degeneration and progressive supranuclear palsy. *Parkinsonism & Related Disorders, 14*(4), 376–378.

Vidailhet, M., & Rivaud-Péchoux, S. (2000). Eye movement disorders in corticobasal degeneration. *Advances in Neurology, 82*, 161–167.

Watts, R. L., Williams, R. S., Growdon, J. D., Young, R. R., Haley, E. C., & Beal, M. F. (1985). Corticobasal ganglionic dengeration [Abstract]. *Neurology, 35*(Suppl 1), 178.

Wenning, G. K., Litvan, I., Jankovic, J., Granata, R., Mangone, C. A., McKee, A.,... Pearce, R. K. (1998). Natural history and survival of 14 patients with corticobasal degeneration confirmed at postmortem examination. *Journal of Neurology, Neurosurgery and Psychiatry, 64*(2), 184–189.

Whitwell, J. L., Jack, C. R., Jr., Boeve, B. F., Parisi, J. E., Ahlskog, J. E., Drubach, D. A.,... Josephs, K. A. (2010). Imaging correlates of pathology in corticobasal syndrome. *Neurology, 75*(21), 1879–1887.

Winter, Y., Bezdolnyy, Y., Katunina, E., Avakjan, G., Reese, J. P., Klotsche, J.,... Gusev, E. (2010). Incidence of Parkinson's disease and atypical parkinsonism: Russian population-based study. *Movement Disorders, 25*(3), 349–356.

Wojcieszek, J., Lang, A. E., Jankovic, J., Greene, P., & Deck, J. (1994). What is it? Case 1, 1994: Rapidly progressive aphasia, apraxia, dementia, myoclonus, and parkinsonism. *Movement Disorders, 9*(3), 358–366.

Yoshida, M. (2006). Cellular tau pathology and immunohistochemical study of tau isoforms in sporadic tauopathies. *Neuropathology, 26*(5), 457–470.

15 Multiple System Atrophy

Kathy Dujardin and Luc Defebvre

INTRODUCTION

The term "multiple system atrophy" (MSA) was introduced in 1969 by Graham and Oppenheimer (Graham & Oppenheimer, 1969). This clinical entity is characterized by a combination (to various degrees) of parkinsonian, cerebellar, dysautonomic, and pyramidal symptoms. In fact, MSA encompasses the nosological set of conditions previously referred to as Shy-Drager syndrome, striatonigral degeneration, and nonfamilial olivopontocerebellar atrophy. These various conditions have some common clinical and neuropathological characteristics, with the presence of hallmark oligodendroglial inclusions containing alpha-synuclein (Papp, Kahn, & Lantos, 1989). Like Parkinson's disease (PD) and dementia with Lewy bodies (DLB), MSA is a synucleinopathy.

Multiple system atrophy is a sporadic, neurodegenerative disease of unknown etiology. It constitutes the most frequent form (5 to 10%) of atypical parkinsonian syndrome. The establishment of consensus diagnostic criteria has enabled better definition of this disease (Gilman et al., 2008). Typically, onset occurs between 45 and 65 years of age. A slight male predominance has often been reported. Clinically, MSA is the most frequent differential diagnosis for PD, with one case of MSA for every 10 to 20 of PD. The mean prevalence is 5 in 100,000 inhabitants. Although familial forms are rare, more cases of parkinsonian syndromes have been reported in the first-degree relatives of patients suffering from MSA than from progressive supranuclear palsy (PSP; Vidal, Vidailhet, Derkinderen, Tzourio, & Alperovitch, 2010). Motor handicap occurs much earlier in MSA than in PD, due to the poor efficacy of antiparkinsonian treatments.

CLINICAL MANIFESTATIONS

The main clinical manifestations of MSA are parkinsonian, cerebellar, pyramidal, and dysautonomic symptoms (Wenning, Tison, Ben Shlomo, Daniel, & Quinn,

1997). The parkinsonian syndrome predominates in the MSA with predominant parkinsonism (MSA-P) subtype, whereas the cerebellar syndrome predominates in the MSA with cerebellar features (MSA-C) subtype. In Europe and the United States, respectively 60% and 75% of MSA cases are type P. In contrast, MSA-C predominates in Japan (Stefanova, Bucke, Duerr, & Wenning, 2009). The prevalence of autonomic dysfunction is pretty much constant from one population to another. The initial presentation varies from one clinical form to another.

The Parkinsonian Syndrome

A parkinsonian syndrome (present by definition in MSA-P) is also present in about half of type C patients (Albanese et al., 1995). It is expressed as sometimes asymmetric akinesia and hypertonia, with axial predominance. Gait disorders may be the initial symptoms. The tremor is often atypical, rapid, and irregular, with a postural myoclonic component. A PD-like rest tremor is present in fewer than 10% of cases (Wenning et al., 1997). Postural instability, falls, hypophonia, and anterocollis appear very early. The postural disorders are sometimes characterized by camptocormia or Pisa syndrome (lateral deviation of the trunk). In general, L-dopa is found to have little or no efficacy (Hughes, Colosimo, Kleedorfer, Daniel, & Lees, 1992) and a significant benefit (lasting for at least 3 to 5 years) only occurs in a small proportion of patients (10%). Dopa-induced, dystonic dyskinesia is less frequent in MSA than in PD (affecting a third of MSA patients after 5 years of treatment; Wenning et al., 1997) but often affects the orofacial and neck muscles. Non-dopa-induced dystonia has also been reported. It is fixed and focal in nature.

The Cerebellar Syndrome

A cerebellar syndrome is observed in 64% of cases (Stefanova et al., 2009; Wenning et al., 1997). It is early and intense in MSA-C but appears later in MSA-P, where it is masked by the parkinsonian syndrome. This results in gait and kinetic limb ataxia. An intention tremor may be present, as well as dysarthria with scanning speech and hypophonia due to parkinsonian dysarthria. Cerebellar oculomotor dysfunctions (such as nystagmus, hypo- or hypermetric saccades and fixation abnormalities) can guide the diagnostic process.

Autonomic Dysfunction

The signs of autonomic dysfunction occur early, are systematically observed, and progress steadily over the course of the disease.

The first clinical manifestations of autonomic dysfunction are usually genito-urinary and sphincter-related disorders (in 83% of cases), such as impotence in men and various urinary disorders in men and women: hypertonia with detrusor instability in two thirds of cases (nocturnal pollakiuria and urge urinary incontinence with incomplete voiding) and detrusor weakness with chronic retention in a third of cases (Beck, Betts, & Fowler, 1994).

In terms of the digestive tract, severe constipation can be related to dystonia and painful spasms of the sphincter. Diarrhea and fecal incontinence have also been reported.

Orthostatic hypotension is observed in 75% of cases and results in feelings of asthenia, dizziness, or near-syncope (faintness without loss of consciousness) during changes in position. Episodes of syncope are rare but possible (in 15% of patients). This hypotension is accompanied by the disappearance of reflex tachycardia. It is defined by a decrease of at least 30 mm Hg in systolic blood pressure and/or a decrease of at least 15 mm Hg in diastolic blood pressure after three minutes of standing. It is often associated with supine hypertension. Orthostatic hypotension occurs much earlier in MSA than in PD and is more severe (Lipp et al., 2009). Other clinical signs of autonomic dysfunction have been reported: vasomotor disorders with cold, purple-colored hands, sweating, and thermoregulatory disorders, pupillary dysfunction, dry eye, and xerostomia.

Pyramidal Symptoms

The pyramidal signs are poorly specific for MSA and are observed in 50% of cases as the Babinski sign and widespread hyperreflexia (Wenning et al., 1997).

Other Clinical Symptoms

Other clinical signs have been described: severe, early-onset anterocollis; early-onset dysarthria combining parkinsonian and cerebellar features (hypophonia, stuttering, scanning, and tremulous speech and early-onset swallowing disorders as a "pseudobulbar syndrome"); nocturnal snoring with paralysis of the abductors of the vocal cords (resulting in stridor via degeneration of the nucleus ambiguus); sleep disorders with snoring, apnea, and rapid eye movement sleep behavior disorders; spontaneous myoclonus or myoclonus triggered by sensory stimuli; limb dystonia; rheumatic pain mainly related to dystonic contractions. The oculomotor disorders are characterized by fixation abnormalities, limited vertical gaze (upward saccades) and, more rarely, limited horizontal gaze.

The symptoms are evaluated on the Unified Multiple System Atrophy Rating Scale (Wenning et al., 2004), which includes questions on activities of daily living (part 1), a motor symptom score (part 2) and screening for orthostatic hypotension (part 3) and invalidity (part 4).

Disease Progression

The disease progression is rapid, with a median survival time from the first signs of less than 10 years (8.6 and 7.3 years for men and women, respectively) (Schrag, Wenning, Quinn, & Ben-Shlomo, 2008). A complete set of MSA symptoms often becomes established within 4 to 5 years. At disease onset, it is sometimes difficult to differentiate between PD and MSA, especially if an initial response to L-dopa is present. There is no significant difference between MSA-P and MSA-C patients in terms of survival. In contrast, patients whose disease starts with severe autonomic dysfunction may not survive as long. The main causes of death are lung disorders and sudden (often nocturnal) death. The most frequently cited negative prognostic factors are age over 60 at onset, stridor, and early-onset autonomic dysfunction.

NEUROPATHOLOGICAL CHARACTERISTICS

Macroscopic examination reveals atrophy of the cerebellum, the olivary and bulbar nuclei, the pons, the locus coeruleus, the substantia nigra, and the putamen (the brownish coloration of which is due to iron overload). *On the microscopic level,* the histopathological lesions include neuron loss and gliosis that affect to varying extents the relays of the basal ganglia (the striatum, and the substantia nigra), the cerebellum (the Purkinje cells, the lower olivary nuclei, and the middle and inferior cerebellar peduncles), the autonomic centers (the nucleus dorsalis nervi vagi, the nucleus ambiguus, the intermediolateral cell column of the spinal cord, and Onuf's nucleus), the pyramidal system and other nuclei (the locus coeruleus and the pontine nuclei) (Ozawa et al., 2004) .

The presence of intracytoplasmic and intranuclear argyrophilic inclusions (revealed by silver impregnation techniques) in oligodendrocytes and, to a lesser extent, in the cytoplasm and nucleus of the neurones is characteristic of MSA (Trojanowski & Revesz, 2007). These inclusions can be labeled with antibodies against alpha-synuclein. The aggregation of alpha-synuclein within the oligodendrocytes is preceded by the accumulation of p25α tubulin polymerisation-promoting protein, which has a role in the myelinization process. These various oligodendrocytic events precede neurodegeneration (Stefanova et al., 2009). Another (parallel) mechanism has an essential role: the formation of alpha-synuclein aggregates in the cytoplasm and nuclei of the neurons and in the neurites (Stefanova et al., 2009).

DIAGNOSTIC CRITERIA

The most recent diagnostic criteria are detailed in Table 15-1 (Gilman et al., 2008). They take account of not only clinical and neuropathological data but also morphological and functional imaging data.

COGNITIVE DISORDERS

Cognitive disorders are not a preponderant component of the clinical picture in MSA. In the current consensus criteria, early-onset severe cognitive decline even constitutes an exclusion criterion for a diagnosis of MSA (Gilman et al., 2008). Nevertheless, extensive assessment of cognitive functions can reveal the existence of a certain number of dysfunctions.

Table 15-1 Diagnostic Criteria for Multiple System Atrophy (MSA)

Definite MSA	– Postmortem confirmation, with detection of cytoplasmic glial inclusions in association with neurodegeneration in striatonigral or olivopontocerebellar structures.
Probable MSA	– Progressive, sporadic damage in adults (age >30) – Autonomic failure involving urinary incontinence plus erectile dysfunction in males, or an orthostatic decrease of blood pressure within 3 minutes of standing by at least 30 mm Hg systolic or 15 mm Hg ***and*** – Poorly levodopa-responsive parkinsonism (bradykinesia with rigidity, tremor, or postural instability) ***or*** – A cerebellar syndrome (gait ataxia with cerebellar dysarthria, limb ataxia, or cerebellar oculomotor dysfunction)
Possible MSA	– Sporadic, progressive damage in adults (after age 30) – At least one feature suggesting autonomic dysfunction (otherwise unexplained urinary urgency, frequency, or incomplete bladder emptying, erectile dysfunction in males, or significant orthostatic hypotension decline that does not meet the level requires in probable MS) ***and*** – Parkinsonian syndrome (bradykinesia with rigidity, tremor, or postural instability) ***or*** – A cerebellar syndrome (gait ataxia with cerebellar dysarthria, limb ataxia, or cerebellar oculomotor dysfunction) ***and*** – At least one of the additional clinical or radiological criteria.
Additional criteria for possible MSA	– ***Possible MSA-P or MSA-C:*** • Babinski sign with hyperreflexia • Stridor – ***Possible MSA-P:*** • Rapidly progressive parkinsonism • Poor response to levodopa • Postural instability within 3 years of motor onset • Gait ataxia with cerebellar dysarthria, limb ataxia, or cerebellar oculomotor dysfunction • Dysphagia within 5 years of motor onset • Atrophy on magnetic resonance imaging (MRI) of putamen, middle cerebellar peduncle, pons, or cerebellum • Hypometabolism on [^{18}F]-fluorodeoxyglucose positron emission tomography (FDG-PET) in putamen, brainstem, or cerebellum – ***Possible MSA-C:*** • Parkinsonism (bradykinesia with rigidity) • Atrophy on the putamen, middle cerebellar peduncle, pons, or cerebellum • Hypometabolism on FDG-PET in the putamen • Presynaptic nigrostriatal dopaminergic denervation in single photon emission computed tomography (SPECT) or PET

(continued)

Table 15-1 Continued

Supporting features	- Orofacial dystonia - Significant anterocollis - Camptocormia (marked anteflexion of the spine) and/or Pisa syndrome (marked lateral flexion of the spine) - Contractions of the hands or feet - Stridor and inspiratory sighs - Recent or worsened snoring - Severe dysphonia - Severe dysarthria - Cold hands or feet - Pathological laughing or crying - Irregular myoclonic (postural or action) tremor
Features suggesting another diagnosis	- Rest tremor - Neuropathy - Onset after age 75 - A family history of ataxia - Dementia (DSM IV) - White matter lesions suggestive of multiple sclerosis - Spontaneous hallucinations

The Prevalence of Cognitive Disorders

Few studies have investigated the frequency of cognitive decline in MSA. In a retrospective study of 38 autopsied cases, Wenning et al. reported that 15.7% of cases developed dementia, always after more than five years of disease progression (Wenning et al., 2000). This late onset was confirmed by O'Sullivan et al., who reported a dementia rate of 14% in a series of 83 autopsied cases (O'Sullivan et al., 2008). However, these studies suffered from bias because cases with dementia at the time of the diagnosis were systematically excluded. This tended to reduce the prevalence of cognitive decline in MSA and lengthen the time to onset. This is why Kitayama et al. deliberately neglected to take account of this criterion at the time of diagnosis in their study of 58 patients with a clinical diagnosis of MSA (Kitayama, Wada-Isoe, Irizawa, & Nakashima, 2009). Dementia was found in ten (17%) of the latter, and the cognitive disorders had appeared before the motor disorders in three cases. In comparison with nondemented patients, the patients with dementia had more marked atrophy of the frontal lobe and reduced brain metabolism in the frontal region. The largest study of cognitive function in MSA to date was that reported by Brown et al. (Brown et al., 2010) as part of the prospective "Neuroprotection and Natural History in Parkinson Plus Syndromes" study performed in 44 specialist movement disorders departments across Europe (Bensimon et al., 2009). Detailed clinical data and additional neuroradiological, cognitive, behavioral and genetic data were collected annually for three years in 760 patients (with a postmortem confirmation of the diagnosis in 20%). A clinical diagnosis of MSA had been made in 398 of these patients, whereas the others had been diagnosed with PSP. The article by Brown et al. (Brown et al., 2010) reported the data collected at the time of study entry (i.e., at the first neuropsychological assessment). Patients with severe cognitive decline (defined as a Mini Mental State Examination (MMSE) score <20) were not included. The examination of cognitive functions included the MMSE, the Frontal Assessment Battery, and the Mattis Dementia Rating Scale (DRS). At study entry, 299 MSA patients (75.1%) had preserved global cognitive function, with a DRS score ≥ 133. Seventy-three (18.3%) had significant cognitive decline (evidenced by a DRS scale ≤ 125). The remainder (6.5%) were in an intermediate situation. On average, the patients with global cognitive decline were older, less educated, and had a longer time since disease onset and a more severe dysexecutive syndrome than patients with preserved global cognitive function. The prevalence of cognitive impairment was similar when comparing patients with early-stage disease (22%) versus advanced disease (24%). The predictive factors for cognitive decline (detailed in Table 15-2) were severe motor impairment, less than 10 years of formal education, male gender, the presence of cardiovascular autonomic dysfunction, and the absence of genito-urinary and bowel disorders. A more detailed analysis of the DRS scores showed that the impairment concerned essentially the "Initiation/Perseveration" subscale, for which 36.8% of the patients obtained a below-normal score. The poor DRS score was mostly due to a reduction in word fluency. In the 44 autopsied MSA patients, 77.1% had no initial cognitive decline and the diagnosis was confirmed in 94.6% of the latter. In the 22.9% with significant cognitive decline at study entry (DRS score ≤ 125 or MMSE score ≤ 24), the diagnosis was confirmed in 64.4% of cases, with a final diagnosis of PSP, DLB. or amyotrophic lateral sclerosis in the others. This study highlighted significant cognitive disorders in a non-negligible proportion of MSA patients— even in early-stage disease. According to Brown et al., these results plead in favor of abandoning cognitive decline as an exclusion criterion in the diagnosis of MSA (Brown et al., 2010).

Table 15-2 Odds ratios and 95% confidence intervals for predictive factors for cognitive decline in MSA, as defined by Brown et al. (2010) in a binary logistic regression.

	Odds ratio	*Confidence interval (95%)*
Severe motor disability*	3.58	1.75–7.29
Formal education < 10 years	2.27	1.10–4.65
Male gender	1.94	1.05–3.56
Presence of cardiovascular dysautonomia	2.64	1.34–5.05
Absence of genitoutinary signs	4.02	1.67–9.60

* The severity of motor disorders was defined by a study-specific motor scale (for details, see Bensimon et al., 2009); a score ≥ 5 corresponded to severe disease.

Anatomical and Functional Correlates

Although Brown et al. acquired neuroimaging data (Brown et al., 2010), they did not correlate their neuroradiologic findings with the patients' cognitive profiles (although this aspect may well be reported on in the future). Brown et al. nevertheless considered that the observed disorders reflected cortical (notably frontal) dysfunction and subcortical dysfunction that are similar to those typically observed in parkinsonian syndromes. The role of frontal and subcortical damage has not necessarily been confirmed by the few neuroimaging studies that have focused on possible links between the cognitive profile and anatomical and/or functional changes. Hence, Paviour et al. (Paviour, Price, Jahanshahi, Lees, & Fox, 2006) reported an association between cognitive decline and the volume of the inferior and posterior brain regions in general (and the pons and the cerebellum in particular). However, only nine patients with very few cognitive disorders had been included in this study; this means that one cannot rule out the involvement of other brain regions in cognitive decline in MSA. Chang et al. administered an extensive battery of cognitive tests and performed MRI in 23 MSA patients (10 MSA-C and 13 MSA-P patients) whose performance levels were compared with those of 37 matched, healthy controls (Chang et al., 2009). The grey matter density was measured with voxel-based morphometry (VBM). The entire MSA group performed worse in executive function tests than controls. On the anatomical level, the researchers found a reduction in grey matter density in the left caudate nucleus, the right hippocampus, and the bilateral insular and frontal regions in the MSA-C group. In the MSA-P group, the grey matter density was reduced in the cerebellum, the insula, the right olfactory lobe and the medial temporal region. There were few significant relationships between the cognitive test scores and the brain atrophy profile. Only Kawai et al. have shown that executive impairment in MSA is related to a reduction in cerebral blood flow in the frontal region, even in the absence of brain atrophy (Kawai et al., 2008).

The Characterization of Cognitive Disorders and Its Role in Differential Diagnosis

Other researchers have tried to specifically characterize the cognitive profile of MSA patients, particularly the nature of the dysexecutive syndrome. Robbins et al. did not observe any learning or long-term memory disorders but did see impairments in all the tests that were sensitive to frontal lobe and basal ganglia lesions (Robbins et al., 1992). In this study, the MSA patients had impairments in visuospatial working memory (relative to matched, healthy controls). They also presented planning disorders in the Tower of London Test and difficulty in alternating between categories in a cognitive-flexibility test. In contrast, their performance levels in associative-learning, object-recognition, and spatial-localization tests were similar to those of controls. The observed performance profile was very similar to that seen for focal lesions of the frontal lobe. Robbins et al. then compared the cognitive disorders observed in MSA with those observed in the other parkinsonian syndromes (Robbins et al., 1994). However, with respect to the tests used in their previous study, the researchers only used those that were sensitive to focal frontal lesions and for which MSA patients showed impairments. They administered the tests to PD, PSP, and MSA patients and strictly matched healthy controls. Compared with the healthy controls, the MSA patients presented impairments in all tests that were sensitive to frontal dysfunction. These impairments were very similar to those in PD patients and less severe than those observed in PSP. The PD and MSA patients differed in terms of the Tower of London Test scores; the MSA profile was closer to that of frontal subjects than that of PD patients. In fact, as seen for the focal frontal lesions, the MSA patients performed the first move as rapidly as the controls but the latency of the subsequent moves was significantly greater. Conversely, in PD, the latency of the first move was longer than normal and that of subsequent moves was normal.

According to Robbins et al., cognitive dysfunction in PD and MSA has the same cause (Robbins et al., 1994). The similarity between cognitive profiles in PD and MSA has also been reported by Testa et al., despite the use of much less specific test procedures (Testa et al., 1993). The researchers reported a marked psychomotor slowing in both diseases, with visuospatial organization disorders and visuoconstructive difficulties. In contrast, other studies have suggested the existence of differences between the respective cognitive profiles. Pillon et al. also compared the dysexecutive syndromes presented by PD, PSP, and MSA patients and found that PSP patients were more severely affected than the other two groups (Pillon et al., 1995). The dysexecutive syndrome in PD and MSA patients was similar, but the condition was more selective in MSA than in PD. In fact, when compared with normative data collected from a control population, the MSA patients showed impairments in word-fluency tests and the Trail-Making Test but performed normally in the Wisconsin Card Sorting Test (WCST) and the Stroop Test. When the MSA patients' performance was compared with that of a group of PD patients, the only intergroup difference concerned the WCST score (worse in PD than in MSA). Pillon et al. (1995) interpreted this result with respect to the distinction drawn between spontaneous and reactive flexibility by Eslinger and Grattan (Eslinger & Grattan, 1993). According to the latter researchers (Eslinger & Grattan, 1993), cognitive flexibility (i.e., the ability to alternate between categories of concepts or action plans) is not a single process. In fact, the cognitive effort is not the same when one compares (a) the ability to internally generate a set of ideas or concepts, and (b) the ability to modify an action plan in response to environmental constraints. Eslinger and Grattan suggested distinguishing between two types of situations: those that require the subject to produce and (sometimes) create various solutions by internally elaborating strategies for alternating between categories of knowledge or answers and those that require modification of a response or behavior when faced with a particular contextual situation. According to Eslinger and Grattan (Eslinger & Grattan, 1993), these two situations involve spontaneous flexibility and reactive flexibility, respectively. Tasks such as verbal or number fluency tests (which require the generation of the largest possible number of items in a category and alternation between subcategories) typically evaluate spontaneous flexibility. In contrast, tests such as the WCST (in which the subject must alternate between response rules as a function of external indicators) evaluate reactive flexibility. Pillon et al. suggested that in MSA, the dysexecutive syndrome may be limited to a loss of spontaneous flexibility (with preservation of reactive flexibility), whereas the opposite is observed in PD (Pillon et al., 1995). Since one of the main practical problems is the early differential diagnosis between PD and MSA, this type of difference may have clinical value. This hypothesis has not been confirmed and contradictory results have even been reported. In fact, Meco et al. found that both MSA and PD patients performed worse than control subjects in executive function tests (Meco, Gasparini, & Doricchi, 1996). Only the Stroop test results enabled differentiation between the two groups of patients; in the interference condition, the MSA patients were significantly slower and made more errors than the PD patients. These results suggest perturbation of the two types of flexibility in both groups but more severe impairment of reactive flexibility in MSA than in PD. Similarly, Dujardin et al. compared the performance levels of MSA patients, PD patients and strictly matched, healthy controls in a set of executive function tests (Dujardin, Defebvre, Krystkowiak, Degreef, & Destee, 2003). Two of the tests involved spontaneous flexibility (a word fluency test and a spatial sequence generation test) and two other tests involved reactive flexibility (the WCST Test and the Stroop Test). Compared with controls, both groups of patients presented executive function disorders but the dysexecutive syndrome in MSA patients was more marked than in PD patients. In fact, the MSA patients presented impairments in all the executive function tasks, whereas the PD patients were impaired in the WCST and the Stroop Test (i.e., the two tests evaluating reactive flexibility). The performance of the two patient groups differed in the word fluency test, in which the MSA patients generated significantly fewer words than PD patients. Hence, there was a difference between spontaneous and reactive flexibilities; these results suggest that both components are affected in MSA, whereas the impairment in PD only concerns situations involving reactive flexibility. In their recent review, Lee et al. also concluded that MSA and PD share a similar cognitive profile, dominated by executive dysfunction, and that cognitive testing contributes little to the differential diagnosis (Lee, Williams, & Storey, 2012).

Neuropathological differences between the two diseases may explain the presence of a more widespread dysexecutive syndrome in MSA. In fact, PD leads to a loss of pigmented neurons in the pars compacta of the substantia nigra. The resulting dopaminergic depletion perturbs the operation of the striatum. The latter's neurons are intact but the lack of dopaminergic inputs causes dysfunction of the circuits linking the striatum to the prefrontal cortex. In MSA, the neurodegeneration affects both the substantia nigra and the striatum, thus inducing both functional and structural impairments. Hence, the more widespread striatal damage in MSA could prompt the more marked executive function disorders and explains the more rapid degradation of the patient's cognitive state as the disease progresses (Soliveri et al., 2000). However, this remains to be confirmed by neuroimaging studies.

Studies that have distinguished between MSA-P and MSA-C have generally found similar cognitive profiles (Burk, Daum, & Rub, 2006; Krishnan, Mathuranath, Sarma, & Kishore, 2006; Lange et al., 2003). This similarity is probably related to the subcortical origin of the cognitive damage in MSA. Very few studies have directly compared the respective cognitive profiles in MSA-P and MSA-C. Kawai et al. found more marked and more widespread impairments in an MSA-P group than in an MSA-C group, for equivalent disease durations (Kawai et al., 2008). This cognitive decline was correlated with a decrease in brain perfusion in the frontal regions. In contrast, Chang et al. reported a more marked impairment in an MSA-C group (Chang et al., 2009).

In summary, even though cognitive disorders are not among the most prominent symptoms, they are present in MSA and mainly affect executive functions. The severity of these disorders varies significantly, even in early-stage disease. The disease degrades cognitive independence and the activities of daily living in some patients but not others. Although cognitive disorders contribute little or nothing to the differential diagnosis of parkinsonian syndromes, these aspects must be taken into consideration and it is advisable to evaluate cognitive function in MSA patients.

BEHAVIORAL DISORDERS

Behavioural disorders have rarely been thoroughly investigated in MSA. An increase in emotional lability and pathologic laughing and crying have been reported (Parvizi, Joseph, Press, & Schmahmann, 2007). In a broad study of 286 patients with a clinical diagnosis of MSA, Schrag et al. observed depressive symptoms in 43% of the participants and anxiety symptoms in 37% (Schrag et al., 2010). Balas et al. compared the severity of depression and anxiety symptoms in the two subtypes of MSA (Balas, Balash, Giladi, & Gurevich, 2010). The anxiety-related and depressive symptoms were markedly more severe in MSA patients than in healthy controls, but there were no significance differences between MSA-P and MSA-C subgroups.

PARACLINICAL EXAMINATIONS

A number of additional investigations can provide evidence for the diagnosis of MSA.

Morphological Imaging

Morphological imaging contributes to the diagnosis of MSA (Schrag et al., 2000; Seppi, Schocke, Wenning, & Poewe, 2005). Magnetic resonance imaging enables visualization of the cerebellar and pontine atrophy that is always present in the C subtype (see Figure 15-1) and putaminal signal hypo-intensity with posterior and lateral predominance in T2-weighted sequences (corresponding to an increase in iron levels in the latter structure). This putaminal T2 signal hypo-intensity is sometimes bordered by a secondary, linear, abnormal hypersignal (see Figure 15-2). A cross-shaped hypersignal within the pons is also very suggestive of MSA (see Figure 15-3). Atrophy of the cerebellar peduncles (with a "cotton wool" appearance and a hyposignal in the dentate nuclei) may also be evidenced.

It should be noted that these abnormalities are not always present and that the MRI dataset is sometimes normal - especially in early-stage MSA.

In the midterm, diffusion tensor imaging and VBM will perhaps facilitate the diagnosis of MSA (Brooks & Seppi, 2009; Tir et al., 2009).

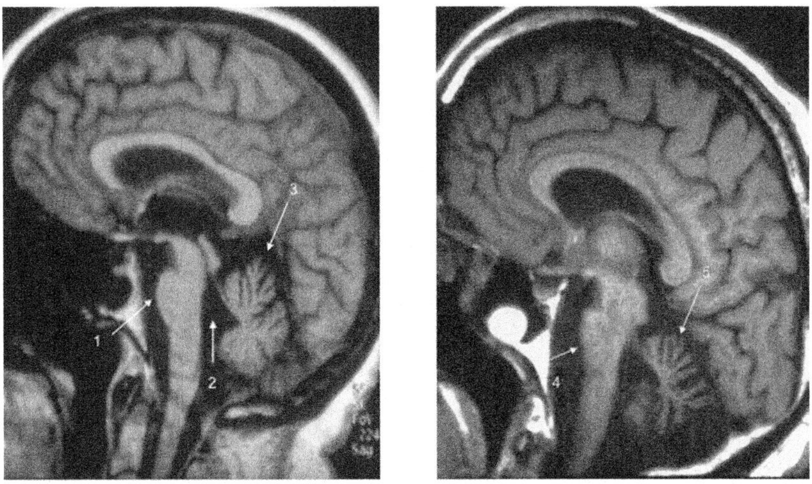

FIGURE 15-1
Brain MRI. T1-weighted sequences, sagittal plane. On the left: moderate pons atrophy *(arrow 1)*, dilatation of the fourth ventricle *(arrow 2)* and cerebellar atrophy *(arrow 3)*. On the right: severe pons and cerebellar atrophy *(arrows 4 and 5)*.

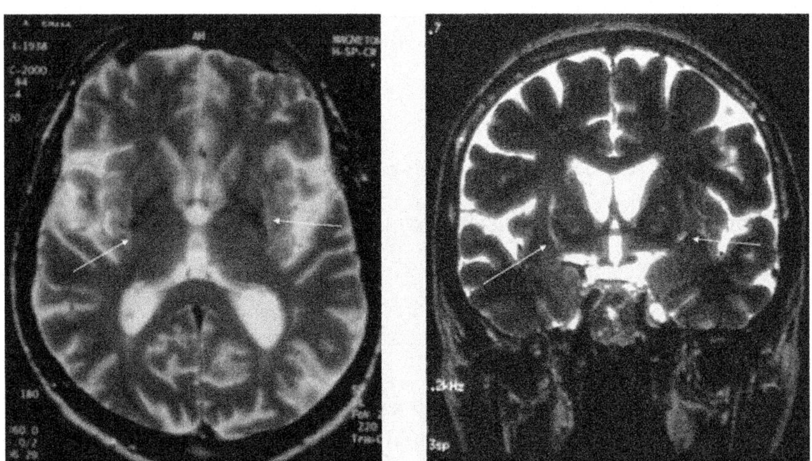

FIGURE 15-2
Brain MRI. T2-weighted sequences. Linear hypersignal of the putamen (arrows). Left: axial plane, right: coronal plane.

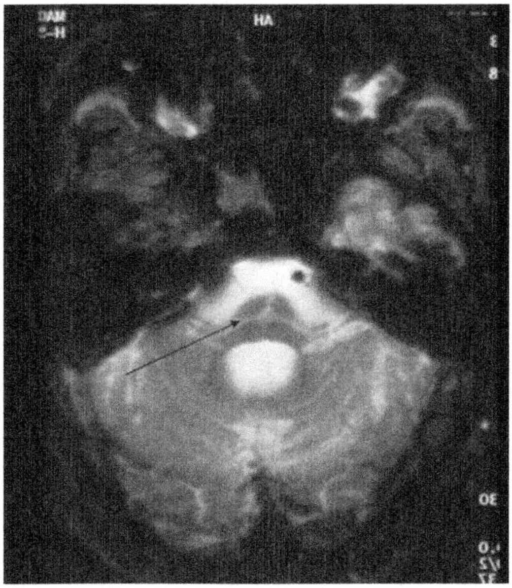

FIGURE 15-3
Brain MRI. T2-weighted sequences, axial plane. Cross-shaped hypersignal within the pons *(arrow)*.

Isotopic Imaging

Isotopic imaging refers here to the images obtained by PET (Gilman, 2005; Gilman et al., 1999) and single-photon tomography (Scherfler et al., 2005).

The metabolic abnormalities reported in MSA can facilitate its diagnosis (see the previously mentioned criteria (Gilman et al., 2008)) and reflect combined damage to the nigrostriatal dopaminergic pathways, the striatum, and the cerebellum. Hence, when faced with an atypical parkinsonian syndrome and the absence of ataxia, the observation of cerebellar hypometabolism suggests MSA-P rather than PD. Similarly, if a cerebellar syndrome is predominant, the presence of striatal hypometabolism argues in favor of MSA-C.

Dopamine transporter imaging (DAT) usually shows striatal decrements in both MSA and PD making it not sensitive for differential diagnosis (Cilia, Marotta, Benti, Pezzoli, & Antonini, 2005). By using the ligand ^{123}I-beta-carboxyindophenyltropane (which binds to the dopamine and serotonin transporters), SPECT reveals the presence of damage to both the caudate nucleus and the brainstem and can help to distinguish between PD patients and early-stage (< 3 years) MSA patients (in 95% of cases; Scherfler et al., 2005). This reduction in ligand binding in the brainstem may be due to damage to the serotoninergic system.

Lastly, cardiac scintigraphy with ^{123}I-meta-iodobenzylguanidine can be used to differentiate between PD (with reduced uptake reflecting postganglial damage) and MSA (normal uptake with preganglial damage; Spiegel, 2010).

Electrophysiology

The investigation of autonomic dysfunction includes a tilt test for orthostatic hypotension. This can be supplemented by an electrocardiographic analysis of the R-R interval in response to standing, deep breathing, or the Valsalva maneuver. These tests must be performed after temporary withdrawal of dopaminergic or anticholinergic medications. Holter blood pressure monitoring is a useful complement to the investigation of autonomic dysfunction (i.e., screening for disease-related nocturnal hypertension).

A urodynamic examination and ultrasound analysis of the bladder (screening for incomplete voiding) may provide a better understanding of urinary disorders and thus guide the therapeutic strategy.

Polysomnography and oxygen saturation monitoring are indicated in cases of suspected sleep apnea and/or stridor.

DRUG TREATMENTS

Although there are few therapeutic possibilities, symptomatic treatments can be evaluated on a case-by-case basis. Neuroprotective treatments are also being studied (for review, see work by Flabeau and colleagues; Flabeau, Meissner, & Tison, 2010). Several clinical trials have evaluated the potential neuroprotective effects of various compounds in MSA (riluzole, minocyclin, growth hormone, oestrogens, lithium, etc.) but have failed to unambiguously demonstrate efficacy. In principle, L-dopa should always be prescribed in an attempt to control the parkinsonian syndrome (see earlier), since a third of MSA patients display transient sensitivity to levodopa (more often in MSA-P). Dopaminergic agonists are no more effective than L-dopa. Amantadine can produce a benefit in 15% of cases. The prescription of dopaminergic medications may be limited by the aggravation of any existing orthostatic hypotension. Domperidone (30 to 60 mg per day) may thus be a useful adjunct. Deep brain stimulation is not recommended because it is inefficient and has adverse effects (Chou, Forman, Trojanowski, Hurtig, & Baltuch, 2004; Tarsy, Apetauerova, Ryan, & Norregaard, 2003).

The medications available for controlling the cerebellar syndrome (clonazepam, baclofen, amantadine, propanolol, buspirone, gabapentine, levotonine, etc.) usually show little or no efficacy. Accordingly, treatment of the cerebellar syndrome is based primarily on physiotherapy.

For controlling orthostatic hypotension, a number of small measures will always be suggested: (a) the withdrawal of any medications with potentially hypotensive effects, (b) restriction of dopaminergic agents, (c) adjunction of domperidone, (d) a sufficient sodium intake to ensure correct blood volume, (e) the use of support stockings, (f) sleeping in a semireclined position, (g) progressive changes of positions, mainly in the morning after waking and after meals (which should not be copious) and (h) limitation of hot baths or showers and exposure to heat. The most effective drug is minodrine (an alpha-1 adrenoreceptor agonist). Fludrocortisone, ephedrine, octreotide, and pyridostigmine can also be prescribed. The potential risk associated with these various drugs is the aggravation of decubitus hypertension, which justifies careful blood pressure monitoring.

The treatment of bladder and bowel disorders depends on their nature: anticholinergic drugs can decrease incontinence but there is a risk of urine retention or an increase in confusion (in patients with cognitive disorders). Nocturnal pollakiuria can be controlled with desmopressin. If the postmictional residual volume is greater than 100 ml, intermittent urinary catheterization should always be prescribed. The potential benefit of botulinum toxin injections into the detrusor or urethral sphincters has yet to be evaluated. Treatment of erectile dysfunction may involve intracavernosal injections of vasodilators (papaverine or prostaglandin E1) and the prescription of sildenafil (although the latter is associated with a risk of blood pressure drops).

For sleep disorders, treatment with positive-pressure night-time ventilation may be justified; this technique is also known to be useful in cases of nocturnal inspiratory stridor, which is likely to lead to sudden death. Tracheotomy can be discussed on a case-by-case basis.

Antispastic agents and botulinum toxin injections can be prescribed for the treatment of dystonic contractions.

CONCLUSION

Multiple system atrophy is a very invalidating movement disorder and has a poor prognosis. The set of symptoms is dominated by motor disorders and autonomic dysfunction. However, the presence of cognitive disorders must not be neglected, since it can lead to dementia and increase the level of handicap.

FUTURE DIRECTIONS

The main challenges for the future are as follows:

- An improvement in early-stage differential diagnosis. At disease onset, it is still difficult to differentiate between MSA and PD. Certain examinations (notably morphological and structural imaging but also functional imaging) help to improve the differential diagnosis but need to become even more discriminant. It is also necessary to develop other approaches, with a view to increasing the sensitivity and specificity of the existing diagnostic criteria.
- The discovery of drugs that not only improve certain symptoms (notably cerebellar syndrome and autonomic dysfunction) but also constitute neuroprotective and disease-modifying treatments that influence the course of the disease and improve the prognosis.
- The implementation of psychological support procedures for the patient and his/her family/carers. This very invalidating disease with a poor prognosis is associated with poor quality of life for the patients and always generates a significant burden for carers. The provision of disease-specific support is preferable in this respect.

REFERENCES

Albanese, A., Colosimo, C., Bentivoglio, A. R., Fenici, R., Melillo, G., & Tonali, P. (1995). Multiple system atrophy presenting as parkinsonism: Clinical features and diagnostic criteria. *Journal of Neurology Neurosurgery and Psychiatry, 59*(2), 144–151.

Balas, M., Balash, Y., Giladi, N., & Gurevich, T. (2010). Cognition in multiple system atrophy: Neuropsychological profile and interaction with mood. *Journal of Neural Transmission, 117*(3), 369–375.

Beck, R. O., Betts, C. D., & Fowler, C. J. (1994). Genitourinary dysfunction in multiple system atrophy: Clinical features and treatment in 62 cases. *Journal of Urology, 151*(5), 1336–1341.

Bensimon, G., Ludolph, A., Agid, Y., Vidailhet, M., Payan, C., & Leigh, P. N. (2009). Riluzole treatment, survival and diagnostic criteria in Parkinson plus disorders: The NNIPPS study. *Brain, 132*(Pt 1), 156–171.

Brooks, D. J., & Seppi, K. (2009). Proposed neuroimaging criteria for the diagnosis of multiple system atrophy. *Movement Disorders, 24*(7), 949–964.

Brown, R. G., Lacomblez, L., Landwehrmeyer, B. G., Bak, T., Uttner, I., Dubois, B., . . . for the NIPPS study group (2010). Cognitive impairment in patients with multiple system atrophy and progressive supranuclear palsy. *Brain, 133*(Pt 8), 2382–2393.

Burk, K., Daum, I., & Rub, U. (2006). Cognitive function in multiple system atrophy of the cerebellar type. *Movement Disorders, 21*(6), 772–776.

Chang, C. C., Chang, Y. Y., Chang, W. N., Lee, Y. C., Wang, Y. L., Lui, C. C., . . . Lui, W. L. (2009). Cognitive deficits in multiple system atrophy correlate with frontal atrophy and disease duration. *European Journal of Neurology, 16*(10), 1144–1150.

Chou, K. L., Forman, M. S., Trojanowski, J. Q., Hurtig, H. I., & Baltuch, G. H. (2004). Subthalamic nucleus deep brain stimulation in a patient with levodopa-responsive multiple system atrophy. Case report. *Journal of Neurosurgery, 100*(3), 553–556.

Cilia, R., Marotta, G., Benti, R., Pezzoli, G., & Antonini, A. (2005). Brain SPECT imaging in multiple system atrophy. *Journal of Neural Transmission, 112*(12), 1635–1645.

Dujardin, K., Defebvre, L., Krystkowiak, P., Degreef, J. F., & Destee, A. (2003). Executive function differences in multiple system atrophy and Parkinson's disease. *Parkinsonism and Related Disorders, 9*(4), 205–211.

Eslinger, P. J., & Grattan, L. M. (1993). Frontal lobe and frontal-striatal substrates for different forms of human cognitive flexibility. *Neuropsychologia, 31*(1), 17–28.

Flabeau, O., Meissner, W. G., & Tison, F. (2010). Multiple system atrophy: Current and future approaches to management. *Therapeutic Advances in Neurological Disorders, 3*(4), 249–263.

Gilman, S. (2005). Functional imaging with positron emission tomography in multiple system atrophy. *Journal of Neural Transmission, 112*(12), 1647–1655.

Gilman, S., Koeppe, R. A., Junck, L., Little, R., Kluin, K. J., Heumann, M., . . . Johanns, J. (1999). Decreased striatal monoaminergic terminals in multiple system atrophy detected with positron emission tomography. *Annals of Neurology, 45*(6), 769–777.

Gilman, S., Wenning, G. K., Low, P. A., Brooks, D. J., Mathias, C. J., Trojanowski, J. Q., . . . Vidailhet, M. (2008). Second consensus statement on the diagnosis of multiple system atrophy. *Neurology, 71*(9), 670–676.

Graham, J. G., & Oppenheimer, D. R. (1969). Orthostatic hypotension and nicotine sensitivity in a case of multiple system atrophy. *Journal of Neurology Neurosurgery and Psychiatry, 32*(1), 28–34.

Hughes, A. J., Colosimo, C., Kleedorfer, B., Daniel, S. E., & Lees, A. J. (1992). The dopaminergic response in multiple system atrophy. *Journal of Neurology Neurosurgery and Psychiatry, 55*(11), 1009–1013.

Kawai, Y., Suenaga, M., Takeda, A., Ito, M., Watanabe, H., Tanaka, F., . . . Sobue, G. (2008). Cognitive impairments in multiple system atrophy: MSA-C vs MSA-P. *Neurology, 70*(16 Pt 2), 1390–1396.

Kitayama, M., Wada-Isoe, K., Irizawa, Y., & Nakashima, K. (2009). Assessment of dementia in patients with multiple system atrophy. *European Journal of Neurology, 16*(5), 589–594.

Krishnan, S., Mathuranath, P. S., Sarma, S., & Kishore, A. (2006). Neuropsychological functions in progressive supranuclear palsy, multiple system atrophy and Parkinson's disease. *Neurology India, 54*(3), 268–272.

Lange, K. W., Tucha, O., Alders, G. L., Preier, M., Csoti, I., Merz, B., . . . Naumann, M. (2003). Differentiation of parkinsonian syndromes according to differences in executive functions. *Journal of Neural Transmission, 110*(9), 983–995.

Lee, W., Williams, D. R., & Storey, E. (2012). Cognitive testing in the diagnosis of parkinsonian disorders: A critical appraisal of the literature. *Movement Disorders, 27*(10), 1243–1254.

Lipp, A., Sandroni, P., Ahlskog, J. E., Fealey, R. D., Kimpinski, K., Iodice, V., . . . Low, P. A. (2009). Prospective differentiation of multiple system atrophy from Parkinson disease, with and without autonomic failure. *Archives of Neurology, 66*(6), 742–750.

Meco, G., Gasparini, M., & Doricchi, F. (1996). Attentional functions in multiple system atrophy and Parkinson's disease. *Journal of Neurology Neurosurgery and Psychiatry, 60*(4), 393–398.

O'Sullivan, S. S., Massey, L. A., Williams, D. R., Silveira-Moriyama, L., Kempster, P. A., Holton, J. L.,. . .Lees, A. J. (2008). Clinical outcomes of progressive supranuclear palsy and multiple system atrophy. *Brain, 131*(Pt 5), 1362–1372.

Ozawa, T., Paviour, D., Quinn, N. P., Josephs, K. A., Sangha, H., Kilford, L., . . . Revesz, T. (2004). The spectrum of pathological involvement of the striatonigral and olivopontocerebellar systems in multiple system atrophy: clinicopathological correlations. *Brain, 127*(Pt 12), 2657–2671.

Papp, M. I., Kahn, J. E., & Lantos, P. L. (1989). Glial cytoplasmic inclusions in the CNS of patients with multiple system atrophy (striatonigral degeneration, olivopontocerebellar atrophy and Shy-Drager syndrome). *Journal of Neurological Sciences, 94*(1–3), 79–100.

Parvizi, J., Joseph, J., Press, D. Z., & Schmahmann, J. D. (2007). Pathological laughter and crying in patients with multiple system atrophy-cerebellar type. *Movement Disorders, 22*(6), 798–803.

Paviour, D. C., Price, S. L., Jahanshahi, M., Lees, A. J., & Fox, N. C. (2006). Regional brain volumes distinguish PSP, MSA-P, and PD: MRI-based clinico-radiological correlations. *Movement Disorders, 21*(7), 989–996.

Pillon, B., Gouider-Khouja, N., Deweer, B., Vidailhet, M., Malapani, C., Dubois, B., Agid, Y. (1995). Neuropsychological pattern of striatonigral degeneration: comparison with Parkinson's disease and progressive supranuclear palsy. *Journal of Neurology Neurosurgery and Psychiatry, 58*(2), 174–179.

Robbins, T. W., James, M., Lange, K. W., Owen, A. M., Quinn, N. P., & Marsden, C. D. (1992). Cognitive performance in multiple system atrophy. *Brain, 115 Pt 1*, 271–291.

Robbins, T. W., James, M., Owen, A. M., Lange, K. W., Lees, A. J., Leigh, P. N., . . . Summers, B. A. (1994). Cognitive deficits in progressive supranuclear palsy, Parkinson's disease, and multiple system atrophy in tests sensitive to frontal lobe dysfunction. *Journal of Neurology Neurosurgery and Psychiatry, 57*(1), 79–88.

Scherfler, C., Seppi, K., Donnemiller, E., Goebel, G., Brenneis, C., Virgolini, I., . . . Poewe, W. (2005). Voxel-wise analysis of [123I]beta-CIT SPECT differentiates the Parkinson variant of multiple system atrophy from idiopathic Parkinson's disease. *Brain, 128*(Pt 7), 1605–1612.

Schrag, A., Good, C. D., Miszkiel, K., Morris, H. R., Mathias, C. J., Lees, A. J., & Quinn NP. (2000). Differentiation of atypical parkinsonian syndromes with routine MRI. *Neurology, 54*(3), 697–702.

Schrag, A., Sheikh, S., Quinn, N. P., Lees, A. J., Selai, C., Mathias, C., . . . Jahanshahi, M. (2010). A comparison of depression, anxiety, and health status in patients with progressive supranuclear palsy and multiple system atrophy. *Movement Disorders, 25*(8), 1077–1081.

Schrag, A., Wenning, G. K., Quinn, N., & Ben-Shlomo, Y. (2008). Survival in multiple system atrophy. *Movement Disorders, 23*(2), 294–296.

Seppi, K., Schocke, M. F., Wenning, G. K., & Poewe, W. (2005). How to diagnose MSA early: The role of magnetic resonance imaging. *Journal of Neural Transmission, 112*(12), 1625–1634.

Soliveri, P., Monza, D., Paridi, D., Carella, F., Genitrini, S., Testa, D., Girotti, F. (2000). Neuropsychological follow up in patients with Parkinson's disease, striatonigral degeneration-type multisystem atrophy, and progressive supranuclear palsy. *Journal of Neurology Neurosurgery and Psychiatry, 69*(3), 313–318.

Spiegel, J. (2010). Diagnostic and pathophysiological impact of myocardial MIBG scintigraphy in Parkinson's disease. *Parkinsons Disease, 2010*, 295346.

Stefanova, N., Bucke, P., Duerr, S., & Wenning, G. K. (2009). Multiple system atrophy: An update. *Lancet Neurology, 8*(12), 1172–1178.

Tarsy, D., Apetauerova, D., Ryan, P., & Norregaard, T. (2003). Adverse effects of subthalamic nucleus DBS in a patient with multiple system atrophy. *Neurology, 61*(2), 247–249.

Testa, D., Fetoni, V., Soliveri, P., Musicco, M., Palazzini, E., & Girotti, F. (1993). Cognitive and motor performance in multiple system atrophy and Parkinson's disease compared. *Neuropsychologia, 31*(2), 207–210.

Tir, M., Delmaire, C., le Thuc, V., Duhamel, A., Destee, A., Pruvo, J. P., & Defebvre L. (2009). Motor-related circuit dysfunction in MSA-P: Usefulness of combined whole-brain imaging analysis. *Movement Disorders, 24*(6), 863–870.

Trojanowski, J. Q., & Revesz, T. (2007). Proposed neuropathological criteria for the post mortem diagnosis of multiple system atrophy. *Neuropathology Applied Neurobiology, 33*(6), 615–620.

Vidal, J. S., Vidailhet, M., Derkinderen, P., Tzourio, C., & Alperovitch, A. (2010). Familial aggregation in atypical Parkinson's disease: A case control study in multiple system atrophy and progressive supranuclear palsy. *Journal of Neurology, 257*(8), 1388–1393.

Wenning, G. K., Ben-Shlomo, Y., Hughes, A., Daniel, S. E., Lees, A., & Quinn, N. P. (2000). What clinical features are most useful to distinguish definite multiple system atrophy from Parkinson's disease? *Journal of Neurology Neurosurgery and Psychiatry, 68*(4), 434–440.

Wenning, G. K., Tison, F., Ben Shlomo, Y., Daniel, S. E., & Quinn, N. P. (1997). Multiple system atrophy: A review of 203 pathologically proven cases. *Movement Disorders, 12*(2), 133–147.

Wenning, G. K., Tison, F., Seppi, K., Sampaio, C., Diem, A., Yekhlef, F.... The Multiple System Atrophy Study Group (2004). Development and validation of the Unified Multiple System Atrophy Rating Scale (UMSARS). *Movement Disorders, 19*(12), 1391–1402.

16 Progressive Supranuclear Palsy

Barbara Borroni and Alessandro Padovani

INTRODUCTION

Progressive supranuclear palsy (PSP) is the second most common parkinsonian neurodegenerative disorder after Parkinson's disease (PD). It was first described as a clinicopathologic entity by Steele, Richardson, and Olszewski (1964) more than 40 years ago. Since then, a giant step forward has been made in carefully defining clinical features and genetic hallmarks. Universally accepted clinical diagnostic criteria and neuropathologic criteria have been established and validated, leading to significant advances in the study of PSP (Houghton & Litvan, 2007).

PSP has an average prevalence of 5.3 per 100.000 (Bower et al., 1997; Nath et al., 2001; Schrag, Ben-Shlomo, & Quinn, 1999) and the mean age at onset is approximately 65 years with a mean survival of almost 10 years from the onset of symptoms (Burn & Lees, 2002; Litvan 2003; Golbe & Ohman-Strickland, 2007). The classical clinical picture of PSP, presenting most frequently with a symmetric, akinetic-rigid syndrome, vertical supranuclear gaze palsy, deficits of executive functions, prominent postural instability and falls, is now referred to as Richardson's syndrome (Stamelou et al., 2010), and seems to comprise about half the patients. However, several variants in the clinical presentation of pathologically confirmed PSP have been described recently, complicating the early differential diagnosis (Stamelou et al., 2010). Advanced neuroimaging techniques have carefully characterized brain features of the disease, helping in the differential diagnosis to other neurodegenerative disorders and in describing PSP clinical subtypes.

Neuropathologically, PSP is a primary tauopathy, as it is defined by the accumulation of tau protein in both brain cortical and subcortical structures. Tau is a protein that is involved in axonal transport and stabilization of neuronal microtubules; tau abnormal phosphorylation can damage microtubule function, axonal transport, and induces tau aggregation into neurofibrillary tangles, which are the most relevant pathologic element of PSP. Genetic background plays a role in PSP pathogenesis, and autosomal dominant forms due to *Microtubule Associated Protein Tau (MAPT)* gene, encoding for tau protein, have been described. Moreover, other genetic and environmental factors have been suggested to take part in disease risk and onset.

All these preceding aspects faced by the recent literature have allowed a better knowledge of this still orphan disease. Up to now, no effective symptomatic or disease-modifying therapy is presently available. As a first step toward the development of future effective treatments, a detailed understanding of the underlying pathophysiology and genotype–phenotype correlations are needed.

NEUROPATHOLOGY

Brain examination in patients with PSP reveals major midbrain and frontal atrophy (Dickson et al., 2007). Distinct microscopic findings allow the neuropathological diagnosis of PSP. The histologic characteristics are neuronal loss, gliosis, and tau-positive filamentous inclusions (neurofibrillary tangles, NFTs) involving astrocytes, oligodendrocytes, and neurons (Kristensen et al., 1985). The most involved sites of pathology are the basal ganglia (i.e., the substantia nigra), subthalamic nucleus, cerebellum (i.e., dentate nucleus), in addition to the brainstem regions (i.e., oculomotor nuclei) and prefrontal cortex (Verny, Duyckaerts, Agid, & Hauw, 1996).

In PSP, tau-positive inclusions present either as coiled bodies or as tufted astrocytes. The former are argyrophilic perinuclear inclusions commonly seen in oligodendrocytes, and these changes often coexist with threadlike processes in white matter, especially in diencephalon and cerebellum. When present in astrocytes, the tau-inclusions are called "tufted astrocytes" (Takahashi Weidenheim, Dickson, & Ksiezak-Reding, 2002). Tufted astrocytes found in motor cortex and striatum are the characteristic features of PSP, and they differ from astrocytic lesions in other neurodegenerative disease as corticobasal degeneration and Pick's disease (Komori, 1999). Involvement of all three cell types, that is, neurons, oligodendrocytes, and astrocytes, makes PSP unique among the tauopathies.

Moreover, tau inclusions in PSP have distinctive biochemical features when compared to other tauopathies. In adult human brain, six tau isoforms that are produced from a single gene by alternative mRNA splicing of exons 2, 3 and 1; moreover, the microtubule-binding domain has either three repeats (3R) or four repeats (4R) on the basis of alternative splicing of exon 10. In PSP, a higher concentration of 4R is present, associated with a 3R:4R ratio fall. The same pattern of 4R prevalence may be found in Corticobasal Degeneration as well. In healthy controls, the concentrations of 3R and 4R are similar, whereas in Pick's disease there is a predominance of 3R tau (Williams & Lees, 2009).

Neurochemical studies indicate that the degenerative process in PSP involves dopaminergic neurons that innervate the striatum (D2 receptors), as well as cholinergic and gamma-aminobutyric acid (GABA) interneurons and efferent neurons, respectively, in the striatum and other basal ganglionic and brainstem nuclei (Warren, Piggott, Lees, & Burn, 2007). Dopamine cell groups involved in PSP are connected with motor and limbic cortical and thalamic regions and are important for motor and executive functions and other cognitive and behavioral features. This is why the destruction of these areas contributes to levodopa nonresponsiveness and frontostriatal cognitive dysfunction in patients with PSP (Sanchez-Gonzalez, Garcia-Cabezas, Rico, & Cavada, 2005).

GENETICS

Large clinical series have reported that about one-third of PSP patients show positive family history for either parkinsonism or dementia (Borroni et al., 2010; Donker Kaat et al., 2009), even though less than 10% had an autosomal dominant inheritance pattern. In autosomal dominant inherited disease, mutations within *MAPT* gene have been seldom associated with PSP phenotype and PSP neuropathology beyond being related to frontotemporal lobar degeneration (Spillantini et al., 1998). As shown in Table 16-1, 9 *MAPT* mutations out of 44 have been currently described associated with PSP (Stanford et al., 2000; Poorkaj et al., 2002; Tsuboi et al., 2002; Delisle et al., 1999; Morris et al., 2003; Rossi et al., 2004; Ros et al., 2005; Spina et al., 2008; Rohrer et al., 2011) (for further details, see http://www.molgen.ua.ac. be/FTDMutations/). Intriguingly, all *MAPT* mutations associated with PSP affect exon 10, increasing the proportion of 4R tau isoforms (Spillantini et al., 1998; Rohrer et al., 2011), which are also found in sporadic forms of the disease. However, reviewing the descriptions of PSP associated with *MAPT* mutations, many cases have fairly atypical signs, but include the classic supranuclear gaze palsy and/or repetitive falls. All described cases had an autosomal inheritance pattern, often with an early-onset, rapidly progressive parkinsonism and impairment of cognitive functions. Almost all the patients developed behavioral abnormalities and frontotemporal dementia during the disease course. Only recently, a sporadic case of early-onset PSP has been associated with the new *MAPT* S285R mutation, resulting in marked increase in exon 10 splicing (Ogaki et al., 2013).

According to the central role of tau protein in PSP pathogenesis, a large number of studies have even shown a significant association between PSP and *MAPT* locus (Baker et al., 1999; De Silva et al., 2003; Rademakers et al., 2005). The *MAPT* locus exists as two major haplotype groups, termed as "H1" and "H2." These haplotypes are defined by at least 100 single nucleotide polymorphisms that are inherited in strong linkage disequilibrium with each other. Inheritance of two copies of the H1 haplotype (H1/H1) has been associated with a major genetic risk factor for PSP (Baker et al., 1999). The most likely explanation of this association is that variants in the H1/H2 haplotypes confer risk/protection against disease by altering expression at the locus, with the H1 haplotype expressing higher levels of *MAPT* (Caffrey, Joachim, Paracchini, Esiri, & Wade-Martins, 2006; Rademakers et al., 2005).

Table 16-1 *MAPT* mutations associated with clinical diagnosis of PSP.

MAPT	*Mutation*	*Clinical features*	*Origin*	*Age atonset*	*Age at death*	*References*
Exon 1	R5L	Falls, dysarthria, micrographia	U.S.A	62	67	Poorkay 2002
Exon 10	N279K	#1 bradyphrenia, parkinsonism, apathy	France	40	47	Delisle 1999
		#2 apathy, attentivedeficits		41	–	
		#3 parkinsonism with tremor, personality change, ocular apraxia, postural instability	Japan	42	54	Ogaki 2013
		#4 parkinsonism, gaze palsy, postural instability		44	56	
		#5 Parkinsonism, gaze palsy, falls		46	–	
		#6 Cognitive impairment, gaze palsy, postural instability, pyramidal signs		41	51	
		#7 Parkinsonism, gaze palsy, falls		42	54	
		#8 Parkinsonism, gaze palsy, falls, pyramidal signs		43	51	
		### 4 families with a common founder, 39 affected members; parkinsonism or dementia associated with behavioural changes	U.S.A (Caucasian)	32–58	6-9 y duration	Tsuboi 2002
		### 1 family, 3 affected members; parkinsonism or dementia associated with behavioural changes	France	38–45	6-8 y duration	
	L284R	#1 multiple falls with progressive dementia	UK	early-40s	48	Rohrer 2011
		#2 personality change, falls, progressive aphasia		mid-40s	52	
		#3 personality change, aphaty, falls, dysarthria		43	47	
	S285R	#1 Sporadic, supranuclear gaze palsy, bradykinesia, falls	Japan	46	49	Ogaki 2013

(*continued*)

Table 16-1 Continued

MAPT	*Mutation*	*Clinical features*	*Origin*	*Age atonset*	*Age at death*	*References*
	ΔN296	#1 gaze palsy, cognitive deficits, emotionallability	Spain	38	–	Pastor 2001
		#2 personality change, parkinsonism		39	–	
		#3 Personality change, cognitive impairment, gaze palsy, falls	Japan	44	–	Ogaki 2013
		#4 Dysarthria, anterocollis, falls, parkinsonism	Italy	39	–	Rossi 2004
	P301L	#1 Parkinsonism not further characterized	Netherland	–	–	Kaat 2009
	G303V	#1 Parkinsonism, falls, gaze palsy, dysarthria	Spain	37	45	Ros 2005
		#2 Not well characterized parkinsonism		41	44	
		#3 Not well characterized parkinsonism		late-30s	–	
		#4Parkinsonsim with tremor and rigidity,	France	41	45	Choumert 2012
		#5Parkinsism, gaze palsy, eye apraxia		37	40	
		#6 Parkinsonism with dystonia, eye apraxia		51	57	
		#7 Parkinsonism with dystonia, gaze palsy		39	44	
		#8 Parkinsonism, gaze palsy, dysphagia		42	46	
		#9 Parkinsonism with dystonia, gaze palsy		32	36	
	S305S	#1Apahty/cognitive deficits	Australia (Caucasian)	55	–	Stanford 2000
		#2 Dementia, apathy, aphasia		48	51	
		#3 Clumsiness, dysarthria, rigidity		49	56	
Intron 10	10+3	#1"atypical PSP-presentation" not further characterized	U.S.A.	47	48	Spina 2009
		#2 "atypical PSP-presentation" not further characterized		52	58	
	10+16	#1 Sporadic parkinsonism qith fatigue, apathy, micrographia, falls	UK	40	45	Morris 2003

Notes: –: not available; #: single patient description; ###: family description

Calculations of population-attributable risk suggest that only about 60% of the risk of PSP can be accounted for by the *MAPT* H1 haplotype, suggesting that there may be additional genetic risk factors involved in PSP. According to this, the first genome-wide association study (GWAS) analysis on autopsy-proven PSP patients identified a new *at-risk* locus on chromosome 11 (Melquist et al., 2007). This locus contains the DNA damage-binding protein 2 (*DDB2*) and lysosomal acid phosphatase 2 (*ACP2*) genes. Since DNA damage and lysosomal dysfunction have been implicated in aging and neurodegenerative processes, both genes were valuable candidates for conferring disease risk. A second GWAS study, carried out both in pathologically proven and clinically diagnosed PSP, confirmed the *MAPT* locus as major genetic risk factor for PSP onset, and identified *STX6, EIF2AK3,* and *MOBP* as associated genes (Höglinger et al., 2011). These genes encode for vesicle-membrane fusion at the Golgi-endosomal interface proteins, for the endoplasmic reticulum unfolded protein response and for a myelin structural component, further extending the complex pathophysiology of PSP (Höglinger et al., 2011).

CLINICAL FEATURES AND PHENOTYPES

According to clinical criteria, PSP is a progressive neurodegenerative disorder with the onset above 40 years of age, presenting with prominent postural instability, supranuclear vertical gaze palsy, and frontal dysfunction (Litvan et al., 1996; Steele et al., 1964).

However, this classical description, recently named as Richardson's syndrome (RS), fails to include all neuropathologically confirmed cases of PSP and does not describe the heterogeneity of clinical PSP phenotypes. To overcome with this, PSP was recently divided clinically and pathologically into two main phenotypes: classical RS and PSP-parkinsonism (PSP-P) (see Table 16-2).

The classical RS has a striking appearance with reduced facial expression, a marked reduction in blink frequency, a wide-eyed stare, axial more than appendicular rigidity, and the tendency to walk, turn, and sit *en bloc* (Boeve, 2011).

Table 16-2 Clinical distinctive features of Richardson's syndrome and PSP-parkinsonsim

Syndrome	*Richardson's syndrome*	*PSP-parkinsonism*
Early falls	Yes	No
Early eye movement abnormalities	Yes	No
Early dementia	Yes	No
Rigidity, symmetry	Yes (axial)	No (limb)
Tremor	No	Often
Response to L-dopa	No	Often
Survival rate	Worse	Better

Unsteadiness of gait with staggering and lurching characteristics, and falls without loss of consciousness are the most common presenting symptoms, occurring in about 60% of patients with PSP (Nath et al., 2003; Williams & Lees, 2009). Poor mobility is probably caused by a combination of bradykinesia, postural instability, retrocollis and supranuclear gaze palsy (Warren & Burn, 2007). Visual and ocular disturbances, giving the syndrome its name, are prominent. Supranuclear gaze palsy with impairment of downward gaze is most specific for underlying PSP, but impairment of upward gaze as well as horizontal gaze is common. Saccades are difficult to initiate, and the eyes can be described as reflecting "saccadic pursuits" when the examiner attempts to have the patient maintain primary gaze on a moving stimulus (Boeve, 2011). Later on, both ocular pursuit and refixation movements are delayed and diminished in amplitude, and eventually all voluntary eye movements are lost. Frequent spilling of food while eating (the dirty-tie phenomenon), problems with reading, and tripping while walking are also common conditions due to the inability to skew gaze downward (Boeve, 2011). Complaints of doubled or blurred vision and sore eyes are common and are related to the dramatic reduction in blink frequency and ophtalmoparesis. The upper eyelids may be retracted, and the wide-eyed, unblinking stare, imparts an expression of perpetual surprise. Apraxia of eyelid opening is not uncommon and can render the patient functionally blind (Nath et al., 2003; Warren & Burn, 2007).

Patients have marked facial dystonia with deep nasolabial folds and furrowed brow (Procerus sign) (Green, 2009). Bulbar symptoms develop early in the course of the disease, producing a characteristic slow, slurred, growling speech and difficulties in swallowing, frequently evolving in dysphagia and aspiration pneumonia (Goetz, Leurgans, Lang, & Litvan, 2003).

More than half of patients with RS will also develop some personality changes or cognitive slowing within the first 2 years (Nath et al., 2007). With the involvement of the fronto-subcortical neural networks, psychomotor slowing, forgetfulness, impaired decision making, and apathy are common. Executive functions can be altered, with difficulties in verbal fluency, working memory, concept formation, planning and execution (Grafman et al., 1995). Motor disinhibition may be demonstrated by the examiner clapping his or her hands three times then asking the patient to emulate the action. PSP patients often continue clapping more than three times ("signe d'applause"). In addition Luria's hand sequence and "go/no-go" tasks may also be impaired (Warren & Burn, 2007). Pseudobulbar disorders, unconcealed obsessive/compulsive features, and disinhibited behavior can also occur (Boeve, 2011).

These symptoms lead to an inexorable decline in functional capacity and quality of life, with increasing motor and mental disability. Most patients become dependent on others for care within 3 to 4 years of diagnosis. Percutaneous gastrostomy is often necessary for recurrent episodes of choking (Nath et al., 2007). Postural instability, motor impairment, and gaze palsy lead to recurrent falls with subsequent fractures and, ineluctably, the patient becomes wheelchair bound.

The classical RS differs from the newly defined small group of patients with PSP-P. These patients have normal eye movements, resting tremor, a positive levodopa response, and focal dementia (Williams et al., 2005). Patients with PSP-P are commonly misdiagnosed with Parkinson's disease. Early clues that might help a clinical diagnosis of PSP-P could consist of rapid progression, prominent axial symptoms, or a poor response to levo-dopa with time, despite clinical features typical of idiopathic Parkinson's disease (Williams & Lees, 2009). RS and PSP-P can be distinguished in the first 2 years according to different clinical features; nevertheless, there is phenotypical overlap, and after 6 years these variants might become similar (Williams et al., 2005). Furthermore, in PSP-P, falls and cognitive dysfunction occur later on than in RS and, as a consequence, survival time is about 3 years longer in PSP-P (O'Sullivan et al., 2008).

Clinical heterogeneity of PSP is furthermore augmented by more atypical cases, presenting as corticobasal syndrome (PSP-CBS), as pure akinesia with gait freezing (PSP-PAGF), or, rarely, associated with progressive nonfluent aphasia (PSP-PNFA) (Williams et al., 2007). These subtypes are not included in the currently used diagnostic criteria.

COGNITIVE AND BEHAVIORAL PROFILE IN PSP

Cognitive impairment, even thought not considered a primary diagnostic criterion for PSP, is currently viewed as a supportive feature in clinical diagnosis (Litvan et al., 1996).

Studies described prominent deficits on tests of attention and executive function, with verbal fluency being particularly severely affected, as well as deficits in both verbal and nonverbal memory with a relative preservation of recognition (Cotelli et al., 2006; Donker Kaat et al., 2007; Borroni et al., 2008). A proper differential diagnosis with other parkinsonisms is still challenging, because, often, comparable profiles of subcortical dementia across neurodegenerative parkinsonisms are reported. Furthermore, it is clearly evident that PSP phenotypes may present neuropsychological heterogeneity.

As described by a recent meta-analysis (Lee, Wiiliams, & Storey, 2012), tests sensitive to executive dysfunction, particularly impaired phonemic verbal fluency, and tests measuring set shifting, such as the Trail Making and the Wisconsin Card Sorting Tests may be useful in differentiating PSP from other parkinsonian syndromes. However, there is increasing recognition of an expanding clinical spectrum that falls under the pathologically defined entity of PSP. For variants with predominant cognitive presentations such as PSP-CBS and PSP–PNFA, the clinical utility of cognitive tests useful in identifying the classic form of PSP (Richardson's syndrome) is likely to be limited. Furthermore, in some cases, PSP presents as the behavioral variant of frontotemporal dementia, with prominent executive deficits and behavioral abnormalities, making differential diagnosis more complex (Hassan, Parisi, & Josephs, 2012).

Estimating dementia prevalence in PSP is hampered by a lack of large-scale prospective studies and frequent failure to report on cognition. These limitations notwithstanding, recent dementia prevalence estimates range from 10% (Josephs & Dickson, 2003) to 52% (O'Sullivan et al., 2008). However, dysexecutive syndrome may occur in up to 80% of PSP patients (Millar, Griffiths, Zermansky, & Burn, 2006).

Behavioral and emotional changes are also key, frequently early, characteristics of PSP. Studies using the Neuropsychiatric Inventory (NPI) or Frontal Behavioural Inventory (FBI) have consistently found apathy (77–91% of cases) as a common behavioral feature in PSP (Borroni et al., 2008). This may be the earliest presenting evidence of neurodegeneration, and can be misdiagnosed as a primary psychiatric disorder rather than a neurodegenerative condition. Moreover, behavioral features such as depression are often overlooked as reactions to learning a new diagnosis of parkinsonism. Other behavioral measures sensitive to frontal lobe damage have found inertia and indifference to be features of PSP (Millar et al., 2006).

In conclusion, incorporating a quantitative neuropsychological and behavioral assessment could enhance the early diagnosis and monitoring disease progression. Further studies, however, are required to develop novel standardized neuropsychological and behavioral tests able to distinguish accurately among the different neurodegenerative parkinsonisms.

NEUROIMAGING HALLMARKS

Although PSP *in vivo* diagnosis, according to current diagnostic criteria (Litvan et al., 1996), relies on clinical evaluation, imaging is often necessary in those cases that exhibit an atypical presentation or in the first phases of pathology, when differential diagnosis with other degenerative movement disorders can be challenging.

Atrophy of the upper brainstem, of the superior cerebellar peduncles and enlargement of third ventricle are the radiological and pathological features of PSP (Aiba et al., 1997; Warmuth-Metz, Naumann, Csoti, & Solymosi, 2001; Steele et al., 1964). Atypical findings on midsagittal view of MR imaging in a large proportion of PSP patients (mainly RS) is the so-called penguin sign or hummingbird sign (Oba et al., 2005; Kato, Arai, & Hattori, 2003). This sign is given by the atrophy of the rostral tegmentum, the pontine base, and the cerebellum. Another feature that is commonly present in PSP and seems related to vertical sopranuclear gaze-palsy, is the morning-glory sign, which is a concavity of the lateral margin of the tegmentum of the midbrain, visible on T2-weighted axial images (Adachi, Kawanami, Ohshima, Sugai, & Hosoya, 2004).

Beyond the visual rating of penguin sign, different quantitative measures of atrophy, to assess an early PSP diagnosis, have been investigated. The area of the midbrain in patients with PSP is about half the area of the midbrain in patients with Parkinson's disease, Multiple System Atrophy-Parkinsonism (MSA-P), and age-matched controls. However, patients with MSA-P usually show some overlap of individual areas with values from patients with PSP (Oba et al., 2005). On the other hand, pons area is smaller in MSA-P, and a reduced midbrain/pons ratio has been proposed as a more sensitive quantitative marker of PSP (Oba et al., 2005). Despite that, other studies failed in replicating the stability of midbrain/pons ratio (Gröschel et al., 2004; Quattrone et al., 2008), and suggested other quantitative approaches, such as the MR parkinsonism index (MRPI, calculated by multiplying the pons area-midbrain area ratio by the middle cerebellar peduncle width-superior cerebellar peduncle width ratio) significantly larger in PSP patients, without overlap of individual values (sensitivity and specificity 100%; Quattrone et al., 2008). It has been reported that MRPI could also predict evolution of clinically unclassifiable parkinsonism (Morelli et al., 2011). The midbrain area in PSP-P patients was intermediate between those from classical RS and Parkinson's disease patients (Longoni et al., 2011). Another quantitative measure reported in literature is the antero–posterior midbrain diameter, but a definite cut-off has not been demonstrated yet (Schrag et al., 2000; Warmuth-Metz et al., 2001).

Functional imaging by means of brain SPECT and PET procedures are not useful in differential diagnosis among neurodegenerative disorders with extrapyramidal features. [^{123}I] FP-CIT (DaTSCAN) SPECT (which labels dopamine transporter) and [^{123}I] IBZM-SPECT (which labels the postsynaptic D2 receptor) are sensible tools to detect parkinsonism at early stages, as first candidate procedures in the differential diagnosis with essential tremor (Berardelli et al., 2013). However, these cannot assess differential diagnosis of PSP with other neurodegenerative parkinsonisms and Parkinson's disease (Brooks, 2010). New tracers targeting tau pathology hold the premises to increase diagnostic accuracy of PSP.

TREATMENT

To date, no effective treatment of PSP is available, and PSP is still considered an orphan disease. Levodopa may have a moderate, but transient response, and it is worthwhile to attempt in the early stages. It has been suggested that Coenzyme Q10, a physiological cofactor of complex I, might significantly improve cerebral energy metabolism (Stamelou et al., 2008); however, more research is required to confirm these preliminary findings and investigate long-term effects. Results from other clinical studies with tau-kinase inhibitors, tau-aggregation inhibitors and microtubule stabilizers will be awaited in the near future.

Relief of symptoms with palliative therapies remains the keystone of disease management and includes different aids and forms of rehabilitation programs for balance, gait, speech, swallowing and vision problems. In later stages however, insertion of PEG may be necessary. Botulinum toxin injections may lead to functional improvement in all forms of dystonia, especially blepharospasm (Muller, Wenning, Wissel, Seppi, & Poewe, 2002).

CONCLUSIONS AND FUTURE DIRECTIONS

Over the last decade, clinical advancements have been achieved by refining the clinical spectrum of PSP into different subtypes, and in studying in deep genetic and biological bases of the disease.

A careful description of different clinical pictures has allowed a better correlation to neuropathology of PSP. However, diagnosis of the disease, especially in the early stages, is still challenging, and biomarkers helping accurate diagnosis in typical and atypical PSP are warranted. A considerable number of PSP cases present with nonclassical symptoms, and for future trials it is important to identify these patients. This would be crucial in light of future treatments targeting tau aggregation and phosphorilation.

ACKNOWLEDGMENTS

The authors thank Drs. A. Benussi, A. Formenti, S. Gazzina, and A. Pilotto.

REFERENCES

Adachi, M., Kawanami, T., Ohshima, H., Sugai, Y., & Hosoya, T. (2004). Morning glory sign: A particular MR finding in progressive supranuclear palsy. *Magnetic Resonance Medical Science, 3*(3), 125–132.

Aiba, I., Hashizume, Y., Yoshida, M., Okuda, S., Murakami, N., & Ujihira, N. (1997). Relationship between brainstem MRI and pathological findings in progressive supranuclear palsy—study in autopsy cases. *Journal of Neurological Science,152*(2), 210–217.

Baker, M., Litvan, I., Houlden, H., Adamson, J., Dickson, D., Perez-Tur, J., . . . Hutton, M. (1999). Association of an extended haplotype in the tau gene with progressive supranuclear palsy. *Humand Molecular Genetics, 8*(4), 711–715.

Berardelli, A., Wenning, G. K., Antonini, A., Berg, D., Bloem B. R., Bonifati V., . . . Vidailhet, M. (2013). EFNS/MDS-ES recommendations for the diagnosis of Parkinson's disease. *European Journal of Neurology, 20*(1), 16–34.

Boeve, B. F. (2011). Progressive supranuclear palsy. *Parkinsonism and Related Disorders, 18*, S192–194.

Borroni, B., Goldwurm, S., Cerini, C., Cosseddu, M., Meucci, N., Mariani, C., . . . Padovani, A. (2010). Familial aggregation in progressive supranuclear palsy and corticobasal syndrome. *European Journal of Neurology* [Epub ahead of print]

Borroni, B., Turla, M., Bertasi, V., Agosti, C., Gilberti, N., & Padovani, A (2008). Cognitive and behavioral assessment in the early stages of neurodegenerative extrapyramidal syndromes. *Archives oof Gerontology and Geriatrics, 47*(1), 53–61.

Bower, J. H., Maraganore, D. M., McDonnell, S. K., & Rocca, W. A. (1997). Incidence of progressive supranuclear palsy and multiple system atrophy in Olmsted County, Minnesota, 1976 to 1990. *Neurology, 49*(5), 1284–1288.

Brooks, D.J. (2010).Imaging approaches to Parkinson disease. *Journal of Nuclear Medicine, 51*(4), 596–609.

Burn, D. J., & Lees, A. J. (2002). Progressive supranuclear palsy: Where are we now? *Lancet Neurol*, 1(6), 359–369.

Caffrey, T. M., Joachim, C., Paracchini, S., Esiri, M. M., & Wade-Martins, R. (2006). Haplotype-specific expression of exon 10 at the human MAPT locus. *Human Molecular Genetics, 15*(24), 3529–3537.

Cotelli, M., Borroni, B., Vanenti, R., Alberaci, A., Calabria, M., Agosti, C., . . . Cappa, S. F. (2006). Action and object naming in frontotemporal dementia, progressive supranuclear palsy, and corticobasal degeneration. *Neuropsychology, 20*(5), 558–565.

Delisle, M. B., Murrell, J. R., Richardson, R., Trofatter, J. A., Rascol, O., Soulages, X., Moh. . . Ghetti, B. (1999). A mutation at codon 279 (N279K) in exon 10 of the Tau gene causes a tauopathy with dementia and supranuclear palsy. *Acta Neuropathologica, 98*, 62–77.

De Silva, R., Hope, A., Pittman, A., Weale, M. E., Morris, H. R., Wood, N. W., & Lees, A. J. (2003). Strong association of the Saitohin gene Q7 variant with progressive supranuclear palsy. *Neurology, 61*, 407–409.

Dickson, D. W., Rademakers, R., & Hutton, M. L. (2007). Progressive supranuclear palsy: Pathology and genetics. *Brain Pathology, 17*(1), 74–82.

Donker Kaat, L., Boon, A. J., Kamphorst, W., Ravid, R., Duivenvoorden, H. J., & van Swieten, J. C. (2007). Frontal presentation in progressive supranuclear palsy. *Neurology, 69*(8), 723–729.

Donker Kaat, L., Boon, A. J., Azmani, A., Kamphorst, W., Breteler, M. M., Anar, B., . . . van Swieten, J. C. (2009). Familial aggregation of parkinsonism in progressive supranuclear palsy. *Neurology, 73*(2), 98–105.

Goetz, C. G., Leurgans, S., Lang, A. E., & Litvan, I. (2003). Progression of gait, speech and swallowing deficits in progressive supranuclear palsy. *Neurology*, 60, 917–922.

Golbe, L. I., & Ohman-Strickland, P. A. (2007). A clinical rating scale for progressive supranuclear palsy. *Brain, 130*(Pt 6), 1552–1565.

Grafman, J., Litvan, I., & Stark, M. (1995). Neuropsychological features of progressive supranuclear palsy. *Brain Cognition, 28*, 311–20.

Green, P. (2009). Parkinson-plus syndromes. In L. P. Rowland and T. A. Pedley (Eds.), *Merritt's neurology*. Philadelphia, PA: Lippincott Williams & Wilkins.

Gröschel, K., Hauser, T. K., Luft, A., Patronas, N., Dichgans, J., Litvan, I., & Schulz, J. B. (2004). Magnetic resonance imaging-based volumetry differentiates progressive supranuclear palsy from corticobasal degeneration. *Neuroimage, 21*(2), 714–724.

Hassan, A., Parisi, J. E., & Josephs, K. A. (2012). Autopsy-proven progressive supranuclear palsy presenting as behavioral variant frontotemporal dementia. *Neurocase, 18*(6), 478–488.

Höglinger, G. U., Melhem, N. M., Dickson, D. W., Sleiman, P. M., Wang, L. S., Klei, L., . . . Schellenberg, G. D. (2011). Identification of common variants influencing risk of the tauopathy progressive supranuclear palsy. *Nature Genetics, 43*(7), 699–705.

Houghton, D., & Litvan, I. (2007). Unraveling progressive supranuclear palsy: from the bedside back to the bench. *Parkinsonism and Related Disorders, 3*, S341–346.

Josephs, K. A., & Dickson, D. W. (2003). Diagnostic accuracy of progressive supranuclear palsy in the Society for Progressive Supranuclear Palsy brain bank. *Movement Disorders, 18*(9), 1018–1026.

Kato, N., Arai, K., & Hattori, T. (2003). Study of the rostral midbrain atrophy in progressive supranuclear palsy. *Journal of Neurological Sciences*, 210(1–2), 57–60.

Komori, T. (1999). Tau-positive glial inclusionsin progressive supranuclear palsy, corticobasaldegeneration and Pick's disease. *Brain Pathology, 9*, 663–679.

Kristensen, M. O. (1985). Progressive supranuclear palsy—20 years later. *Acta Neurologica Scandinavica*, 71(3):, 177–189.

Lee, W., Williams, D. R., & Storey, E. (2012). Cognitive testing in the diagnosis of parkinsonian disorders: a critical appraisal of the literature. *Movement Disorders, 27*(10), 1243–54.

Litvan, I., Agid, Y., Calne, D., Campbell, G., Dubois, B., Duvoisin, R. C., . . . Zee, D. S. (1996). Clinical research criteria for the diagnosis of progressive supranuclear palsy

(Steele-Richardson-Olszewski syndrome): report of the NINDS-SPSP international workshop. *Neurology*, 47, 1–9.

Litvan, I. (2003). Update on epidemiological aspects of progressive supranuclear palsy. *Mov Disorders*, *18* (Suppl 6), S43–50.

Longoni, G., Agosta, F., Kostić, V. S., Stojković, T., Pagani, E., Stošić-Opinćal, T., & Filippi, M. (2011). MRI measurements of brainstem structures in patients with Richardson's syndrome, progressive supranuclear palsy-parkinsonism, and Parkinson's disease. *Movement Disorders*, *26*(2), 247–255.

Melquist, S., Craig, D. W., Huentelman, M. J., Crook, R., Pearson, J. V., Baker, M., . . . Stephan, D. A. (2007). Identification of a novel risk locus for progressive supranuclear palsy by a pooled genomewide scan of 500,288 singlenucleotide polymorphisms. *American Journal of Human Genetics*, *80*, 769–778.

Millar, D., Griffiths, P., Zermansky, A. J., & Burn, D. J. (2006). Characterizing behavioral and cognitive dysexecutive changes in progressive supranuclear palsy. *Movement Disorders*, *21*(2), 199–207.

Morelli, M., Arabia, G., Novellino, F., Salsone, M., Giofrè, L., Condino, F., Messina, D., & Quattrone, A. (2011). MRI measurements predict PSP in unclassifiable parkinsonisms: a cohort study. *Neurology*, 77(11), 1042–1047.

Morris, H. R., Osaki, Y., Holton, J., Lees, A. J., Wood, N. W., Revesz, T., & Quinn, N. (2003). Tau exon 10 +16 mutation FTDP-17 presenting clinically as sporadic young-onset PSP. *Neurology*, *61*, 102–104.

Muller, J., Wenning, G. K., Wissel, J., Seppi, K., & Poewe, W. (2002). Botulinum toxin treatment in atypical parkinsonian disorders associated with disabling focal dystonia. *Journal of Neurology*, *249*, 300–304.

Nath, U., Ben-Shlomo, Y., Thomson, R.G., Lees, A. J., & Burn, D. J. (2003). Clinical features and natural history of progressive supranuclear palsy: A clinical cohort study. *Neurology*, *60*, 910–916.

Nath, U., Ben-Shlomo, Y., Thomson, R. G., Morris, H. R., Wood, N. W., Lees, A. J., & Burn, D. J. (2001). The prevalence of progressive supranuclear palsy (Steele-Richardson-Olszewski syndrome) in the UK. *Brain*, *124*(Pt 7), 1438–1449.

Nath, U., Donker Kaat, L., Boon, A., Kamphorst, W., Ravid, R., Duivenvoorden, H. J., & van Swieten, J. C. (2007). Frontal presentation in progressive supranuclear palsy. *Neurology*, *69*, 723–729.

Oba, H., Yagishita, A., Terada, H., Barkovich, A. J., Kutomi, K., Yamauchi, T., . . . Suzuki, S. (2005). New and reliable MRI diagnosis for progressive supranuclear palsy. *Neurology*, *64*(12), 2050–5.

Ogaki, K., Li, Y., Takanashi, M., Ishikawa, K., Kobayashi, T., Nonaka, T., . . . Hattori, N. (2013). Analyses of the MAPT, PGRN, and C9orf72 mutations in Japanese patients with FTLD, PSP, and CBS. *Parkinsonism and Related Disorders*, *19*(1), 15–20.

O'Sullivan, S. S., Massey, L.A., Williams, D. R., Silveira-Moriyama, L., Kempster, P. A., Holton, J. L., . . . & Lees, A. J. (2008). Clinical outcomes of progressive supranuclear palsy and multiple system atrophy. *Brain*, *131*, 1362–1372.

Poorkaj, P., Muma, N. A., Zhukareva, V., Cochran, E. J., Shannon, K. M., Hurtig, H., . . . Schellenberg, G. D. (2002). An R5L tau mutation in a subject with a progressive supranuclear palsy phenotype. *Annals of Neurology*, *52*(4), 511–516.

Quattrone, A., Nicoletti, G., Messina, D., Fera, F., Condino, F., Pugliese, P., . . . Gallo, O. (2008). MR imaging index for differentiation of progressive supranuclear palsy from Parkinson disease and the Parkinson variant of multiple system atrophy. *Radiology*, *246*(1), 214–221.

Rademakers, R., Melquist, S., Cruts, M., Theuns, J., Del-Favero, J., Poorkaj, P., . . . Hutton, M. L. (2005). High-density SNP haplotyping suggests altered regulation of tau gene expression in progressive supranuclear palsy. *Human Molecular Genetics, 14,* 3281–3292.

Rohrer, J. D., Paviour, D., Vandrovcova, J., Hodges, J., de Silva, R., & Rossor, M. N. (2011). Novel L284R MAPT mutation in a family with an autosomal dominant progressive supranuclear palsy syndrome. *Neurodegenerative Diseases, 8*(3), 149–152.

Ros, R., Thobois, S., Streichenberger, N., Kopp, N., Sánchez, M. P., Pérez, M., . . . de Yébenes, J. G. (2005). A new mutation of the tau gene, G303V, in early-onset familial progressive supranuclear palsy. *Archives of Neurology, 62,* 1444–1450.

Rossi, G., Gasparoli, E., Pasquali, C., Di Fede, G., Testa, D., Albanese, A., Bracco, F., & Tagliavini, F. (2004). Progressive supranuclear palsy and Parkinson's disease in a family with a new mutation in the tau gene. *Annals of Neurology, 55,* 448.

Sanchez-Gonzalez, M. A., Garcia-Cabezas, M. A., Rico, B., & Cavada, C. (2005). The primate thalamus is a key target for brain dopamine. *Journal of Neuroscience, 25,* 6076–6083.

Schrag, A., Ben-Shlomo, Y., & Quinn, N. P. (1999). Prevalence of progressive supranuclear palsy and multiple system atrophy: a cross-sectional study. *Lancet, 354*(9192), 1771–1775.

Schrag, A., Good, C. D., Miszkiel, K., Morris, H. R., Mathias, C. J., Lees, A. J., & Quinn, N. P. (2000). Differentiation of atypical parkinsonian syndromes with routine MRI. *Neurology, 54*(3), 697–702.

Spillantini, M. G., Murrell, J. R., Goedert, M., Farlow, M. R., Klug, A., & Ghetti, B. (1998). Mutation in the tau gene in familial multiple system tauopathy with presenile dementia. *Proceedings of the National Academy of Sciences USA, 95*(13), 7737–7741.

Spina, S., Farlow, M. R., Unverzagt, F. W., Kareken, D. A., Murrell, J. R., Fraser, G., . . . Ghetti, B. (2008). The tauopathy associated with mutation +3 in intron 10 of Tau: characterization of the MSTD family. *Brain, 131*(Pt 1), 72–89.

Stamelou, M., De Silva, R., Arias-Carrión, O., Boura, E., Höllerhage, M., Oertel, W. H., . . . Höglinger, G. U. (2010). Rational therapeutic approaches to progressive supranuclear palsy. *Brain, 133*(Pt 6), 1578–1590.

Stamelou, M., Reuss, A., Pilatus, U., Magerkurth, J., Niklowitz, P., Eggert, K. M., . . . Höglinger, G. U. (2008). Short-term effects of coenzyme Q10 in progressive supranuclear palsy: a randomized, placebo-controlled trial. *Movement Disorders, 23*(7), 942–949.

Stanford, P. M., Halliday, G. M., Brooks, W. S., Kwok, J. B., Storey, C. E., Creasey, H., . . . Schofield, P. R. (2000). Progressive supranuclear palsy pathology caused by a novel silent mutation in exon 10 of the tau gene: expansion of the disease phenotype caused by tau gene mutations. *Brain, 123*(Pt 5), 880–893.

Steele, J. C., Richardson, J. C., & Olszewski, J. (1964). Progressive supranuclear palsy. *Archives of Neurology, 10,* 333–359.

Takahashi, M., Weidenheim, K. M., Dickson, D. W., & Ksiezak-Reding, H. (2002). Morphological and biochemical correlations of abnormal tau filaments in progressive supranuclear palsy. *Journal of Neuropathology and Experimental Neurology, 61*(1), 33.

Tsuboi, Y., Uitti, R. J., Delisle, M. B., Ferreira, J. J., Brefel-Courbon, C., Rascol, O., . . . Wszolek, Z. K. (2002). Clinical features and disease haplotypes of individuals with the N279K tau gene mutation: a comparison of the pallidopontonigral degeneration kindred and a French family. *Archives of Neurology, 59,* 943–950.

Verny, M., Duyckaerts, C., Agid, Y., & Hauw, J. J. (1996). The significance of cortical pathology in progressive supranuclear palsy. Clinico-pathological data in 10 cases. *Brain, 119*(Pt 4), 1123.

Warmuth-Metz, M., Naumann, M., Csoti, I., & Solymosi, L. (2001). Measurement of the midbrain diameter on routine magnetic resonance imaging: a simple and accurate method of differentiating between Parkinson disease and progressive supranuclear palsy. *Archives of Neurology, 58*(7), 1076–1079.

Warren, N. M., & Burn, D. J. (2007). Progressive supranuclear palsy. *Practical Neurology, 7*, 16–23.

Warren, N. M., Piggott, M. A., Lees, A. J., & Burn, D. J. (2007). The basal ganglia cholinergic neurochemistry of PSP and other neurodegenerative diseases. *Journal of Neurology, Neurosurgery and Psychiatry, 78*(6), 571.

Williams, D. R., De Silva, R., Paviour, D. C., Pittman, A., Watt, H. C., Kilford, L., . . . Lees, A. J. (2005). Characteristics of two distinct clinical phenotypes in pathologically proven progressive supranuclear palsy: Richardson's syndrome and PSP-parkinsonism. *Brain 128*, 1247–1258.

Williams, D. R., Holton, J. L., Strand, C., Pittman. A., De Silva. R., Lees, A. J., & Revesz, T. (2007). Pathological tau burden and distribution distinguishes progressive supranuclear palsy-parkinsonism from Richardson's syndrome. *Brain, 130*, 1566–1576.

Williams, D. R., & Lees, A. J. (2009). Progressive supranuclear palsy: Clinicopathological concepts and diagnostic challenges. *Lancet Neurology, 8*(3), 270–279.

17 Neuropsychological and Neuropsychiatric Features of Dystonia and the Impact of Medical and Surgical Treatment

Mariam Torkamani and Marjan Jahanshahi

INTRODUCTION TO DYSTONIA

Dystonia is a movement disorder associated with sustained or intermittent muscle contractions, abnormal postures, and involuntary movements (Albanese et al., 2013). Dystonia is the third most common movement disorder after Parkinson's disease (PD) and essential tremor. According to the Epidemiological Study of Dystonia in Europe, around 75,000 people have Dystonia in Europe and the annual period prevalence of primary dystonia was 152 per million (Epidemiological Study of Dystonia in Europe, 2000). This disfiguring, disabling and often painful condition can affect various aspects of the patient's life. The muscle contractions can be painful and dystonia can make participation in simple daily activities difficult, and the outward disfiguring nature of the condition can have a negative impact on various aspects of the patient's life.

Classification of Dystonia

Until recently, dystonia was classified by etiology (e.g., primary versus secondary), bodily distribution (focal, multifocal, segmental, hemidystonia, generalized) and age of onset (early vs. late onset). A recent expert review of the classification of dystonia has proposed two major axes, the first based on clinical characteristics and the second based on etiology (Albanese et al., 2013). However, as most of the existing literature use previous classifications, we have used these in structuring the current chapter.

The primary form is diagnosed when dystonia is the only symptom present (other than tremor) and no structural brain abnormality can be identified by imaging. The majority of cases of primary dystonia are idiopathic, with the cause unknown, and a large proportion likely to have a genetic origin. In contrast, secondary dystonia is related to identifiable causes such as structural brain pathology, or are medication-induced such as by neuroleptics (tardive dystonia) or develops in association with a degenerative disorder (e.g., PD) or secondary to psychological factors (psychogenic dystonia). In addition, Fahn, Bressman, and Marsden (1998) also distinguished dystonia plus syndromes (e.g., dystonia plus parkinsonism or dystonia plus myoclonus and dopa responsive dystonia-DRD) and heredodegenerative dystonia. Dystonia commonly affects a single body part in isolation (focal), or two or more unrelated body parts (mulitfocal). Segmental dystonia is diagnosed when two adjacent body parts are involved whereas generalized dystonia affects the legs and one or more parts of the body. Dystonia can affect muscles of the neck (cervical dystonia [CD] or torticollis), eyes (blepharospasm), face (hemifacial), larynx (laryngeal or spasmodic dysphonia), mouth, tongue, and jaw muscles (oromandibular, which, in combination with blepharospam, is labeled as Meige's disease) or the hand (focal hand). Writer's cramp is the most common focal hand dystonia; others include typist's, musician's, and pianist's cramps (Frucht, 2004). The new classification, distinguishes five categories based on age of onset: infancy (birth to 2 years), childhood (3–12 years), adolescence (13–20 years), early adulthood (21–40 years), late adulthood (>40 years) (Albanese et al., 2013). The age of onset of dystonia and the particular body part first affected have prognostic implications. Early-onset dystonia, particularly in the legs, is likely to spread to other parts of the body and to become generalized. In contrast, late-onset dystonia, particularly in the upper parts of the body, is likely to remain focal or segmental.

Pathophysiology of Dystonia

The exact cause of dystonia is not known. Dystonia is considered a movement disorder associated with dysfunction of the basal ganglia (Berardelli et al., 1998; Marsden, 1976), although more recently, cerebellar involvement in the disorder has also been documented (Argyelan, 2009; Delmaire et al., 2007; Jinnah & Hess, 2006; Neychev, Fan, Mitev, Hess, & Jinnah, 2008). Enlarged putamina in patients with CD or focal hand dystonia (Black, Ongur, & Perlmutter, 1998), increased gray matter volume in the internal segment of the globus pallidus (GPi) in CD (Draganski, Thun-Hohenstein, Bogdahn, Winkler, & May, 2003), and hyperechogenic basal ganglia lesions particularly in the lenticular nucleus have been documented in patients with CD (75%) or focal hand dystonia (83%) (Becker et al., 1997). Structural abnormality in the cerebellar cortex, particularly lobules V and VI, have been reported in writer's cramp (Delmaire et al., 2007) and CD (Draganski et al., 2003). Imaging studies have shown movement-related overactivity of the dorsolateral prefrontal cortex, the anterior cingulate, the SMA and the lenticular nuclei, and underactivation of the primary motor cortex (e.g., Ceballos-Baumann et al., 1995; Dresel, Haslinger, Castrop, Wohlschlaeger, & Ceballos-Baumann, 2006). Genetic studies have now identified many different genetic forms associated with various types of primary or dystonia plus syndromes or secondary heredodegenerative dystonia, with the *DYT1* gene mutation in chromosome 9q34 associated with primary generalized dystonia being the first discovered (see Nemeth, 2002).

Furthermore, according to the De Long (1990) and Albin, Reiner, Anderson, Penney, and Young (1990) models, hyperkinetic movement disorders such as dystonia are associated with reduced inhibitory output from the GPi, which gives rise to increased thalamic and cortical activation. There is some support for this model from hyperkinetic transgenic mice model of *DYT1* dystonia (e.g., Chiken, Shashidharan, & Nambu, 2008) and neuronal recordings from the GPi of patients with dystonia undergoing deep brain stimulation (DBS) surgery (e.g., Vitek et al., 1999), but the improvement of dystonia with GPi DBS, which reduces the activity of the GPi are not consistent with these "rate" models. Using different TMS protocols, reduced cortico–cortical inhibition (Edwards, Huang, Wood, Rothwell, & Bhatia, 2003; Ridding, Sheean, Rothwell, Inzelberg, & Kujiral, 1995) and increased plasticity (e.g., Quartarone et al., 2003) have been demonstrated in dystonia. A further abnormality documented is increased temporal and spatial discrimination thresholds (Bara-Jimenez, Shelton, & Hallett, 2000; Tinazzi et al., 2002). Furthermore, since not all carriers of the dystonia genes develop the dystonic symptoms, and task-specific dystonias such as writer's cramp and musician's dystonia have been associated with hours spent writing/practicing (Roze et al., 2009; Schmidt et al., 2009) and are often preceded by some specific trauma/insult (e.g., Defazio et al., 1998), the importance of environmental factors in the onset of dystonia in genetically predisposed and vulnerable individuals is highlighted.

COGNITIVE FUNCTION IN DYSTONIA

Cognitive deficits are not considered part of the initial clinical presentation or disease progression in primary dystonia. This clinical impression is largely confirmed by the handful of studies that have investigated cognitive function in primary dystonia (see Table 17-1). The picture is different in dystonia plus syndromes, which are commonly associated with cognitive deficits.

Cognition in Primary Dystonia

A number of early studies focused on specific aspects of cognition and established three main findings. First, children with dystonia were not intellectually

Table 17-1 Investigations of cognitive function in primary dystonia, describing sample characteristics, the cognitive tests administered and the specific deficits found

Author	*N*	*Sample characteristics*	*Measures*		*Main findings*
Jahanshahi 2003	10 12	Various (3 generalized, 5 cervical and 2 focal arm) Age and IQ matched controls	– Dual task performance; tapping and pegboard – Missing Digit Test – NART – PVSAT – RNG – Word fluency test	– Self ordered random number sequences – Stroop – Visual–visual conditional associative learning – WCST	Poorer category word fluency and dual task performance relative to controls
Scott 2003	14	Various (11 generalized, 2 focal and 1 segmental)	– CANTAB: ID/ED set shifting; reaction time; spatial working memory; spatial span; stockings of Cambridge; rapid visual information processing test	– Functional Limitations Profile – HADS – SF36	Greater deficits on attentional set shifting relative to normative data
Balas 2006	28 28	Generalized (20 manifesting and 8 non–manifesting DYT1 gene carriers) Education, gender, and IQ matched controls	– Raven's matrices – RAVLT – Rey complex figure – Verbal fluency (phonemic and semantic) – TMT – CANTAB ID/ED set shifting; stockings of Cambridge; spatial working memory; spatial span; spatial span reverse	– Stroop – WAIS–III digit span; similarities; symbol search – Judgment of line orientation – Purdue pegboard, beck questionnaire – STAI – Visual analogue scale	Increased verbal memory retroactive interference in symptomatic DYT1 group relative to controls

Allam 2007	9	Blepharospasm	– RAVLT – Toulouse Pieron Test – Stroop	– SAT – WMS–R: digit and digit symbol subtests	Deficits in sustained attention
	9	Age and education matched controls			
Bugalho 2008	45	Various (15 Blepharospasm 15 Cervical dystonia 15 Writer's cramp)	– WCST – Stroop – Benton visual retention test	– WAIS–Block assembly test – Y–BOCS	More perseverative errors on WCST relative to controls
	27	Age, gender, and education matched controls			
Aleman 2009	20	Blepharospasm	– Raven's matrices – WAIS–I: five digits test manual sequences – WMS: – lists of words I and II Spatial location – WCST	– Purdue pegboard test – Oral making trails – Digital recognition – Tactile denomination – Tapping test – BAI – BDI	More impairments in complex movement planning, motor dexterity, visuospatial working memory, and tactile object recognition relative to controls
	17	Age, gender and education matched controls			
Dias 2009	22	Blepharospasm	– MMSE – FAB		No difference between groups in MMSE or FAB. Concluded that blepharospasm patients do not have executive dysfunction.
	29	Age, gender, education and duration of illness matched patients with hemifacial spasm			

NART: National Adult Reading Test; PVSAT: Paced Visual Serial Addition Test; RNG: Random Number Generation; WCST: Wisconsin Card Sorting Test; CANTAB: Cambridge Neuropsychological Test Automated Battery; ID/ED: Intra/Extra dimensional; HADS: Hospital Anxiety and Depression Scale; SF-36: Short Form 36; RAVLT: Rey Auditory Verbal Learning Test; TMT: Trials Making Test; WAIS: Wechsler Adult Intelligence Scale; STAI: Spielberger State and Trait Anxiety Inventory; SAT: Sustained Attention Test; WMS: Wechsler Memory Test; Y-BOCS; R: Revised: Yale-Brown Obsessive Compulsive Scale; BAI: Beck Anxiety Inventory; BDI: Beck Depression Inventory; MMSE: Mini Mental State Examination; FAB: Frontal Assessment Battery impaired and, in fact, had higher IQs than controls (Riklan, Cullinan, & Cooper, 1976). Second, although some report normal perception of egocentric space (Anastasopoulos et al., 1998), others documented significantly worse manipulation of personal space but not spatial perception (Hinse et al., 1996) or deficits in extrapersonal orientation in dystonia (Leplow & Stubinger, 1994). Third, treatment of dystonia with high-dose anticholinergics produces impairment on a test of explicit memory and the Stroop task (Taylor, Lang, Saint-Cyr, Riley, & Ranawaya, 1991).

Recent studies that have investigated cognition in primary dystonia have used relatively extensive batteries of standardized neuropsychological tests assessing various domains of cognition (see Table 17-1).

In 2003, Jahanshahi and colleagues assessed executive function, working memory, and attention (see Table 17-1) in a sample of 10 patients with generalized or focal dystonias and compared their performance with age and IQ matched healthy controls. The patients only performed significantly worse than healthy controls on category word fluency and concurrent performance of finger tapping and peg placement under dual task conditions. However, when the significance threshold was adjusted to account for the number of comparisons, these group differences were no longer significant. In the same year, Scott and colleagues (2003) found that patients with dystonia differed from the normative data only on a single test, the extra-dimensional set-shifting subtest of the Cambridge Neuropsychological Test Automated Battery (CANTAB) (see Table 17-1). Patients with clinical depression often fail this subtest (Purcell, Maruff, Kyrios, & Pantelis, 1997), but the dystonia patients who failed the subtest did not differ from those who passed it in terms of depression. This dysfunction in set shifting has been subsequently reported in some (Bugalho, Correa, Guimarraes, & Xavier, 2008; Aleman, de Erausquin, & Mitchell, 2009), but not all (Balas, Peretz, Badarny, Scott, & Giladi, 2006) studies (see Table 17-1).

Bugalho and colleagues (2008) found greater perseverative errors on the Wisconsin Card Sorting test (WCST), suggesting a disturbance in set shifting in patients with focal and segmental dystonia relative to controls. Patients with blepharospasm also showed more preservative errors on the WCST than matched healthy controls, suggestive of deficits in set shifting (Aleman et al., 2009). These patients with blepharospasm also had more difficulties with planning complex movements requiring coordination of both hands, tactile identification of objects, and reverse visuospatial span. Since the patients and controls were matched in terms of mood as well as age and IQ, it was concluded that the cognitive deficits were independent of mood disturbance in dystonia. Patients with blepharospasm had similar scores on measures of global cognitive and frontal lobe functioning to a matched control group with hemifacial spasm (HFS; Dias et al., 2009). Balas et al. (2006) compared cognition in manifesting and nonmanifesting *DYT1* gene carriers relative to healthy controls. They found a significant difference in retroactive interference on a test of verbal memory in manifesting *DYT1* gene carriers relative to controls, but not between nonmanifesting *DYT1* gene carries and controls. Furthermore, the manifesting gene carriers did not show any deficits on the set shifting subtest from the CANTAB battery or any of the other measures of cognition (see Table 17-1) relative to healthy controls.

It is likely that the patient's motor symptoms and their conscious attempts to control these during cognitive assessment interferes with performance on some cognitive tests (Jahanshahi, Rowe, & Fuller, 2003). For example, Allam, Frank, Pereira, and Tomaz (2007) found deficits on a test of sustained attention in patients with blepharospasm, which improved following symptomatic improvement with botullinum toxin (Botox), such that after treatment the patients did not differ from the controls (see Figure 17-1).

A number of studies have assessed other aspects of cognitive function. Hoffland and colleagues (2011) found deficits in praxis in patients with CD relative to matched healthy controls. The patients made more errors and were slower in copying meaningless gestures, but not in copying meaningful gestures. Fiorio, Tinazzi, and Aglioti (2006) found slower mental rotation of the hands, but not feet, in patients with writer's cramp relative to matched healthy controls. Ploner, Stenz, Fassdorf, and Arnold (2005) investigated egocentric and allocentric spatial memory in CD and found no significant differences between patients and controls, although unlike controls, the patients seemed to use a single strategy in completing different spatial tasks. Ghilardi and colleagues (2003) assessed sequence learning in nonmanifesting (NMC) *DYT1* gene carriers and healthy controls, and found significantly reduced sequence learning in NMC *DYT1* gene carriers relative to healthy controls, with the former group showing a different time course of learning. The impaired learning in the NMC group was associated with significant increased activation in the presupplementary motor area and the lateral cerebellum and reduced activation in the left cingulate gyrus relative to the controls. In a later study, Carbon et al. (2011) investigated behavioral deficits and differences in patterns of brain activation in manifesting carriers (MC) of the *DYT1* gene as well as carriers of other primary dystonia mutations such as *DYT6*. Although both the MC and NMC of the *DYT1* gene showed similar deficits in sequence learning, DYT6 carriers had no such deficits. Furthermore,

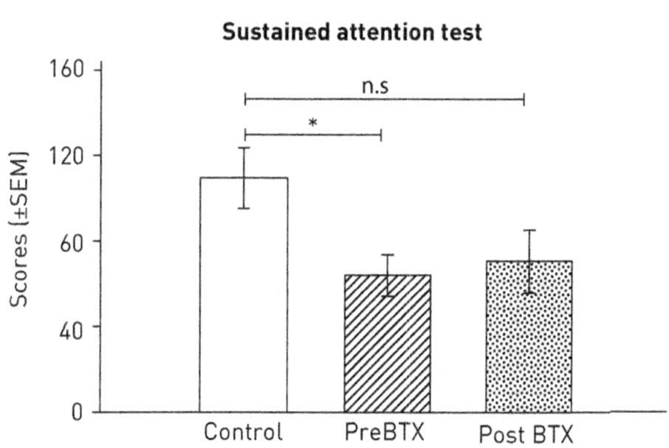

FIGURE 17-1
Scores on a sustained attention test for controls and patients with blepharospasm before and after Botulinum toxin (BTX) injections in the study of Allam et al. (2007).

MC of *DYT1* gene showed significant increases in sequence learning-related activation of the lateral cerebellum and right premortor and inferior partietal areas, indicating that deficits in explicit sequence learning may be specific to the *DYT1* genotype.

Cognition in Dystonia Plus Syndromes

Details of the studies that have investigated cognitive function in patients with dystonia plus syndromes are listed in Table 17-2 and considered next.

Cognition in Myoclonus Dystonia

Myoclonus dystonia (MD) is characterized by jerklike myoclonic movements in the face, neck, or limbs combined with dystonia, usually CD and writer's cramp. MD has an autosomal dominant mode of inheritance and is associated with mutation of the *SGCE* gene, and two loci have been identified on the *DYT11* at 7q21 and *DYT15* 15 18p11. Studies examining cognitive function in MD have provided mixed evidence. Doheny et al. (2002) completed a comprehensive genetic, neurological, motor, psychiatric, and neuropsychological assessment on 50 individuals from three families with MD (see Table 17-1). In all three families, mutation carriers had IQs in the average or high-average ranges, but deficits in verbal learning and memory were noted in one family, impaired memory was reported in another family, whereas no deficits were found in the third family. Deficits in processing speed were also found particularly in MC in one family, and to a lesser extent in another family. In contrast, Foncke and colleagues (2009) assessed cognition in 27 patients with MD and found no significant differences between the patients and controls or between the symptomatic and asymptomatic mutation carriers (see Table 17-2 for details). Klempir, Klempiroca, and Roth (2010) examined five members of a family with MD, and although details of the cognitive assessment were not provided, deficits in selective attention particularly on the Stroop and mild deficits in working memory were noted in three of the patients.

In a more recent study that compared MC and NC of the *DYT11* gene, and healthy controls, some differences between the three groups were found (van Tricht et al., 2012). The results showed that only MC showed executive dysfunction. With the exception of deficits on semantic verbal fluency, no other cognitive impairments were found in NC. There was no association between the severity of dystonia and cognitive performance, but patients with more severe myoclonus had lower semantic fluency scores. Patients who had experienced an anxiety disorder (N=23) performed significantly worse on the WAIS-III letter-number sequencing subtest, but, otherwise, psychiatric disorder was not associated with any effects on cognition. These results suggest that MC and NC not only differ in terms of genotype but also with respect to the cognitive phenotype.

Table 17-2 Investigations of cognitive function in dystonia plus syndromes

Author	*N*	*Sample characteristics*	*Measures*	*Main findings*
			i) Moyoclonous dystonia	
Doheny et al., 2002	50	Myoclonous dystonia (members of 3 families)	– WAIS–II Information; digit span; arithmetic; comprehension; similarities; letter–number sequencing; picture completion; matrix reasoning – CVLT – WMS–II – Visual reproduction Stroop – WCST – TMT – Verbal fluency (semantic & phonemic) – Shipley Institute of Living Scale	Results from three families with myoclonous. Average or high average IQ, impaired verbal learning and memory in one family, impaired memory in the second family, and no cognitive deficits in the third family. Deficits in processing speed in two of the families
Foncke 2009	27 42	Myoclonous dystonia (14 symptomatic, 13 asymptomatic) Healthy controls	– The Dutch Adult Reading Test – WAIS–II and III – Spatial reasoning – Stroop – TMT – Boston naming test – WMS–III – Fluency (phonemic and category) – Visual memory (Immediate and delayed recognition of faces) – RAVLT – Verbal memory (immediate and delayed recall)	No significant differences between patients and controls on any of the tests
Van Tricht et al., 2012	51 36	Myoclonous dystonia (31 DYT11 mutation carrying and 20 DYT11 non–mutation carrying) Healthy controls	– WAIS–III – Similarities – Matric reasoning – Stroop – TMT – Letter–number sequencing – Fluency (phonemic and semantic) – Rivermead behavioural memory test Paragraph recall subtest – RAVLT – Vienna test system – Dysexecutive Questionnaire – CFQ	Mild executive dysfunction in mutation carrying MD patients and impairment of verbal fluency in non–mutation carrying MD patients. Modest association of severity of myoclonous and executive function

(continued)

Table 17-2 Continued

Author	*N*	*Sample characteristics*	*Measures*	*Main findings*
			ii) Dopa Responsive dystonia	
Nitschke et al., 1998	3	Dopa responsive dystonia	– WAIS – WCST	Improvement in concept formation and performance of set shifting abilities under levodopa treatment
Lopez–Laso et al., 2011	14	Dopa responsive dystonia (7 adults and 7 children)	– WAIS–III – WISC–R	IQ in the borderline to extremely low ranges. Only 3 cases had received levodopa before age 10, had normal IQ.
			iii) X–linked parkinsonism dystonia	
Howe et al., 2009; Kemmotsu et al., 2011	1	X–linked dystonia–parkinsonism	– WASI: Vocabulary; similarities; block design; matrix reasoning subtests – MMSE – DRS–2 – WAIS: Attention; executive monitoring; digit span; digit symbol) – TMT – PASAT – Hopkins Verbal Learning Test–Revised – WMS: logical memory and face memory subtests – Boston naming test – Controlled Oral Word Association – Stroop – Category Fluency (Animals) – Benton Judgment of Line – Benton Facial Recognition Test – WCST – Luria Recursive Writing – Reading index, processing speed and working memory index – Wechsler Test of Adult – WAIS–III – Colour Trails Test – Test for Reception of Grammar – Benton Visual Form Discrimination	Impairment in memory, visuospatial language, executive function. Cognitive and motor slowing, reduced mental flexibility and impaired problem solving, which were improved after GPi–DBS.

WAIS: Wechsler Adult Intelligence Scale; CVLT: California Verbal Learning Test; WMS-R: Wechsler Memory Test; WCST: Wisconsin Card Sorting Test; TMT: Trail Making Test; RAVLT: Rey Auditory Verbal Learning Test; CFQ: Cognitive Failures Questionnaire; WISC-R: Wechsler Intelligence Scale for Children-Revised; DRS-2: Dementia Rating Scale 2, GPI-DBS: deep brain stimulation of internal segment of globus pallidus

Cognition in Dopa-Responsive Dystonia

Dopa-responsive dystonia (DRD) (sometimes referred to as Segawa disease) is in the majority of cases due to autosomal dominant guanosine triphosphate cyclohydrolase I (GTPCH) deficiency, affecting dopamine and serotonin synthesis and is the form of dystonia that responds to dopamine medication. DRD typically begins in early childhood with gait instability, and the disease may progress to become generalized (Segawa, Nomura, & Nishiyama, 2003). In the original descriptions of patients with DRD due to GTPCH I deficiency, no mental abnormalities were noted (Segawa et al., 2003; Segawa, Ohmi, Itoh, Aoyama, & Hayakawa, 1971). In a study reporting on three cases with DRD from the same family, Nitschke and colleagues (1998) found IQs in the low-average to average ranges, and impaired performance on the WCST. Levodopa treatment resulted in improved performance IQ, and fewer errors and perseverations and more categories correctly sorted on the WCST. From the retrospective inspection of the medical records and prospective neurological examination of 34 patients with genetically verified GTPCH deficiency, Trender-Gerhard et al. (2009) documented concentration problems and verbal memory deficits. More recently, Lopez-Laso and colleagues (2011) studied 14 patients (7 adult and 7 children). Nine of the 14 patients had IQs in the 59 to 84 range, which is lower than average. In fact, 6 of the 7 adults and 3 of the 7 children obtained IQs in the borderline to extremely low ranges.

Cognition in X-Linked Dystonia Parkinsonism

X-linked dystonia-parkinsonism (XDP), also known as Lubag's disease, is a progressive neurodegenerative disorder, that is initially highly characteristic of dystonia, but as the disease progresses, parkinsonian symptoms emerge while the dystonic symptoms lessen (Evidente, Gwinn-Hardy, Hardy, Hernandez, & Singleton, 2002; Lee et al., 2002). In a case report considering the suitability of a 67-year old male patient for DBS, Howe, Kellison, Fernandez, Okun, and Bowers (2009) assessed cognitive status using an extensive neuropsychological battery (see Table 17-2). On the Mini-Mental State Examination and Dementia Rating Scale, the patient was noted to be demented. He had a performance IQ in the borderline range and verbal IQ in the low-average range. Impairment in memory, visuospatial function, language, and executive functioning was reported. His overall cognitive performance remained in the impaired and demented range after withdrawal of anticholinergic medication. Patients with such extensive cognitive deficits are usually not considered suitable for DBS; however, due to the severity of his movement disorder, this case had GPi-DBS. Twenty-seven months following surgery, Kemmotsu et al. (2011) found mild improvements in memory and problem-solving abilities, no changes in cognitive status, language, and performance on a visuo-spatial task, but processing speed was reduced.

In summary, the existing evidence indicates that the main aspects of cognition are intact in primary dystonia, with only isolated deficits documented. Based on available evidence, it is not clear if cognitive impairment is a feature of the clinical presentation of MD, although at least those with gene mutations appear to have deficits in executive function. DRD can be associated with IQs below average, executive dysfunction and deficits in attention and memory. However, early treatment with levodopa appears to have a protective effect on cognitive function in DRD. XDP is associated with cognitive impairment and dementia.

PSYCHIATRIC FEATURES OF DYSTONIA

A common method employed in assessing psychiatric disorders in dystonia has been through the use of the structured clinical interview and the application of the criteria from various versions of the *Diagnostic Statistical Manual (DSM)*. Other studies have relied on the use of a range of validated self-report measures such as the Beck Depression Inventory, Beck Anxiety Inventory, and Yale Brown Obsessive-Compulsive Scale (YBOCS). Other key methodological differences between studies include the sample size and use of healthy participants or a disease control group. Furthermore, with notable exceptions (e.g., Dias et al., 2011), most studies failed to specify what percent of the samples were taking psychoactive medication for treatment of their dystonia or psychiatric disorders.

Psychiatric Features of Primary Dystonia

A large literature on psychiatric disorders in primary dystonia exists, which we will review by body parts affected.

Cervical Dystonia

There is ample evidence suggesting high rates of psychiatric disorder in CD. In one of the earliest studies of psychiatric features of CD, Patterson and Little (1943) reported psychiatric disorder in 21 of their 83 (25.3%) patients. Two of the 29 patients in the sample of Mathews et al. (1978) had had psychiatric treatment for depression prior to the onset of CD. Jahanshahi and Marsden (1988a) studied a sample of 100 patients with CD and a control group of 49 patients with cervical spondylosis (CS); 17% of CD and 27% of the CS patients had past or present psychiatric disorders, a difference that was not significant. In both groups, depression and anxiety were the most common psychiatric diagnoses (in 21 of 23 CD patients). The remaining two CD patients either had OCD or personality disorder. Moderate to severe depression affected 29% of CD and 15% of CS patients, but the differences between the groups in trait anxiety and obsessionality were not significant. Later studies confirmed moderate to severe depression, with the cognitive elements of depression distinguishing the CD and CS groups (Jahanshahi & Marsden, 1988b, 1990). The most striking difference was related to body image, with the responses of 39% of the CD and only 4% of the CS suggestive of a negative body image (Jahanshahi & Marsden, 1988a). Naber, Weinberger, Bullinger, Polsby, and Chase (1988) studied 32 patients with CD, and found mild depression in 25% of the sample, anxiety in only one patient, previous history of depression in three, and current psychiatric disorder in two patients only. In a study with 44 CD patients, 66% fulfilled the criteria for at least one diagnosis of current or lifetime psychiatric disorder (Wenzel et al., 1998). Among 40 patients with CD, 55% had at least one lifetime or current psychiatric disorder. 40% met the *DSM-III-R* criteria for anxiety and 37.5% met the criteria for major depressive disorder (MDD). In 42.5% of these patients, at least one lifetime diagnosis was made prior to the onset of their dystonia (Moraru et al., 2002).

In a study with one of the largest CD samples, Gundel, Wolf, Xidara, Busch, and Ceballos-Baumann (2001) assessed 116 patients with CD and found that both lifetime and current rates of mood and anxiety disorders were significantly elevated relative to the data from the general population, with lifetime mood disorders in 53.5% and anxiety disorders in 83.6%. Current social phobia showed a 10-fold increase in CD, whereas current mood disorders were increased by 2.4 times, and all lifetime psychiatric morbidity by 2.6 times in CD compared to the representative general population sample. In a further study, Gundel and colleagues (2003) compared psychiatric morbidity in 48 patients with CD and 48 patients with alopecia areta (AA), which results in hair loss from scalp. Compared to the German general population data, both CD and AA patients had significantly higher current and lifetime psychiatric morbidity. Mood disorders, anxiety disorders, and social phobia were the most common diagnoses in both groups. Most importantly, current psychiatric disorder was significantly higher in CD (77%) than in AA (42%). Lencer et al. (2009) assessed 70 patients with CD and 16 with blepharospasm. Compared to a population-based sample (N=3943), the dystonia patients had a 4.5-fold increased chance of a psychiatric disorder, and their lifetime prevalence of psychiatric or personality disorder was 70.9%; with rates of anxiety and major depression being high.

OCD is a frequent psychiatric feature in most types of dystonia. Bugalho, Correa, Guimaraes, and Xavier (2006) reported two cases with Meige syndrome and CD and writer's cramp, both of whom fulfilled *DSM-IV* criteria for OCD. Cavallaro et al. (2002) specifically investigated OCD in 76 patients with various types of primary focal dystonia. Twenty percent of their sample met *DSM-IV* criteria for OCD, and 3.5% for obsessive-compulsive spectrum disorders, and 10.5% were diagnosed with subclinical OCD. The prevalence of OCD in dystonia patients was significantly higher than healthy controls, and the patients had a significantly higher family morbidity risk for OCD than that found in the general population. Interestingly, in another study, Fabbrini et al. (2010) found high rates (57%) of psychiatric diagnosis in 89 patients with various forms of focal dystonia than those with hemifacial spasm (HFS), and healthy controls, but the incidence of anxiety or OCD was comparable between the three groups.

Blepharospasm

Blepharospam is frequently associated with depression and OCD. Compared to patients with HFS, the 159 cases with blepharospam assessed by Hall et al. (2005) were more than two times more likely to meet the criteria for generalized anxiety disorder, and had significantly higher depression scores, though they did not differ in terms of obsessivecompulsive symptoms. The study of Lencer et al. (2009) considered earlier, which showed a 4.5-fold increased rate of psychiatric morbidity in dystonia relative to the general population, also included patients with blepharospasm; as did the report by Fabbrini et al. (2010) who found mood and anxiety disorders in 67.7% of their sample. A similar rate of 71% with a current or lifetime psychiatric diagnosis was reported by Wenzel et al. (1998), with depression and phobias being the most common diagnoses.

In comparison to healthy controls, patients with blepharospasm have been shown to have higher rates of OCD and self-reported depression (Bihari, Hill,& Murphy, 1992). In a subsequent study, Broocks, Thiel, Angerstein, and Dressler (1998) found that although none of the patients with blepharospasm met the diagnostic criteria for OCD, they had significantly higher scores on the Hamburg Obsession-Compulsion Inventory than an HFS control group. In contrast, Munhoz et al. (2005) found high rates of OCD in both patients with blepharospasm and those with HFS. 67% of patients with blepharospasm and 70% of those with HFS met the *DSM-IV* criteria for OCD, and, although this difference was not significant, the severity of the obsessive compulsiveness was greater in patients with blepharospasm. Similarly, Mula et al. (2012) found equivalent rates of OCD in 26% of patients with focal dystonia (8 blepharospasm and 11 CD) and 28% of HFS, which were higher than in healthy controls; however, the rates of depression or anxiety did not differ from healthy controls. Furthermore, in their sample of 15 patients with CD, 15 with blepharospasm and 15 with writer's cramp, Bugalho et al. (2008) reported that only three fulfilled the *DSM-IV* criteria for clinical OCD, but significantly more patients scored above the cut-off score on the Yale-Brown Obsessive Compulsive Scale (YBOCS) than healthy controls. In Fabbrini et al.'s (2010) sample, only 1 in the 28 cases with blepharospasm (3.57%) had OCD, whereas 9.6% of the sample of Wenzel et al. (1998) met *DSM-III-R* criteria for OCD. Cavallaro et al. (2002) reported OCD in 20% of their sample with various types of focal dystonia, including blepharospam. These studies are consistent in suggesting that, although the rates of OCD in blepharospasm are significantly higher than healthy controls, they are similar to disease control groups such as patients with HFS. The differing rates ranging from none to 67% may partly result from the use of different assessment tools and criteria for diagnosis of OCD.

Spasmodic Dysphonia

In a study comparing patients with spasmodic dysphonia and matched healthy controls, 39% of the patients reported depression and anxiety on self-rating scales, which was significantly higher than controls (Cannito, 1991). Whurr, Lorch, and Nye (1998) found a similar rate of 37% for mild to moderate depression in patients with spasmodic dysphonia. More recently, in a sample of 48 patients with spasmodic dysphonia, 42% met the *DSM-IV* criteria for current psychiatric disorder, which was significantly higher than a control group with vocal fold paralysis (20%) (Gundel, Busch, Ceballos-Baumann, & Seifert, 2007). Fabbrini et al. (2010) also examined 16 patients with laryngeal dystonia and found mood disorders in 12.5%, anxiety disorders in 18.7%, and adjustment disorders in 18.7%, but no OCD. However, the frequency of these psychiatric disorders was not significantly different from healthy controls.

Focal Hand Dystonia and Writer's Cramp

In one of the earliest studies of writer's cramp, based on clinical observation, Bindman and Tibbetts (1977) reported that 9 of the 10 patients with writer's cramp displayed obsessive personalities. In a study that compared anxiety in writer's cramp patients with healthy controls, no significant differences were found (Harrington, Wieck, Marks, & Marsden, 1988), and only 3 of the 22 patients (13.6%) had general anxiety disorder. Kubota and colleagues (2001) compared 12 patients with writer's cramp and found significantly higher obsessive-compulsive symptoms in the patients compared to a group of individuals with writing impairments due to peripheral nerve lesions and compared to healthy controls. Grafman, Cohen, and Hallett (1991) studied 20 cases with focal hand dystonia using the MMPI, the STAI and the Beck Depression Inventory, and, other than mild depression in 20%, the scores on the personality scales were within the normal range and none of the patients had a remarkable psychiatric history. It was concluded that focal hand dystonia is not associated with psychopathology. In contrast, Voon and colleagues (2010) studied 39 patients with focal hand dystonia, and found that 13% of the patients met the criteria for OCD compared with 2% in the general population. Recurrent depression was present in 18% of the patients and current or previous depression in 33%, 41% of whom had a family history of depression. Anxiety disorders affected 26% of the sample. None of the 11 patients with arm dystonia assessed by Fabbrini et al. (2010) had mood or anxiety disorders, and only 1 patient had OCD, and another had adjustment disorder. These rates were not different from their healthy control group. As noted by Fabbrini et al. (2011), the differences from the rates reported by Voon and colleagues may relate to the fact that although all their cases with focal hand dystonia had writer's cramp, the Voon sample consisted of people with musician's dystonia. Thus, although it seems that musician's dystonia is associated with psychiatric morbidity (Voon et al., 2010), other forms of focal hand dystonia, particularly writer's cramp, are not (Harrington et al., 1988; Grafman et al., 1991; Fabbrini et al., 2010).

Generalized Dystonia

In the sample of 329 community dwelling patients with dystonia of various presentations, studied by Lewis, Butler, and Jahanshahi (2008), 10.4% had generalized dystonia and 30% had moderate to severe depression. The extent of dystonia had a significant effect on depression scores, which was due to patients with focal dystonia having lower scores. Around 54% of the participants were critical of their appearance, and 25% felt that there were permanent (negative) changes in their appearance. The body part associated with the highest level of depression was the neck, and patients with CD had the highest depressive scores, whereas depression was lower in patients with generalized dystonia. These results suggest that since postural abnormality is most visible in patients with CD, it is associated with high levels of perceived stigma (Papathanasiou, MacDonald, Whurr, & Jahanshahi, 2001). Similarly since generalized dystonia is usually early onset, patients are more likely to have adjusted better over time. In this sample, self-esteem, body concept, disfigurement, and quality of life were significant predictors of depression.

There is evidence for the association of recurrent MDD with the *DYT1* mutation. Heiman et al. (2004) studied a large group of patients with the *DYT1* gene mutation and compared manifesting carriers (MC), nonmanifesting carriers (NMC), and noncarriers (NC). They found that the risk of recurrent MDD was increased in both MC and NMC compared to NC. The prevalence of early-onset recurrent MDD was 12.5% in MC, 10% in NMC and 1.5% in NC group. The severity of dystonia was not associated with the risk of recurrent MDD. It was concluded that the psychiatric expression of *DYT1* appears to be limited to recurrent early-onset MDD because carriers were not at increased risk for other affective disorders. Similarly, early-onset recurrent MDD was associated with the *DYT1* mutation, and this association was independent of motor manifestations of dystonia. The same group (Heiman et al., 2007) subsequently investigated rates of OCD in their sample. There were no significant differences in OCD between the three groups, with the OCD rates of 3% in MC, 2% in NMC, and 5% in NC. Therefore, unlike early-onset MDD, which is associated with the *DYT1* gene, no association was found with OCD.

Psychiatric Features of Dystonia Plus Syndromes

Myoclonus Dystonia

In a study of 50 individuals from three families with MD, Doheny et al. (2002) found occurrence of depression in all three families, and OCD, substance abuse, anxiety disorders, and psychosis in two of the three families.

In their sample of MC and NMC carriers of the *DYT11* mutation, Foncke et al. (2009) reported that significantly more of the MC had *DSM-IV* diagnoses (11 of 27 patients) relative to the controls (6 of 42). The severity of dystonia in MC significantly correlated with anxiety and depression. In contrast, the NMC did not have any significant psychiatric morbidity, with the exception of OCD in one case. The rates of OCD in both groups were not elevated relative to controls. Studies comparing people who are MC, NMC, as well as NC of the MD mutation have found interesting results. Saunders-Pullman et al. (2002) noted that the rate of OCD was significantly greater in carriers than noncarriers and also greater in MC than in NMC. No association was found between the severity of MD and OCD. In contrast, alcohol dependence was increased for MC only but not in the carrier group overall. Generalized anxiety disorder was also higher in the MC than the NMC group and also in all carriers relative to NC, but neither of these differences was significant. In a further study by the same group, the authors found increased rates of OCD among members of both the MC and NMC groups relative to the NCs, but increased alcohol dependence only in the MC group (Hess et al., 2007). Thus, in MD, OCD does not appear to be reactive but rather an expression of the *DYT11* gene, whereas alcohol dependence, which was more prevalent only among MCs, may be reactive.

Depression, anxiety, social phobia, agoraphobia, panic attacks, and alcohol abuse were reported as common psychiatric disorders, and mild OCD, borderline personality disorder, and emotional instability were also noted in some cases of MD (Ritz et al., 2009; Klempir et al., 2010). Others have shown presence of psychiatric disorders in MD prior to surgical treatment with DBS (Contarino et al., 2011). Depression in MD can be severe as in the two familial cases with a novel SGCE mutation reported by Misbahuddin, Placzek, Lennox, Taanman, and Warner (2007), one of whom committed suicide. Van Tricht et al. (2012) found increased rates of depression in patients with MD regardless of mutation status, but increased rates of anxiety only in the MC group, particularly social phobia. OCD was rare, and alcohol dependence was also low. They suggested that depression may be secondary to the disease, but that anxiety may be a clinical phenotype of *DYT11* as it was only present in the MC group. In a more recent study of 10 mutation carrying MD patients, Weissbach et al. (2013) found a psychiatric diagnosis in 70% of the sample, with anxiety being the most common disorder affecting 60%. They also reviewed the evidence on psychiatric comorbidity from 23 studies and found that psychiatric disorder was more common in MC (71%) than in NC (42%) of the MD gene mutation.

Thus, although there seems to be consensus across studies that MD is associated with increased psychiatric morbidity, whether rates of OCD are elevated in MD is inconsistent. This may relate to differences in the samples, whether participants were all from the same families, and the proportion of mutation carriers included, as well as the method of assessment. In a review of the results of 22 reports of psychiatric symptoms in MD, including some of the studies considered earlier, Peall, Waite, Blake, Owen, and Morris (2011) concluded that psychiatric morbidity is higher in MCs than asymptomatic individuals (NMCs and NCs), suggesting that psychiatric morbidity is associated with presence of the motor disease. They also concluded that rates of OCD were particularly different between MC and asymptomatic individuals (NMC and NC), suggesting that it may be part of the phenotype of MD. Finally, contrary to previous conclusions (Saunders-Pullman et al., 2002; Hess et al., 2007), Peall et al. (2011) also found that the rate of alcohol dependence was not significantly different between MC and NMC, but it was significantly higher in NMC than NC, suggesting that alcohol dependence may correlate with presence of the SGCE mutation regardless of whether MD symptoms developed or not. Further studies with larger samples are necessary to examine this issue.

Dopa Responsive Dystonia

The original descriptions of dopa-responsive dystonia (DRD) noted that there were no mental or psychological abnormalities (Segawa et al., 1971; 2003). However, subsequent studies have revealed a number of associated psychiatric problems. In a family with 11 members carrying the DRD GCH I mutation, psychiatric problems, particularly depression and anxiety, was reported in half and OCD in one case (Hahn et al., 2001). Others reported increased rates of depression, anxiety, OCD, and other disorders such as sleep disturbance, mood swings, or migraine, in patients with DRD (Van Hove et al., 2006; Trender-Gerhard et al., 2009; Tadic et al., 2012). However, in another study with 14 patients suffering from DRD, Lopez-Laso et al. (2011) did not find any depression or OCD, and they found anxiety in only one case.

X-Linked Dystonia-Parkinsonism

In the case report of a patient with x-linked dystonia–parkinsonism (XDP), Howe and colleagues (2009) did not find any significant depression or apathy on self-report measures. However, when this patient was assessed following GPi-DBS surgery (Kemmotsu et al., 2011), the patient experienced moderate depression, increased levels of apathy, and some anxiety.

Are Psychiatric Disorders in Dystonia Primary or Secondary?

Psychiatric disorder in dystonia can be either primary, and have a biological basis, or it can be secondary to the onset and experience of living with dystonia. There is evidence supporting both sides of the debate. Several lines of evidence support the primary nature of psychiatric disorder in dystonia. For instance, in a proportion of cases, the onset of psychiatric disorder precedes the development of dystonia (Lauterbach et al., 2004; Wenzel et al., 1998; Moraru et al., 2002), and in some studies this rate has been noted to be as high as 69% (Fabbrini et al., 2010), whereas in another study, the mean age at which psychiatric disorder was identified preceded the average age of onset of dystonia (Lencer et al., 2009). Further evidence comes from a study that showed higher rates of recurrent MDD in both MC and NMC of the *DYT1* gene than NC (Heiman et al., 2004). Evidence supporting the secondary nature of psychiatric disorders in dystonia also exists. Some studies have found that depression and anxiety are significantly associated with dystonia severity (e.g., Naber et al., 1988; Lewis et al., 2008; Scheidt et al., 1996), whereas others have shown negative perceptions, coping strategies, social support, and life events to be key predictors of psychiatric comorbidity in CD (Jahanshahi & Marsden, 1990; Jahanshahi, 1991; Lewis et al., 2008; Gundel et al., 2001; 2003). Furthermore, a longitudinal study showed that changes in mood tracked changes in severity of CD (Jahanshahi & Marsden, 1990). Elsewhere, significant improvement of depression and anxiety have been noted when dystonia improves with Botox (e.g., Jahanshahi & Marsden, 1992; Whurr et al., 1998; Murry, Cannito, & Woodson, 1994) or DBS (e.g., Halbig et al., 2005; Kiss, 2007).

In summary, a considerable proportion of patients with various forms of primary focal, segmental, or generalized dystonia or dystonia plus syndromes experience psychiatric disorders, with depression, anxiety, and OCD being the most common. In fact, a 4.5-fold increase in psychiatric morbidity in CD and blepharospasm (Lencer et al., 2009) and a 10-fold increase in social phobia in CD (Gundel et al., 2001) relative to the general population make these pressing aspects of dystonia with regards to clinical management. This evidence underlines the necessity of identifying and treating psychiatric disorder in dystonia patients, particularly because depression and anxiety are the strongest predictors of quality of life in CD (Ben-Sholmo Camfield, & Warner, 2002) and depression, disability, disfigurement, and body concept predict quality of life in other forms of focal, segmental, and generalized dystonia (Page, Butler, & Jahanshahi, 2007).

IMPACT OF MEDICAL AND SURGICAL TREATMENT OF DYSTONIA ON COGNITION AND PSYCHIATRIC MORBIDITY

The first and most common approach to the treatment of primary dystonia is medication, usually anticholinergics, GABA-derivatives or benzodiazepines. Botox into the affected muscles to induce temporary paralysis can also result in symptomatic relief of dystonia. Surgical interventions such as GPi DBS result in an average symptomatic improvement ranging from 55–73% (Tagliati et al., 2011). Other targets such as the subthalamic nucleus (Kleiner-Fisman et al., 2007) or the Voa (Ghika et al., 2002) or vental intermediate thalamic nucleus (Trottenberg et al., 2001) have also been used. Jahanshahi, Czernecki, and Zurowski (2011) recently reviewed the evidence on the impact of DBS treatment of primary and secondary dystonia on cognition, psychiatric morbidity, and quality of life.

Cognition

Taylor and colleagues (1991) studied the effect of high-dose anticholinergic medication on cognitive function in adults with dystonia, and found poorer performance on explicit memory and worse performance on the Stroop in patients with dystonia compared to matched healthy controls after treatment initiation. As noted earlier attempts to consciously control the symptoms may influence cognitive performance (Jahanshahi et al., 2003) and in support of this, Allam et al. (2007) found that sustained attention deficits improved substantially with the improvement of blepharospasm following administration of Botox. Three studies have specifically examined changes in cognition following bilateral DBS of GPi or STN in primary dystonia (Halbig et al., 2005; Pillon et al., 2006; Jahanshahi et al., 2014), and others present results of clinical investigations (Vidailhet et al., 2007; Kupsch et al., 2006; Hung et al., 2007; Valldeoriola et al., 2010; Kleiner-Fisman et al., 2007; Ostrem et al., 2011). These indicate that DBS treatment of primary dystonia is not associated with change in major domains of cognition, other than a deficit on a test of sustained attention. However, individual patients show postoperative decline on specific tests (e.g., Halbig et al., 2005; Kiss, 2007; Kleiner-Fisman et al., 2007; Jahanshahi et al., 2013). In the absence of control groups or failure to use parallel versions of cognitive tests, practice effects, postsurgical reduction of anticholinergic medication, and improved motor symptoms are potential confounding factors. GPi-DBS has been associated with stable and even improved postoperative cognition in XDP (Howe et al., 2009; Kommotsu et al., 2011), and in 10 patients with MD followed for periods of 6, 12, and 62 months after GPi or VIM DBS, Gruber et al. (2010) found no change in cognition, assessed on a relatively extensive battery of tests. Despite the fact that the majority of studies have found that DBS surgery does not produce any cognitive change in primary or dystonia plus syndromes, since all brain surgeries carry a risk of cognitive adverse effects, Jahanshahi et al. (2011) recommended a cautious approach and inclusion of a brief cognitive assessment before and after DBS surgery in dystonia.

Psychiatric Morbidity

Symptomatic treatment of dystonia with Botox results in improvement of mood. Following Botox, improvements in depression and functional ability have been reported in CD (Jahanshahi & Marsden, 1992) and improvements in depression and anxiety in spasmodic dysphonia (e.g., Murry et al., 1994; Whurr et al., 1998).

Assessing patients' psychiatric status prior to surgery is essential. Since suitability for DBS requires exclusion of patients with major psychiatric disorders, the evidence on the impact of DBS surgery on psychiatric comorbidity may not be fully representative of the range or severity of psychiatric disorders associated with dystonia (Jahanshahi et al., 2011). These studies generally show that mild to moderate depression is significantly improved after GPi-DBS in primary dystonia (Krauss et al., 2006; Halbig et al., 2005; Kupsch et al., 2006; Kiss 2007, Valderiorla et al., 2010). These same studies show that anxiety tends to remain stable after surgery (see Jahanshahi et al., 2011 for review). GPi-DBS is associated with less clear psychiatric benefits in dystonia plus syndromes. In 5 patients with MD and SGCE mutation who had DBS of the GPi, Contarino et al. (2011) noted that psychiatric problems, mainly depression, social anxiety, and OCD were unchanged or worsened following GPi-DBS, despite functional improvement of dystonia. Following GPi-DBS, a patient with XDP experienced moderate depression, increased and clinically significant levels of apathy, and also increased state of anxiety compared to the pre-operative baseline (Kemmotsu et al., 2011). Other case reports of symptomatic benefits of GPi-DBS for Lubag disease, have not included any information on psychiatric status (Martinez-Torres et al., 2009).

Although OCD is another common psychiatric disorder in dystonia, to date, none of the studies have reported the impact of DBS surgery on obsessive-compulsive symptoms. There has been one case report of migration of the implanted electrode to the region of the amygdala causing depression with delusions and severe apathy (Piacentini et al., 2008). The most serious psychiatric adverse effect of DBS surgery in primary dystonia has been suicide. Two of the 16 dystonia cases (12.5%) in the sample of Foncke et al. (2006) committed suicide. Suicide is a multifactorially determined behavior, and it remains unclear whether suicide post-DBS is a result of the stimulation spreading to limbic circuits or reflects problems with readjustment to change following surgery. Suicide is a preventable adverse effect of DBS surgery, and careful pre-operative psychiatric screening and frequent postoperative follow-up can be valuable in this regard (Jahanshahi et al., 2011).

CONCLUSIONS AND FUTURE DIRECTIONS

In primary dystonia, most cognitive domains including IQ, memory, and language are intact and isolated deficits in executive function, set shifting, visuo-spatial processing, praxis, mental rotation, and sequence learning have been reported. In contrast, cognitive deficits ranging from mild impairment to dementia seem to be characteristic of dystonia plus syndromes. Psychiatric disorders, particularly depression, anxiety, and OCD are common in primary and secondary dystonia. It is unclear whether psychiatric co-morbidity in dystonia is a primary feature of the illness or a secondary reaction to the disabling and disfiguring movement disorder, and there is currently scant evidence supporting both possibilities. It is likely that other genetic mutations associated with dystonia will be discovered in future. To address the primary versus secondary question, further studies examining associations between presence of specific dystonia genetic mutations and psychiatric disorders would be informative. Furthermore, the relation of the severity of the dystonia symptoms to psychiatric comorbidity and cognitive impairment has not been extensively examined and could be a topic for future investigation. This coupled with longitudinal studies of changes in dystonia symptoms, cognition, and psychiatric comorbidity over time from the early stages of the illness, can clarify any synchrony or temporal dissociation between these various aspects of the disorder. Imaging studies comparing dystonia patients with or without cognitive deficits and psychiatric disorders would also help clarify the neural substrates of these nonmotor symptoms. The evidence reviewed here shows that, similar to Parkinson's disease, dystonia is also a movement disorder with prominent nonmotor features. Furthermore, nonmotor features such as depression and anxiety have been shown to have a major influence on the quality of life of patients with primary dystonia (Ben-Shlomo et al., 2002; Page et al., 2006), which suggests that they should also be the focus of clinical management in dystonia alongside the movement disorder.

ACKNOWLEDGMENTS

Mariam Torkamani was funded by a grant from the European Commission Ambient Assisted Living.

REFERENCES

Albanese, A., Bhatia, K., Bressman, S. B., Delong, M. R., Fahn, S., Fung, V. S., . . . Teller, J. K. (2013). Phenomenology and classification of dystonia: A consensus update. *Movement Disorders*, 28(7), 863–873.

Albin, R. L., Reiner, A., Anderson, K. D., Penney, J. B., & Young, A. B. (1990). Striatal and nigral neuron subpopulations in rigid Huntington's disease: implications for the functional anatomy of chorea and rigidity-akinesia. *Annals of Neurology*, 27(4), 357–365.

Aleman, G. G., de Erausquin, G. A., & Micheli, F. (2009). Cognitive disturbances in primary blepharospasm. *Movement Disorders*, 24, 2112–2120.

Allam, N., Frank, J. E., Pereira, C., & Tomaz, C. (2007). Sustained attention in cranial dystonia patients treated with botulinum toxin. *Acta Neurologica Scandinavica*, 116, 196–200.

Anastasopoulos, D., Nasios, G., Psilas, K., Mergner, T., Maurer, C., & Lücking, C. H. (1998). What is straight ahead to a patient with torticollis? *Brain, 121,* 91–101.

Argyelan, M., Carbon, M., Niethammer, M., Ulug, A. M., Voss, H. U., Bressman, S. B., . . . Eidelberg, D. (2009). Cerebellothalamocortical connectivity regulates penetrance in dystonia. *Journal of Neuroscience*, 29(31), 9740–9747.

Balas, M., Peretz, C., Badarny, S., Scott, R. B., & Giladi, N. (2006). Neuropsychological profile of DYT1 dystonia. *Movement Disorders*, 21, 2073–2077.

Bara-Jimenez, W., Shelton, P., & Hallett, M. (2000). Spatial discrimination is abnormal in focal hand dystonia. *Neurology*, 55, 1869–1873.

Becker, G., Naumann, M., Scheubeck, M., Hofmann, E., Deimling, M., Lindner, A., . . . Reiners, K. (1997). Comparison of transcranial sonography, magnetic resonance imaging, and single photon emission computed tomography findings in idiopathic spasmodic torticollis. *Movement Disorders*, 12, 79–88.

Ben-Shlomo, Y., Camfield, L., & Warner, T. (2002). What are the determinants of quality of life in people with cervical dystonia? *Journal of Neurology, Neurosurgery and Psychiatry*, 72, 608–614.

Berardelli, A., Rothwell, J. C., Hallett, M., Thompson, P. D., Manfredi, M., & Marsden, C. D. (1998). The pathophysiology of primary dystonia. *Brain*, 121, 1195–1212.

Bihari, K., Hill, J. L., & Murphy, D. L. (1992). Obsessive-compulsive characteristics in patients with idiopathic spasmodic torticollis. *Psychiatry Research*, 42, 267–272.

Bindman, E., & Tibbetts, R. W. (1977). Writer's cramp—a rational approach to treatment? *British Journal of Psychiatry*, 131, 143–148.

Black, J., Ongur, D., & Perlmutter, J. S. (1998). Putamen volume in idiopathic focal dystonia. *Neurology*, 51, 819–824.

Broocks, A., Thiel, A., Angerstein, D., & Dressler, D. (1998). Higher prevalence of obsessive-compulsive symptoms in patients with blepharospasm than in patients with hemifacial spasm. *American Journal of Psychiatry*, 155(4), 555–557.

Bugalho, P., Correa, B., Guimarães, J., & Xavier, M. (2006). Obsessive-compulsive disorder and executive deficits in two patients with primary dystonia. *Parkinsonism & Related Disorders*, 12(6), 388–391.

Bugalho, P., Correa, B., Guimaraes, J., & Xavier, M. (2008). Set-shifting and behavioral dysfunction in primary focal dystonia. *Movement Disorders*, 23, 200–206.

Cannito, M. P. (1991) Emotional considerations in spasmodic dysphonia: psychometric quantification. *Journal of Communication Disorders*, 24, 313–329.

Carbon, M., Argyelan, M., Ghilardi, M.F., Mattis, P., Dhawan, V., Bressman, S., Eidelberg, D. (2011). Impaired sequence learning in dystonia mutation carriers: a genotypic effect. *Brain*, 134, 1416–1427.

Cavallaro, R., Galardi, G., Cavallini, M. C., Henin, M., Amodio, S., Bellodi, L., & Comi, G. (2002). Obsessive compulsive disorder among idiopathic focal dystonia patients: an epidemiological and family study. *Biological Psychiatry*, 52, 356–361.

Ceballos-Baumann, A. O., Passingham, R. E., Warner, T., Playford, E. D., Marsden, C. D., & Brooks, D. J. (1995). Overactive prefrontal and underactive motor cortical areas in idiopathic dystonia. *Annals of Neurology*, 37, 363–372.

Chiken, S., Shashidharan, P., & Nambu, A. (2008). Cortically evoked long-lasting inhibition of pallidal neurons in a transgenic mouse model of dystonia. *Journal of Neuroscience*, 28, 13967–13977.

Contarino, M. F., Foncke, E. M., Cath, D. C., Schuurman, P. R., Speelman, J. D., & Tijssen, M. A. J. (2011). Effect of pallidal deep brain stimulation on psychiatric symptoms in myoclonus-dystonia due to ε- arcoglycan mutations. *Archives of Neurology*, 68(8), 1087–1089.

Defazio, G., Berardelli, A., Abbruzzese, G., Lepore, V., Coviello, V., Acquistapace, D., . . . Livrea, P. (1998). Possible risk factors for primary adult onset dystonia, a case-control investigation by the Italian Movement Disorders Study Group. *Journal of Neurology, Neurosurgery and Psychiatry*, 64(1), 25–32.

Delmaire, C., Vidailhet, M., Elbaz, A., Bourdain, F., Bleton, J. P., Sangla, S., . . . Lehericy, S. (2007). Structural abnormalities in the cerebellum and sensorimotor circuit in writer's cramp. *Neurology*, 69, 376–380.

DeLong, M. R. (1990). Primate models of movement disorders of basal ganglia origin. *Trends in Neuroscience*, 13, 281–285.

Dias, F. M., Doyle, F. C., Kummer, A., Cardoso, F., Caramelli, P., & Teixeira, A. L. (2009). Executive functioning in patients with blepharospasm in comparison with patients with hemifacial spasm. *Arquivos Neuropsiquiatria*, 67(1), 12–15.

Dias, F. M., Kummer, A., Doyle, F. C., Harsányi, E., Cardoso, F., Fontenelle, L. F., & Teixeira, A. L. (2011). Psychiatric disorders in primary focal dystonia and in Parkinson's disease. *Journal of Neuropsychiatric Disease and Treatment*, 7, 111–116.

Doheny, D. O., Brin, M. F., Morrison, C. E., Smith, C. J, Walker, R. H., Abbasi, S., . . . Silverman, J. M. (2002). Phenotypic features of myoclonus- dystonia in three kindreds. *Neurology*, 59, 1187–1196.

Draganski, B., Thun-Hohenstein, C., Bogdahn, U., Winkler, J., & May, A. (2003). "Motor circuit" gray matter changes in idiopathic cervical dystonia. *Neurology*, 11, 1228–1231.

Dresel, C., Haslinger, B., Castrop, F., Wohlschlaeger, A. M., & Ceballos-Baumann, A. O. (2006). Silent event-related fMRI reveals deficient motor and enhanced somatosensory activation in orofacial dystonia. *Brain*, 129, 36–46.

Edwards, M. J., Huang, Y. Z., Wood, N. W., Rothwell, J. C., & Bhatia, K. P. (2003). Different patterns of electrophysiological deficits in manifesting and non-manifesting carriers of the DYT1 gene mutation. *Brain*, 126(9), 2074–2080.

Epidemiological Study of Dystonia in Europe (ESDE). (2000). A prevalence study of primary dystonia in eight European countries. *Journal of Neurology*, 247(10), 787–792.

Evidente, V. G., Gwinn-Hardy, K., Hardy, J., Hernandez, D., Singleton, A. (2002). X-linked dystonia ("Lubag") presenting predominantly with parkinsonism: a more benign phenotype? *Movement Disorders*, 17, 200–202.

Fabbrini, G., Berardelli, I., Moretti, G., Pasquini, M., Bloise, M., Colosimo C., . . . Beradelli, A. (2010). Psychiatric disorders in adult-onset focal dystonia: a case-control study. *Movement Disorders, 25*, 459–465.

Fabbrini, G., Berardelli, I., Moretti, G., Pasquini, M., Colosimo, C., & Berardelli, A. (2011). Nonmotor symptoms in adult-onset focal dystonia: psychiatric abnormalities. *Movement Disorders, 26*, 1764–1765.

Fahn, S., Bressman, S. B., & Marsden, C. D. (1998). Classification of dystonia. *Advances of Neurology, 78*, 1–10.

Fiorio, M., Tinazzi, M., & Aglioti, S. M. (2006). Selective impairment of hand mental rotation in patients with focal hand dystonia. *Brain, 129*, 47–54.

Foncke, E. M., Schuurman, P. R., & Speelman, J. D. (2006). Suicide after deep brain stimulation of the internal globus pallidus for dystonia. *Neurology, 66*, 142–143.

Foncke, E. M., Cath, D., Zwinderman, K., Smit, J., Schmand, B., & Tijssen, M. (2009). Is psychopathology part of the phenotypic spectrum of myoclonus-dystonia?: a study of a large Dutch M-D family. *Cognitive & Behavioral Neurology, 22*, 127–133.

Frucht, S. J. (2004). Focal task-specific dystonia in musicians. *Advances in Neurology, 94*, 225–230.

Ghika, J., Villemure, J. G., Miklossy, J., Temperli, P., Praglong, E., Christen-Zaech, S., . . . Vingerhoets, F. (2002). Postanoxic generalized dystonia improved by bilateral Voa thalamic deep brain stimulation. *Neurology, 58*, 311–313.

Ghilardi, M. F., Carbon, M., Silvestri, G., Dhawan, V., Tagliati, M., Bressman, S., . . . Eidelberg, D. (2003). Impaired sequence learning in carriers of the DYT1 dystonia mutation. *Annals of Neurology, 54*, 102–109.

Grafman, J., Cohen, L. G., & Hallett, M. (1991). Is focal hand dystonia associated with psychopathology? *Movement Disorders, 6*, 29–35.

Gruber, D., Kühn, A. A., Schoenecker, T., Kivi, A., Trottenberg, T., Hoffmann, K. T., . . . Kupsch, A. (2010). Pallidal and thalamic deep brain stimulation in myoclonus-dystonia. *Movement Disorders, 25*(11), 1733–1743.

Gundel, H., Busch, R., Ceballos-Baumann, A., & Seifert, E. (2007). Psychiatric comorbidity in patients with spasmodic dysphonia: a controlled study. *Journal of Neurology, Neurosurgery and Psychiatry, 78*, 1398–400.

Gundel, H., Wolf, A., Xidara, V., Busch, R., & Ceballos-Baumann, A. O. (2001). Social phobia in spasmodic torticollis. *Journal of Neurology, Neurosurgery and Psychiatry, 71*, 499–504.

Gundel, H., Wolf, A., Xidara, V., Busch, R., Ladwig, K. H., Jacobi, F., . . . Cebballos-Baumann, A. O. (2003). High psychiatric comorbidity in spasmodic torticollis: a controlled study. *Journal of Nervous and Mental Disease, 191*, 465–473.

Hahn, H., Trant, M. R., Brownstein, M. J., Harper, R. A., Milstien, S., & Butler, I. J. (2001). Neurologic and psychiatric manifestations in a family with a mutation in exon 2 of the guanosine triphosphate-cyclohydrolase gene. *Archives of Neurology, 58*(5), 749–755.

Halbig, T. D., Gruber, D., Kopp, U. A., Schneider, G. H., Trottenberg, T., & Kupsch, A. (2005). Pallidal stimulation in dystonia: effects on cognition, mood, and quality of life. *Journal of Neurology, Neurosurgery and Psychiatry, 76*, 1713–1716.

Hall, T. A., McGwin, G. Jr., Searcey, K., Xie, A., Hupp, S. L., Owsley, C., & Kline, L. B. (2005). Benign essential blepharospasm: risk factors with reference to hemifacial spasm. *Journal of Neuro-Ophthalmology, 25*, 280–285.

Harrington, R. C., Wieck, A., Marks, I. M., & Marsden, C. D. (1988). Writer's cramp: not associated with anxiety. *Movement Disorders, 3*(3), 195–200.

Heiman, G. A., Ottman, R., Saunders-Pullman, R.J., Ozelius, L. J., Risch, N. J., Bressman, S. B. (2007). Obsessive compulsive disorder is not a clinical manifestation of the DYT1 dystonia gene. *American Journal of Medical Genetics Part B: Neuropsychiatric Genetics*, 144B, 361–364.

Heiman, G. A., Ottman, R., Saunders-Pullman, R. J., Ozelius, L. J., Risch, N. J., & Bressman, S. B. (2004). Increased risk for recurrent major depression in DYT1 dystonia mutation carriers. *Neurology*, 63(4), 631–617.

Hess, C. W., Raymond, D., Aguiar Pde, C., Frucht, S., Shriberg, J., Heiman, G. A., . . . Saunders-Pullman, R. (2007). Myoclonus-dystonia, obsessive-compulsive disorder, and alcohol dependence in SGCE mutation carriers. *Neurology*, 68, 522–524.

Hinse, P., Leplow, B., Humbert, T., Lamparter, U., Junge, A., & Emskotter, T. (1996). Impairment of visuospatial function in idiopathic spasmodic torticollis. *Journal of Neurology*, 243, 29–33.

Hoffland, B. S., Snik, D., Bhatia, K. P., Baratelli, E., Katschnig, P., Schwingenschuh, P., . . . Edwards, M. J. (2011). Patients with primary cervical dystonia have evidence of discrete deficits in praxis. *Journal of Neurology, Neurosurgery and Psychiatry*, 82(6), 615–619.

Howe, L. L., Kellison, I. L., Fernandez, H. H., Okun, M. S., & Bowers, D. (2009). Neuropsychological profile of a Filipino gentleman with X-linked dystonia-parkinsonism: a case report of Lubag disease. *Clinical Neuropsychology*, 23(1),100–117.

Hung, S. W., Hamani, C., Lozano, A. M., Poon, Y. Y., Piboolnurak, P., Miyasaki, J. M., . . . Moro, E. (2007). Long-term outcome of bilateral pallidal deep brain stimulation for primary cervical dystonia. *Neurology*, 68(6), 457–459.

Jahanshahi, M. (1991). Psychosocial correlates of depression in torticollis. *Journal of Psychosomatic Research*, 35, 1–15.

Jahanshahi, M., & Marsden, C. D. (1988a). Depression in torticollis: a controlled study. *Psychological Medicine*, 18, 925–933.

Jahanshahi, M., & Marsden, C. D. (1988b). Personality in torticollis: a controlled study. *Psychological Medicine*, 18, 375–387.

Jahanshahi, M., & Marsden, C. D. (1992). Psychological functioning before and after treatment of torticollis with botulinum toxin. *Journal of Neurology, Neurosurgery and Psychiatry*, 55(3), 229–231.

Jahanshahi, M., & Marsden, D. (1990). A longitudinal follow-up study of depression, disability and body concept in torticollis. *Behavioural Neurology*, 3, 233–246.

Jahanshahi, M., Czernecki, V., & Zurowski, A.M. (2011). Neuropsychological, neuropsychiatric, and quality of life issues in DBS for dystonia. *Movement Disorders*, 26(1), S63–S78.

Jahanshahi, M., Rowe, J., & Fuller, R. (2003). Cognitive executive function in dystonia. *Movement Disorders*, 18, 1470–1481.

Jahanshahi, M., Torkamani, M., Beigi, M., Wilkinson, L., Page, D., Madeley, L., . . . Tisch, S. (2014). Pallidal stimulation for primary generalised dystonia: Effect on cognition, mood and quality of life. *Journal of Neurology*, 261, 164–173.

Jinnah, H. A., & Hess, E. J. (2006). A new twist on the anatomy of dystonia: the basal ganglia and the cerebellum. *Neurology*, 67, 1740–1741.

Kemmotsu, N., Price, C. C., Oyama, G., Okun, M. S., Foote, K. D., Howe, L. L., Bowers, D. (2011). Pre- and post- GPi DBS neuropsychological profiles in a case of X-linked dystonia-Parkinsonism. *Clinical Neuropsychology*, 25(1), 141–159.

Kiss, Z. H. (2007). Bilateral pallidal neurostimulation—long-term motor and cognitive effects in primary generalized dystonia. *Nature Clinical Practice Neurology*, 3, 482–483.

Kleiner-Fisman, G., Liang, G. S., Moberg, P. J., Ruocco, A. C., Hurtig, H. I., Baltuch, G. H., . . . Stern, M. B. (2007). Subthalamic nucleus deep brain stimulation for severe idiopathic dystonia: impact on severity, neuropsychological status, and quality of life. *Journal of Neurosurgery*, 107, 29–36.

Klempir, J., Klempiroca, O., Roth, J. (2010). Influence of emotional instability on behavioral disorders in DYT11. *Movement Disorders*, 25(6), 798–804.

Krauss, J. K., Loher, T. J., Weigel, R., Capelle, H. H., Weber, S., & Burgunder, J. M. (2003). Chronic stimulation of the globus pallidus internus for treatment of non-dYT1 generalized dystonia and choreoathetosis: 2- year follow up. *Journal of Neurosurgery*, 98, 785–792.

Kubota, Y., Murai, T., Okada, T., Hayashi, A., Toichi, M., Sakihama, M., . . . Kaji, R. (2001). Obsessive-compulsive characteristics in patients with writer's cramp. *Journal of Neurology, Neurosurgery and Psychiatry*, 71, 413–414.

Kupsch, A., Benecke, R., Muller, J., Trottenberg, T., Schneider G-H., Poewe, W., . . . Volkmann, J. (2006). Pallidal deep-brain stimulation in primary generalized or segmental dystonia. *New England Journal of Medicine*, 355, 1978–1990.

Lauterbach, E. C., Freeman, A., & Vogel, R. L. (2004). Differential DSM-III psychiatric disorder prevalence profiles in dystonia and Parkinso's disease. *Journal of Neuropsychiatry and Clinical Neuroscience*, 16, 29–36.

Lee, L.V., Maranon, E., Demaisip, C., Peralta, O., Borres-Icasiano, R., Arancillo, J., . . . Reyes, M. T. (2002). The natural history of sex-linked recessive dystonia parkinsonism of Panay, Philippines (XDP). *Parkinsonism & Related Disorders*, 9(10), 29–38.

Lencer, R., Steinlechner, S., Stahlberg, J., Rehling, H., Orth, M., Baeumer, T., . . . Hagenah, J. (2009). Primary focal dystonia: evidence for distinct neuropsychiatric and personality profiles. *Journal of Neurolofy, Neurosurgery and Psychiatry*, 80, 1176–1179.

Leplow, B., & Stubinger, C. (1994). Visuospatial functions in patients with spasmodic torticollis. *Perceptual and Motor Skills*, 78, 1363–1375.

Lewis, L., Butler, A., & Jahanshahi, M. (2008). Depression in focal, segmental and generalized dystonia. *Journal of Neurology*, 255, 1750–1755.

López-Laso, E., Sánchez-Raya, A., Moriana, J. A., Martínez-Gual, E., Camino-León, R., Mateos-González, M. E., . . . Artuch, R. (2011). Neuropsychiatric symptoms and intelligence quotient in autosomal dominant Segawa disease. *Journal of Neurology*, 258(12), 2155–2162.

Marsden, C. D. (1976). The problem of adult-onset idiopathic torsion dystonia and other isolated dyskinesias in adult life (including blepharospasm, oromandibular dystonia, dystonic writer's cramp, and torticollis or axial dystonia). In R. Eldridge and S. Fahn (Eds.). (1976). *Dystonia*. New York, NY: Raven Press.

Martinez-Torres, I., Limousin, P., Tisch, S., Page, R., Pinto, A., . . . Zrinzo, L. (2009). Early and marked benefit with GPi DBS for Lubag syndrome presenting with rapidly progressive life-threatening dystonia. *Movement Disorders*, 24(11), 1710–1712.

Matthews, W. B., Beasley, P., Parry-Jones, W., & Garland, G. (1978). Spasmodic torticollis: a combined clinical study. *Journal of Neurology Neurosurgery & Psychiatry*, 41, 485–492.

Misbahuddin, A., Placzek M., Lennox G., Taanman J. W., & Warner T. T. (2007) Myoclonus-dystonia syndrome with severe depression is caused by an exon-skipping mutation in the epsilon-sarcoglycan gene. *Movement Disorders*, 22, 1173–1175.

Moraru, E., Schnider, P., Wimmer, A., Wenzel, T., Birner, P., Griengl, H., & Auff, E. (2002). Relation between depression and anxiety in dystonic patients: implications for clinical management. *Depression and Anxiety*, 16, 100–103.

Mula, M., Strigaro, G., Marotta, A.E., Ruggerone, S., Tribolo, A., Monaco, R., & Cantello, F. (2012). Obsessive-compulsive-spectrum symptoms in patients with focal dystonia, hemifacial spasm, and healthy subjects. *Winter*, 24(1), 81–86.

Munhoz, R. P., Teive, H. A., Della Coletta, M. V., Germiniani, F. M., Iwamoto, F. M., Camargo, C. H., & Werneck, L. C. (2005). Frequency of obsessive and compulsive symptoms in patients with blepharospasm and hemifacial spasm. *Arq Neuropsiquiatr*, 63(2A), 213–216.

Murry, T., Cannito, M. P., & Woodson, G. E. (1994). Spasmodic dysphonia. Emotional status and botulinum toxin treatment. *Archives of Otolaryngology–Head and Neck Surgery*, 120, 310–316.

Naber, D., Weinberger, D. R., Bullinger, M., Polsby, M., & Chase, T. N. (1988). Personality variables, neurological and psychopathological symptoms in patients suffering from spasmodic torticollis. *Comprehensive Psychiatry*, 29, 182–187.

Nemeth AH (2002) The genetics of primary dystonias and related disorders. *Brain*, 125, 695–721.

Neychev, V. K., Fan, X., Mitev, V. I., Hess, E. J., & Jinnah, H. A. (2008). The basal ganglia and cerebellum interact in the expression of dystonic movement. *Brain*, 131(9), 2499–2509.

Nitschke, M., Steinberger, D., Heberlein, I., Otto, V., Müller, U., & Vieregge, P. (1998). Dopa responsive dystonia with Turner's syndrome: clinical, genetic, and neuropsychological studies in a family with a new mutation in the GTP-cyclohydrolase I gene. *Journal of Neurology, Neurosurgery and Psychiatry*, 64(6), 806–808.

Ostrem, J. L., Racine, C. A., Glass, G. A., Grace, J. K., Volz, M. M., Heath, S. L., & Starr, P. A. (2011) Subthalamic nucleus deep brain stimulation in primary cervical dystonia. *Neurology*, 76, 870–878.

Page, D., Butler, A., & Jahanshahi, M. (2007). Quality of life in focal, segmental, and generalized dystonia. *Movement Disorders*, 22, 341–347.

Papathanasiou, I., MacDonald, L., Whurr, R., & Jahanshahi, M. (2001). Perceived stigma in spasmodic torticollis. *Movement Disorders*, 16, 280–285.

Patterson, R. M. & Little, S. C. (1943). Spasmodic torticollis. *Journal of Nervous and Mental Disorders*, 98, 571–599.

Peall, K. J., Waite, A. J., Blake, D. J., Owen, M. J., & Morris, H. R. (2011). Psychiatric disorders, myoclonus dystonia, and the epsilon-sarcoglycan gene: a systematic review. *Movement Disorders*, 26(10), 1939–1942.

Piacentini, S., Romito, L., Franzini, A., Granato, A., Broggi, G., & Albanese, A. (2008). Mood disorder following DBS of the left amygdaloid region in a dystonia patient with a dislodged electrode. *Movement Disorders*, 23(1), 147–150.

Pillon, B., Ardouin, C., Dujardin, K., Vittini, P., Pelissolo, A., Correncin, O., . . . Vidailhet, M; & French SPIDY Study Group. (2006). Preservation of cognitive function in dystonia treated by pallidal stimulation. *Neurology*, 66(10), 1556–1558.

Ploner, C. J., Stenz, U., Fassdorf, K., & Arnold, G. (2005). Egocentric and allocentric spatial memory in idiopathic cervical dystonia. *Neurology*, 64, 1733–1738.

Purcell, R., Maruff, P., Kyrios, M., & Pantelis, C. (1997). Neuropsychological function in young patients with unipolar major depression. *Psychological Medicine*, 27, 1277–1285.

Quartarone, A., Bagnato, S., Rizzo, V., Siebner, H. R., Dattola, V., Scalari, A., . . . Girlanda, P. (2003). Abnormal associative plasticity of the human motor cortex in writer's cramp. *Brain*, 126, 2586–2596.

Ridding, M. C., Sheean, G., Rothwell, J. C., Inzelberg, R., & Kujirai, T. (1995). Changes in the balance between motor cortical excitation and inhibition in focal, task specific dystonia. *Journal of Neurology, Neurosurgery and Psychiatry*, 59, 493–498.

Riklan, M., Cullinan, T., & Cooper, I. S. (1976). Psychological studies in dystonia musculorum deformans. *Advances in Neurology*, 14, 189–200.

Ritz K., Gerrits M. C., Foncke E.M., van Ruissen F., van der Linden C., Vergouwen M. D., . . . Tijssen, M. A. (2009). Myoclonus-dystonia: clinical and genetic evaluation of a large cohort. *Journal of Neurology, Neurosurgery and Psychiatry*, 80, 653–658.

Roze, E., Soumare, A, Pironneau, I., Sangla, S., de Cock, V.C., Teixeira, A., . . . Elbaz, A. (2009). Case-control study of writer's cramp. *Brain*, 132, 756–764.

Saunders-Pullman, R., Shriberg, J., Heiman, G., Raymond, D., Wendt, K., Kramer, P., . . . Bressman, S.B. (2002). Myoclonus dystonia: possible association with obsessive-compulsive disorder and alcohol dependence. *Neurology*, 58, 242–245.

Scheidt, C.E., Heinen, F., Nickel, T., Heinen, F., Wissel, J., Poewe, W., . . . Deuschl, G. (1996). Spasmodic torticollis—a multicentre study on behavioural aspects IV: Psychopathology. *Behavioural Neurology*, 9, 97–103.

Schmidt, A., Jabusch, H. C., Altenmüller, E., Hagenah, J., Brüggemann, N., Lohmann, K., . . . Klein, C. (2009). Etiology of musician's dystonia: familial or environmental? *Neurology*, 72(14), 1248–1254.

Scott, R., Gregory, R., Wilson, J., Banks, S., Turner, A., Parkin, S., . . . Aziz, T. (2003). Executive cognitive deficits in primary dystonia. *Movement Disorders*, 18, 539–550.

Segawa, M., Nomura, Y., & Nishiyama, N. (2003). Autosomal dominant guanosine triphosphate cyclohydrolase I deficiency (Segawa disease). *Annals of Neurology*, 54(6), S32–S45.

Segawa, M., Ohmi, K., Itoh, S., Aoyama, M., & Hayakawa, H. (1971). Childhood basal ganglia disease with remarkable response to L-dopa: hereditary basal ganglia disease with marked diurnal fluctuation. *Shinryo*, 24, 667–672.

Tadic, V., Kasten, M., Brüggemann, N., Stiller, S., Hagenah, J., & Klein, C. (2012). Dopa-Responsive Dystonia Revisited: Diagnostic Delay, Residual Signs, and Non-motor Signs. *Archives of Neurology*, 69(12), 1558–1562.

Tagliati, M., Krack, P., Volkmann, J., Aziz, T., Krauss, J. K., Kupsch, A., & Vidailhet, A. M. (2011). Long Term management of DBS in dystonia: Response to stimulation, adverse events, battery changes, and special considerations. *Movement Disorders*, 26, S54–S62.

Taylor, A. E., Lang, A. E., Saint-Cyr, J. A., Riley, D. E., & Ranawaya, R. (1991). Cognitive processes in idiopathic dystonia treated with high-dose anticholinergic therapy: implications for treatment strategies. *Clinical Neuropharmacology*, 14, 62–77.

Tinazzi, M., Fiaschi, A., Frasson, E., Fiorio, M., Cortese, F., & Aglioti, S.M. (2002). Deficits of temporal discrimination in dystonia are independent from the spatial distance between the loci of tactile stimulation. *Movement Disorders*, 17, 333–338.

Trender-Gerhard, I., Sweeney, M. G., Schwingenschuh, P., Mir, P., Edwards, M.J., Gerhard, A., . . . Bhatia, K. P. (2009). Autosomal-dominant GTPCH1-deficient DRD: clinical characteristics and long-term outcome of 34 patients. *Journal of Neurology, Neurosurgery and Psychiatry*, 80(8), 839–845.

Trottenberg, T., Meissner, W., Kabus, C., Arnold, G., Funk, T., Einhaupl, K.M., & Kupsch, A. (2001). Neurostimulation of the ventral intermediate thalamic nucleus in inherited myoclonus-dystonia syndrome. *Movement Disorders*, 16, 769–771.

Valldeoriola, F., Regidor, I., Minguez-Castellanos, A., Lezcano, E., Garcia-Ruiz, P., Rojo, A., . . . Grupo ESpañol para el EStudio de la EStimulación PALidal en la

DIStonía. (2010). Efficacy and safety of pallidal stimulation in primary dystonia: results of the Spanish multicentric study. *Journal of Neurology, Neurosurgery and Psychiatry*, 81, 65–69.

Van Hove, J. L., Steyaert, J., Matthijs, G., Legius, E., Theys, P., Wevers, R., . . . Casaer, P. (2006). Expanded motor and psychiatric phenotype in autosomal dominant Segawa syndrome due to GTP cyclohydrolase deficiency. *Journal of Neurology, Neurosurgery and Psychiatry*, 77, 18–23.

van Tricht, M. J. V, Dreissen, Y. E. M., Cath, D., Dijk, J. M., Contarino, M. F., van der Salm, S. M., . . . Tijssen, M. A. (2012). Cognition and psychopathology in myoclonus-dystonia. *Journal of Neurology, Neurosurgery and Psychiatry* ,83, 814–820.

Vidailhet, M., Vercueil, L., Houeto, J. L., Krystkowiak, P., Lagrange, C., Yelnik, J., . . . French SPIDY Study Group. (2007). Bilateral, pallidal, deep brain stimulation in primary generalized dystonia: a prospective 3 year follow-up study. *Lancet Neurology*, 6, 223–229.

Vitek, J. L., Chockkan, V., Zhang, J. Y., Kaneoke, Y., Evatt, M., DeLong, M. R., . . . Bakay, R. A. (1999). Neuronal activity in the basal ganglia in patients with generalized dystonia and hemiballismus. *Annals of Neurology*, 46, 22–35.

Voon, V., Butler, T. R., Ekanayake, V., Gallea, C., Ameli, R., Murphy, D. L., & Hallett, M. (2010). Psychiatric symptoms associated with focal hand dystonia. *Movement Disorders*, 25, 2249–2252.

Weissbach, A., Kasten, M., Grünewald, A., Brüggemann, N., Trillenberg, P., Klein, C., & Hagenah, J. (2013). Prominent psychiatric comorbidity in the dominantly inherited movement disorder myoclonus-dystonia. *Parkinsonism & Related Disorders*, 19(4), 422–425.

Wenzel, T., Schnider, P., Wimmer, A., Steinhoff, N., Moraru, E., & Auff, E. (1998). Psychiatric comorbidity in patients with spasmodic torticollis. *Journal of Psychosomatic Research*, 44, 687–690.

Whurr, R., Loch, M., & Nye, C. (1998). The treatment of spasmodic dysphonia with botulinum toxin. *Neurology Review International*, 2, 11–15.

18 Essential Tremor

Kelly E. Lyons and Alexander I. Tröster

INTRODUCTION

Essential tremor (ET) is one of the most common movement disorders. Worldwide prevalence estimates vary dramatically, ranging from 0.01% to 20.5% of the population in reports from 19 countries, with the average being 0.9% for the total population and 4.6% for those 65 years of age and older (Louis & Ferreira, 2010). ET is characterized by a postural tremor apparent when the limbs are held against gravity such as when the arms are outstretched in front of the body or a kinetic tremor occurring during action such as writing, typing, drinking, eating, and so forth. The tremor is generally bilateral and most commonly affects the upper extremities (95%), although the head (30%), voice (20%), tongue (20%), jaw (10%), lower extremities (10%) and trunk (5%) can also be affected (Deuschl & Elble, 2009). ET is hereditary in about half of all cases; two genes have been implicated in ET (*FET1* or *ETM1*, which maps to a region on the long arm of chromosome 3 and the *ETM2* gene, which maps to a region on the short arm of chromosome 2). Mutations in these genes are rare, however, and leave unexplained many cases of familial tremor, usually transmitted in an autosomal dominant fashion. In addition, many patients report no family history (Zeuner & Deuschl, 2012). Therefore, the cause of ET is currently unknown and there is debate regarding the neuropathological changes associated with ET. The impact of ET on the performance of activities of daily living (ADLs) and consequently quality of life is variable with some patients having little to no disability and no need for treatment. Others have disability associated primarily with anxiety provoking situations, requiring treatment only as needed. In other cases, ET can lead to significant disability, making ADLs difficult or even impossible and significantly impacting quality of life, requiring regular medical or surgical treatment to control the tremor (Lyons et al., 2003). Regardless of severity, tremor can lead to significant embarrassment and negatively impact social and emotional well-being (Louis & Rios, 2009). Studies have also revealed neuropsychological symptoms associated with ET that significantly impact quality of life, including cognitive impairment, anxiety, and depression.

NEUROPATHOLOGY

The cause of ET is unknown and there is currently great debate regarding the specific neuropathological changes associated with ET. It is generally accepted that the cerebellum is involved in ET; however, early studies found no neuropathological changes specific to ET (A. Rajput, Robinson, & Rajput, 2004). Louis and colleagues, in a study of 33 ET brains, reported that 76% had changes in the cerebellum, including a reduction in Purkinje cells as well as an increase in Purkinje cell torpedoes (axonal swellings) when compared to controls, and 24% had Lewy bodies in the brainstem, primarily in the locus coeruleus. Based on these findings, the authors suggested that ET seems to be neurodegenerative (Louis, Faust, et al., 2007). In contrast, Rajput and colleagues did not find an increase in Purkinje cell torpedoes (A. H. Rajput, Robinson, Rajput, & Rajput, 2011) and neither Rajput and colleagues nor Shill and colleagues found a reduced number of Purkinje cells or increased Lewy bodies in ET compared to controls (A. H. Rajput et al., 2011; Shill et al., 2008). However, Shill et al. did find increased cerebellar gliosis and a decrease in pigmented neurons in the locus coeruleus (Shill et al., 2008). Further research is needed to confirm the neuropathological changes in ET and to determine whether ET is a neurodegenerative disease. If, as has been suggested, ET is associated with increased risk of also developing Parkinson's disease (PD) or Alzheimer's disease (AD), then neuropsychological studies, which yield different profiles in PD and AD, might inform whether these comorbid conditions account for some of the cognitive changes in ET.

NEUROCHEMISTRY

Biochemical analyses have also been completed in an attempt to explain the neuropathological basis of ET. To date, the GABAergic system has been shown to have the greatest implication in ET. This is consistent with the beneficial effects seen with benzodiazepines, ethanol, and gabapentin, which increase GABA activity (Zesiewicz et al., 2011). In a study of 10 ET brains, there was a 35% decrease in $GABA_A$ and a 22% decrease of $GABA_B$ receptors in the dentate nucleus of the cerebellum compared to controls (Paris-Robidas et al., 2012). These differences were not seen in the molecular or granular layers of the cerebellar cortex. The number of $GABA_B$ receptors in the dentate nucleus was negatively correlated with the duration of ET. The authors suggest that the decrease in GABA receptors in the dentate nucleus is related to the disinhibition of cerebellar output along the cerebello–thalamo–cortical pathway leading to tremor. This interpretation is consistent with the neuropsychological findings of Tröster et al. suggesting that the pattern of cognitive deficits, primarily subtle changes in attention, and executive function, are consistent with dysfunction in the cerebello–thalamo–cortical pathway (Tröster et al., 2002).

In another study of 23 ET brains, parvalbumin, which is a marker of GABAergic activity, was significantly reduced in the locus coeruleus in ET versus controls, but no difference was seen in the cerebellum. There were no differences in striatal tyrosine hydroxylase (marker for dopamine neurons) or locus coeruleus dopamine beta-hydroxylase (marker for noradrenergic neurons) between ET and control brains (Shill et al., 2012). A more detailed analysis of these data revealed that the decrease in parvalbumin in the locus coeruleus was found primarily in patients diagnosed at an older age (mean 80 years) with shorter disease duration (mean 6 years) (Deuschl, 2012). This finding is counterintuitive because if GABAergic changes indexed by parvalbumin were related to the cause of ET, one might expect that persons with the longest disease duration would have the greatest decrease in parvalbumin. It was suggested that late-onset, short-duration ET may not be classic ET, but instead represents senile tremor with different neuropathological changes.

NEUROIMAGING

Structural Neuroimaging Studies

A review of structural neuroimaging studies found that the majority of studies reported findings consistent with the hypothesis that the cerebellum is involved in the pathophysiology of ET (Passamonti, Cerasa, & Quattrone, 2012). Voxel-based morphometry (VBM) studies revealed inconsistent changes compared to controls including no changes (Daniels et al., 2006); gray matter loss in the cerebellar vermis in ET patients with both hand and head tremor, but no significant differences in those with just hand tremor (Quattrone et al., 2008); white and gray matter loss in the bilateral cerebellum, right frontal lobe, left medulla, parietal lobes, right insula and right limbic lobe (Benito-Leon et al., 2009); and gray matter loss in the cerebellum, vermis, frontal and occipital lobes, left middle temporal gyrus, and right superior parietal lobule (Bagepally et al., 2012). In the latter study, gray matter atrophy in the frontal, temporal, and parietal cortex as well as the thalamus and caudate nucleus was correlated with tremor severity. In addition, when those with and without head tremor were compared, those with head tremor had more extensive atrophy, but not in the cerebellum.

Diffusion tensor imaging (DTI) studies, measuring white matter differences between ET and control subjects, have also reported somewhat inconsistent findings. Studies have reported no differences (Martinelli et al., 2007); reduced fractional anisotropy in the cerebellum, pons, midbrain and frontal, parietal, and temporal cortex (Shin, Han, Kim, & Lee, 2008); reduced fractional anisotropy in the dentate nucleus and superior cerebellar peduncle (Nicoletti et al., 2010); and an increased apparent diffusion coefficient of the red nucleus (Jia, Jia-Lin, Qin, Qing, & Yan, 2011).

Although most structural imaging studies report changes in the cerebellum in ET patients, there are inconsistent findings about which parts of the cerebellum and other brain regions are affected. This inconsistency could be due to differences in study methodology as well as clinical and demographic characteristics of the subjects. Unfortunately, studies that have reported changes in the motor and cognitive areas of the cerebellum or cortex, failed to evaluate the neuropsychological status of the patients, which is a critical shortcoming when attempting to draw inferences about the neuronanatomical basis of cognitive alterations in ET.

Functional Neuroimaging Studies

Multiple positron emission tomography (PET) studies have demonstrated increased bilateral activation of the cerebellum with ET. Several studies have reported increased blood flow bilaterally in the cerebellum during postural tremor (arms held in front of body) compared to a resting state (Colebatch, Findley, Frackowiak, Marsden, & Brooks, 1990; Jenkins et al., 1993; Wills, Jenkins, Thompson, Findley, & Brooks, 1994, 1995). In another PET study, ET patients had increased bilateral cerebellar activity including the vermis when compared to controls and when given ethanol there was a decrease in activity in the cerebellum bilaterally for both ET cases and controls; however, this caused an increase in activation of the inferior olive in only the ET patients (Boecker et al., 1996). Finally, two PET studies used a GABA ligand to examine the involvement of GABA in ET. In one study, there was decreased $GABA_A$ binding in the dentate nucleus, ventrolateral thalamus and lateral premotor cortex (Boecker et al., 2010). In the second study, there was decreased $GABA_A$ binding in the cerebellum, including the vermis, posterior lobes, and right anterior lobe (Gironell et al., 2012). In the latter study, researchers also measured serotonin binding and found no abnormalities in ET. These findings are consistent with the biochemical studies suggesting the involvement of GABA in the pathophysiology of ET.

Functional magnetic resonance imaging (fMRI) has also been used to examine changes in ET patients while performing cognitive tasks to determine if ET has a neuropsychological impact. In one study, 12 ET patients and 12 matched controls completed a Stroop task (Cerasa et al., 2010). The two groups performed similarly on the task; however, the ET group had an increased brain response in the dorsolateral prefrontal cortex and the inferior parietal cortex. Given that the Stroop task is a measure of attention, the authors concluded that ET patients need greater cognitive effort than controls to maintain the same level of attentional control.

A second fMRI study of 15 mild ET patients and 15 controls matched for age, education, and gender examined brain changes during a verbal working memory task with low, medium, and high memory load (Passamonti et al., 2011). The task included six trials of each difficulty level, and reaction time and accuracy were measured. The ET group and controls completed extensive neuropsychological testing prior to the fMRI. There were no differences between the two groups in terms of flexible behavior, short-term verbal memory, attention, verbal fluency, visuospatial skills, anxiety, or depression. However, the ET group scored lower than controls on cognitive control (Frontal Assessment Battery), long-term verbal memory, and language comprehension. ET and control groups performed similarly on the study task, with increased working-memory load resulting in increased reaction time and decreased accuracy. The fMRI results indicated that there was an increased cerebellar response in the posterior lobules (crus I/lobule VI) during the high-memory-load task in ET patients compared to controls, again suggesting that increased cognitive effort is required in order for ET patients to have performance comparable to that of controls. In ET patients, the functional connectivity was altered between the posterior lobules and the executive control circuit including the dorsolateral prefrontal cortex, inferior parietal lobule, and the thalamus and also between the posterior lobules and the default mode network including the hippocampus, precuneus, and ventromedial prefrontal cortex, which controls the generation of distracting thoughts. Finally, individual differences in neuropsychological status were related to imaging findings, with low cognitive scores associated with greater imaging abnormalities. In general, the structural and functional neuroimaging studies support the involvement of the cerebellum in ET and also the presence of neuropsychological changes. Further research is necessary to better understand what parts of the cerebellum and other brain structures are involved in ET.

ACTIVITIES OF DAILY LIVING

Several factors contribute to the impact of ET on the performance of ADLs including tremor severity, body parts affected, and type of tremor. Kinetic tremor, which occurs during voluntary movement, can make ADLs such as writing, typing, dressing, personal hygiene, eating, and drinking very difficult to complete (Lyons & Pahwa, 2008). The Fahn, Tolosa, Marin Tremor Rating Scale is most commonly used in clinical settings to measure the impact of ET on ADLs as well as the severity and distribution of tremor (Fahn, Tolosa, & Marin, 1988). In addition to the clinician's assessment of tremor (items 1-10), this scale includes four tasks involving drawing and pouring, and seven historical ADL questions about speaking, feeding, drinking, hygiene, dressing, writing, and working. Each item is scored from 0 (not present) to 4 (severe). The Tremor Research Group (TRG) Tremor Rating Assessment Scale (TETRAS) was developed with the goals of having an ET specific rating scale that could be done quickly (< 10 minutes) and requires no materials other than a pen and paper to complete (Elble et al., 2012). The scale consists of 9 clinician-assessed items of tremor distribution and severity and 12 items related to ADLs including speaking, eating with a spoon, drinking from a glass, hygiene, dressing, pouring, carrying food trays/plates/other items, using keys, writing, working, social impact, and a question asking the most affected task due to tremor. Each question is scored from 0 (normal) to 4 (severe). The Tremor Activities of Daily Living Scale (TADLS) focuses more specifically on ADLs and includes 30 activities that are often difficult for patients with ET to perform, including feeding (drinking, eating), grooming (brushing teeth, shaving), manipulating household objects (unlocking a door, using a telephone, washing dishes, using a television remote), and work-related activities (writing, typing on a computer keyboard) (Lyons et al., 1998).

In addition to the physical limitations imposed by ET, embarrassment or self-consciousness can impact ADLs by increasing avoidance of performing tasks in front of others, relationships and social activities (Velickovic & Gracies, 2002). A sample of 106 population-based ET patients and 349 ET patients from a clinical center were asked "Does your tremor often embarrass you?" (Louis & Rios, 2009) In the population-based sample, 19% of ET patients indicated they were embarrassed by their tremor compared to 58% in the clinic-based sample. In the clinic sample, it was determined that females were twice as likely as males to report embarrassment due to tremor. In addition, younger patients, those with an earlier age of onset, longer disease duration, positive family history, increased disability, voice tremor, lower educational levels, and greater medication use were more likely to report tremor-related embarrassment. In fact, there was an 86% increase in the odds of using medication in those reporting embarrassment, which did not appear to be related solely to disability as 47.5% of ET patients with mild upper extremity tremor and no head tremor reported embarrassment. In an attempt to better assess embarrassment in ET patients, the Essential Tremor Embarrassment Assessment (ETEA) was created (Traub, Gerbin, Mullaney, & Louis, 2010). The ETEA is a patient-completed assessment that consists of 14 questions. Responses for each question range from 0 (disagree) to 5 (agree strongly). The ETEA items "My tremor is embarrassing to me," "I am embarrassed by my tremor when I eat or drink in public," and "I sometimes try to hide my tremor" were the items with the most positive responses; however, greater than 50% of patients responded positively to 7 of the 14 questions.

In a study on the impact of ET on professional and daily activities, 35.6% of patients reported at least moderate impairment in their job due to tremor, 28.8% reported negative reactions to their tremor from colleagues, and 23.7% reported that they were at least moderately bothered by their colleagues' reactions (Lorenz, Poremba, Papengut, Schreiber, & Deuschl, 2011). In the same study, regarding the impact of tremor on everyday life, 26.3% reported at least moderate impairment, 5.3% frequently needed help with ADLs, 18.4% reported negative reactions from persons in their personal life that lead to avoidance of ADLs in 17%, 14.5% reported at least moderate disturbance of hobbies, and 14.5% indicated that they try to conceal their tremor. Together, these studies demonstrate that physical limitations and emotional issues, including embarrassment, are common in ET, can significantly impact ADLs, and both should be assessed in clinical and neuropsychological examinations.

QUALITY OF LIFE

Quality of life is a subjective sense of well-being that is influenced by multiple factors. In ET, quality of life is related to the ability to perform physical and instrumental ADLs that allow a person to remain independent in their home and community, emotional well-being and social stigma (Tröster et al., 1999) In a study of 32 newly diagnosed ET patients and matched controls, according to the SF-36 generic quality-of-life assessment, ET patients had lower scores on physical function, role limitation due to physical function, pain, role limitation due to emotional problems, and energy/vitality. There were no differences in emotional well-being, social function, or general health (Nguyen, Ngian, Cordato, Shen, & Chan, 2007). In a study of 102 moderate to severe ET patients, results from the SF-36 indicated that compared to the normal population, ET patients scored worse on all eight domains. However, the greatest differences were for physical-function role limitation and mental health. Further, differences were greater for the mental component than the physical component score (Lorenz, Schwieger, Moises, & Deuschl, 2006). These studies demonstrate that both physical and emotional issues are related to quality of life in ET patients.

Qality of life in ET is often measured by either generic measures or measures developed for other movement disorders such as PD. Although some information can be gained from these instruments, generic measures are often not sensitive enough to account for the specific issues related to ET, and measures for other disease states often include items that are not relevant to ET. To better measure quality of life in ET patients, Tröster and colleagues developed an ET-specific quality of life assessment, the Quality of Life in Essential Tremor Questionnaire (QUEST) (Tröster, Pahwa, Fields, Tanner, & Lyons, 2005). The QUEST is a 30-item, patient-completed assessment yielding a total score and five subscores including physical, psychosocial, communication, hobbies/leisure, and work/finance. Each question is scored on a scale of 0–4 (never, rarely, sometimes, frequently, always). In addition, there are several items that are not scored, included general ratings of overall health status and overall quality of life on a scale from 0–100, number of hours per day with tremor (0–24), and patient self-ratings of tremor severity (none, mild, moderate, marked, severe) in the head, voice, upper extremities, and lower extremities). The initial validity evaluation in a sample of 200 ET patients indicated that the scale had good to excellent internal consistency ranging from 0.79 to 0.95. In addition, correlations among patient-rated tremor severity and quality of life domains suggested good construct and face validity. For instance, communication was most strongly related to voice and head tremor, whereas physical aspects of quality of life were most strongly related to upper extremity tremor, especially of the dominant hand. An independent validation of the QUEST Spanish version found that the total score had a marginal floor or ceiling effect and good internal consistency and reproducibility (0.73-0.86) (Martinez-Martin et al., 2010). QUEST was also correlated with the EQ-5D measure of health status (0.40), Hospital Anxiety and Depression Scale–Depression (0.39), Clinical Global Impression of Severity (0.39), and QUEST patient-rated tremor severity (0.63).

A study that used QUEST to measure quality of life in 50 ET patients examined responses to each of the 30 items (Chandran & Pal, 2013). There were positive responses to each of the 30 items; however, those with greater than 50% of the sample responding positively included interference with job/profession, writing, drinking, negative feelings about self, embarrassment, depression, worrying about the future, and anxiety. The majority of these items were in the psychosocial domain. The QUEST total score was significantly correlated with perceived health status, perceived quality of life, Hamilton Depression and Anxiety scales, and a modified Fahn, Tolosa, Marin tremor rating scale. Quality of life was not correlated with age, age of tremor onset, or duration of tremor.

NEUROPSYCHOLOGICAL SYMPTOMS

Anxiety

Anxiety has been shown to be more common in ET patients than normal controls. In a study comparing 84 ET patients and 78 controls using the SCL-90R, a 90-item self-report measure of psychological symptoms, ET patients had significantly higher scores for anxiety (0.93 versus 0.43) and phobic anxiety (0.41 versus 0.25) compared to controls (Tan et al., 2005). In this study, anxiety was correlated with tremor severity, but not with tremor duration. In another study, 50 ET patients were compared with 50 matched controls using the Hamilton Anxiety Rating Scale (Chandran et al., 2012). Anxiety scores were significantly higher in ET patients (7.4) compared to controls (0.7), and 66% of ET patients were anxious compared to 18% of controls. Anxiety was correlated with Fahn, Tolosa, Marin Tremor Rating Scale scores and depression, but not with age, age of tremor onset, or duration of tremor. These studies suggest that anxiety is relatively common in ET and should be assessed when patients are evaluated.

Depression

Depression has also been reported to be more common in ET patients than healthy controls. In a study of 235 ET patients and 4,379 controls, 44% of ET patients compared to 26% of controls reported depression (Louis, Benito-Leon, & Bermejo-Pareja, 2007). In addition, ET patients were more likely to be taking antidepressant medications (6.8% vs. 2.6%). In a study of 50 ET patients and 50 matched controls, 44% of ET patients were depressed versus 8% of controls as measured by the Hamilton Depression Rating Scale (HDRS scores 7.8 vs. 1.7) (Chandran et al., 2012). Depression scores were correlated with tremor rating scale scores, but not age, age of tremor onset, or tremor duration. In addition, depression scores were the only variable in the study that significantly contributed to quality of life as measured by the QUEST. A study using *DSM-IV* interviews (SCID-I and SCID-II) compared 37 ET patients and 34 controls (Fabbrini et al., 2012). The most common psychiatric disorders in ET patients were depressive disorders, which occurred in 27% of ET patients and 9% of controls. These disorders were not related to age at tremor onset, tremor duration, tremor severity, or ADL scores; however, depression was more common in ET patients with a family history. Finally, to more closely assess the impact of depression in ET patients, Louis and colleagues (Louis, Huey, Gerbin, & Viner, 2012) used the Center for Epidemiological Studies Depression Scale (CESD-10), a 10-item, self-report measure, to stratify 70 depressed ET patients into those with minimal depression ($n = 41$), moderate depression ($n = 24$) and severe depression ($n = 5$). Total tremor score and tremor duration did not differ between the groups. The CESD scores were correlated with quality of life as evidenced by marked associations with the total QUEST score and all subscales. Further, the minimally depressed group had the best quality of life followed by the moderate group and, finally, the most severe group. CESD was not correlated with total tremor score. CESD was also the main predictor of quality of life (QUEST) followed by disability due to tremor, age, and total tremor score. In addition, in the minimally depressed group, 7.3% were taking antidepressants, 4.2% of the moderate group, and none of the most severe group. Tremor medication compliance also declined as depression increased. In total, these studies suggest that depression is common in ET and has a significant impact on quality of life, yet few ET patients are taking anti-depressants. Therefore, depression should be assessed in all ET patients and treatment should be recommended if warranted.

Cognition

In one of the first studies of neuropsychological functioning in ET, Gasparini et al. (Gasparini et al., 2001) compared 27 ET patients to 15 PD patients and 15 healthy controls. ET patients were significantly worse than controls on response inhibition and problem solving (Stroop Color-Word and Wisconsin Card Sorting (WCST) tests). The authors concluded that ET patients have a disruption of frontal lobe functions, similar to PD patients, that may reflect a common dysregulation of dopamine pathways; however, they did not examine neuropsychological functions related to other brain regions. In another study, neuropsychological testing was performed in 18 ET and 18 PD patients who presented for surgical treatment of tremor. The battery of tests included measures of vocabulary, language, visuospatial processes, verbal and visual reasoning, attention/concentration, learning, memory, executive functions, and mood (Lombardi, Woolston, Roberts, & Gross, 2001). In comparison to a normative sample, the ET patients performed significantly worse on measures of verbal fluency (FAS, Animals) and had significantly more depressive symptoms; however, there was not a significant correlation between depressive symptoms and neuropsychological test performance. In addition, the ET sample obtained scores lower than, but not significantly different from controls on measures of object naming (Boston Naming Test - BNT), attention/concentration (Digit Span, Letter-Number Sequencing), executive functioning (WCST–number of errors, perseverative responses), and measures of learning and memory (California Verbal Learning Test–CVLT list-learning, delayed recall and recognition). In comparison to PD patients, ET patients scored significantly worse on tests of lexical verbal fluency and attention/concentration. PD patients were worse than ET patients on a task requiring facial recognition. The authors concluded that the difficulties ET patients demonstrated were suggestive of frontosubcortical dysfunction. They also noted that the cognitive declines demonstrated by the ET patients resembled those of patients with cerebellar lesions (e.g., deficits of working memory, executive functioning, verbal fluency).

Tröster and colleagues assessed 101 ET patients referred for thalamotomy or thalamic deep brain stimulation (DBS) (Tröster et al., 2002). ET patients had significant deficits compared to test normative samples on measures of auditory selective attention (Brief Test of Attention), response inhibition (Stroop Color-Word interference condition), manual dexterity bilaterally (Grooved Pegboard), verbal fluency (FAS, Animals), object naming (BNT), visuoperceptual functions (Hooper Visual Organization Test, Facial Recognition Test), and learning/memory (CVLT). The deficits were mild for attention, response inhibition, and letter fluency; moderate for manual dexterity; and subtle on tasks involving categorical fluency, object naming, visuoperceptual functions, and learning/memory. These results are consistent with those noted in other studies, with the exception of deficits on the WCST. This difference may be related to Tröster et al.'s exclusion of patients with concomitant medical conditions and depression that were not controlled well with medication or to a lower mean tremor duration compared to previous studies. It is possible that patients with ET demonstrate a progression of deficits affecting motor skills, verbal fluency, and attention that does not include executive functioning until later in the course of the disease. The independent effects of tremor severity and duration on neuropsychological functioning need further investigation. Tröster et al. concluded that the deficits demonstrated by the ET patients were suggestive of difficulty with the initiation and maintenance of efficient information processing strategies, and that some of these deficits were similar to those with cerebellar dysfunction. Overall, the studies of neuropsychological functioning in ET suggest that the most consistent deficits occur in verbal fluency, particularly lexical fluency. Milder declines are seen in object naming, attention/concentration, learning/memory, and executive and visuoperceptual functions.

PHARMACOTHERAPY

There are currently no medications that were developed specifically for ET; therefore, all medications were found to improve tremor when being used for other conditions. According to the American Academy of Neurology (AAN) guidelines for the treatment of ET, propranolol, propranolol long acting, and primidone are recommended in the treatment of ET (Zesiewicz et al., 2005). Propranolol or primidone should be initiated as monotherapy, and if tremor is not adequately controlled, they can be tried in combination. Benzodiazepines have been shown to reduce tremor and are particularly helpful in ET patients with anxiety. Gabapentin and topiramate may also be efficacious in the treatment of ET, but topiramate should be used with caution due to side effects related to confusion (Lyons et al., 2003) and potential dysnomia. Multiple other medications have been examined for ET, but there is currently either inconclusive or insufficient evidence to recommend their use. In general, current medications for ET improve tremor by approximately 30–50% in 50% of ET patients (Zesiewicz et al., 2011). No studies have specifically compared neuropsychological, ADL, or quality of life changes associated with the various pharmacological treatments for ET.

DEEP BRAIN STIMULATION

Deep brain stimulation (DBS) of the ventral intermediate (Vim) nucleus of the thalamus is currently the preferred surgical treatment for ET. Many studies have confirmed a mean improvement in upper limb tremor from 60–90% after Vim

DBS, with associated improvements in daily functioning (Zesiewicz et al., 2005). Head and voice tremor outcomes have been less consistent, with improvement after unilateral DBS ranging from 15%–51% and 39%–100% after bilateral procedures (Lyons & Pahwa, 2008). The short- and long-term effects of Vim DBS have been well documented in ET, with benefit in tremor control reported up to 12 years after surgery (Nazzaro, Pahwa, & Lyons, 2012).

Activities of Daily Living and Quality of Life

Hariz and colleagues (Hariz, Blomstedt, & Koskinen, 2008) reported 19 ET patients up to 7 years after unilateral Vim DBS. There was a 49% improvement in total tremor scores at 1 year, which was reduced to 18% at 7 years. ADL scores were improved by 62% at 1 year and 5% at 7 years, which was not significantly different from presurgical scores, but was significantly improved compared to the stimulation off condition. The ADL Taxonomy Scale revealed improvements in the personal and instrumental ADLs of eating, drinking, cutting food, shaving/makeup, pedicuring, using a phone, heating up liquid or preparing food, and weekly or large shopping 1 year after surgery, but only eating was significantly improved 7 years after surgery. The Nottingham Health Profile (NHP), a general measure of health-related quality of life that measures emotional reactions, sleep, energy level, pain, physical mobility, and social isolation in Part 1 and in Part 2 evaluates aspects of daily life including occupation, household management, social life, family life, sex life, hobbies/interests, and holidays was also examined. In general there were no changes in Part I one year after surgery, but scores had declined by 7 years. Improvements in social life, interests/hobbies, and looking after the home were sustained long term in males but not in females. However, social life measured by a visual analog scale was improved after 7 years for all patients.

Nazzaro and colleagues (Nazzaro et al., 2012) evaluated tremor control and quality of life up to 12 years after unilateral Vim DBS. One year after surgery (n = 78) there was a 55% reduction in total tremor, an 85% reduction in targeted upper limb tremor, and a 73% improvement in ADLs compared to presurgery. An average of 4 years after surgery (range 2–7 years; n = 42), total tremor was reduced by 44%, targeted tremor by 71%, and ADLs by 52% compared to presurgery. Finally, after an average of 9 years (range 7–12 years), total tremor was improved by 31%, targeted tremor by 68%, and ADLs by 37% compared to presurgery. The PDQ-39 was used to measure quality of life and results indicated that the total score and dimensions of ADLs, emotional well-being and stigma were significantly improved for up to 7 years compared to presurgery. However, after 7 years, only stigma remained significantly improved compared to presurgery, although the dimensions of ADLs and emotional well-being were still better than presurgery scores. In addition, the mobility scores were significantly worsened only at the longest follow-up compared to presurgery.

The reduction in tremor control and worsening of ADLs and quality of life long term may be related to several factors. In both studies, unilateral Vim DBS was performed and, given that ET is generally bilateral, worsening of tremor in the other limb and other body parts such as the head or voice, may be occurring. Worsening in targeted tremor suggests that either disease progression or tolerance to stimulation may be impacting tremor control. Finally, aging and comorbidities could also be impacting the successful completion of ADLs and quality of life, evidenced by the significant worsening in mobility, which would not necessarily be expected with ET or as a long-term complication of unilateral Vim DBS.

Neuropsychological Changes

Only a few studies have examined neuropsychological changes after Vim DBS for ET. In a study of 40 ET patients three months after unilateral Vim DBS (Tröster et al., 1999), significant but modest improvements were reported in verbal memory (Wechsler Memory Scale-Revised: Logical Memory II; CVLT: Recognition), visual attention (Spatial Span Backwards), visual Gestalt formation (Hooper Visual Organization Test), visual construction (Dementia Rating Scale-DRS Construction), and dominant hand dexterity (Grooved Pegboard). Verbal fluency was the only measure that declined. These patients were also examined 12 months after surgery with similar outcomes (Fields et al., 2003). In comparison to presurgery, subjects maintained improvements in delayed verbal memory, visual construction, visual perception, and dominant-hand manual dexterity. There was also improvement in verbal learning (CVLT: Immediate Recall), perhaps reflecting a practice effect. Significant improvements were reported from the three to 12-month evaluations in verbal learning and concept formation (DRS: Conceptualization). There were no significant declines in any measures 12 months after surgery. However, four patients with baseline deficits in verbal fluency showed further decrements following surgery, suggesting exacerbation of verbal fluency deficits after Vim DBS.

In another study, 27 ET patients with mild cognitive declines following surgery were compared to 22 ET patients without declines (Woods, Fields, Lyons, Pahwa, & Tröster, 2003). There were no significant differences in neuropsychological performance, tremor, or demographics presurgery, or in postoperative motor functioning. However, a larger proportion of patients with cognitive declines underwent left, rather than right, thalamic DBS, and ET onset after age 37 was a significant predictor of cognitive status postsurgery. A significantly higher pulse width was used in the group with cognitive declines in comparison to the stable group and there was a significant association between cognitive decline and pulse width greater than 119 microseconds. In conclusion, although data are limited, there does not appear to be any significant decline in neuropsychological status following Vim DBS; however, presurgical deficits may be worsened, particularly verbal fluency.

CONCLUSIONS

Essential tremor is one of the most prevalent movement disorders, yet the cause is currently unknown. The majority of the neuropathological findings to date confirm the involvement of the cerebellum in ET, but further research is necessary to determine the extent of involvement within the cerebellum as well as in other brain structures. Neurochemical studies suggest the involvement of the GABAergic system. Neuroimaging studies have also suggested the involvement of the cerebellum but have also pointed to more widespread changes throughout the brain suggesting a basis for both a motor and cognitive component to ET. ADLs and quality of life can be significantly impaired by tremor and the impact of embarrassment and the neuropsychological symptoms of anxiety, depression, and cognitive changes should not be underestimated.

FUTURE DIRECTIONS

Several questions are important to address:

- What is the extent of involvement of the cerebellum in ET and what other brain structures are affected that lead to both the motor and neuropsychological changes associated with ET?
- Further neurochemical studies are needed to further define the GABAergic changes associated with ET and determine if other brain chemicals are affected.
- Additional well-controlled neuroimaging studies accounting for disease severity, disease duration and neuropsychological status need to be done.
- Additional, large, well-controlled studies examining the neuropsychological symptoms of ET need to be completed to better understand the potential changes in neuropsychological status of ET patients throughout the disease course.

REFERENCES

Bagepally, B. S., Bhatt, M. D., Chandran, V., Saini, J., Bharath, R. D., Vasudev, M. K., . . . Pal, P. K. (2012). Decrease in cerebral and cerebellar gray matter in essential tremor: a voxel-based morphometric analysis under 3T MRI. *Journal of Neuroimaging, 22*(3), 275–278. doi: 10.1111/j.1552–6569.2011.00598.x

Benito-Leon, J., Alvarez-Linera, J., Hernandez-Tamames, J. A., Alonso-Navarro, H., Jimenez-Jimenez, F. J., & Louis, E. D. (2009). Brain structural changes in essential tremor: voxel-based morphometry at 3-Tesla. *Journal of Neurological Sciences, 287*(1-2), 138–142. doi: 10.1016/j.jns.2009.08.037

Boecker, H., Weindl, A., Brooks, D. J., Ceballos-Baumann, A. O., Liedtke, C., Miederer, M., . . . Miederer, I. (2010). GABAergic dysfunction in essential tremor: an 11C-flumazenil PET study. *Journal of Nuclear Medicine, 51*(7), 1030–1035. doi: 10.2967/jnumed.109.074120

Boecker, H., Wills, A. J., Ceballos-Baumann, A., Samuel, M., Thompson, P. D., Findley, L. J., & Brooks, D. J. (1996). The effect of ethanol on alcohol-responsive essential tremor: a positron emission tomography study. *Annals of Neurology, 39*(5), 650–658.

Cerasa, A., Passamonti, L., Novellino, F., Salsone, M., Gioia, M. C., Morelli, M., . . . Quattrone, A. (2010). Fronto-parietal overactivation in patients with essential tremor during Stroop task. *Neuroreport, 21*(2), 148–151. doi: 10.1097/WNR.0b013e328335b42c

Chandran, V., & Pal, P. K. (2013). Quality of life and its determinants in essential tremor. *Parkinsonism & Related Disorders, 19*(1), 62–65. doi: 10.1016/j.parkreldis.2012.06.011

Chandran, V., Pal, P. K., Reddy, J. Y., Thennarasu, K., Yadav, R., & Shivashankar, N. (2012). Non-motor features in essential tremor. *Acta Neurologica Scandinavica, 125*(5), 332–337. doi: 10.1111/j.1600-0404.2011.01573.x

Colebatch, J. G., Findley, L. J., Frackowiak, R. S., Marsden, C. D., & Brooks, D. J. (1990). Preliminary report: activation of the cerebellum in essential tremor. *Lancet, 336*(8722), 1028–1030.

Daniels, C., Peller, M., Wolff, S., Alfke, K., Witt, K., Gaser, C., . . . Deuschl, G. (2006). Voxel-based morphometry shows no decreases in cerebellar gray matter volume in essential tremor. *Neurology, 67*(8), 1452–1456.

Deuschl, G. (2012). Locus coeruleus dysfunction: a feature of essential or senile tremor? *Movement Disorders, 27*(1), 1–2. doi: 10.1002/mds.24885

Deuschl, G., & Elble, R. (2009). Essential tremor--neurodegenerative or nondegenerative disease towards a working definition of ET. *Movement Disorders, 24*(14), 2033–2041. doi: 10.1002/mds.22755

Elble, R., Comella, C., Fahn, S., Hallett, M., Jankovic, J., Juncos, J. L., . . . Zesiewicz, T. (2012). Reliability of a new scale for essential tremor. *Movement Disorders, 27*(12), 1567–1569. doi: 10.1002/mds.25162

Fabbrini, G., Berardelli, I., Falla, M., Moretti, G., Pasquini, M., Altieri, M., . . . Berardelli, A. (2012). Psychiatric disorders in patients with essential tremor. *Parkinsonism & Related Disorders, 18*(8), 971–973. doi: 10.1016/j.parkreldis.2012.05.005

Fahn, S., Tolosa, E., & Marin, C. (1988). Clinical rating scale for tremor. In J. Jankovic & E. Tolosa (Eds.), *Parkinson's disease and movement disorders* (pp. 225–234). Baltimore, MD-Munich, Germany: Urban & Schwarzenberg.

Fields, J. A., Troster, A. I., Woods, S. P., Higginson, C. I., Wilkinson, S. B., Lyons, K. E., . . . Pahwa, R. (2003). Neuropsychological and quality of life outcomes 12 months after unilateral thalamic stimulation for essential tremor. *Journal of Neurology, Neurosurgery and Psychiatry, 74*(3), 305–311.

Gasparini, M., Bonifati, V., Fabrizio, E., Fabbrini, G., Brusa, L., Lenzi, G. L., & Meco, G. (2001). Frontal lobe dysfunction in essential tremor: a preliminary study. *Journal of Neurology, 248*(5), 399–402.

Gironell, A., Figueiras, F. P., Pagonabarraga, J., Herance, J. R., Pascual-Sedano, B., Trampal, C., & Gispert, J. D. (2012). Gaba and serotonin molecular neuroimaging in essential tremor: a clinical correlation study. *Parkinsonism & Related Disorders, 18*(7), 876–880. doi: 10.1016/j.parkreldis.2012.04.024

Hariz, G. M., Blomstedt, P., & Koskinen, L. O. (2008). Long-term effect of deep brain stimulation for essential tremor on activities of daily living and health-related quality of life. *Acta Neurologica Scandinavica, 118*(6), 387–394. doi: 10.1111/j.1600-0404.2008.01065.x

Jenkins, I. H., Bain, P. G., Colebatch, J. G., Thompson, P. D., Findley, L. J., Frackowiak, R. S., . . . Brooks, D. J. (1993). A positron emission tomography study of essential tremor: evidence for overactivity of cerebellar connections. *Annals of Neurology, 34*(1), 82–90.

Jia, L., Jia-Lin, S., Qin, D., Qing, L., & Yan, Z. (2011). A diffusion tensor imaging study in essential tremor. *Journal of Neuroimaging, 21*(4), 370–374. doi: 10.1111/j.1552-6569.2010.00535.x

Lombardi, W. J., Woolston, D. J., Roberts, J. W., & Gross, R. E. (2001). Cognitive deficits in patients with essential tremor. *Neurology, 57*(5), 785–790.

Lorenz, D., Poremba, C., Papengut, F., Schreiber, S., & Deuschl, G. (2011). The psychosocial burden of essential tremor in an outpatient- and a community-based cohort. *European Journal of Neurology, 18*(7), 972–979. doi: 10.1111/j.1468-1331.2010.03295.x

Lorenz, D., Schwieger, D., Moises, H., & Deuschl, G. (2006). Quality of life and personality in essential tremor patients. *Movement Disorders, 21*(8), 1114–1118.

Louis, E. D., Benito-Leon, J., & Bermejo-Pareja, F. (2007). Self-reported depression and anti-depressant medication use in essential tremor: cross-sectional and prospective analyses in a population-based study. *European Journal of Neurology, 14*(10), 1138–1146.

Louis, E. D., Faust, P. L., Vonsattel, J. P., Honig, L. S., Rajput, A., Robinson, C. A., . . . Hernandez, N. (2007). Neuropathological changes in essential tremor: 33 cases compared with 21 controls. *Brain, 130*(Pt 12), 3297–3307.

Louis, E. D., & Ferreira, J. J. (2010). How common is the most common adult movement disorder? Update on the worldwide prevalence of essential tremor. *Movement Disorders, 25*(5), 534–541. doi: 10.1002/mds.22838

Louis, E. D., Huey, E. D., Gerbin, M., & Viner, A. S. (2012). Depressive traits in essential tremor: impact on disability, quality of life, and medication adherence. *European Journal of Neurology, 19*(10), 1349–1354. doi: 10.1111/j.1468-1331.2012.03774.x

Louis, E. D., & Rios, E. (2009). Embarrassment in essential tremor: prevalence, clinical correlates and therapeutic implications. *Parkinsonism & Related Disorders, 15*(7), 535–538. doi: S1353-8020(08)00301-5 [pii] 10.1016/j.parkreldis.2008.10.006

Lyons, K. E., & Pahwa, R. (2008). Deep brain stimulation and tremor. *Neurotherapeutics, 5*(2), 331–338.

Lyons, K. E., Pahwa, R., Busenbark, K. L., Troster, A. I., Wilkinson, S., & Koller, W. C. (1998). Improvements in daily functioning after deep brain stimulation of the thalamus for intractable tremor. *Movement Disorders, 13*(4), 690–692. doi: 10.1002/mds.870130414

Lyons, K. E., Pahwa, R., Comella, C. L., Eisa, M. S., Elble, R. J., Fahn, S., . . . Watts, R. L. (2003). Benefits and risks of pharmacological treatments for essential tremor. *Drug Safety, 26*(7), 461–481.

Martinelli, P., Rizzo, G., Manners, D., Tonon, C., Pizza, F., Testa, C., . . . Lodi, R. (2007). Diffusion-weighted imaging study of patients with essential tremor. *Movement Disorders, 22*(8), 1182–1185.

Martinez-Martin, P., Jimenez-Jimenez, F. J., Carroza Garcia, E., Alonso-Navarro, H., Rubio, L., Calleja, P., . . . Benito-Leon, J. (2010). Most of the Quality of Life in Essential Tremor Questionnaire (QUEST) psychometric properties resulted in satisfactory values. *Journal of Clinical Epidemiology, 63*(7), 767–773. doi: 10.1016/j.jclinepi.2009.09.001

Nazzaro, J. M., Pahwa, R., & Lyons, K. E. (2012). Long-term benefits in quality of life after unilateral thalamic deep brain stimulation for essential tremor. *Journal of Neurosurgery, 117*(1), 156–161. doi: 10.3171/2012.3.JNS112316

Nguyen, H. V., Ngian, V., Cordato, D., Shen, Q., & Chan, D. K. (2007). Quality of life in a random sample of community dwelling older patients with essential tremor. *Acta Neurologica Scandinavica, 116*(5), 289–292.

Nicoletti, G., Manners, D., Novellino, F., Condino, F., Malucelli, E., Barbiroli, B., . . . Quattrone, A. (2010). Diffusion tensor MRI changes in cerebellar structures of patients with familial essential tremor. *Neurology, 74*(12), 988–994. doi: 10.1212/WNL.0b013e3181d5a460

Paris-Robidas, S., Brochu, E., Sintes, M., Emond, V., Bousquet, M., Vandal, M., . . . Calon, F. (2012). Defective dentate nucleus GABA receptors in essential tremor. *Brain, 135*(Pt 1), 105–116. doi: 10.1093/brain/awr301

Passamonti, L., Cerasa, A., & Quattrone, A. (2012). Neuroimaging of Essential Tremor: What is the Evidence for Cerebellar Involvement? *Tremor & Other Hyperkinetic Movements (N Y), 2.*

Passamonti, L., Novellino, F., Cerasa, A., Chiriaco, C., Rocca, F., Matina, M. S., . . . Quattrone, A. (2011). Altered cortical-cerebellar circuits during verbal working memory in essential tremor. *Brain, 134*(Pt 8), 2274–2286. doi: 10.1093/brain/awr164

Quattrone, A., Cerasa, A., Messina, D., Nicoletti, G., Hagberg, G. E., Lemieux, L., . . . Salsone, M. (2008). Essential head tremor is associated with cerebellar vermis atrophy: a volumetric and voxel-based morphometry MR imaging study. *AJNR American Journal of Neuroradiology, 29*(9), 1692–1697. doi: 10.3174/ajnr.A1190

Rajput, A. H., Robinson, C. A., Rajput, M. L., & Rajput, A. (2011). Cerebellar Purkinje cell loss is not pathognomonic of essential tremor. *Parkinsonism & Related Disorders, 17*(1), 16–21. doi: 10.1016/j.parkreldis.2010.08.009

Rajput, A., Robinson, C. A., & Rajput, A. H. (2004). Essential tremor course and disability: A clinicopathologic study of 20 cases. *Neurology, 62*(6), 932–936.

Shill, H. A., Adler, C. H., Beach, T. G., Lue, L. F., Caviness, J. N., Sabbagh, M. N., . . . Walker, D. G. (2012). Brain biochemistry in autopsied patients with essential tremor. *Movement Disorders, 27*(1), 113–117. doi: 10.1002/mds.24004

Shill, H. A., Adler, C. H., Sabbagh, M. N., Connor, D. J., Caviness, J. N., Hentz, J. G., & Beach, T. G. (2008). Pathologic findings in prospectively ascertained essential tremor subjects. *Neurology, 70*(16 Pt 2), 1452–1455.

Shin, D. H., Han, B. S., Kim, H. S., & Lee, P. H. (2008). Diffusion tensor imaging in patients with essential tremor. *AJNR American Journal of Neuroradiology, 29*(1), 151–153. doi: 10.3174/ajnr.A0744

Tan, E. K., Fook-Chong, S., Lum, S. Y., Gabriel, C., Koh, K. K., Prakash, K. M., & Louis, E. D. (2005). Non-motor manifestations in essential tremor: use of a validated instrument to evaluate a wide spectrum of symptoms. *Parkinsonism & Related Disorders, 11*(6), 375–380.

Traub, R. E., Gerbin, M., Mullaney, M. M., & Louis, E. D. (2010). Development of an essential tremor embarrassment assessment. *Parkinsonism & Related Disorders, 16*(10), 661–665. doi: 10.1016/j.parkreldis.2010.08.017

Tröster, A. I., Fields, J. A., Pahwa, R., Wilkinson, S. B., Strait-Troster, K. A., Lyons, K., . . . Koller, W. C. (1999). Neuropsychological and quality of life outcome after thalamic stimulation for essential tremor. *Neurology, 53*(8), 1774–1780.

Tröster, A. I., Pahwa, R., Fields, J. A., Tanner, C. M., & Lyons, K. E. (2005). Quality of life in Essential Tremor Questionnaire (QUEST): development and initial validation. *Parkinsonism & Related Disorders, 11*(6), 367–373.

Tröster, A. I., Woods, S. P., Fields, J. A., Lyons, K. E., Pahwa, R., Higginson, C. I., & Koller, W. C. (2002). Neuropsychological deficits in essential tremor: an expression of cerebello-thalamo-cortical pathophysiology? *European Journal of Neurology, 9*(2), 143–151.

Velickovic, M., & Gracies, J. M. (2002). Movement disorders. Keys to identifying and treating tremor. *Geriatrics, 57*(7), 32–36.

Wills, A. J., Jenkins, I. H., Thompson, P. D., Findley, L. J., & Brooks, D. J. (1994). Red nuclear and cerebellar but no olivary activation associated with essential tremor: a positron emission tomographic study. *Annals of Neurology, 36*(4), 636–642.

Wills, A. J., Jenkins, I. H., Thompson, P. D., Findley, L. J., & Brooks, D. J. (1995). A positron emission tomography study of cerebral activation associated with essential and writing tremor. *Archives of Neurology, 52*(3), 299–305.

Woods, S. P., Fields, J. A., Lyons, K. E., Pahwa, R., & Troster, A. I. (2003). Pulse width is associated with cognitive decline after thalamic stimulation for essential tremor. *Parkinsonism & Related Disorders, 9*(5), 295–300.

Zesiewicz, T. A., Elble, R. J., Louis, E. D., Gronseth, G. S., Ondo, W. G., Dewey, R. B., Jr., . . . Weiner, W. J. (2011). Evidence-based guideline update: treatment of essential tremor: report of the Quality Standards subcommittee of the American Academy of Neurology. *Neurology, 77*(19), 1752–1755. doi: 10.1212/WNL.0b013e318236f0fd

Zesiewicz, T. A., Elble, R., Louis, E. D., Hauser, R. A., Sullivan, K. L., Dewey, R. B., Jr., . . . Weiner, W. J. (2005). Practice parameter: therapies for essential tremor: report of the Quality Standards Subcommittee of the American Academy of Neurology. *Neurology, 64*(12), 2008–2020.

Zeuner, K. E., & Deuschl, G. (2012). An update on tremors. *Current Opinions in Neurology, 25*(4), 475–482. doi: 10.1097/WCO.0b013e3283550c7e

Name Index

Subject Index

CPSIA information can be obtained
at www.ICGtesting.com
Printed in the USA
BVOW06*1431030617
485812BV00004B/4/P

9 780199 812370